Statistics for Biology and Health

Series Editors
K. Dietz, M. Gail, K. Krickeberg, A. Tsiatis, J. Samet

Springer
New York
Berlin
Heidelberg
Barcelona
Hong Kong
London
Milan
Paris
Singapore
Tokyo

Statistics for Biology and Health

Philip Hougaard

Analysis of Multivariate Survival Data

With 118 Illustrations

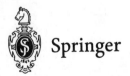 Springer

Philip Hougaard
Department of Statistics
Novo Nordisk A/S
Novo Alle Bldg. 9F2
DK-2880 Bagsvaerd
DENMARK
pho@novo.dk

Series Editors

K. Dietz
Institut für Medizinische Biometrie
Universität Tübingen
West Bahnhofstrasse 55
D-72070 Tübingen
GERMANY

M. Gail
National Cancer Institute
Rockville, MD 20892
USA

K. Krickeberg
Le Chatelet
F-63270 Manglieu
FRANCE

A. Tsiatis
Department of Statistics
North Carolina State University
Raleigh, NC 27695
USA

J. Samet
School of Public Health
Department of Epidemiology
Johns Hopkins University
615 Wolfe St.
Baltimore, MD 21205-2103
USA

Library of Congress Cataloging-in-Publication Data
Hougaard, Philip.
 Analysis of multivariate survival data / Philip Hougaard.
  p. cm. — (Statistics for biology and health)
 Includes bibliographical references and index.
 ISBN 0-387-98873-4 (alk. paper)
  1. Medicine—Research—Statistical methods. 2. Multivariate analysis. 3. Survival
analysis (Biometry) I. Title. II. Series.
 R853.S7 H68 2000
 610'.7'27—dc21   00-040047

Printed on acid-free paper.

Production managed by MaryAnn Brickner; manufacturing supervised by Jerome Basma.
Camera-ready copy prepared from the author's LaTeX files.
Printed and bound by Edwards Brothers, Inc., Ann Arbor, MI.
Printed in the United States of America.

9 8 7 6 5 4 3 2 1

ISBN 0-387-98873-4   SPIN 10729868

Springer-Verlag New York Berlin Heidelberg
A member of BertelsmannSpringer Science+Business Media GmbH

Preface

There are many books covering survival data, that is, data concerning the time to some event. In the standard case, the event is death, but the topic is much broader. This book, however, covers the extension to multivariate survival data. In popular terms, this means everything where more than one time is involved. One such type is the survival times of several individuals, which are related in some way, and where independence cannot be assumed. Another type of data is multiple data, where we study repeated occurrences of the same event. A further type is the times to several events for the same persons, like outbreak of disease, time to complication and death. Analysis of such types of data is only briefly covered by other books. Most of the material in this book is only available in journal papers; some of it is not available in writing at all.

This field is still in its infancy, and this is one reason for it's being exciting. On the one hand, it implies that we don't know how far the theory can be developed. On the negative side is that it implies that in some cases this book treats models that the future will realize are not sensible. In that case, please bear with me. I think it is a necessity to explore a large number of models in a new field, in order to understand which properties are the most important. Then, when a sufficient amount of experience has been gathered, we may be able to separate the good from the bad. It is my hope that this book can help the field to mature.

The field of application is the biological and medical field, but the theory is also applicable to technical reliability, demography, actuarial science and other fields, where multivariate times are observed.

This book is intended for persons, who already have some experience with survival data. This means that the introductory chapters are somewhat short, but contain the material needed for the rest of the chapters. It puts particular emphasis on some topics needed later, like mixture models, time-dependent covariates, and estimation of non-parametric hazard functions.

This book is a tool box rather than a cook book, meaning that a major aim is to help consider what kind of problem and what kind of data are being studied, in order to choose a model that is as good as possible for the problem at hand. Thus the aim is not just to present a few standard solutions to be applied for all kinds of data. The model building part of the material (Chapters 1, 3, Section 5.3 and many other places) is less technical, and can therefore be read by non-specialists. All chapters start with an introduction, which is less technical than the rest of the chapter and ends with a summary of what has been found.

The book starts with an introduction to survival data, and to the various types of data to be considered as multivariate survival data, Chapter 1, which also lists a number of examples. Some time is spent on clarifying the concepts, which is particularly important as the field is rather new. Standard methods for univariate survival data are described in Chapter 2. The various mechanisms that create dependence in multivariate survival data are discussed in Chapter 3. Model-independent measures of dependence for bivariate data are described in Chapter 4. Multi-state models, the most classical way of analyzing life history data, are described in Chapter 5. The statistical inference for such models is described in Chapter 6. Shared frailty models are random effects models (that is, survival data models similar in concepts to the normal distribution one-way variance components models) and described in Chapter 7. The statistical inference is described in Chapter 8. Special aspects for the analysis of recurrent events are described in Chapter 9. Extensions of the shared frailty model are described in Chapters 10 and 11. Competing risks models (that is, models for data on cause of death) are considered as a special case in Chapter 12. Regression models emphasizing the marginal distributions, allowing for dependence as described by some nuisance parameters, are described in Chapter 13, together with the copula approach, modeling the dependence for fixed marginals. The most general bivariate non-parametric methods are described in Chapter 14. Finally, Chapter 15 gives a summary of the theory and an overview of the most relevant method for each of the major applications discussed.

This book was started as a set of notes prepared for a course on advanced survival analysis, arranged by the Biostatistics Section of the Belgian Statistical Society. For this course, I wanted to present the types of complicated survival data, and their analysis. Over a one year period, I presented the material to my colleagues at Novo Nordisk. Furthermore, I presented a part of the material at a course at the Laboratory of Actuarial Mathematics at the University of Copenhagen. It has also been presented at conferences of the Nordic Region of the Biometric Society and of the International Society for Clinical Biostatistics.

The comments from my colleagues at Novo Nordisk and others, who have seen some of the chapters, are greatly appreciated. In particular, valuable comments have been received from Odd Aalen, Per Kragh Andersen, Kim Knudsen and Mei-Ling Ting Lee.

Furthermore, the persons who have presented interesting data to me should be thanked. Many of the data sets are taken from the literature, but there also are a number of data sets that I have worked on myself. In particular, the twin data set, kindly delivered by Niels V. Holm, of the University of Odense.

Philip Hougaard
March 6, 2000
e-mail: pho@novo.dk

Contents

1
Introduction

The overall purpose of this book is to present four approaches to handle multivariate survival data, but before doing that we start by clarifying the concepts both for simple survival data and multivariate survival data.

This chapter starts with an introduction to survival data, describing what survival data is, Section 1.1. The chapter then discusses the various kinds of data, to be considered. This serves a triple purpose. It gives an introduction to which kinds of data are considered in this book, it is an introduction to the actual data sets used later in the book, and third, it is a classification that helps in finding the most appropriate model for a specific kind of data set. First we describe the ordinary univariate data, Section 1.2, where for each person a single time is recorded and persons are assumed independent. The time may correspond to an event (like death, or outbreak of disease), or the event might not happen within the observation period, in which case, we say the time is censored. Although the analysis of such data is briefly described in Chapter 2, this just serves as a starting point for the more advanced types of data. Interval censored data are data, where the times are not known precisely, because the status is only studied at a few time points. Each event time is then only known to lie in some interval. Such data are considered in Section 1.3 in the univariate case. Then multivariate survival data, the real topic of this book, are studied. First two kinds of data structures, parallel and longitudinal, are introduced (Section 1.4). In the case of parallel data, the number of times is known from the beginning (although the number of these times corresponding to events respectively censorings is not fixed), whereas for longitudinal data, the number of times is a consequence of the development of the process over time. Then we discuss six different types of multivariate survival data (Sections 1.5 to 1.10). As will be demonstrated, these classifications are not in all cases mutually exclusive, and combinations are also possible. We introduce the classification in order to emphasize key differences and similarities. There are the basic parallel data, following several individuals or specified components to a given type of event (Sections 1.5 and 1.6). We might study repeated cases of the same event (Section 1.7). Then we have repeated measurements, where we, in a designed study, consider the time to some event under a planned set of circumstances (Section 1.8). Furthermore, we might study different events as they develop over time (Section 1.9). Finally, there are cause of death data, where there is only one time variable involved, but we consider the cause among a set of possible causes (Section 1.10). This consideration should help in choosing the most relevant model for a given data set. In all cases, some specific data sets are described. Some, but not all, of these data sets are analyzed in this work. The various types are summarized in Section 1.15.

There is a short introduction to the multivariate censoring types considered (Section 1.11). Truncation in the multivariate case is discussed in Section 1.12. A classification of covariates is described in Section 1.13. Finally, the various aims for an analysis of multivariate survival data are discussed in Section 1.14.

For all real applications we will assume that we have data on an individual level. This is necessary in order to make the detailed evaluations of dependence in the models. In the case of summary data for populations, it is much more difficult to make the same considerations.

1.1   What is survival data?

This section describes basic aspects of survival data, and therefore might be skipped by experienced readers. *Survival data* is a term used for describing data that measure the time to some event. In the case that has given this field its name, the event is death, but the term is also used with other events, like occurrence of a disease or a complication. It can be the time to an epileptic seizure. In industrial applications, it is typically time to failure of a unit, or some component in a unit. Within economics, it can be the time to acceptance of a job offer for an unemployed person. In demography, the event can be entering marriage. In many cases, the event is a transition from one state to another. But we will also see cases where it is not an advantage to introduce states. In the cases above, death is a transition from the state alive to the state dead (Figure 1.1). Occurrence of disease is a transition from a state of being healthy to a state of presence of disease (Figure 1.2). In the economic example, it is a transition from a state unemployed to a state employed. In the demographic example, it

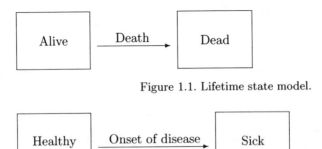

Figure 1.1. Lifetime state model.

Figure 1.2. Disease state model.

is a transition from being unmarried to being married. For the epileptic seizure the strict definition of an event is a transition from the seizure-free state to the state of active seizure, but for practical purposes the duration of a seizure is short compared to the time studied and therefore we might consider the whole seizure an event, rather than just the start of the seizure. In Figures 1.1 and 1.2, the name of the transition is included above the arrow. This will not be done later, as the transition is defined by the names of the states it goes from and comes to. Depending on the context, we will use words like *death, event, failure* and *transition* to cover the same thing – namely, what happens at the response time. In some cases, the interesting aspect is the transition, corresponding to the incidence in the disease state model. In other cases, the interesting aspect is the state, corresponding to the prevalence in the disease state model (the proportion being sick in a given age).

In order to discuss these aspects, we need to define the time. Time to an event is considered a positive real valued variable having a continuous distribution. It is necessary to define a time point, say, time 0, from which times are measured. In most cases, the defining time point will be the time of some event, i.e., a transition. When we measure time as age, the defining time point is birth. This can be considered as a time of transition from a state fetus to a state human being. For studying the occurrence of complications for a disease, the natural time scale is the duration of the disease, but for many diseases this is not possible, because the exact time of occurrence of disease is unknown. Instead we have to make do with the time since diagnosis of the disease (the known duration), which is operational, but not always scientifically satisfactory. For a drug trial, the natural time 0 is the time of start of treatment. Generally, there does not need to be an individual event to define time 0. For example, an observational study might follow a group of individuals during a period in calendar time. In that case we can define time as age for each individual, but it might make more sense to let time 0 be the calendar time of start of observation. The time 0 does not need to be identical to the time of start of observation; when it

Time 0	Time scale
Birth	Age
Diagnosis of disease	Duration
Entry into state	Waiting time
Bleeding	Duration of pregnancy
Start of treatment	Length of treatment
Baseline measurement	Calendar time

Table 1.1. Possible choices of time scale.

is not, the data are truncated (see Section 2.1.2). Table 1.1 gives a list of possible definitions of time 0. As an example of entry into a state, consider occupational mortality, where time 0 is the time of start within the occupation. As another example, the female risk of heart disease is known to increase after menopause, not only owing to the age. In that case it might be natural to define time 0 as the time of menopause. Duration of pregnancy is traditionally measured since start of the last menstrual bleeding, because this time is well-defined and known. However, the term appears to be in conflict with common sense, as conception takes place something like day 10–14 within the pregnancy. As a time scale it is acceptable, because when a woman is considered within the state pregnant, time 0 is known. It is, however, necessary to be careful in the early phase of this time scale; for example, it makes no sense to consider mortality for women within the first week of pregnancy. The time 0 point needs to be known at the start of observation. As a counter example, take a medical doctor, who might be inclined to define time 0 as the time of diagnosis of the disease under study, in order to evaluate how long the patients have had symptoms before the diagnosis. Thus his time scale covers negative times. However, this does not work, one reason being that individuals who have symptoms but do not develop disease are implicitly ruled out from being included. In order to study the problem, a completely different study is needed, one where a group of individuals is followed, and the response time is the time to diagnosis, measured in relation to their age, letting symptoms be described by a time-dependent explanatory variable. Many medical studies are centered around a baseline measurement on a group of people having a given disease at some point in time. From a scientific point of view, it can be natural to use age or duration of the disease as time scale, with truncation, but in some cases we might prefer to define time as the time since the baseline measurement. For most models, the definition of time 0 is crucial, the only exception being constant hazards models (see Section 2.2.1).

In order to use survival data methods, the state must be known at all times, until censoring (end of observation). This is to be understood so that the current state must be known at all times and this is certainly not trivial. For example, menopause is defined as the time of the last menstrual bleeding. This is illustrated in Figure 1.3. It is clear that A marks the time

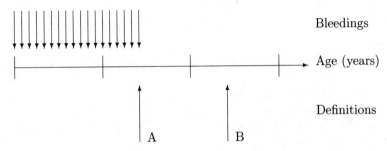

Figure 1.3. Menopausal model.

of the last bleeding. But at time A we do not know this. It is not possible to say whether an occurrence of bleeding is the last unless you have a whole lifespan. To make an operational definition, we wait for one year (time B) before it is said we know for sure that the bleeding was the last. In the period from A to B, we do not know the current state, because it depends on whether the woman will get more bleedings. At time B we conclude that menopause happened at time A. The strict consequence is that any woman who has had a bleeding within the last year does not know whether she has obtained menopause, even if she is only 20 years old. To modify the definition to become an acceptable definition from a survival data viewpoint, menopause must be defined as the end of the bleeding-free year (time B), so that menopause is the first time she has had a year without bleedings. Using definition B, we can at any time tell whether the woman has passed menopause at that time. It appears easy to add or subtract one year to go from one definition to the other, but this is not possible for all women. It is necessary to have a strict definition on this point as the woman might die between time A and B, in which case it is unknown whether she should count as having obtained menopause. Within the statistical field of stochastic processes, the acceptable times are known as stopping times.

Some extension on the state being known at all times is possible, for example, interval censoring, where the state is only known at some time points and hidden states (Section 5.10), where some states cannot be separated. For some cases of recurrent events, we might not know the exact time of each event but only the total number of events within certain time intervals.

Survival data consider only a single or a few types of states and events. This rules out the possibility of continuous measurements of, for example, quality of life. If such a concept should be included, it would need to be grouped into a few well-defined groups. On the other hand, the time to the event is considered in great detail in survival analysis, sometimes much more than relevant for the application. The biostatistical tradition for times for human beings is to measure time in days, and then analyze the effect of explanatory factors by rank-based methods. For example, for studies of cancer, this does not make sense from a medical point of view, because they can be developing for up to 20 years before being diagnosed and the rank-based methods may imply large differences for small changes in the time value; for an example see Section 2.4. Similarly, in the economic example above, the hourly payment might be of higher importance to the individual than the time of obtaining the job, but survival analysis methods put the emphasis on the time to obtaining the job, and can, at most, classify the salary into a few groups.

Having these limitations in mind, we are ready to exploit the potential in analysis of survival data.

1.2 Univariate data

This term means that all time variables describing the time to the same type of event and individuals are assumed to be independent. The event considered will be called death for theoretical evaluations, even though it also can be other events. Therefore, the data consist of n independent times, $T_1, ..., T_n$, with corresponding death indicators $D_1, ..., D_n$. Thus, in the case of death, $D = 1$, T is time to death; in the case of censoring $D = 0$, and T is the observation time. A subscript i is used to denote the individuals. There might be explanatory variables $z_1, ..., z_n$, which may be of vector form. These may be fixed or time-dependent, if the time courses are known from the beginning. Data with general time-dependent covariates will be considered as multivariate data, in the cases where we might consider modeling the covariate development as a stochastic process. Univariate data are included here only for comparison and for building a basis for discussing the more advanced types of data.

1.2.1 Population data

This example is included in order to discuss full lifetimes of ordinary individuals. These data describing the survival of the population of Denmark, are from the Statistical Yearbook of Denmark (1996). This book gives a table, where for each sex, the survivor function (the proportion alive) at each birthday from 0 to 100 years is shown. We have extrapolated the data by assuming constant hazard up to 110 years, using the value for persons 99 years of age. For evaluating moments we use the midpoint in each age class. There is no indication of the variability of these estimates. The data are not given in sufficient detail to make it possible to perform the evaluations suggested in this book, and, in fact, are not covering lifetimes from birth to death. Instead the data include the survival experience during the

years 1993–94. However, the data are very good at illustrating considerations about theoretical features of lifetime distributions. They are used
to discuss why special statistical methods are needed for survival data in
Sections 2.1.2 and 2.1.3. The data will be used for illustration of Weibull
models in Section 2.2.2, Gompertz models in Section 2.2.3, truncated distributions in Section 2.2.6, to compare parametric methods in Section 2.2.8,
and to compare proportional hazards and accelerated failure time models
in Section 2.5.1. Hougaard (1999) applied a normal distribution to these
data, in order to show the shortcomings of that approach.

1.2.2 Survival of diabetics

Green and Hougaard (1984) study the survival among insulin-dependent
diabetic patients in the county of Funen, Denmark. The diabetic population
as of July 1, 1973, was ascertained by obtaining copies of all prescriptions
in the county during a five-month period. A total of 1499 patients were
studied. This version of the data has follow-up until July 1, 1980, and 395
patients died before that date. As the natural time scale is either age or
duration of diabetes, the data are truncated. To avoid truncation, the time
scale should be calendar time, that is, time since July 1, 1973; and this
time scale is probably not of sufficient importance for a non-parametric
model. The individuals start observation at whatever age (duration) they
were on July 1, 1973. The data are used to illustrate multiple time scales
in Section 2.4.8. The patients have later been followed up, until 1982 (see
Green et al., 1985).

1.3 Interval censored data

In this case, the exact time of an event is not known, but it is known to lie
in some interval. The intervals are generally different for the individuals.
The main reason for data being of this kind is that knowing the state requires a detailed examination, for example, a blood sample for determining
HIV status, a urine sample for determining albumin status (Section 1.9.1),
or a mammography to examine the presence of breast cancer. The event
considered is an irreversible event, so that whenever it has happened it
can be detected by the actual examination procedure. It is assumed that
the state is examined at a number of time points. Because the condition
is irreversible, it is sufficient to record the last time the person is seen before the event, L_i, and the first time after the event R_i. The status at all
other inspection times is then a consequence of these numbers. Thus, the
ith observation is in the interval $(L_i, R_i]$. Some observations may be exact,
which can be included by letting $L_i = R_i - \epsilon$ for some small choice of ϵ.
Ordinary right censored data correspond to $R_i = \infty$.

Interval censored data are common but often not analyzed in a satisfactory way. Non-parametric methods for univariate interval censored observations show some overlap to non-parametric methods for ordinarily censored multivariate survival data. Owing to lack of space, methods for interval censored data are not described in this book.

1.3.1 Diabetic nephropathy

This data set contains all the insulin-dependent diabetic patients treated at the Steno Diabetes Center, Denmark, since it opened in 1933 until 1972. The data have been studied by Borch-Johnsen, Andersen and Deckert (1985), Ramlau-Hansen et al. (1987) and Hougaard, Myglegaard, and Borch-Johnsen (1994). The patients were diagnosed between 1933 and 1972, and started treatment at the hospital between 1933 and 1981. They were followed from first visit at the hospital until death, emigration, or January 1, 1984. Thus data are left truncated, both when age and duration of diabetes are used as time scales. There were 2890 such patients.

The main purpose in this analysis is to study the occurrence of the complication diabetic nephropathy. It is the most serious diabetes complication, starting with the kidneys leaking protein and leading ultimately to renal failure, in which case the patient needs either a kidney transplant or dialysis. For studying the occurrence we need to exclude 163 patients for which there were no data on examination for nephropathy. Furthermore, 115 patients who had nephropathy at the first examination have been excluded. That leaves 2612 patients. In the first part of the period, nephropathy was detected by a stix, a prepared stick, which after being dipped in the patient's urine gave a positive response, when the protein content was high (comparable to saying that the daily excretion is above 0.5 g). The more modern technique is determination of albumin (the main component of the protein), and the corresponding limit is 300 mg pr day. The modern assay is more precise and can determine the actual content in the urine. Therefore, today one further splits into normo-albuminuria (below 30 mg/day) and micro-albuminuria (30–300 mg/day). The modern methods were not used for this data set, but we also include a data set where they are used (see Section 1.9.1). The day-to-day variation in protein and albumin excretion is, however, quite large, and therefore several positive samples are necessary to give the diagnosis of nephropathy. Therefore in this analysis only the year of onset of nephropathy is considered. For 508 patients, the year of onset of nephropathy is known. For 1996 patients, the complication is not observed; that is right censoring. For the remaining 108 patients, it is known that they developed the complication, but the actual year is not known. These are the real interval censored observations. The time scale used for these data is duration of diabetes. The data are used in Section 2.2.7 to illustrate mixture models and in Section 2.5.3 to illustrate neglected covariates in accelerated failure time models.

1.4 Multivariate data structures

The term *multivariate survival data* covers the field where independence between survival times cannot be assumed. The dependence can occur for very different kinds of data. Before we define the various kinds of data, we will consider two main types of data structures. The difference between the two types of data structures to be introduced, parallel and longitudinal, is that for parallel data, the number of times is fixed by the design, whereas the longitudinal data are allowed to show a random number of times. We believe that it is useful to make this distinction, as the parallel data can be considered the truly multivariate time data, and the longitudinal data perhaps should rather be considered stochastic process data, or multiple time data. In this book both types will, however, be called multivariate survival data. The probability mechanisms that can create dependence is considered in Chapter 3.

One advantage of considering these cases independently is that it is common to use different words for the two cases. For example, a high-risk group in the parallel case will have *early* events, whereas a high-risk patient in the longitudinal case will have *frequent* events. Similarly, for covariates, we can discuss whether they are *common*, in the case of parallel data, or *constant*, in the case of longitudinal data.

It is common to apply a term like *correlated survival times*. This term will not be used here, for two reasons. One is that it suggests it makes sense to evaluate the correlation coefficient; and as will be demonstrated, this is only relevant in a few special cases. The other reason is that it is only applicable for parallel data; as for longitudinal data, even when events happen independently of each other, there will typically be correlation between the recorded times, because they are ordered. An illustration of this problem is presented in Section 5.5.2. Also the term *clustered data* has been used for such data. This is in conflict with the term *cluster analysis*, which covers data where the responses cluster, but the objects are not known to be related beforehand. Thus, I think, it is confusing to use this term for the data considered, which are clustered by design.

It is, of course, also possible to have more advanced types of data, obtained by combining several of the types described. In that case, the classification should be considered as establishing the concepts needed for describing the types of data.

1.4.1 Parallel data

In this case several items (individuals, or units of a system) are followed simultaneously. The simplest case to consider is the pair of lifetimes of a set of twins. This gives data sets of matrix form, which in the standard case have time responses of the form T_{ij}, $i = 1, ..., n$, $j = 1, ..., k$, where i denotes group, and j denotes an individual within the group. There is a corresponding set of failure indicators, D_{ij}, $i = 1, ..., n$, $j = 1, ..., k$. Table 1.5 shows an example. It is assumed that there is independence between different values of i, and, possibly, dependence between the times for the same value of i. The number of times (k) in a group is assumed to be pre-specified, but as some of them correspond to failures, and, possibly, some of them to censorings, the number of events $(\sum_j D_{ij})$ is not specified. Of course, the number of events is at most k. Furthermore, there should not be ordering restrictions for these data, like a requirement that $T_{i1} < T_{i2}$. If there are such restrictions, the data should be considered as longitudinal data. In a computer, such data are sometimes naturally considered as one record for each value of i, sometimes for each combination of i and j.

Such data can be extended to allow for a varying (but prespecified) number of times for each value of i, for truncation, and covariates, which may be common to all times in a group (depend on i only), be of the matched pairs type (depend on j only), or be allowed different for each observation (depend on both i and j). The latter are called general covariates (see Section 1.13).

As all data can be considered as longitudinal using calendar time as the time scale, it is fair to ask, why introduce the concept of parallel data? The reason is that parallel data are simpler, we can use other approaches to them, and the interpretation is simpler. For example, the measures of dependence, described in Chapter 4, are only applicable for parallel data; and the non-parametric estimation methods of Chapter 14 are also developed for parallel data only.

1.4.2 Longitudinal data

In this case, we assume that we observe stochastic processes, one for each value of i, and we observe the events or transitions over time. Typically, for human data, there will be one process for each person. This is also called life history analysis. Independence over i will be assumed. Thus the times of transition will be an increasing sequence of times, and, in the simplest cases, only the last time can be a censoring, all the others are events (times of transitions). The number of times, say, K_i, is random. Some models will have a maximum possible number of events, some will not. The times may correspond to recurrent similar events, or it may be transitions between various states, in which case, the data include not only the time, but also the name of the transition taking place. Thus it is known that the process i is followed over the interval $(0, C_i)$, where C_i is a fixed or random time, and the times of events are of the form T_{ij}, $i = 1, ..., n$, $j = 1, ..., K_i$. Depending on the circumstances, we might let the times be the pure event times, using C_i as the end of observation, or we might let the times consist of the event times plus a censoring at time C_i. In the first case, it is possible that $K_i = 0$. It follows from the definition that $T_{ij} \leq T_{i,j+1}$. The cases with equality will need special consideration. That is, the model should be specifically constructed to allow for equality. If it is a process with several possible events, we further need to know the initial state S_{i0}, and the observed transition types, which can be described by the names of the states the transitions lead to, S_{ij}, $i = 1, ..., n$, $j = 1, ..., K_i$. For example, we can name the states as $1, ..., m$, and let the value 0 correspond to censoring. If the initial state is common to all individuals, it might be preferable to call it state number 1. In a computer this is naturally considered as one record per time variable, owing to the random number of times for each individual. In the very simple models, it can be described as one record per person.

There may be covariates, which can be constant (i.e., person specific) or time-dependent. Conceptually, there are two types of time-dependent covariates. There are those that are used to make the hazard model depend on the past development of the process and those that vary owing to factors not considered in the statistical model, that is, external to the process studied.

The model can be extended to account for holes (lapses) in the data – that is, that the same process is followed for several non-connected periods – but this will rarely be necessary. Often, however, we might concentrate on a subset of the possible transitions.

In some cases, we might not have the exact time of each event, but only the number of events within selected time intervals.

1.5   Several individuals

A standard example of parallel data is the lifetimes of several individuals, which cannot be assumed to be independent, because they are related in some way. A prototype bivariate example is twins (see Section 1.5.1), where the monozygotic (identical) twins have all their genetic material in common, and the dizygotic (fraternal) twins have a part of their genetic material in common, like other siblings. However, both types of twins share the childhood environment, including, in particular the pre-birth period, and therefore are more like each other than other siblings. We will use twins as a generic example of bivariate parallel data. Another example is ordinary sibships, where the siblings share some genes, and part of the childhood environment. Klein (1992) studies the survival of whole families from the Framingham study. Other examples could be married couples, group life insurance of employees sharing a common environment at their workplace, and matched pairs experiments (see Section 1.5.4). The field also covers random center effects in a multi-center clinical trial. Multi-state models for such data are considered in Section 5.3.3. Random effects models are described in Chapters 7, 10, and 11. Other models are described in Chapters 13 and 14.

Zygosity	Males	Females
MZ	1366	1448
DZ	2488	2756
UZ	415	512
Total	4269	4716

Table 1.2. Zygosity distribution of Danish twin data (from Hougaard, Harvald, and Holm, 1992). MZ, monozygotic, DZ, dizygotic, UZ, unknown zygosity.

Survival status	Males	Females
Both dead	1150	997
One dead	1106	1118
No deaths	2013	2601

Table 1.3. Survival status of Danish twin pairs in 1980.

1.5.1   Danish twins

This will be a main example in this book. This data set covers a part of the Danish twin register (Hauge *et al.*, 1968; Hauge, 1981). It consists of the twins born in the period 1881–1930 in Denmark of like sex, and where both members are known to be alive at age 15 years. As they are all truncated at the same time, it is only necessary specifically to account for the truncation in some models. The individuals are followed up until 1980. The mortality has been analyzed by Hougaard, Harvald, and Holm (1992a–c). This data set includes 8985 pairs of twins. The zygosity distribution is given in Table 1.2. Most twins are dizygotic. Unfortunately, about 10 % are of unknown zygosity. We have included them separately in the data set to make this problem more visible. The survival status as of 1980 is given in Table 1.3. There were a total of 6518 deaths. The requirement that both twins be alive at age 15 leads to exclusion of about two-thirds of the twin pairs born. There was a very high infant mortality for these twins, firstly because they were born in a period with high infant mortality (1881–1930), and secondly because twins are smaller at birth than other children, and have a higher infant mortality owing to their birth weight. It has been necessary to exclude the early deaths, because zygosity information is difficult to obtain if one or both twins died as infants. As these data will be considered separately for each sex, and, in most models, separately for each zygosity group, the only covariate available is date of birth. These data are used in Section 4.2.1 to illustrate general estimation of Kendall's coefficient of concordance, and in Section 6.7.2 to illustrate multi-state models. There are a number of analyses in Section 8.12.5 to illustrate various features of frailty models. They will be analyzed by bivariate frailty models in Section 10.1.2, 10.4.6, and 10.5.9. They are studied by a short-term frailty model in Section 11.3.3. They are analyzed by marginal modelling approaches in Sections 13.1.4, 13.2.3, and 13.6.3. They are used in Section

Sex	Data set	# deaths	# death times
Males	MZ	1069	1045
	DZ	1999	1916
	MZ+DZ	3068	2846
	UZ	338	334
Females	MZ	904	880
	DZ	1761	1700
	MZ+DZ	2665	2498
	UZ	447	436

Table 1.4. Number of deaths and number of different death times, in days, for Danish twins.

14.11 to illustrate non-parametric estimates. A summary of the applications is given in Section 15.3.1.

Whenever possible, these data will be analyzed by non-parametric methods, to illustrate that this is possible, even though the number of events is very large. This implies a parameter for each death time and therefore the number of event times are described in Table 1.4. Grouping of the times into weekly, monthly, or even yearly data would be possible, and would simplify the analysis. This is specifically considered in Sections 8.12.5 and 14.11.1.

1.5.2 Adoption study

Sørensen et al. (1988) study the relation in lifetime between adoptees and their biological and adoptive parents. The data were considered by means of frailty models for multivariate survival data by Nielsen et al. (1992). The data included 960 Danish adoptees, born 1924–1926, all of whom were alive on their 16th birthday. This means that the data are truncated at this time. Biological mothers were considered at risk from delivery, biological fathers from 280 days before delivery, and the adoptive parents from the formal time of adoption. Their results are described in Section 8.12.6.

1.5.3 Litter-matched tumorigenesis experiment

Mantel, Bohidar, and Ciminera (1977) report data on 50 male and 50 females litters, each of three rats. One rat in each litter was drug-treated and the other two served as control animals. The time to tumor appearance was registered with death of other causes considered as censoring. The study was ended after 104 weeks. The data are shown in Table 1.5. There were only two tumor deaths for male rats, and therefore these data are not included. These data are used as a main example for the univariate methods, by not accounting for the litter effect. This is done for Weibull models (Section 2.2.2), Gompertz models (Section 2.2.3), non-parametric

Drug	Control1	Control2	Drug	Control1	Control2
101+	49	104+	104+	102+	104+
104+	104+	104+	77+	97+	79+
89+	104+	104+	88	96	104+
104	94+	77	96	104+	104+
82+	77+	104+	70	104+	77+
89	91+	90+	91+	70+	92+
39	45+	50	103	69+	91+
93+	104+	103+	85+	72+	104+
104+	63+	104+	104+	104+	74+
81+	104+	69+	67	104+	68
104+	104+	104+	104+	104+	104+
104+	83+	40	87+	104+	104+
104+	104+	104+	89+	104+	104+
78+	104+	104+	104+	81	64
86	55	94+	34	104+	54
76+	87+	74+	103	73	84
102	104+	80+	80	104+	73+
45	79+	104+	94	104+	104+
104+	104+	104+	104+	101	94+
76+	84	78	80	81	76+
72	95+	104+	73	104+	66
92	104+	102	104+	98+	73+
55+	104+	104+	49+	83+	77+
89	104+	104+	88+	79+	99+
103	91+	104+	104+	104+	79

Table 1.5. Time to tumor (weeks) for female rats. Fifty pairs of one drug treated and two control animals. Data of Mantel, Bohidar, and Ciminera (1977). + denotes censoring.

Status	Placebo	6-MP
P	1	10
C	22	7
C	3	32+
C	12	23
C	8	22
P	17	6
C	2	16
C	11	34+
C	8	32+
C	12	25+
C	2	11+
P	5	20+
C	4	19+
C	15	6
C	8	17+
P	23	35+
P	5	6
C	11	13
C	4	9+
C	1	6+
C	8	10+

Table 1.6. Remission length (weeks) for 21 leukemia patients. P, partial remission; C, complete remission. Data of Freireich (1963).

estimation of the integrated hazard function (Section 2.3.2), the proportional hazards model (Section 2.4.8), and accelerated failure time models (Section 2.5.3). The data are analyzed as multivariate data by means of shared frailty models in Section 8.12.1, and by multivariate frailty models in Sections 10.3.1, 10.4.6 and 10.5.9. Marginal models for these data are discussed in Sections 13.2.3 and 13.6.3.

1.5.4 Length of leukemia remission

This is a drug treatment trial, comparing 6-MP with placebo for 21 matched pairs of leukemia patients, published by Freireich (1963). The patients were matched according to center and remission status, either partial or complete. Thus one in each pair received 6-MP and one placebo. The response was the time to remission of leukemia (in weeks). Besides treatment, the only variable known is remission status. The data are listed in Table 1.6. They have been used in many other papers, but in most cases neglecting the pairing. They have, however, been analyzed by means of a frailty model by Andersen et al. (1993). The data are used to evaluate Kendall's τ in Section 4.2.1, and analyzed as multivariate data, by means of a frailty model in Section 8.12.6. Marginal models for these data are discussed in Section 13.2.3 and 13.6.3. A summary of the applications is in Section 15.3.2.

1.6   Similar organs

Another case of parallel data is the times to failure for several similar human organs, like time to blindness of the right and left eye. The same situation arises for kidneys, although it is more difficult to follow the individual status for each kidney. Such data are not common in medicine, but similar data are particularly relevant in industrial applications, where the different times will be failure times for components of a system. A key question in industrial applications is to which extent any part of the system should be duplicated in order to improve reliability of the whole system. Large systems have been designed where reliability is examined assuming that the different units behave independently. However, as the construction implies that the units share the local environment, there is typically a positive dependence between the units of a system. This markedly influences the reliability of the whole system. One probability model for such data is a shock model, where the system is subject to damage caused by successive shocks that may be fatal to one or more of the components. This gives a positive probability of several components' failing simultaneously.

There are clear similarities between the structures for data on different individuals and data on different organs, as they both consider the same type of event for several objects. It is a matter of taste whether one would consider these classes of data as one or two types. The reason we have chosen to consider it as two different types is that there are very large differences in the structure of the dependence we can expect. This topic is further discussed in Section 3.1.1. Censoring is typically homogeneous in such cases (see Section 1.11).

1.6.1   Diabetic retinopathy

This is a treatment comparison study of the time to blindness (severe visual loss) for a set of 197 diabetic patients. One eye for each patient is randomized to laser photocoagulation treatment and the other serves as a control. Thus it allows for within-patient evaluation of the treatment effect. There are two covariates, the type of diabetes (insulin-dependent or non-insulin-dependent) and treatment. This data set was described by Huster, Brookmeyer, and Self (1989). Further analyses of the same data are described by Liang, Self, and Chang (1993) and many others. In this book this data set is only discussed in exercises (Section 1.17 and 15.5).

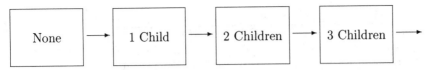

Figure 1.4. Fertility model for a woman.

1.6.2   Amalgam fillings

Aalen, Bjertness and Sønju (1995) consider the problem of the lifetime of amalgam fillings. They have data on all amalgam fillings for 32 persons made during a 17-year period by six dentists. There are from 4 to 38 fillings for each person, giving a total of 566 fillings, of which 143 fail during the observation period. Covariates available are sex and age (quoted as age in 1987). For each filling, time 0 is defined as the time of insertion of the filling. The age of insertion of each filling is not part of the data set, which limits the possible models that can be applied. Times are measured in years. The dependence structure for such data is considered in Section 3.3.8. It is studied by a shared frailty model in Section 8.12.4. The results are summarized in Section 15.3.6.

1.7   Recurrent events

In the previous sections, we have a prespecified number of items, which are followed individually until failure. On the other hand, we can have a single individual who can experience the same event several times. These are longitudinal data. An example is the study of fertility histories for women (see Figure 1.4). There is a state corresponding to the number of children she at any time has given birth to. For each birth, she moves to the next state. We may assume some structure on the hazard function to describe differences in fertility on the one hand, and feedback (stopping when the desired number of children is obtained), on the other hand. The figure does not account for the possibility of twin births, but such a feature could be included by inserting arrows corresponding to jumping over a state. Fertility histories are further discussed in Sections 3.3.1 and 5.3.1. Also multiple cases of adverse events for a patient in a drug clinical trial are covered by this case. This includes, for example, hypoglycemic events for a diabetic patient. There can be only one type of event, as in the fertility model, or the process might be alternating between two states. For example, menstrual bleeding patterns might be considered either bleeding or not bleeding. The number of events for each individual may be low, for example, childbirths, or high, for example, for epileptic seizures or menstrual bleedings.

Somewhat similar problems arise for times to tumor appearance, as each organ may experience multiple tumors. However, it might be difficult to identify the separate tumors.

Retinoid	Control
182	63 102 119 161 161 172 179
No events	88 91 95 105 112 119 119 137 145 167 172
63 68	91 98 108 112 134 137 161 161 179
152	71 174
130 134 145 152	95 105 134 137 140 145 150 150
98 152 182	66 68 130 137
88 95 105 130 137 167	77 85 112 137 161 174
152	81 84 126 134 161 161 174
81	66 77 98 102 102 102
71 84 126 134 152	112
116 130	88 88 91 98 112 134 134 137 137 140 140 152 152
91	77 179
63 68 84 95 152	112
105 152	71 71 74 77 112 116 116 140 140 167
63 102 152	77 95 126 150
63 77 112 140	88 126 130 130 134
77 119 152 161 167	63 74 84 84 88 91 95 108 134 137 179
105 112 145 161 182	81 88 105 116 123 140 145 152 161 161 179
152	88 95 112 119 126 126 150 157 179
81 95	68 68 84 102 105 119 123 123 137 161 179
84 91 102 108 130 134	140
No events	152 182 182
91	81
	63 88 134
	84 134 182

Table 1.7. Times to mammary tumor appearance (days) after retinoid treatment (23 rats) and control treatment (25 rats). Data of Gail, Santner, and Brown (1980).

1.7.1 Mammary tumors

Gail, Santner, and Brown (1980) described a data set of multiple instances of mammary tumors for 48 female rats. The experiment was based on 76 animals, which were injected with a carcinogen at day 0, and treated with retinyl acetate for 60 days. At day 60, the 48 animals, which were tumor free were randomized to continued retinoid prophylaxis (treatment 1), or control (treatment 2). Only the 48 animals are considered. All animals are followed until 182 days after the initial injection. The times are listed in Table 1.7. In some cases, there are multiple tumors detected by the same day. These data are used to illustrate frailty models for recurrent events in Section 9.8.

Age	Baseline	Period 1	Period 2	Period 3	Period 4
31	11	5	3	3	3
30	11	3	5	3	3
25	6	2	4	0	5
36	8	4	4	1	4
22	66	7	18	9	21
29	27	5	2	8	7
31	12	6	4	0	2
42	52	40	20	23	12
37	23	5	6	6	5
28	10	14	13	6	0
36	52	26	12	6	22
24	33	12	6	8	4
23	18	4	4	6	2
36	42	7	9	12	14
26	87	16	24	10	9
26	50	11	0	0	5
28	18	0	0	3	3
31	111	37	29	28	29
32	18	3	5	2	5
21	20	3	0	6	7
29	12	3	4	3	4
21	9	3	4	3	4
32	17	2	3	3	5
25	28	8	12	2	8
30	55	18	24	76	25
40	9	2	1	2	1
19	10	3	1	4	2
22	47	13	15	13	12

Table 1.8. Epileptic count data of Thall and Vail (1990). Placebo treated.

1.7.2 Epileptic seizures

Epileptic seizures make a typical example of recurrent events, but as an individual can experience several thousand seizures over a lifetime, each lasting at most a few minutes, we cannot keep track of the total number of seizures. This makes it impossible to analyze the data in similar detail as fertility data. We will typically assume that the hazard does not depend on the previous number of seizures. Therefore we use the model of Figure 2.2, but only consider the start of seizures and not the duration. We typically count the number of seizures within prespecified time intervals. Thall and Vail (1990) present data of this type, where the number of events within four successive two-week periods are given. This was an add-on experiment, meaning that the patients received their usual anti-epileptic medication plus progabide or placebo. These data are listed in Table 1.8 for the placebo

Age	Baseline	Period 1	Period 2	Period 3	Period 4
18	76	11	14	9	8
32	38	8	7	9	4
20	19	0	4	3	0
30	10	3	6	1	3
18	19	2	6	7	4
24	24	4	3	1	3
30	31	22	17	19	16
35	14	5	4	7	4
27	11	2	4	0	4
20	67	3	7	7	7
22	41	4	18	2	5
28	7	2	1	1	0
23	22	0	2	4	0
40	13	5	4	0	3
33	46	11	14	25	15
21	36	10	5	3	8
35	38	19	7	6	7
25	7	1	1	2	3
26	36	6	10	8	8
25	11	2	1	0	0
22	151	102	65	72	63
32	22	4	3	2	4
25	41	8	6	5	7
35	32	1	3	1	5
21	56	18	11	28	13
41	24	6	3	4	0
32	16	3	5	4	3
26	22	1	23	19	8
21	25	2	3	0	1
36	13	0	0	0	0
37	12	1	4	3	2

Table 1.9. Epileptic count data of Thall and Vail (1990). Progabide treated.

treatment group, and Table 1.9 for the added treatment. Also included in the tables are baseline values covering the number of seizures for the 8 weeks prior to the study, and the age of the patients. These data have been analyzed in Hougaard, Lee, and Whitmore (1997). They are used for illustration of shared frailty models for recurrent events in Section 9.8, independent increments frailty models in Section 11.1.6, and short-term frailty models in Section 11.2.1. A summary of the applications is presented in Section 15.3.5.

1.7.3   Infections in catheters for patients on dialysis

These data describe the time from insertion of catheter into dialysis patients until it has to be removed owing to infection. There were 82 patients enrolled in the study and they had from one to eight observation periods. A subset of the data covering the first two observation periods for 38 patients was published by McGilchrist and Aisbett (1991). The time scale used is time since insertion for each catheter. This, unfortunately, restricts the set of possible models we might apply as we cannot obtain data on how long patients had been without a catheter. It would have been preferable to record data using calendar time, or age in days. We only know that there were at least ten weeks between successive periods. It is possible that the catheters were removed for other reasons, and thus there can be more than one censoring. The published data thus present themselves like parallel data, as we have designed the data set to include the same number of times for all persons, but they are really longitudinal data. There are three covariates. The age at the time of insertion, which may be the same, or may be increased from period 1 to 2. The sex is given as 1 for males and 2 for females. The type of disease is specified as 0=GN, 1=AN, 2=PKD, and 3=other. These abbreviations were not explained in the paper, but they probably mean glumerulonephritis, acute tubular nephropathy, and polycystic kidney disease. The data are given in Table 1.10. They are used to create a standard proportional hazards model in Section 2.4.8 and to illustrate Kendall's τ in Section 4.2.1, frailty models in Section 8.12.3, and bivariate frailty models in Section 10.5.9. Marginal models for these data are considered in Sections 13.1.4, 13.2.3, and 13.6.3, and general non-parametric methods in Section 14.11.2. A summary of the applications is presented in Section 15.3.4.

1.7.4   Insurance claims

Gossiaux and Lemaire (1981) collected six data sets from the literature on the number of automobile insurance claims per policy over a fixed time period. Two data sets are given in Table 1.11, a Swiss data set of Bichsel (1964) and a British data set of Johnson and Hey (1971). These data were analyzed by Willmot (1987) by means of Poisson overdisper-

Times	Event	Age	Sex	Type	Times	Event	Age	Sex	Type
8, 16	1, 1	28	1	3	23, 13	1, 0	48	2	0
22, 28	1, 1	32	1	3	447, 318	1, 1	31, 32	2	3
30, 12	1, 1	10	1	3	24, 245	1, 1	16, 17	2	3
7, 9	1, 1	51	1	0	511, 30	1, 1	55, 56	2	0
53, 196	1, 1	69	2	1	15, 154	1, 1	51, 52	1	0
7, 333	1, 1	44	2	1	141, 8	1, 0	34	2	3
96, 38	1, 1	35	2	1	149, 70	0, 0	42	2	1
536, 25	1, 0	17	2	3	17, 4	1, 0	60	1	1
185, 177	1, 1	60	2	3	292, 114	1, 1	43, 44	2	3
22, 159	0, 0	53	2	0	15, 108	1, 0	44	2	3
152, 562	1, 1	46, 47	1	2	402, 24	1, 0	30	2	3
13, 66	1, 1	62, 63	2	1	39, 46	1, 0	42, 43	2	1
12, 40	1, 1	43	1	1	113, 201	0, 1	57, 58	2	1
132, 156	1, 1	10	2	0	34, 30	1, 1	52	2	1
2, 25	1, 1	53	1	0	130, 26	1, 1	54	2	0
27, 58	1, 1	56	2	1	5, 43	0, 1	50, 51	2	1
152, 30	1, 1	57	2	2	190, 5	1, 0	44, 45	2	0
119, 8	1, 1	22	2	3	54, 16	0, 0	42	2	3
6, 78	0, 1	52	2	2	63, 8	1, 0	60	1	2

Table 1.10. Time (days) to infection in kidney catheters for 38 patients on dialysis. Data of McGilchrist and Aisbett (1991).

sion model. They will also be analyzed by Poisson overdispersion models in Section 9.8.1.

1.8 Repeated measurements

Such data are typically results of a designed experiment. The standard case is a cross-over experiment. The time to the same type of event is studied for a fixed number of times for the individuals. It is similar to the recurrent events in the sense that we study the same type of event and it is done at longitudinal time points. The data structure is parallel, because the number of observation times is fixed. For each spell we define a start time of 0, but there will be holes in the physical time. There is no overlap in the physical time between the coordinates. It is also necessary to have a maximum time allowed after which the observation will be censored. For example, this model can be used for measuring the time to a short-term effect of a drug and if the effect does not show up within a given period, the time is censored, corresponding to no effect of the drug. For example, within anesthesia one can make a cross-over experiment of two drugs, applied on separate days. If the person does not become unconscious, one has to give up following the process and censor the observation after

No. of claims	CH 1961	UK 1968
0	103704	370412
1	14075	46545
2	1766	3935
3	255	317
4	45	28
5	6	3
6	2	0
Total	119 853	421240

Table 1.11. Automobile claims data. CH, Switzerland (Bichsel, 1964) and UK, United Kingdom (Johnson and Hey, 1971).

some prespecified time. It is a prerequisite that there be no damage caused by the event, because if there were, we could not be sure that we could get the desired number of response times in each case. Therefore, it would not work to evaluate a drug like glucagon to increase blood glucose after a hypoglycemic attack, because we do no want to induce hypoglycemic attacks and thus we cannot be sure of obtaining the desired number of sessions in each individual. The multi-state models do not make sense in this case, because a given time point corresponds to several different points in physical time. The most relevant models are the shared frailty models of Chapter 7.

1.8.1 Watermaze

The Morris watermaze is a memory and learning model. One such application is described in Rasmussen *et al.* (1996). Rats are put into a pool filled with a liquid that is not transparent. There is an underwater (and thus invisible) platform that the rat has to find. The first time, the platform is found by coincidence, but later the rat learns where the platform is and is able to find it faster. The interesting aspect is how much faster the rat can locate the platform. If the platform is not found within a short period (2 or 4 minutes) the rat is taken up to avoid drowning. This ensures that we obtain the required number of sessions for each rat.

1.8.2 Exercise test times

Danahy *et al.* (1977) study the time to angina before and after treatment with isosorbide dinitrate, nitroglycerin, and placebo. Parts of these data have been analyzed using multivariate survival data methods by Pickles and Chrouchley (1994a,b). There were 21 patients undergoing ten exercise tests, one immediately before treatment and three after treatment, at 1, 3 and 5 hours, respectively. The exercise tests lasted until the patients had angina pectoris or censoring (14 occasions). The observation times

SLP	SLT	OP0	OP1	OP3	OP5	OI0	OI1	OI3	OI5
155	431	150	172	118	143	136	445+	393+	226
269	259	205	287	211	207	250	306	206	224
408	446	221	244	147	250	215	232	258	268
308	349	150	290	205	210	235	248	298	207
135	175	87	157	135	105	129	121	110	102
409	523	301	357	388	388	425	580	613	514
455	488	342	390	441	468	441	504+	519+	484+
182	227	215	210	188	189	208	264	210	172
141	102	131	125	99	115	154	110	123	105
104	231	108	114	136	111	89	145	172	123
207	249	228	224	251	206	250	230	264	216
198	247	190	199	243	222	147	403	290	208
274	397	234	249	267	241	231	540+	370	316
191	251	218	194	197	223	224	432	291	212
156	401	199	329	197	176	152	733+	492	303
458	766	406	431	448	328	417	743+	566	391
188	199	194	168	168	159	213	250	150	180
258	566+	277	264	276	251	490	559+	557+	439
437	552	424	512	560	478	406	651	624	554
115	237	234	232	281	237	229	327	280	321
200	387	227	199	223	227	265	565+	504+	517+

Table 1.12. Exercise times to angina pectoris (seconds). SL: sublingual, O: Oral, T: nitroglycerin, P: Placebo, I: isosorbide dinitrate. 0: Before intake, 1,3,5: Time (hours) after intake. Data of Danahy *et al.* (1977).

ranged from 110 to 743 seconds and thus there was sufficient time between the occasions as there were at least 1 hour between tests. The purpose of the study is to evaluate the treatment effect. The data are listed in Table 1.12. They are used to illustrate frailty models in Section 8.12.2. Whether there is a varying degree of dependence is considered in Sections 10.3.1 and 10.4.6. Marginal models are used to evaluate the treatment effect in Sections 13.2.3 and 13.6.3. They are used to discuss the limitations of non-parametric methods in Section 14.11.3. A summary of the applications is presented in Section 15.3.3.

1.9   Different events

In the previous sections, there have been some similarities between the events. This, of course, might not be the case. For example, we might have a structure where a person is followed in three states, healthy, disabled and dead (see Figure 1.5). This does have many of the same problems as in the case of several individuals; but, for example, symmetry is not an option

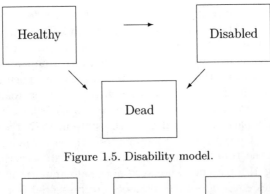

Figure 1.5. Disability model.

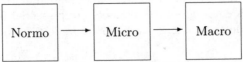

Figure 1.6. Albuminuria model.

and it is particularly relevant to consider how the various events influence the future course for that person. For such data, the multi-state models of Chapter 6 are particularly relevant. The disability model is further discussed in Section 5.3.2. Typically, there are only few possible events.

A famous example is the survival-sacrifice experiments, where some animals are killed in order to determine the probability of having experienced a tumor at selected time points. More comments on this model can be found in Section 5.10.

1.9.1 Albuminuria

Another example, in Section 1.3.1, is the albumin status for diabetic patients. Albumin is a protein that is excreted in the urine in amounts of less than 10 mg/24 h for healthy persons. As the kidneys for a diabetic patient deteriorate, the amount excreted can increase up to 10 g/24 h. It is a tradition to use limits of 30 and 300 mg/24 h to define normoalbuminuria (<30), microalbuminuria (30–300), and macroalbuminuria (>300 mg/24 h). The latter is also termed nephropathy. This model is depicted in Figure 1.6. Major physical exercise and diseases like the flu might produce random fluctuations and blood-pressure-lowering agents can reduce the excretion, but generally the excretion increases over time and therefore the process is irreversible. In actually studying this process, data are collected based on urine samples, and therefore interval censored. There is a major day-to-day variation in excretion and the clinical definition therefore requires that two of three consecutive measurements are above 30 mg/24 h in order to diagnose the complication microalbuminuria as persistent. Similarly, two of three must be above 300 mg/24 h for macroalbuminuria to be persistent. For the applications in this book, the diagnosis is considered to be at the first measurement above the respective limit. It is outside the scope of this book to analyze the data as interval censored data. The figure has similarities to the structure of Figure 1.4 on the birth histories for women, but because birth is the same event it makes sense to compare the intensity for getting the first and the second child, and it makes much less sense to compare the hazard of microalbuminuria with that of macroalbuminuria.

This data set was studied by Gall *et al.* (1995), who considered the mortality for 328 patients, according to the state in 1987, the start of the study (baseline). During the follow-up period, 51 patients died. Gall *et al.* (1997) studied the time to microalbuminuria, a state experienced by 72 patients among 191 patients who were normoalbuminuric in 1987. More detailed analyses covering all 328 patients are presented in Section 6.7.4. A summary of the applications can be found in Section 15.3.7.

1.9.2 Colon cancer

This is a clinical trial including 929 stage C colon cancer patients enrolled between March 1984 and October 1987. They were randomized to observation, levamisole alone, or levamisole combined with fluorouracil. The study was done by Moertel *et al.* (1990) and also considered by Fleming (1992). The aim was to study both the time to cancer recurrence and death.

1.9.3 Survival after myocardial infarction

This data set on the short-term mortality after myocardial infarction was considered by Madsen, Hougaard, and Gilpin (1983), Hougaard and Madsen (1985), and Hougaard (1986a) and covers 1140 admissions to a hospital for 1059 patients suffering an infarction. The mortality for one year was considered with special emphasis on the first six weeks in order to discharge patients early, if the risk of death or complications was low. Of particular importance are the complications cardiac arrest, which can be effectively treated at the coronary care unit, and cardiogenic shock, which is connected with a very large mortality.

Owing to lack of data, it is, unfortunately, not possible to consider the dependence between multiple admissions.

These data are considered in Section 2.2.7 for illustrating mixture models and in Section 2.4.8 to illustrate interpretation of regression coefficients. The analysis describing the time to the various events is performed by means of a multi-state model in Section 6.7.3.

1.9.4 Stanford heart transplant data

This is one of the most widely used examples of survival data. It includes the patients enrolled in the Stanford Heart transplant program, from entry

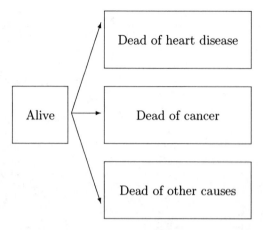

Figure 1.7. Competing risks model with three causes of death.

into the program, until death. It is listed by Crowley and Hu (1977), and further analyzed by Kalbfleisch and Prentice (1980) and Allison (1995). It covers 103 patients. Some of them (69) underwent a heart transplantation. The number of deaths was 75. The interesting question is whether their survival was improved by transplantation. These data are used in Section 2.4.8 to illustrate what it means that the explanatory variables should be known at all times. A more correct analysis with state-dependent mortality is performed in Section 6.7.1. A non-parametric analysis is performed in Section 14.11.4.

1.10   Competing risks

This term covers cause of death data, corresponding to the various causes of death "competing" to end the life of a given person. Such data are also called multiple decrement data. Say there are k causes of death. The data structure is the lifetime T_i with cause of death indicators $D_{i1}, ..., D_{ik}$. At most one of the indicators equals 1. Alternatively, we can have a single variable, S_i, with the cause of death, being equal to j, when $D_{ij} = 1$, and zero for censorings. This model is considered as longitudinal data, as depicted in Figure 1.7. There is one difference compared to the other cases, and that is that there is at most one event within each structure. This seriously limits what we can estimate, as will be illustrated below, but we have included this case because we can borrow some knowledge from the other cases in order to illustrate the problems with such data (see Chapter 12). Strictly speaking, competing risks data are not truly multivariate data. It is included because the field can benefit from the general theory. A detailed consideration of competing risks is, however,

Cause of death

	Conventional mice
Thymic lymphoma	159 189 191 198 200 207 220 235 245 250 256
	261 265 266 280 343 356 383 403 414 428 432
Recticulum cell sarcoma	317 318 399 495 525 536 549 552 554 557 558
	571 586 594 596 605 612 621 628 631 636 643
	647 648 649 661 663 666 670 695 697 700 705
	712 713 738 748 753
Other causes	163 179 206 222 228 249 252 282 324 333 341
	366 385 407 420 431 441 461 462 482 517 517
	524 564 567 586 619 620 621 622 647 651 686
	761 763
	Germ-free mice
Thymic lymphoma	158 192 193 194 195 202 212 215 229 230 237
	240 244 247 259 300 301 321 337 415 434 444
	485 496 529 537 624 707 800
Recticulum cell sarcoma	430 590 606 638 655 679 691 693 696 747 752
	760 778 821 986
Other causes	136 246 255 376 421 565 616 617 652 655 658
	660 662 675 681 734 736 737 757 769 777 800
	807 825 855 857 864 868 870 870 873 882 895
	910 934 942 1015 1019

Table 1.13. Necropsy data for RFM mice (days) of Hoel and Walburg (1972).

also useful for other cases, as similar problems arise for the time to the first event in the different events case.

This case is not considered as parallel data, even though a commonly used approach is to define identical cause-specific lifetimes $T_{ij} = T_i$, in which case, the data appear like our standard parallel setup. In popular terms, the reason for not doing so is that nothing is run in parallel. More specifically, the cause-specific lifetime approach suggests that we meaningfully can discuss a lifetime of heart disease. We cannot do so, as will be elaborated upon in Chapter 12.

1.10.1   Radiation-exposed mice

These data, which are described in Hoel and Walburg (1972), consider the lifetimes of two types of male mice (conventional and germ-free), who are exposed to 300 rads of X-radiation at 5–6 weeks of age. There are 95 conventional mice and 82 germ-free mice. The cause of death is described as three possibilities, thymic lymphoma, recticulum cell sarcoma, and other causes. The data are given in Table 1.13 and are considered in Section 12.7 to illustrate competing risks models.

1.10.2 Malignant melanoma

This data set, originally presented by Drzewiecki, Ladefoged, and Christensen (1980) and later listed in Andersen *et al.* (1993), concerns 205 patients who had a radical operation for malignant melanoma (cancer of the skin) at the Department of Plastic Surgery, University Hospital of Odense, Denmark. The time since operation is measured. They were followed up until the end of 1977. The cause of death is considered as either death from malignant melanoma or death of other causes. There were 57 deaths from malignant melanoma and 14 from other causes. The covariates known are level of invasion (values 1, 2 or 3), inflammatory cell infiltration (ICI), (values 1, 2, 3 or 4), melanoma in mucous membrane (indicator), presence of epithelioid cells (indicator), presence of ulceration (indicator), tumor thickness (in 1/100 mm), sex, (1=F, 2=M), age at operation (years) and biopsy taken before operation, (indicator). These data are considered in Section 2.3.1 to illustrate the Kaplan-Meier estimate, in Section 2.3.2 to illustrate the Nelson-Aalen estimate, and in Section 2.4.8 to illustrate the Cox model. Finally, they are considered as competing risks data in Section 12.7. A summary of the applications is presented in Section 15.3.8.

1.11 Types of censoring

For univariate data the standard type of censoring is right censoring, which is further subclassified according to whether the time is fixed by design or is considered random. We might further experience interval censoring, as described in Section 1.3. For multivariate longitudinal data the standard is to study processes from time 0 until some time C, which is often different from process to process. For parallel data, there are two standard cases, homogeneous and heterogeneous censoring. Homogeneous censoring, which is also called univariate censoring, corresponds to observing the whole group as a stochastic process, and is the standard for data on similar organs. End of study or death of the individual leads to simultaneous censoring for both eyes. For twins, end of study happens at the same age, which also corresponds to homogeneous censoring. However, in other cases this might not be so. For example, for twins, a single individual can be lost to follow-up during the study, even though the other is still followed. In a study of the failure of the kidneys of persons, a healthy individual may donate a kidney to a sick family member. In this case, it is preferable to censor both kidneys at the time of removal of one kidney, unless one is specifically interested in the post-removal period. For studying the familial dependence for lifetimes of fathers and sons using individual age as the time scale, end of study happens at different time points. In this case, one should either consider this as a parallel data set with a common risk dependence, or if an event-related mechanism is relevant, choose the age of the son as a common time scale, with fathers age at birth of the son as an explanatory variable. Heterogeneous censoring applies when each individual has a separate censoring time.

The above examples have all had censoring times that are independent of the survival time. In some models also more advanced censoring patterns are acceptable. This will be called process-dependent censoring. This allows censoring at time t to depend on the observed process up to time t. The classical example of this is a study of the lifetimes of electric bulbs. A number of bulbs are turned on simultaneously and the experiment continues until a pre-specified number of them have burned out. This is denoted as type II censoring. In this book, the examples will rather concern the events for the same group or individual. The most extreme case is censoring at the time of the first event, which leads to competing risks data. In that case, there is a limit to what can be identified, as described in Chapter 12. As another example, one can suggest that in a study of adverse events as recurrent events in a clinical trial of a new drug, each event leads to a probability p of withdrawal from the study and thus censoring. In some models, this will be acceptable.

When there are no censorings, we call data complete. In almost all cases in survival data, censoring is right censoring, i.e., observations are known to be larger than some given value.

To describe calculations with right censored observations, we use an indicator variable, D, being 1 if the observation is an event and 0 when it is a censoring. For listing censored data we use the symbol $+$, so that $t+$ denotes a censoring at time t. This is more in line with common language than the symbol * used by many authors, and it will not be used when it can be confused with the mathematical addition operator.

1.12   Types of truncation

Truncation is a well-defined concept in univariate survival data. There it is just conditional on the event's not having happened at the relevant time. In the simplest case it is just specifying that the person is alive at the relevant age. For multivariate data, there are more ways in which truncation can occur. The most simple is the parallel case, where it is assumed that there have been no events until the relevant day, as for the twin data set, where both twins should be alive at the age of 15 years. In other cases, it might mean that we only include individuals that satisfy some requirement; for example, a company might give pension insurance for employees who are above 25 years old. For longitudinal data, we may or may not have information on what has happened previously. For example, for fertility data, we typically can get information on how many children the woman has, whereas for epileptic patients, it is impossible to find out how many seizures the patient has had at the time of inclusion in a study.

Truncation may relate to several different events. For example, for fertility data, we may restrict attention to women who are alive and have no children at age 25 years. This truncation not only refers to the event under study (child birth), but also to survival.

1.13   Explanatory variables

As seen above, there are, in many cases, some explanatory factors or covariates available. This might be factors that are of intrinsic importance for the application, like treatment in a drug trial, or factors that are known or suspected to influence the hazard of event, but not interesting per se. The notation used in the parallel case is that there is a p-vector of covariates for the i, j-th object denoted z_{ij}, and the components of it z_{ijm}. Two important special cases stand out, the common covariates and the matched pairs covariates. *Common covariates* mean covariates that are common for all members of the group in the case of parallel data. For longitudinal data, these are more correctly termed constant covariates. They do not change as the process develops. In both cases, a simple description is that the covariates depend on i only. For monozygotic twins, examples are sex and any other genetically based covariate. Both monozygotic and dizygotic twins share year of birth and the common pre-birth environment. For litters in general, any variable that relates to the mother is common for the litter members. In principle, the same applies to the father, but it can be more difficult to document the father of each animal. On the other hand, *matched pairs* covariates is a term for covariates that only depend on j. This makes sense for parallel data, but not for longitudinal data, as we cannot be sure of having the same number of observations for each individual. The typical example of a matched pairs covariate is a drug trial, where individuals are paired and then one in each pair receives each treatment. We use this in the strict sense, so that coordinate $j = 1$ corresponds to one treatment and $j = 2$ to the other. This is also the reason for the name chosen (matched pairs). Also the case of more than two treatments is covered by this approach. The effect of matched pairs covariates can be evaluated within groups. Of course, we also allow for more general covariates, but the special cases are better at showing perspectives and limitations of the approaches considered.

In a cross-over repeated measurements study of two treatments — say, A and B — it is common to randomize half the individuals to the order AB and the other half to the order BA. This gives a matched pairs covariate, when j indexes the treatment. If instead j indexes the period, this will not give a matched pairs covariate according to our definition. Some of the considerations for matched pairs covariates will still apply when j indexes the period. Some other considerations will not apply and this is the reason for using the strict definition.

A special point is that we will also consider unobserved or neglected covariates. In particular, unobserved common covariates lead to dependence between the individuals in a group. In the univariate case, unobserved covariates are considered in Sections 2.2.7 and 2.4.6; and in the multivariate case, this is discussed in Section 3.1.2 and treated mathematically in Chapter 7.

1.14   Purpose of multivariate survival studies

Typically, the subject matter problem directly presents the aim of the whole study. In this section, we will rather consider the aim in a more technical statistical frame. For example, for the subject matter problem, the aim can be to quantify the effect of a covariate, and in that case, it is very important whether the covariate is fixed by the design (like treatment in a randomized study) or uncontrolled. As another example, in an epidemiological study, it is very important whether a variable is modifiable, like smoking, or not modifiable, like sex, because a modifiable variable immediately implies a suggestion on how to change the risk in the future. These aspects are very important for the interpretation from the statistical point of view, but for the technical computational point of view presented here, it is more important whether they vary within or between observational units, as described in the previous section. This section will also consider the purpose of a statistical analysis rather than a whole study. A study will typically consist of a number of analyses to illustrate various aspects of the problem, including for example effect of secondary variables and checking of the main model.

On the general level, we will consider five different aims of an analysis of multivariate survival data. A major aim is to evaluate the effect of some covariate, in general. This will, however, be considered as two different aims, depending on whether the covariate is a common covariate or a matched pairs covariate. The reason for this is that some procedures only make sense for one of these methods, so we need this splitting in order to recognize the differences. This can be illustrated by normally distributed data, where the paired t-test only makes sense for matched pairs covariates. Of course, we might also be interested in the effect of general covariates, that is, covariates that are neither of the common nor of the matched pairs type. This is not described as a separate aim, because the two simple types of covariates well illustrate problems with such a design. A third aim is to evaluate the dependence between the various responses in the data, for example the dependence between twins, or in the case of data on different

Purposes
Effect of common covariates
Effect of matched pairs covariates
Assessment of dependence
Prediction (evaluation of probabilities)
Model checking (for another model)

Table 1.14. Purposes of a model for multivariate survival data. For comments, see text.

events, the effect of, say, myocardial infarction on death. As a longitudinal example, we can consider recurrent events of myocardial infarctions. There the dependence leads to the risk of a future attack being higher, when the person already has suffered such an event. The interest in the dependence relies on determining by how much the risk is increased. The fourth aim considered is prediction, that is, determining the probability of some event or events happening for a single group or individual, based on information collected before (that can be an overall probability or based on some covariates) or during the study (that is, conditional probabilities given the responses for other individuals or early observation for the actual individual). In other words, this aim concerns absolute risks, where the first three concern relative risks. Evaluating the median is also included in the prediction purpose. Finally, the aim can be to study the goodness-of-fit, which we will also call model checking. In this case the model is considered in order to evaluate whether a simpler model is a satisfactory description. A model to test goodness-of-fit might not in itself be satisfactory from a theoretical point of view. In fact, the actual model might not be specified, as in a standard normal distribution, where one studies the residuals in some way. The five purposes are summarized in Table 1.14.

The overall basis for this book is that we have multivariate data showing dependence. Correspondingly, simple (or unspecific) methods for testing independence are not covered. This purpose, which in our terminology is model checking of an independence model, is only covered by using a specific dependence model and then testing independence in this frame.

1.15   Chapter summary

Survival data concern times to some events. An event is typically defined as a transition from one of a few states to another state. The main emphasis is the timing of this event. It is a standard requirement that at any one time, we observe whether the event has happened at that specific time point. This should be satisfied for all times, until a time of end of observation (censoring). The time is measured from some specific time point, but observation does not need to start at that time (truncation).

	Parallel Long.	Objects	Event types	Number of times (k)	Number of events (e)
Individuals	P	Several	1	Fixed	$\leq k$
Similar organs	P	Several	1	Fixed	$\leq k$
Different events	L	1	Several	Random	$\leq k$
Recurrent events	L	1	1	Random	$k-1 \leq e \leq k$
Repeated meas.	P	1	1	Fixed	$\leq k$
Competing risks	L	1	Several	1	≤ 1

Table 1.15. Key properties of the various data types.

We have classified multivariate data into two data structures, which are further subdivided into six different types. The advantage of this classification is that it helps choosing the most appropriate model. A summary of the properties of the various types is given in Table 1.15. Based on the number of objects, the number of event types and whether the number of times is fixed or random, it is possible to classify most of the data types. Basically, the first three columns describe the differences. The last two columns are consequences of whether the data are parallel or longitudinal. The only types that cannot be discriminated by these aspects are the first two. In fact, it is a matter of taste whether they should be considered as one or two classes. Whether a set of data belongs to the individuals or similar organs classes depends on how physically close the objects are. Similar organs are physically related and share the environment at any time instance. Several individuals might share risk factors, but only share the environment at some moments. Repeated measurements data are special in the sense that even though the experiment is done over time, it is designed so that all individuals are secured to experience the pre-specified treatments.

In many cases, there are covariates available. It is important to consider whether these covariates have the same value for all individuals in a group for parallel data (are constant for longitudinal data), or as another special case, each group have the same set of covariates, as this places some restrictions on the models that can be applied. Truncation is much more important for multivariate data than for univariate and needs to be taken seriously. The purpose of a study can be to evaluate the effect of a given covariate, or to evaluate the degree of dependence, to determine a probability or to check the assumptions of a simpler model.

1.16 Bibliographic comments

There are many interesting books on univariate survival data methods with varying amounts of material within the field we call multivariate survival (Kalbfleisch and Prentice, 1980; Cox and Oakes, 1984). More recent books based on the theory of counting processes are Andersen *et al.* (1993) and

Fleming and Harrington (1991). There are also several more applied books, for example, Klein and Moeschberger (1997). For a description of how to do the analyses in SAS, see Allison (1995).

Section 1.1 is based on Hougaard (1999). Some of the classifications of data types have been introduced and discussed by Hougaard (1987). There is a major discussion of various kinds of data in Hutchinson and Lai (1991). Regarding the data sets, references have been included at the introduction of the data.

Table 1.1 and Figures 1.1, 1.2 and 1.3 first appeared in Hougaard (1999). Table 1.2 first appeared in Hougaard, Harvald, and Holm (1992a). Table 1.5 is a transcript from Mantel, Bohidar, and Ciminera (1977). Table 1.6 is a transcript from Freireich *et al.* (1963). Table 1.7 is a transcript from Gail, Santner, and Brown (1980). Table 1.8 and 1.9 are transcripts from Thall and Vail (1990). Table 1.10 is a transcript from McGilchrist and Aisbett (1991). Table 1.11 contains transcripts from Bichsel (1964) and Johnson and Hey (1971). Table 1.12 is a transcript from Danahy *et al.* (1977). Table 1.13 is a transcript from Hoel and Walburg (1972), by permission of Oxford University Press.

1.17   Exercises

Exercise 1.1 Mammary tumors

Describe the truncation and censoring present in the data of Section 1.7.1. Is the covariate of the common or matched pairs type? What is the purpose of this study?

Exercise 1.2 Diabetic retinopathy

Consider the diabetic retinopathy data of Section 1.6.1. Is the type of diabetes a common covariate, a matched pairs covariate, or a general covariate? Which kind of covariate is treatment? Which kind of covariate is the interaction of type of diabetes and treatment? What kind of censoring would you imagine there could be for such data?

Exercise 1.3 Tumorigenesis data

Consider the data of Section 1.5.3. Is the covariate treatment of the common or matched pairs type? What is the purpose of the experiment? Is the censoring homogeneous?

2
Univariate survival data

This chapter gives a description of univariate survival data methods. The topic is also described in many other books. Thus, it is not absolutely necessary for persons experienced in survival analysis to read it, but it does contain notation and key results that will be needed later. Furthermore, some aspects are treated in more detail than elsewhere, in order to create a basis for understanding specific points in later chapters.

First as an introduction to survival data, we consider the fundamental question, What makes this type of data different from all other types of data? Or, in other words, why does this subject need a special statistical theory? The answer is given in Section 2.1. The reason is, of course, that we observe something that develops dynamically over time. There are two aspects to this; one is that the data are special in the sense that they are only partially observed as we only know the time of death after it has happened and that might happen after the time of evaluating the data. Consequently, at the time of evaluation, all we know is that the person is still alive. In that case, we say that data are censored. The other aspect is that many evaluations should be made conditional on what is known presently and this may well change over time. This appears extremely natural; we only consider the risk of death for persons who are still alive, but it implies that many standard statistical approaches cannot be used. As an extra result of these considerations, we get the answers to two other questions: Why is the hazard function so important in this case? Why are non-parametric methods so popular?

Theory for the univariate case will be considered, first the classical parametric methods, the exponential, the Weibull and the Gompertz distribution and the piecewise constant hazards model (Section 2.2). Mixture models are treated in detail, because they are needed for the frailty models and more generally for understanding random effects concepts. Understanding the univariate case in depth is necessary in order to apply the approach to multivariate observations. Parametric models allow for rather specific evaluations and for interpreting survival patterns, but are often more restrictive than desired. In biostatistics, non-parametric methods are now the standard in survival analysis and the most basic methods, the Kaplan-Meier estimate of the survivor function and the Nelson-Aalen estimate of the integrated hazard function, are considered in Section 2.3. How covariates and risk factors can be included in a proportional hazards regression model is described in Section 2.4. This covers the standard partial likelihood approach suggested by Cox (1972). Time-dependent covariates are treated in detail, because they are needed for fitting the more advanced multi-state models. The effect of neglected covariates, which can lead to non-proportional hazards, is also treated in more detail than is usual. This is in order better to understand random effects models. An alternative model for the effect of covariates is the accelerated failure times model (Section 2.5). This model is more restrictive owing to lack of suitable estimation routines in the non-parametric case, but it allows for a more direct random effects interpretation and avoids some of the problems with neglected covariates. Finally, there are a few words on counting processes (Section 2.6).

At least a cursory reading of this chapter is recommended. For the multi-state models, Section 2.4.4 is a key section. Similarly for frailty models, Sections 2.2.7 and 2.4.6 must be read. For marginal modeling, Section 2.4.5 must be read. For non-parametric models, Section 2.3 is useful.

2.1   Special features of survival data

In broad terms what makes survival data special is that the responses are times and times are not measured in the same way as other variables. Other variables are measured almost instantaneously, and independently of the response size. In survival data, the largest observations require longer time to observe than the shortest observations. Time is observed sequentially. This does have several consequences. Probably most statisticians will mention the presence of censored data (Section 2.1.1), as the most special feature in survival analysis. I think, however, that the concept of conditioning (Section 2.1.2) is much more fundamental. Other, less important, reasons include the choice of parametric models (Section 2.1.3) and the possibility of having no or multiple events (Section 2.1.4).

2.1.1 Censored data

Censored data means that the observations are only partially known. One major reason for this is that the person studied is alive when the data are evaluated, and thus his complete lifetime is not known at that time. All that is known is that his lifetime exceeds his age at the time of evaluation. The presence of censored data is a major technical problem. First, we have to make some assumptions about the mechanisms behind censoring. Censoring has to be unrelated to the future lifetime. This requirement has to be made explicit. The probability distribution of the residual lifetime for those censored must equal that of those who are not censored. If there are any explanatory variables, the probability distribution of the residual lifetime of those censored must equal that of those who are not censored, having the same value of the explanatory variables. At a first glance, it seems complicated to analyze such data, but it turns out that this is not the case. The key point is that the likelihood function should include terms corresponding to what we observe, and this means that if an exact lifetime is observed, it should contribute with its density, and if it is censored at some time t, it should contribute with the probability that the lifetime exceeds t.

There are many other reasons for censoring than just the individual's being alive at the time of evaluating the data. The person can be lost to follow-up, for example; if a person emigrates, it may be impossible to keep track of the person. However, even if it is possible to track the person, it can be irrelevant to study that person if we study some risk factor related to the area that he moved from. It might be decided in the protocol that observation should stop at some pre-specified time. For example, we might be particularly interested in the mortality before age 70, and then decide to censor the survivors at that age. In industrial applications it is common to have type II censoring, where the study is stopped after a fixed number of events. If the aim is to study death from cardiovascular disease, the person needs to be censored if he dies from cancer.

Censoring is not only a problem for survival data. Just about any measurement device has a range within which it can function and outside of which it only says that the result is outside of the range. For example, a thermometer can only measure the temperature within a given range. This is also a common problem in assay methods for measurement of the concentration of some substance in blood, where there is a detection limit, under which we just know that the concentration is small. For some assays, a large proportion of healthy individuals has so small concentration that a value cannot be assessed.

2.1.2 Conditioning

This problem is most easily introduced by an example. We study the mortality data of the Statistical Yearbook (1996) of Denmark, with a few approximations, like assuming constant density within each year, and extrapolation above 100 years. According to this table, the median lifetime of a Danish male is 75 years and 80 days, meaning that 50 % of the males die before they reach that age, and 50 % after, based on the mortality experience in 1993–94. Can a person celebrating his 75'th years birthday utilize this information, suggesting that he only has 80 days left, evaluated by the median? No, the death pattern from age 0 to age 74 years is irrelevant for his consideration. The natural approach is to take his present state as known, that is, to condition on his being alive at age 75. It is then possible to evaluate the conditional probability that he will die within the coming 80 days (1.4 %); or he might be more interested in the conditional median given survival until age 75, and this quantity is 82 years 294 days. In contrast, if he had died at age 70, say, we would never ask the question of his lifetime, because we already know the answer. What is appropriate for this person is the truncated distribution of the lifetime after age 75 years, i.e., the distribution given that the lifetime is at least 75 years. It is slightly more precise to say left-truncated; but as only left-truncation is considered here, it will just be called truncation. This aspect has enormous consequences for the approach to survival data. One logical consequence is to discuss the distribution of the lifetime, say, T, by means of the hazard function defined at any time point t as the probability of death within a short interval, given that the person was alive at the beginning of the interval. That is,

$$\lambda(t) = \lim_{\Delta t \searrow 0} \frac{Pr(t \leq T < t + \Delta t \mid t \leq T)}{\Delta t}, \tag{2.1}$$

which equals $-d \log S(t)/dt$, where $S(t)$ is the survivor function, i.e., $S(t) = Pr(T > t)$, the probability of the lifetime being longer than t. We only consider continuous distributions and thus the hazard function is well defined.

For survival data, the survivor function is more convenient than the ordinary distribution function $F(t) = 1 - S(t)$. The density is $f(t) = -dS(t)/dt$. The relations between the density and the hazard function are $\lambda(t) = f(t)/S(t)$ and $f(t) = \lambda(t) \exp\{-\Lambda(t)\}$, where $\Lambda(t) = \int_0^t \lambda(u)du$ is the integrated hazard function. Table 2.1 shows how the density, the survivor function, and the hazard are changed by truncation at time v, i.e., conditioning on $T > v$. This shows the advantage of the hazard, which, unlike the other quantities, is not changed by the conditioning. This is, of course, because it is already conditioned on survival until time t, and therefore it makes no difference to also condition on survival until time v ($v < t$).

Quantity	In full distribution	In truncated distribution given survival to time v
Survivor function	$S(t)$	$S(t)/S(v)$
Density	$f(t)$	$f(t)/S(v)$
Hazard function	$\lambda(t)$	$\lambda(t)$

Table 2.1. The influence of truncation $(t > v)$ on distributional quantities.

This conditioning corresponds to the concept of being at risk, that is, before the event, the individual has to be in a state from where the relevant transition is possible. For example, you are only at risk of death if you are alive at present. You cannot contract a disease if you already have it. You cannot marry if you are already married. Technically, you cannot start an epileptic seizure if you are presently having an epileptic seizure; but again the duration of a seizure is so short that we, for practical purposes, will consider an epileptic to be at risk of having an epileptic seizure continuously.

From a mathematical point of view, this is naturally analyzed as a random process developing over time, that is, a stochastic process, with one realization of the process for each individual. As the event is just a time of transition, the stochastic process to choose is a counting process, being 0 before the event, and 1 at and after the event. This can appear as a rather complicated way of describing a single random variable, but it is necessary in order to accommodate the special features of survival data.

Some of the non-parametric estimation methods will highlight the conditioning principle, as a successive conditioning, where at each time of event, the method will condition on the person's being alive immediately before the time point.

The discussion above on truncation has been concerned with which quantities we would like to estimate. But truncation is also relevant for the data. Very often the time of start of observation will be denoted time 0, and thus truncation is not a problem, but it might be more relevant to let the time be described by the age, and then start observation at whatever age the person has at the time, when the study starts, say t_0. This is truncation at time t_0, and alternatively called late entry. Also for the more complicated models and data sets, which will be discussed later, it is necessary to handle truncated data.

2.1.3   Choice of parametric/non-parametric models

The standard distributions, we usually apply to other types of data, are, in most cases, not relevant as models for survival data. We will not here try to fit such distributions to lifetimes, but this has been done by Hougaard (1999). As described above, the survival time is necessarily positive. For many other types of positive data, we will apply the normal distribution, even though we know that it is in conflict with the data's being positive.

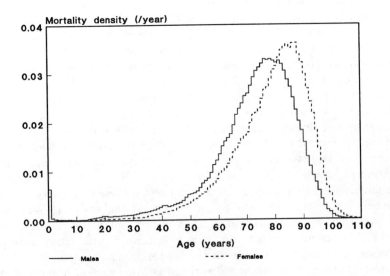

Figure 2.1. Density of lifetimes in the Danish population.

One such example is the height of human beings. With the relevant values of the mean and variances, the probability that the normal distribution suggests a negative height is so small that we need not care. It may or may not be the same for survival data, but the possibility of negative values seems particularly awkward in this case.

Non-parametric methods

Non-parametric methods have turned very popular within survival analysis, for several reasons. One is that often data have some features that are not easily obtained by parametric models. For example, human lifetimes show a decreasing hazard the first 5 years of life. This feature is relevant for some considerations but irrelevant for others, but by assuming a non-parametric hazard function, one avoids having to think about this problem. Similarly, there is an increased hazard a few years around the legal driving age (18 years in the country studied). For many other types of data, there are also some areas where we know that the fit of a parametric model is bad, but in survival data, these are tied up to particular ages, and therefore we find it more inconvenient. A more important reason is related to the conditioning aspect discussed above. Consider again the 75-year-old male. How should we evaluate his chance of surviving to age 76? It is natural to say that this should be based on the survival experience of previous males of age 75. In a parametric model, this will, however, be based on all the information in the data set, including, for example, males who died at age 20. In that sense, the non-parametric methods can be considered the logical consequence of the conditioning principle applied to the data. Above, the conditioning principle was used to illustrate which quantities were relevant, and it leads to parametrizing the lifetime distribution by means of the hazard function. Now, it has further consequences, as it tells us how to make inferences on these parameters. For discussing mortality of persons aged 75 years, only the mortality experience of persons aged 75 years should be considered. In other words, it should be irrelevant whether we study 500 persons aged 75, or 1000 persons followed from birth, of which 500 survive to age 75 years. However, the world is not that simple for all survival data methods. When we get to the regression models (Section 2.4), we are back to having all data contributing to the estimates of all parameters. Non-parametric methods also have several shortcomings. If the data set on these males aged 75 only includes one death before the age of 76, say, at the age of 75 years and 10 days, then we estimate that it is absolutely impossible to die at the age of 75 years and 11 days, and this is in conflict with common sense. A reasonable compromise between the simple parametric models and the completely non-parametric models is the piecewise constant hazards model (see Section 2.2.4). Similar considerations apply to data more generally than survival data; each time you apply a model, observations in one group will have influence on the estimates for other groups. But the successive development over time makes it particular important for survival data.

Within industrial applications and demography, it is common to evaluate the mean lifetime, as we have done above. However, within biostatistics, this is considered unacceptable. One reason for this is that censoring generally makes it difficult to estimate the right tail, and this tail can have a marked influence on the mean. As can be seen in Figure 2.1, the population data are left-skewed, implying that assumptions made about the right tail have smaller influence. This argument does not carry over to other times. A second reason is that evaluation of moments immediately make many people think of the response as normally distributed, which can be quite misleading. Finally as described below, for some types of events there is a proportion never experiencing the event, which invalidates the use of moments. For illustrating probability distributions we use moments, because they are good to demonstrate whether a distribution has a long tail.

2.1.4 Multiple events

In order to apply ordinary methods for survival data, we need to define some random variables. For true lifetimes, this is easy, because we know that the lifetime is well defined, even when it is not observed owing to the presence of censored data. All people will die eventually. However, for many other events, we cannot be sure that the event will ever happen. If we study some disease, the person may or may not develop the disease under study even with long observation time. In order to define a random variable

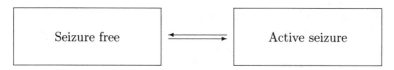

Figure 2.2. Epileptic seizure model.

corresponding to that disease, we must allow a value of infinity. This is not appropriate for standard models. For other diseases, an individual might get multiple attacks of the same disease, making it impossible to fit into a standard setup of a designed experiment. The hazard based setup for survival data allows the possibility of there being zero or many events for each individual. For example, if we study recurrent epileptic seizures (see Figure 2.2), the number of inter-seizure times cannot be specified in advance, and it is relevant to make a model that can accommodate any number of events, i.e., a stochastic process model.

2.2   Parametric methods

In this section, various parametric models that are commonly applied to survival data are considered. Furthermore, some less common extensions are described. The exponential distribution is a basic building block for survival data, and is needed for understanding all other survival distributions. In some cases, like for modeling epileptic seizures, this distribution can be relevant. However, it is rare that data on lifetimes satisfy this distribution. The actuarial tradition is to use the Gompertz or Gompertz-Makeham distribution. The industrial tradition is to use the Weibull distribution for studying reliability. The demographic and epidemiological tradition is to use piecewise constant hazards models. The biostatistical tradition is more along the non-parametric methods, which are considered later. We will treat all these, emphasizing similarities and differences. Furthermore, we will consider mixture models, truncation models, and hidden cause of death models. The distributions will be studied in the simplest case, with n independent identically distributed variables. In this and the following sections we let U denote the lifetime and T the observed time, influenced by censoring, to make it clear which is which. Later, T will be used for both. Let the lifetimes be $U_1, ..., U_n$. We denote the random variables by upper-case letters and the realized values by the corresponding lowercase letters. We describe the survivor function by $S(u)$, the density by $f(u)$, the hazard function by $\lambda(u)$, and the integrated hazard function by $\Lambda(u)$. Regarding censoring, we first assume type I (fixed) censoring, where there are known censoring times, $c_1, ..., c_n$, which may be common to the individuals, but for comparison to later results, they are allowed to differ between individuals. What we observe for the ith individual is survival until time c_i if $U_i > c_i$, and death at time U_i if $U_i \leq c_i$. Thus, we observe the individual only until the earliest time, either death or censoring. For evaluating the likelihood function, it is convenient to define the observed lifetime $T_i = \min\{U_i, c_i\}$ and an indicator of death, $D_i = 1\{T_i = U_i\}$. The symbol $1A$ is used to denote the indicator function of the set A. Thus D_i is 1 for deaths and 0 for censorings. Below we neglect the subscript i. In case of observing a death, the likelihood should include the density $f(U)$, which is written as $\lambda(U) \exp\{-\Lambda(U)\}$, and utilizing that $U = T$ in this case gives a contribution to the likelihood of $\lambda(T) \exp\{-\Lambda(T)\}$. The probability of getting a censoring equals $S(c)$, as the individual has to survive to time c, and using that $c = T$ in this case, the contribution to the likelihood is $\exp\{-\Lambda(T)\}$. By means of the death indicator, these two expressions can be united in a single expression

$$L(\lambda) = \lambda(T)^D \exp\{-\Lambda(T)\}. \tag{2.2}$$

The appearance of this single expression is the advantage of using T and D as variables. Even though we have defined censoring times for all individuals, the likelihood only depends on the censoring time for the individuals that were actually censored. Similar expressions are obtained for other censoring patterns. Consider instead the case of random censoring, that is, $C_1, ..., C_n$ are assumed independent and random, following some distribution, independently of the lifetime. For convenience of the formula, it is assumed that the distribution is continuous with density $g(c)$ and survivor function $G(c)$, but discrete or partially discrete distributions can easily be included. The distribution $G(.)$ must not have common parameters with the lifetime distribution, because otherwise the censoring times would carry information on the interesting parameters. Furthermore, we do not attempt to estimate the parameters of $G(.)$. The probability of observing a death time at t is then $f(t)G(t)$, because it is necessary that there is a death at that time and that censoring happens after that time, and we will assume that we do not know the censoring time, unless the individual is actually censored. Similarly, the probability of observing a censoring at time t is $g(t)S(t)$. These two expressions can be united into a single likelihood formula

$$\lambda(T)^D \exp\{-\Lambda(T)\}g(T)^{1-D}G(T)^D. \tag{2.3}$$

This expression is not the same as Equation (2.2), but the difference is a factor $g(T)^{1-D}G(T)^D$, which depends only on the observations and the censoring distribution, and thus is independent of the parameters of the lifetime distribution. That is, the log likelihood function ℓ considers the term as an additive constant. This implies that the derivative of the likelihood function is the same whether censoring is fixed or random independent, and thus the estimation equation is the same under the two censoring patterns. It also implies that the second derivative of the log likelihood function is the same. The negative inverse of this can be used to evaluate the variance of the estimates. This is an advantage, because it means that we can perform asymptotical statistical inference without considering whether censoring is fixed or random. It should, however, be emphasized that the exact distribution of the estimates will depend on the censoring pattern, and that if we want to evaluate the Fisher information, by the expected value of the second derivative of the log likelihood function, we need to make specific assumptions regarding the censoring pattern. This is the reason why asymptotic inference for survival data is nearly always based on the observed information, that is, the second derivative, without taking mean values. In the following, we use the likelihood version of Equation (2.2).

For data truncated at time v, both the density and survivor function are divided by $S(v)$, as described in Table 2.1. This implies that if we define the term in Equation (2.2) as $p(T, D)$, the contribution to the likelihood of an observation of (T, D) after truncation at time v is $p(T, D)/p(v, 0)$. In the log likelihood this will be a difference of terms corresponding to the event/censorings and a term mathematically identical to censoring at the time of truncation. This implies that if one has access to the code of a computer program that handles right-censored data for a parametric model, it is easily modified to handle left truncated data as well.

2.2.1   The exponential distribution

By far the simplest parametric model is the exponential distribution, which has only a single parameter and is characterized by a constant hazard, say, λ. The parameter can attain all positive values. If $\lambda = 1$, we say the distribution is unit exponential. The lifetime can also attain all positive values. The density is $f(u) = \lambda \exp(-\lambda u)$, the survivor function $S(u) = \exp(-\lambda u)$, and the integrated hazard $\Lambda(u) = \lambda u$. The exponential distribution is the only one that has the lack of memory property that the distribution of the residual lifetime, after truncation, is the same as the original distribution. That is, the distribution of $U - v$ conditional on $U > v$ is the same as the original distribution of U. A consequence of this result is that the exponential is the only distribution that is not influenced by the definition of time 0. What matters is the length of the observation period, i.e., $U - v$. Thus, it is trivial to handle truncation. The mean lifetime is

$$EU = 1/\lambda,$$

where E denotes the expected value and the variance is

$$Var(U) = 1/\lambda^2,$$

so that the standard deviation is $1/\lambda$, that is, equal to the mean. This is a special case of the Weibull distribution to be described below, and more general moments will be specified in that case. The distribution of cU, where c is a positive constant, is still exponential, and the hazard is λ/c.

Method (scale)	Confidence interval for λ
λ	−0.96–2.96
$\log \lambda$	0.14–7.10
$\lambda^{1/2}$	0.0004–3.92
$\lambda^{1/3}$	0.04–4.52
$-2 \log Q$	0.06–4.40
Exact (no censoring)	0.03-3.69

Table 2.2. Asymptotic and exact confidence intervals, for $D. = T. = 1$.

The minimum of n independent exponential random variables with hazard λ will also have an exponential distribution, with parameter $n\lambda$.

With censored data, the likelihood function in the i.i.d. (independent identically distributed) case reduces to

$$\lambda^{D.} \exp(-\lambda T.), \tag{2.4}$$

using $D. = \sum D_i$, and $T. = \sum T_i$. Generally, we use the dots (.) to denote summation over that index. It is easily seen that $D.$, the total number of events and $T.$, the total observation time, are jointly sufficient. This formulation makes the expression independent of the number of individuals, n. The derivative of the log likelihood function is

$$d\ell/d\lambda = D./\lambda - T..$$

It follows that when $D. > 0$, there is a unique maximum at $\lambda = D./T..$ This equation has a strong interpretation, as it is just the ratio of the number of events to the total observation time. This ratio is called the occurrence-exposure rate. In the case of $D. = 0$ (no observed deaths), the likelihood function is decreasing in λ, and the natural solution is to let λ take the boundary value 0. The second derivative is $-D./\lambda^2$, making it possible to estimate the variance by $D./T.^2$, which is obtained by evaluating the second derivative at $\hat{\lambda}$. A 95 % confidence interval based on the Wald test statistic can then be given by

$$\hat{\lambda} \pm 1.96\hat{\lambda}/D.^{\frac{1}{2}}.$$

The lower limit is negative as long as $D. < 4$, and much better coverage probabilities are obtained by transforming to the scale of $\lambda^{1/2}$ or $\lambda^{1/3}$ for evaluation of the asymptotic normal approximation, which give the following confidence intervals for λ

$$\hat{\lambda}\{1 \pm 1.96/(2D.^{\frac{1}{2}})\}^2,$$

and

$$\hat{\lambda}\{1 \pm 1.96/(3D.^{\frac{1}{2}})\}^3.$$

To illustrate the differences between these parametrizations, confidence intervals based on various asymptotic approximations are shown in Table 2.2, for the extreme case of one event. For higher values of $d.$, the differences are smaller. The first three are based on an asymptotic normal distribution, and clearly the one based on $\lambda^{1/3}$ is close to the interval based on the likelihood ratio test statistic $(-2 \log Q)$. The reason is that this parameter transformation makes the third derivative of the log likelihood function vanish at the estimate, thus making the log likelihood function closer to a quadratic function. The interval based on the square root is designed to make the tail probabilities well approximated by 2.5 % in each tail. The final interval is not correct under censoring, but shows the exact interval based on complete observation of a single individual, using the exponential distribution. In all other cases, n does not enter the formula. All that is sufficient to know is $D.$ and $T..$.

The Fisher information is the negative mean of the second derivative, which is easily seen to be $\lambda^{-2} \sum ED_i$. In particular, in the uncensored case, we find that the information is $n\lambda^{-2}$. If there is a common and known censoring time c, the information is $n\lambda^{-2}\{1 - \exp(-\lambda c)\}$. If instead, there is random independent censoring with a distribution of c_i being exponential with hazard μ, the information is $n\{\lambda(\lambda + \mu)\}^{-1}$. By varying the parameters c and μ, we can get any degree of censoring and any value for the information between 0 and $n\lambda^{-2}$. The exact distributions will be different between the two censoring patterns, but by basing inference on the observed second derivative instead of the expected information, we can avoid having to consider the censoring pattern, and this is a great simplification. The consequence of this is that more detailed evaluations of the asymptotic distribution, for example, an expansion giving correction terms to the asymptotic distribution is only possible, if one chooses a specific censoring pattern, and thus only valid under exactly those circumstances.

2.2.2   The Weibull distribution

This distribution has two parameters, which we denote λ and γ, and they are both positive. The hazard at time u is $\lambda(u) = \lambda\gamma u^{\gamma-1}$. We abbreviate the distribution as Weibull(λ, γ). In the case of $\gamma > 1$, the hazard is increasing, from a value of 0 at time 0 to a value of ∞ at time ∞. In the case of $\gamma = 1$, the exponential distribution is obtained, and the hazard is constant. In the case of $\gamma < 1$ a decreasing hazard is obtained. It decreases from a value of ∞ at time 0 to a value of 0 at time ∞. The integrated hazard function is

$$\Lambda(u) = \lambda u^\gamma, \tag{2.5}$$

and the survivor function is $S(u) = \exp(-\lambda u^\gamma)$. The distribution of U^γ is exponential. A lot of results for the Weibull distribution can be obtained by utilizing this result. For example, the qth moment is $EU^q = \lambda^{-q/\gamma}\Gamma(1 + q/\gamma)$. This expression is valid for all real $q > -\gamma$. For $q \leq -\gamma$, the moment

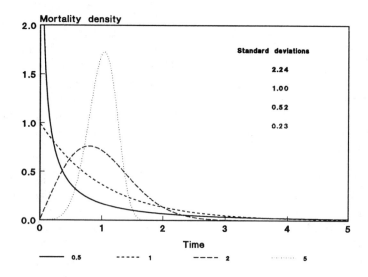

Figure 2.3. Weibull densities with mean 1. The values of γ are 0.5, 1, 2 and 5. The values of λ are 1.41, 1, 0.785 and 0.623, respectively.

is infinite. Thus, the mean is

$$EU = \lambda^{-1/\gamma}\Gamma(1 + 1/\gamma)$$

and the variance is

$$Var(U) = \lambda^{-2/\gamma}\{\Gamma(1 + 2/\gamma) - \Gamma(1 + 1/\gamma)^2\}.$$

All moments can be evaluated by this approach. This distribution can describe both positively and negatively skewed distributions. The skewness is positive in the case of large relative variability and negative in the case of small relative variability. The skewness is negative for γ large, an approximate limit is 3.6. The skewness will be illustrated later, in Figure 2.11. Also the moments on the logarithmic scale can be found. The logarithmic mean is $E\log U = \{\psi(1) - \log\lambda\}/\gamma$ and the variance is

$$Var(\log U) = \psi'(1)/\gamma^2, \tag{2.6}$$

where $\psi(\cdot)$ denotes the digamma function $\psi(x) = \Gamma'(x)/\Gamma(x)$. Figure 2.3 shows the density for various choices of γ and values of λ chosen so that the mean lifetime equals 1. Figure 2.4 similarly shows the hazard function.

This is a very nice distribution from a probability point of view. It has a scale parameter (λ) in the hazard, but it also accepts a scale factor on the time axis, as

$$U \sim \text{Weibull}(\lambda, \gamma) \Rightarrow cU \sim \text{Weibull}(\lambda c^{-\gamma}, \gamma), \tag{2.7}$$

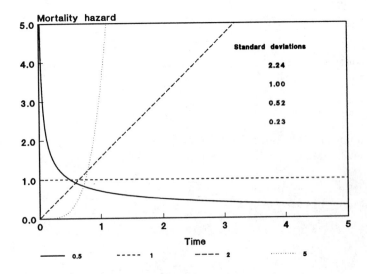

Figure 2.4. Weibull hazard functions with mean 1. The values of γ are 0.5, 1, 2 and 5.

when c is a positive constant. The symbol $U \sim F$ means that the random variable U follows the distribution F. Furthermore, the distribution of U^c is Weibull$(\lambda, \gamma/c)$, for c a positive constant. The distribution of the minimum of n i.i.d. variables from this distribution is Weibull$(n\lambda, \gamma)$. This implies that the distribution is minimum stable. That the distribution is minimum stable, means that the distribution of the minimum of n i.i.d. variables is the same as a scale transformation of one of the variables. It can be derived in cancer models as the result of a biological model assuming that tumors are created by a cell damaged by several hits.

Likelihood function

In the i.i.d. case with censoring, the log likelihood function is

$$\log L = \sum_i D_i \log(\lambda\gamma) + (\gamma - 1)D_i \log T_i - \lambda T_i^\gamma. \qquad (2.8)$$

In this case, there are no simple sufficient statistics, and this makes the model difficult from a statistical point of view. The derivatives with respect to the parameters are

$$d\ell/d\lambda = D./\lambda - \sum_i T_i^\gamma,$$

and

$$d\ell/d\gamma = D./\gamma + \sum_i D_i \log T_i - \lambda T_i^\gamma \log T_i.$$

The equation for λ has a very simple structure, which means that whenever γ is known, $\hat{\lambda}$ is easily found to be

$$\hat{\lambda} = D./\sum_i T_i^\gamma. \tag{2.9}$$

A similar equation can be derived for general hazard models, when there is a scale parameter in the hazard function. The second derivatives are

$$d^2\ell/d\lambda^2 = -D./\lambda^2$$

$$d^2\ell/d\gamma^2 = -D./\gamma^2 - \lambda \sum_i T_i^\gamma (\log T_i)^2$$

$$d^2\ell/d\lambda d\gamma = -\sum_i T_i^\gamma \log T_i.$$

In the case of complete data, we can calculate the expected information, which for a single observation is

$$-Ed^2\ell/d\lambda^2 = 1/\lambda^2$$

$$-Ed^2\ell/d\gamma^2 = \{1 + \Gamma''(2) - 2\Gamma'(2)\log\lambda + (\log\lambda)^2\}/\gamma^2$$

$$-Ed^2\ell/d\lambda d\gamma = \{\Gamma'(2) - \log\lambda\}/\lambda\gamma.$$

From this we can evaluate that the asymptotic variance of $\hat{\gamma}$ is of the form $q\gamma^2$ for some q, and thus independent of λ.

It can be difficult to fit the Weibull directly by Newton-Raphson iteration, because λ describes the hazard at $t = 1$, and this is, in many cases, an extrapolation from the main body of the deaths. This might lead to the second derivative matrix's not being negative definite when evaluated during the iteration phase, that is, away from the maximum likelihood estimation. Furthermore, the suggested improvements during the iteration do not necessarily increase the likelihood. The model can be fitted by SAS as will be described below, and that takes care of these problems; but here the difficulties will be described, as a practical description of what can be done for such problems. There are at least three ways to simplify the problems. The most basic is to divide all times by some constant c, chosen as a typical lifetime. This is a reparametrization of λ, using Equation (2.7), and can make λ and γ approximately independent. A second approach is to evaluate the profile likelihood, where the estimate, Equation (2.9), of λ is inserted into the likelihood function, Equation (2.8), making it a one-parameter function to maximize. That gives a profile log likelihood, which,

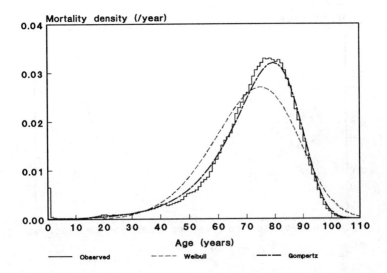

Figure 2.5. Fitted Weibull and Gompertz densities for lifetimes in the Danish male population.

apart from a constant is

$$\ell(\gamma) = D.\log\gamma - D.\log\sum T_i^\gamma + \gamma\sum(D_i\log T_i). \qquad (2.10)$$

In this way we reduce a two-parameter likelihood to a one-parameter (but slightly more complicated) likelihood. The real advantage is that it is much easier to make the iterative solution converge for the profile likelihood. The profile likelihood approach removes (or reduces) the problem that the second derivative is not necessarily negative definite far from the maximum likelihood estimate. A disadvantage of the profile method is that the asymptotic variance is only found for $\hat{\gamma}$, in the ordinary way from the second derivative of the profile log likelihood. Extra calculations are needed to evaluate the variance for $\hat{\lambda}$ and the covariance. The third possibility to improve on the convergence method, is simply to utilize Equation (2.9) by including an extra step in the Newton iteration, based on that equation. Thus the iteration would go along the line.

1. Suggest initial estimate for the shape parameter (γ).
2. Use Equation (2.9) to find the scale parameter (λ).
3. Calculate the derivatives of ℓ with respect to both λ and γ, say, F and the matrix H of second derivatives.
4. Find new values of λ and γ by the formula

$$\begin{pmatrix} \lambda \\ \gamma \end{pmatrix} - FH^{-1}.$$

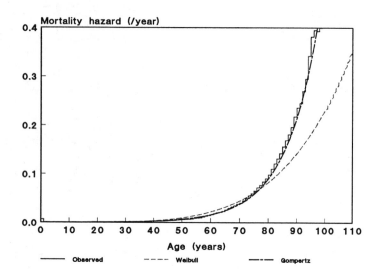

Figure 2.6. Fitted Weibull and Gompertz hazard functions for lifetimes in the Danish male population.

5. If the change in parameters is sufficiently small you are finished.
6. Discard the value of λ.
7. Go to step 2.

Without steps 2 and 6, this is an ordinary Newton-Raphson iteration of the bivariate problem, as described in Appendix B. Steps 2 and 6 speed up convergence, when the initial estimate is far from the maximum likelihood estimate. It is not advisable to change steps 3 and 4 into univariate iteration based on γ only, because that would seriously slow the convergence, by not satisfactorily accounting for the dependence between λ and γ.

Application

Applied to the population data on Danish males, the estimates are $\hat{\lambda} = 2.5 \cdot 10^{-11}$/year and $\hat{\gamma} = 5.28$. The mean in this distribution is 71.8 years, and the standard deviation 14.8 years. The density is illustrated in Figure 2.5 and the hazard function in Figure 2.6. The hazard plot puts more emphasis on the late part of the curve, where there are only few observations.

Evaluation and application in SAS

The Weibull model can be fitted by SAS by means of proc lifereg, using the following program

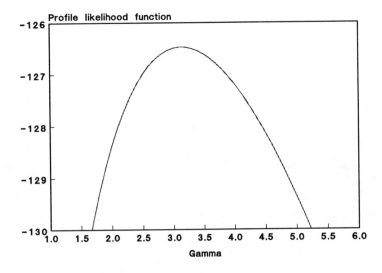

Figure 2.7. Weibull profile likelihood for tumorigenesis data.

data lifetime;
 infile *filename*;
 input time death;
 proc lifereg;
 model time*death(0)=;

The 0 value in parenthesis denotes the levels of the variable implying censoring. SAS uses a different parametrization than ours. The estimates from the procedure are a scale parameter, say, σ, which equals $1/\gamma$ and an intercept parameter, say, ν. The parameters used here can be found from $\gamma = 1/\sigma$ and $\lambda = \exp(-\nu/\sigma)$. The likelihood function is evaluated for the logarithm to the times, which means that in order to obtain the log likelihood function for the observed times, one should add $\sum D_i \log T_i$. This is applied to the female control rats of the tumorigenesis data set (Section 1.5), neglecting the litter effect. In this case, SAS gives the estimates $\hat{\sigma} = 0.3187$ and $\hat{\nu} = 5.067$, based on the 19 events among the 100 rats, and from this we derive $\hat{\gamma} = 3.14$ and $\hat{\lambda} = 1.24 \cdot 10^{-7}$. The standard error of $\hat{\gamma}$ is 0.67, and that of $\hat{\lambda}$ is $3.81 \cdot 10^{-7}$, and thus three times higher than the estimate. The likelihood for the log times, quoted by SAS, is -45.60, which can be transformed to the likelihood of the observations of -126.47. The profile likelihood approach is illustrated in Figure 2.7. For each value of γ, the best-fitting value of λ, Equation (2.9), is inserted into the likelihood. Clearly, this is a well-behaved likelihood function.

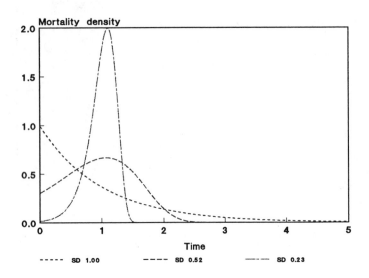

Figure 2.8. Gompertz densities with mean 1. The values of (λ, φ) are $(1,1)$, $(0.3025,4.377)$ and $(0.01366,226.4)$.

2.2.3   The Gompertz distribution

This distribution also has two parameters and has been used in actuarial science since 1825. The hazard is $\lambda(u) = \lambda\varphi^u$. All positive values of λ are acceptable. For $\varphi > 1$, the hazard is increasing, from λ at time 0 to ∞ at time ∞. For $\varphi = 1$, the exponential distribution is obtained. For $\varphi < 1$, the hazard is decreasing and does not integrate to ∞, so that a proportion of the population cannot experience the event under study. This is acceptable in some circumstances, but not in general. The integrated hazard is

$$\Lambda(u) = \lambda(\varphi^u - 1)/\log\varphi, \tag{2.11}$$

for $\varphi \neq 1$. If the random variable U is multiplied by a positive constant, say c, the distribution stays within the Gompertz family, and the parameters are $\tilde{\lambda} = \lambda/c$ and $\tilde{\varphi} = \varphi^{1/c}$. The non-linear transformation of φ makes it important to make clear the unit in which time is measured. The minimum of n independent identically distributed copies is Gompertz, with parameters $n\lambda$ and φ. Even though both a scale factor on the time and minimum operation gives another distribution within the Gompertz family, the distributions are not minimum stable. For being minimum stable, each distribution should transform in the same way by the two approaches, which they do not as the scale transformation modifies φ and the minimum operation does not. Moments can be found by numerical integration. For $\varphi > 1$, the standard deviation is lower than the mean. If the distribution is

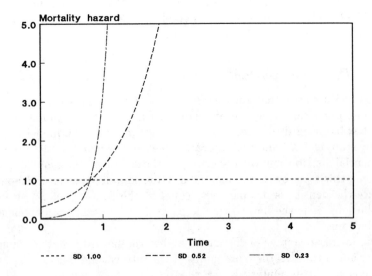

Figure 2.9. Gompertz hazard functions with mean 1.

truncated, that is, we consider U conditional on $U > v$ and study the residual lifetime, $U - v$, for some fixed v, the distribution is again Gompertz,
with the same value of φ, and λ exchanged by $\lambda\varphi^v$.

The density is illustrated in Figure 2.8 for cases that match the moments
of the Weibull distributions in Figure 2.3. There are no Gompertz distributions that match the moments of Weibull distributions with shapes (γ)
below 1. The Gompertz distributions are more left skewed than the Weibull
distributions. Similarly, Figure 2.9 shows the hazard functions.

The likelihood derivation is similar to the case above and will not be
shown here.

Applications

Applied to the population data for Danish males, the estimates are $\hat{\lambda} =$
$8.7 \cdot 10^{-5}$/year and $\hat{\varphi}=1.091$, when the time is measured in years. The
value of φ has an interpretation that for each increase in age by 1 year,
the hazard increases by 9 %. The distribution is also depicted in Figure 2.5
and 2.6. The mean is 73.0 years and the standard deviation is 14.5 years.
It has an excellent fit, except for describing the infant mortality. It can be
generalized to the Gompertz-Makeham distribution by adding a constant
hazard, see Section 2.2.5. This improves the fit at young ages.

Applied to the tumorigenesis data set, of Section 1.5.3, the estimates are
$\hat{\lambda} = 2.46 \cdot 10^{-4}$ $(1.83 \cdot 10^{-4})$, and $\hat{\varphi} = 1.036$ (0.010). Generally, the standard

error (SE) is reported in a parenthesis after the estimate. The log likelihood is -127.99, and thus the fit is not as good as that of the Weibull hazard.

2.2.4 Piecewise constant hazards

This model assumes that the hazard is constant within some time intervals. The practical advantage of this model is that it is a simple way to get a flexible hazard function, with simple estimation. The model implies that by studying each interval separately, we can use many results from the exponential distribution, with censoring at the end of the interval. Some authors call this a piecewise exponential distribution, but that is a misnomer, because the density is not piecewise equal to the densities of exponential distributions, it is the hazard that is piecewise the hazard of exponential distributions.

A major disadvantage of the model is that the hazard is not continuous as function of time, as there are jumps at the interval end points. First, the time axis is split into intervals $0 = x_0 < x_1 < ... < x_m$, where x_m is larger than the largest observation time, and possibly infinite. The hazard in the interval $(x_{q-1}, x_q]$ is λ_q. Thus the hazard function can be described as

$$\lambda(t) = \sum_{q=1}^{m} \lambda_q 1\{x_{q-1} < t \le x_q\}. \tag{2.12}$$

It is important to put the equality sign on the right end point, in order to make the formulas agree with later formulas for non-parametric estimates. A special case is the equidistant case, that is, where $x_q = qh$, $q = 1, ..., m$, where h is the common interval length. The number of intervals can be as low as 2, and as high as any finite number. The minimum of several observations with piecewise constant hazards having the same intervals, will also follow a piecewise constant hazards distributions. Multiplying by a factor on the time scale will lead to a piecewise constant hazards distribution, but the intervals will change.

It turns out that the likelihood function can be easily formulated by means of an indicator $D_{iq} = D_i 1\{x_{q-1} < T_i \le x_q\}$ of death of the ith individual in the qth interval, and the observation time T_{iq} in the interval. This quantity equals

$$T_{iq} = \begin{cases} 0 & \text{if } T_i \le x_{q-1} \\ T_i - x_{q-1} & \text{if } x_{q-1} < T_i \le x_q \\ x_q - x_{q-1} & \text{if } x_q < T_i \end{cases}$$

An alternative formulation, more suited for calculations, is

$$T_{iq} = \min\{T_i, x_q\} - \min\{T_i, x_{q-1}\}. \tag{2.13}$$

By means of these quantities, the likelihood function can be described as a product over i (individuals) and q (intervals), as

$$\prod_i \prod_q \lambda_q^{D_{iq}} \exp(-\lambda_q T_{iq}). \qquad (2.14)$$

By reversing the order of multiplication, and gathering terms by summing over i, we obtain the likelihood function

$$\prod_q \lambda_q^{D_{\cdot q}} \exp(-\lambda_q T_{\cdot q}), \qquad (2.15)$$

using $D_{\cdot q} = \sum_i D_{iq}$, and $T_{\cdot q} = \sum_i T_{iq}$. It is easily seen that the set of $D_{\cdot q}$, the number of deaths in the intervals, and $T_{\cdot q}$, the observation times in the interval, are jointly sufficient. The derivation of estimates follows that of the exponential distribution, and the formula for the estimate becomes $\hat{\lambda}_q = D_{\cdot q}/T_{\cdot q}$. The diagonal of the second derivative matrix becomes $-D_{\cdot q}/\lambda_q^2$. The mixed derivatives are all zero, showing that asymptotically the estimated hazard values are independent. However, they are only asymptotically independent, as can be illustrated by the fact that if all individuals die in the first interval, there is no information left to determine the hazard in the other intervals. The formula for the estimate is also valid in the boundary case, with no events in the interval, but the second derivative is not finite.

An interesting extension is to piecewise linear functions. By adding a single parameter, the model can be extended to a continuous model, thus avoiding the jumps at the interval end points. However, the fitting of this model is much more complicated, which will be demonstrated in an exercise.

Evaluation in SAS

This model can be fitted in SAS, in the sense that proc lifereg can handle the exponential distribution, by defining the observed lifetimes in the various intervals and the corresponding death indicators. If the interval length is 30 days, the program can look like

```
data a;
  infile filename;
  input time death;
  month=ceil(time/30);
do monthj=1 to month;
  timej=30;
  deathj=0;
  if monthj=month then do;
    deathj=death;
    timej=time-30*(month-1);
  end;
  output;
end;
proc lifereg;
class monthj;
model timej*deathj(0)=monthj/dist=exponential;
```
An alternative is to use proc genmod.

2.2.5 Hidden causes of death

This corresponds to the competing risks model of Section 1.10 and Chapter 12, but where the actual cause of death is not known. Thus we assume that there is one cause of death having a hazard function $\lambda_1(u)$ and another having hazard function $\lambda_2(u)$. The hazard function for the lifetime (that is, corresponding to the total mortality) is the sum $\lambda_1(u) + \lambda_2(u)$. Only the total mortality is observed. If $\lambda_1(u)$ is constant, maybe corresponding to the risk of accidents, and $\lambda_2(u)$ a Gompertz distribution, corresponding to age-related causes like cancer and heart disease, the lifetime follows a Gompertz-Makeham distribution. The same idea can be used for $\lambda_2(u)$ corresponding to a Weibull distribution, and this can remove the restriction of the initial hazard being zero, for $\gamma > 1$. This model has the inconvenience that under certain parameter restrictions, the model collapses, for example, if $\varphi = 1$ in the Gompertz-Makeham model, or $\gamma = 1$ in the similar Weibull model, the hazard is a sum of two constants, in which case the parameters cannot be identified, only the sum of them.

2.2.6 Truncated distributions

One way to make more general distributions is to introduce truncation at a known time v, and consider the residual lifetime at time v. One could argue that such mechanisms always are present. For example, a lifetime is measured since the time of birth, but even in this case, the time is truncated because before birth the individual has been a fetus for 9 months, a period during which a number of individuals have been lost. In industrial applications the failure time is measured since the product is released, but this is after some items have been removed owing to quality control. It has been shown that truncation makes no change for an exponential distribution, and that for a Gompertz distribution it leads to a Gompertz distribution, with the same value of φ, but a changed value of λ. For a Weibull distribution, however, it leads to a different distribution, where the hazard at time u is $\lambda(u) = \lambda\gamma(u + v)^{\gamma-1}$. This can be considered a modification that generalizes a Weibull model into a Weibull-like model with non-zero initial hazard. For estimation, it is still possible to make use of a generalization of Equation (2.9).

This does appear as a very attractive distribution, but as for many other extensions of simple distributions, there are problems in fitting them to data. For the Danish population data, the iteration moves toward high values of v and γ, that is, to the boundary estimate corresponding to the Gompertz distribution. For the control part of the tumorigenesis data, the iterative procedure suggests a negative value of v, which is impossible. Thus the suggestion for these data is to use an ordinary Weibull distribution.

2.2.7 Mixture distributions

One way to make parametric models give a better fit is to consider some sort of mixture model. On the general level, it is based on a chosen parametric model and assumes that one of the parameters varies between individuals, but as the value is not described by known explanatory variables, it has to be assumed to be random; that is, it is assumed to follow some distribution. Furthermore, as the value is unknown, it has to be integrated out. This can have two purposes in univariate models, one can use the approach as a way of generating more general distribution families or one can think of it as a heterogeneity model, where we interpret the population as a mixture of persons with different risks. This approach is also called compounding.

There are two simple ways to make such mixtures for survival models. One is to assume that there is a scale factor on the hazard. This factor has been denoted λ in the distributions described above. This approach corresponds to a univariate version of the frailty model described in Chapter 7. The other possibility is to assume that there is a scale factor on the lifetime, rather than on the hazard. This has been denoted c in the descriptions above. It turns out that for Weibull models, the two approaches give the same result, but in all other cases, the approaches give different distributions.

Binary mixtures

A simple explanation of the idea is to consider the population as consisting of two subpopulations with different risks. This could, for example, correspond to men and women. When this is the case, we should preferably analyze them separately, or suggest a model that relates the parameters for women to those of men. If, however, we have no information on the sex of each person, these approaches are impossible and instead we have to consider the sex as random. This means that if the proportion of men in the population is p, we have to consider that there is a chance p, that a randomly selected person is a man and then $1 - p$ that the person is a woman. This, of course, leads to an increased variation in the response time compared to the case where the sex is known, but in most cases, it also leads to invalidation of the assumed probability distribution. If, for example, the hazard for each sex is constant, the hazard in the whole population decreases. The reason is that as time passes, the proportion of men changes, so that at old ages, the proportion of women is higher, owing to their lower risk. For the sex example, it is obvious that we should collect information on the sex of each individual, as it is a basic variable and easily obtained, but if the population consists of carriers and non-carriers of a specific gene, it can be difficult or impossible to collect this information. In fact, it is still possible to make this consideration even when it is not known which gene is the relevant one. A binary distribution like the one presented here or more generally a discrete mixture distribution is good for explaining the idea, but it has some more technical disadvantages. It is implicitly assumed that there is a single factor explaining all of the heterogeneity. That is, there is only a single gene influencing mortality. Instead we prefer a multifactorial model corresponding to there being many genes influencing mortality and this requires that the mixture distribution is continuous. Binary mixtures are considered in an exercise; but otherwise, we will emphasize the use of continuous mixture distributions.

The hazard-based model

First, we consider the hazard-based model. To emphasize that it is a random mixture, we exchange λ for Y and assume that the hazard conditionally on Y has the form

$$Y\mu(t), \tag{2.16}$$

where $\mu(t)$ is 1 in the exponential case, $\gamma t^{\gamma-1}$ in the Weibull case, and φ^t in the Gompertz case. The variable Y is called the frailty and describes the individual unobserved risk. The distribution of Y is denoted the mixture distribution and the distribution when Y is fixed is denoted the conditional distribution. The observed distribution, i.e., when Y is integrated out, is called the marginal distribution. The hazard in this distribution is called the marginal hazard and denoted $\omega(t)$. A general formula for the marginal distribution can be obtained by means of the Laplace transform of the mixture distribution. The Laplace transform of a random variable Y is defined as $L(s) = E\exp(-sY)$. Laplace transforms are described in the Appendix (Section A.1). From the model, it is found that the conditional

Conditional distribution	Mixture distribution	Marginal distribution	
Exponential	Gamma	Pareto	
Exponential	PVF	Truncated Weibull	
Weibull	Gamma	Pareto power	
Weibull	Stable	Weibull	
Weibull	PVF		
Gompertz	PVF submodel	Gompertz	

Table 2.3. Some hazard based mixture distributions.

survivor function is

$$S(t \mid Y) = \exp\{-YM(t)\}, \tag{2.17}$$

where $M(t) = \int_0^t \mu(u)du$. The marginal survivor function can then be evaluated by

$$S(t) = ES(t \mid Y) = E\exp\{-YM(t)\} = L(M(t)). \tag{2.18}$$

Thus, when the Laplace transform of the mixture distribution is simple, it is easy to perform this calculation. Furthermore, if the distribution of Y is from a natural exponential family, it is easy to express these results by means of the normalizing constant, because the Laplace transform is a ratio of normalizing constants. Some such distributions are described in Appendix A. A list of models where the conditional distribution is chosen to be exponential, Weibull, or Gompertz is shown in Table 2.3. In general, when the conditional distribution is exponential, the marginal distribution has a decreasing hazard. A gamma distribution of parameters (δ, θ) has Laplace transform $\theta^\delta/(\theta + s)^\delta$. If this is used together with an exponential conditional distribution, the marginal survivor function is

$$S(t) = (1 + t/\theta)^{-\delta}, \tag{2.19}$$

which is the Pareto distribution, with hazard $\omega(t) = \delta/(\theta + t)$. The moment ET^q exists only when $-1 < q < \delta$, showing that this distribution has a fairly long tail. The value of ET^q is $\theta^q\Gamma(1 + q)\Gamma(\delta - q)/\Gamma(\delta)$. The gamma mixture of Weibull distributions gives a three-parameter model corresponding to a power transformation of a Pareto random variable. An alternative family of mixture distributions is the positive stable distributions, which are also described in Appendix A. The distribution with parameters (α, δ) has Laplace transform $\exp(-\delta s^\alpha/\alpha)$, implying that if the conditional distribution is Weibull of shape γ, the marginal distribution is Weibull $(\delta/\alpha, \alpha\gamma)$, and thus the approach can lead to any shape parameter lower than the original. The family of distributions does not become larger in this way. The variation is, of course, increased by introducing an extra random variable, a fact that is most clearly shown on the logarithmic scale. Using Equation (2.6), it is seen that the variance is increased by a factor of α^{-2}. An extended family of distributions, including both the gamma and the positive stable distributions, is the power variance function (PVF) distributions (see the Appendix, Section A.3.4). A PVF mixture of exponentials gives a distribution with hazard $w(t) = \delta(\theta + t)^{\alpha-1}$. This distribution is the same as the truncated Weibull (Section 2.2.6), with $\gamma < 1$. By a suitable choice of parameters, a mixture distribution from the power variance function family can turn a conditional Gompertz distribution into a marginal Gompertz, with a lower value of φ. To find the restriction on the parameters needed, we need to combine the integrated hazard of Equation (2.11) with the Laplace transform of the PVF distribution (Equation (A.17)). This gives the restriction $\theta = 1/\log\varphi$. To be specific, this means that if the conditional hazard is $Y\varphi^t$, and Y follows $\text{PVF}(\alpha, \delta, 1/\log\varphi)$, the marginal distribution of T has hazard $\lambda\tilde{\varphi}^t$, with $\lambda = \delta(\log\varphi)^{1-\alpha}$ and $\tilde{\varphi} = \varphi^\alpha$.

Under the heterogeneity interpretation it makes sense to discuss updating the distribution of Y. First, we study the frailty distribution among the surviving individuals. As the group under study contains people of different risks, the composition of the group changes over time, owing to the faster removal of the high-risk individuals. The conditional density of Y given survival to time t is found by taking the expression in Equation (2.17), multiplying by the density of Y, say, $g(y)$, and dividing by the expression in Equation (2.18). This turns out to be a member of the exponential family generated by $g(y)$. The formula is

$$\exp(-\theta y)g(y)/\int_0^\infty \exp(-\theta u)g(u)du, \qquad (2.20)$$

where $\theta = M(t)$. The denominator in the expression is $L(\theta)$. These evaluations suggest an advantage of using exponential families for the frailty distribution when truncation is experienced. For example, for the gamma model, only the θ parameter is changed, implying a change of scale, but apart from this the frailty distribution is unchanged. Generally, an exponential family frailty model is not in conflict with truncation. In other cases, the chosen family of frailty distributions might not be applicable. For example, if the frailty at birth follows a positive stable distribution, the distribution after truncation will not be of the same form, but included in the PVF family of distributions. The relation between the marginal and the conditional hazard can be described as

$$w(t) = \mu(t)E(Y \mid T > t), \qquad (2.21)$$

which has the strong interpretation as the observed hazard being equal to the mean hazard, evaluated among the survivors at the time of study.

It is also possible to update the distribution, when the lifetime is known. That is, to evaluate the conditional distribution of Y given T. This is done later, see Equation (7.13).

Performing mixtures has a number of consequences that must be understood, before it is relevant to apply the approach to generate dependence in multivariate survival models. First of all, the approach increases the variance, which is the main idea, by including several sources of variation. This is the cause for a constant conditional hazard being turned into a decreasing marginal hazard. Secondly, a key point is whether the family of distributions of the marginals is extended compared to the family of conditional distributions. From a theoretical (random effects) point of view it is an advantage, when the family is not extended, because this implies that a given marginal distribution can be obtained in many ways. That is, the total variation can be split in a continuum of ways into contributions from the mixture distribution and the conditional distribution. However, from a fitting point of view, it is an advantage when the family of distributions is extended, because then a better fit can be obtained. Thirdly, the effect of explanatory factors is modified in a non-trivial way, which will be considered later (Section 2.4.6).

In the case of hidden causes of death, one could suggest a model where the jth cause of death has frailty Y_j and hazard $\mu_j(t)$. In the special case where all the hazards functions are the same, this leads to a model of the total hazard of $(Y_1 + ... + Y_k)\mu(t)$, which means that it is a simple frailty model with frailty $Y = Y_1 + ... + Y_k$ and hazard $\mu(t)$. This evaluation can alternatively be interpreted so that if one starts with a simple frailty model, where the distribution of Y is infinite divisible, the model allows for such a splitting into several causes of death. The gamma, the stable, and the PVF function family are infinite divisible. A binary mixture distribution is not infinitely divisible.

The time scale model

The alternative mixture method is to let the time scale change by assuming that c in Equation (2.7), in the Weibull case, is random. This leads to exactly the same distributions as the hazard based case above, by letting $c = Y^{-1/\gamma}$. Thus the lifetime T can be described as

$$Y^{-1/\gamma}W, \tag{2.22}$$

where W is Weibull$(1,\gamma)$ distributed. This relation can immediately be used to evaluate moments and other properties. We simply find $ET = E(Y^{-1/\gamma})EW$. A similar model can be made for the Gompertz case, but no simple results are known in this case. The problem with interpretation of this result is that the parameter γ of the Weibull term enters in the power of the other term, implying that there is an inconvenient parameter restriction for such models.

A time-based model can be defined more generally than in the Weibull and Gompertz distribution, by just $T = ZW$, where Z and W are positive-valued random variables, with Z acting as a random variable for the scale factor c. Table 2.4 lists some well-known cases. The exponential model is the same as the hazard based model with gamma mixture distribution. The two other models are not standard survival data models.

Conditional (W) distribution	Scale (Z) distribution	Marginal (T) distribution
Exponential	Reciprocal gamma	Pareto
Lognormal	Lognormal	Lognormal
Gamma	Reciprocal gamma	F with scale

Table 2.4. Some time-based mixture distributions.

Applications

The approach can be illustrated by some applications. The hazard of death after a myocardial infarction is very high the first days and then decreases markedly. The mixture model assumes that the hazard is constant for each person, but owing to differences between individuals, the marginal hazard decreases. We use the one-year survival data described in Section 1.9.3. It was found in Hougaard (1986b) that the estimates in the PVF mixture of exponentials model are $\hat{\alpha} = 0.116$ (SE 0.038), $\hat{\delta} = 0.040$ (0.006), and $\hat{\theta} = 0.07$ (0.05), with a log likelihood value of -2424.64. It appears from the estimates that θ could be 0, corresponding to a positive stable mixture and a Weibull distribution for the lifetime, but the fit is significantly worse judged by the likelihood ratio test statistic. The estimates under this hypothesis are $\hat{\alpha} = 0.241$ (0.013) and $\hat{\delta}=0.0254$ (0.0013), and the log likelihood is -2431.67. A main difference between the general model and the model under the hypothesis is the initial hazard, which is infinite under the hypothesis and finite under the alternative. It follows from the results above in Section 2.2.6 that the general model is identical to using the residual lifetime after truncation in a Weibull model, in the case $\gamma < 1$. From the value of $\hat{\theta}$, we conclude that the truncation time is only 0.07 days, and thus in fact it is comparable to the time from the actual attack until admission to the hospital. This means that it is possible that the survival time after the attack follows a Weibull distribution, but the requirement that they are admitted alive to the hospital leads to the truncated distribution. In practice, this is an overinterpretation of the data. Admission times differ between individuals, and hospital time is quoted in days. The analysis treated the times as grouped in 24 hour time periods and therefore a time period of 0.07 days is very short. However, the example illustrates the idea that the observed pattern could be due to a positive stable mixture of exponential times, combined with truncation. Under the assumption of a Pareto distribution, we find estimates of $\hat{\delta} = 0.0598$ (0.0037) and $\hat{\theta} = 0.28$ (0.06), with a log likelihood value of -2428.67, which is also significantly worse than the full model. A frailty model can not be used to conclude whether the conditional hazard is constant or decreasing; it can only tell that the observed decreasing hazard can be explained by constant individual hazards and heterogeneity between individuals.

For the data on time to diabetic nephropathy of Section 1.3.1, we have applied various Weibull mixture models, using both a gamma and a general

Model	Parameter	Males	Females
Gamma	δ	0.100 (0.015)	0.087 (0.017)
	θ	3,344,482	16,795
	γ	5.82 (0.61)	4.00 (0.51)
	$\log L$	$-1,628.25$	$-1,183.51$
PVF	α	-0.58 (0.24)	-1.09 (0.64)
	δ	0.212 (0.069)	0.196 (0.122)
	θ	1,640,869 (1,720,073)	34,353 (26,503)
	γ	4.92 (0.48)	3.49 (0.40)
	$\log L$	$-1,617.65$	$-1,178.44$

Table 2.5. Estimates for parametric mixture models for the incidence of diabetic nephropathy.

PVF mixture distribution. The form of the hazard function becomes $\delta\gamma(\theta + t^{\gamma})^{\alpha-1}t^{\gamma-1}$. Table 2.5 gives the results for males and females separately. The marginal incidences are depicted in Figure 2.10, and it is clear that they increase for the first 15–20 years, after which they decrease toward 0. The gamma and the PVF model give similar estimates for the first 15 years, but the terminal courses are different. According to the gamma model, all individuals are susceptible, and therefore, there is a marked long-term incidence. According to the PVF model, which gives a better fit, a proportion (52 % for males, 66 % for females) is not susceptible at all. This explains that the hazard is virtually zero at long durations. So the overall interpretation is that the individual (or conditional) hazard increases, and this effect is also seen for the observed hazard initially, but after 15–20 years the variation between individuals forces the marginal hazard to decrease.

2.2.8 Comparison of parametric models

The key question is which distribution family to select in a specific case. Table 2.6 summarizes the major qualitative differences between the distributions. Some comments on the table are appropriate. For human lifetimes we observe an increasing hazard, and therefore the exponential model is not satisfactory. It is inconvenient that the piecewise constant hazard function is not continuous. Unless we have an idea that the hazard is not monotone, it is inconvenient that the piecewise constant model does not secure a monotone estimate. Often, the estimate in the piecewise constant model will go up and down, and we do not know whether this is real effect, or a consequence of random error. A non-zero initial hazard is possible for the Weibull model, when $\gamma < 1$, in which case the hazard is infinite initially and decreases over the whole lifespan. What the table refers to by saying that non-zero initial is impossible means that we cannot have a non-zero initial hazard together with an increasing hazard. The hazard function for a failure related to wear can be 0 near the time origin, making a Weibull dis-

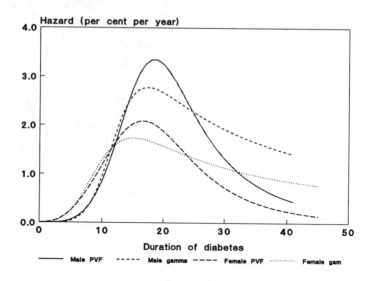

Figure 2.10. Estimates for diabetic nephropathy using Weibull mixture models based on gamma and PVF mixture distributions, for males and females separately.

Property	Exponential	Weibull	Gompertz	Piecewise constant
Increasing hazard possible	No	Yes	Yes	Yes
Continuous hazard	Yes	Yes	Yes	No
Estimate monotone	(Constant)	Yes	Yes	No
Non-zero initial hazard	Yes	No	Yes	Yes
Minimum stable	Yes	Yes	No	No
Explicit estimation	Yes	No	No	Yes
Needs choice of intervals	No	No	No	Yes
No. of parameters	1	2	2	m
Dimension of sufficient statistic:				
Complete data	1	n	n	$2m-1$
Censored data	2	$2n$	$2n$	$2m$

Table 2.6. Comparison of parametric models. Qualitative properties.

Distribution	Deaths before 20 years (%)	Deaths after 110 years (%)
Observed	1.3	0.002*
Normal	0.04	0.8
Weibull	0.05	0.09
Gompertz	0.5	0.00008

Table 2.7. Estimated proportion of early deaths and long-term survivors in various distributions. Danish population data, males. *Extrapolated.

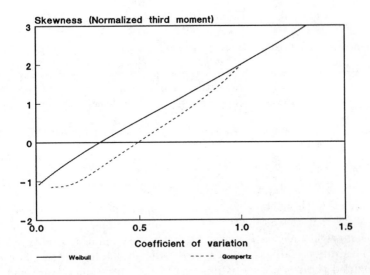

Figure 2.11. Skewness as a function of the coefficient of variation in Weibull and Gompertz distributions.

tribution relevant, for example, a car does not fail from rust the first year. However, if failure of the car owing to traffic accidents is included, a non-zero initial hazard is needed. Similarly, for human lifetimes, the Weibull model might give a good description of mortality of some cancers, because for many cancer types, the risk is essentially zero during childhood. However, the total mortality needs a model where the initial hazard is positive. Thus, even though some cause-specific hazards can be 0 initially, the total initial hazard is typically strictly positive. For the Weibull and Gompertz models the tails are illustrated in Table 2.7, based on the population data of Section 1.2.1. Also included are the values for a normal distribution, which would have given a symmetric distribution in Figure 2.5. Regarding the mass below 20 years, the Gompertz makes an almost even distribution, whereas the Weibull puts most of the mass near age 20. The different initial

Property	Exponential	Weibull	Gompertz
Hazard	λ	$\lambda\gamma t^{\gamma-1}$	$\lambda\varphi^t$
Parameters	$\lambda > 0$	$\lambda > 0, \gamma > 0$	$\lambda > 0, \varphi \geq 1$
Exponential submodel	Full model	$\gamma = 1$	$\varphi = 1$
Mean(μ)	λ^{-1}	$\lambda^{-1/\gamma}g_1(\gamma)$	
Range for μ	R_+	R_+	R_+
Variance (σ^2)	λ^{-2}	$\lambda^{-2/\gamma}g_2(\gamma)$	
Restriction	$\sigma = \mu$	$0 < \sigma$	$0 < \sigma \leq \mu$
cT	Exponential	Weibull[γ]	Gompertz
T^c	Weibull	Weibull[λ]	
$\min(T_1, ..., T_n)$	Exponential	Weibull[γ]	Gompertz[φ]
Residual lifetime	Exponential[λ]		Gompertz[φ]
Connected mixture distribution	None	Positive stable	PVF submodel

Table 2.8. Comparison of parametric models. Quantitative properties. Blank means no simple result. Parameters in [ ] are unchanged by the operation. Connected mixture distribution means the frailty mixture distribution giving a marginal distribution within the same family. $g_1(\gamma)$ and $g_2(\gamma)$ refer to functions only depending on γ.

hazards mean that the Gompertz has a longer left tail than the Weibull. It is clear that the normal is not good at describing the tails and that the Gompertz is reasonably good (except for the infant mortality). A further illustration of differences can be done by evaluating the skewness (the normalized third moment) as function of the coefficient of variation (see Figure 2.11). As both distributions include a scale parameter, this parameter is removed by normalizing with respect to the scale parameter. Both distributions have negative skewness when the variability is low. For the Weibull, this happens when $\gamma > 3.6$, corresponding to the coefficient of variation being below 0.308. For the Gompertz, we cannot specify a similar simple parameter relation, but the skewness is negative when the coefficient of variation is below 0.495. The exponential distribution is the point $(1,2)$ where the two curves cross. The piecewise constant hazard model has a further advantage in the bounded influence (see Section 2.1.3). The Weibull and Gompertz distributions are difficult to handle for large data sets, because there are no sufficient reductions of the data.

Table 2.8 summarizes the quantitative properties derived earlier for the exponential, Weibull, and Gompertz distributions. Clearly, these distributions have many nice properties from a survival data point of view. The Weibull distribution is nicer than the Gompertz, from a theoretical point of view, owing to it's being a location-scale model on the logarithmic scale. The relation between the Weibull and the Gompertz family is described in an exercise.

Property	Parametric	Non-parametric
Estimated distribution	Continuous	Discrete
Hazard estimation	Yes	No
Monotone hazard	Possible	Not relevant
Biological interpretation	Possible	No
Result	A few numbers	Table or figure
Explicit estimation		
Right censored data	Piecewise constant	Yes
Fit	Restricted	Good
Precision	Generally good	Poor

Table 2.9. Comparison of parametric and non-parametric models.

2.3   Simple non-parametric methods

In order to avoid assuming that some parametric model is correct, it is common to use non-parametric methods. In this section, we consider the case of independent, identically distributed data. The simplest non-parametric estimate of a distribution function is the empirical distribution; that is, the distribution is assumed equal to the observed distribution. This is the non-parametric maximum likelihood estimate for complete observations. Thus, even though we assume that the true distribution is continuous, we estimate it by a discrete distribution. Kaplan and Meier (1958) suggested an extension to censored data, formulated by means of the survivor function, and described in Section 2.3.1. From this, an estimate of the integrated hazard function can be derived using the relation $\Lambda(t) = -\log S(t)$, but if one starts by considering the integrated hazard function, a slightly different estimate is obtained, the Nelson-Aalen estimate of Section 2.3.2.

A key question is whether we should apply a parametric or a non-parametric model. A comparison between the parametric models described above and the non-parametric methods of Kaplan-Meier and Nelson-Aalen is made in Table 2.9. It is clear that the real advantage of the non-parametric models is the fit, which can handle any distribution, but there is a large price to pay for this good fit. It is much more difficult to report a non-parametric estimate, as the results must be shown in a figure or a table, whereas a parametric model can be described by the values of a few parameters. A major disadvantage of the non-parametric procedures is that the hazard function cannot be estimated; it is not even defined, as the distribution is discrete. For some purposes, the hazard function is much more interesting and relevant to estimate than the survivor function and the integrated hazard function, but it is also more challenging to estimate. It is more complicated as it is necessary to smoothen out the discrete masses of the Kaplan-Meier and the Nelson-Aalen estimates to make a continuous distribution. One such method is kernel function smoothing (see Müller and Wang, 1994).

2.3.1   The Kaplan-Meier estimate

The aim of this procedure is to estimate a survivor function non-parametrically in the presence of right censoring. This estimator is also called the product limit estimator owing to its derivation, as a limit, when the time is split into intervals, and the interval length goes to 0.

Suppose we have independent observation times $T_1, ..., T_n$ and corresponding death indicators $D_1, ..., D_n$. For each time point t, we define the size of the risk set as $R(t) = \sum_i 1\{T_i \geq t\}$. This has an interpretation as the number of persons under observation at time t. It is a left continuous decreasing step function. Like for the piecewise constant hazards model, we start by a set of intervals $0 = x_0 < x_1 < ... < x_m = \infty$. For convenience, we assume that censoring only takes place at the interval end points, or in intervals without deaths. For convenience, we may restrict the time points to be equidistant (except the last interval, which is taken up to ∞). We now parametrize the distribution by the conditional probabilities of death within the intervals, given that the individual was alive at the beginning of the actual interval, say, $p_j = Pr(x_{j-1} < T \leq x_j \mid x_{j-1} < T)$. This parametrization corresponds to the conditioning of Section 2.1.2; that is, it is a discrete version of the hazard function. Thus when data are available, we have the number of individuals alive at the beginning of the interval, $R(x_{j-1})$, and the number of deaths within interval j. Conditional on $R(x_{j-1})$, the number of deaths follows a binomial distribution with probability parameter p_j. To spell this out, the assumption is that for any individual alive at the beginning of the interval, there is a random variable D_{ij}, with the binomial distribution

$$Pr(D_{ij} = 1) = p_j, \ Pr(D_{ij} = 0) = 1 - p_j. \tag{2.23}$$

The natural estimate of p_j is then $D_{.j} = \sum_i D_{ij}$ divided by $R(x_{j-1})$, that is, $\hat{p}_j = D_{.j}/R(x_{j-1})$. To estimate the value of the survivor function at some interval endpoint, say, x_q, we first notice that $S(x_q) = \prod_{j=1}^q (1 - p_j)$. Inserting estimates gives

$$\hat{S}(x_q) = \prod_{j=1}^q \{1 - D_{.j}/R(x_{j-1})\}. \tag{2.24}$$

To make it a non-parametric estimate, let the intervals be finer and finer. Then q is no longer defined, but suppose we want to estimate the value at some given t. Then, if t is not an interval end point we consider the last end point before t. If the intervals are sufficiently fine, there will not be deaths between these two points unless there is a death exactly at t. By studying the terms, we see that most terms actually correspond to intervals with no deaths, and these intervals contribute to the product by factors of 1 in Equation (2.24). These terms can be removed, and thus there are only factors corresponding to the times of observed deaths before t, say $t_1, ..., t_q$. Each of these death times, $t_r, r = 1, ..., q$, will be contained in one interval,

Time	R(t)	N	Factor	$\hat{S}(t)$
(0)	5			1
2	5	1	0.8	0.8
3	4	0	1	0.8
5	3	2	1/3	0.267
7	1	0	1	0.267
(After 7)	0			Undefined

Table 2.10. Example showing the Kaplan-Meier calculations for a data set of 2, 3+, 5, 5, and 7+.

say, interval $j(r)$. Assuming a continuous distribution, there will be only one death at each of these times. Therefore, the estimate of the survivor function will be

$$\hat{S}(t) = \prod_{r=1}^{q} \{1 - 1/R(x_{j(r)-1})\}.$$

Now, it is clear that there is a contribution at each death time, and the only resemblance with the set of intervals is the function $j(r)$, but it can be seen that $R(x_{j(r)-1})$ just describes the number at risk immediately before time t_r, and we can therefore exchange the term $R(x_{j(r)-1})$ with $R(t_r)$. In practice, there might be several observations at the same time point, that is, ties, so that at time t_r, there are N_r deaths. Then the formula for the Kaplan-Meier estimate is

$$\hat{S}(t) = \prod_{r=1}^{q} \{1 - N_r/R(t_r)\}. \tag{2.25}$$

This function is a right continuous decreasing step function, with changes at the death times. If the largest time value corresponds to a death, $\hat{S}(t)$ becomes 0 eventually. If the largest time value corresponds to a censoring, the function will have a non-zero value at that time point and be undefined afterward. One consequence of this is that the mean lifetime cannot be estimated. A solution is to calculate the mean restricted to the observation period, which is obtained by assuming that the survivor function is 0 after the largest time. This is the lower bound corresponding to the observations, and thus obviously biased. The upper bound for the mean lifetime will be infinite. A better solution is to evaluate the median, which can be determined, when the observation period is long enough for the survivor function to cross 1/2.

If there are ties, the result is the same as if the deaths occurred at different times immediately after each other.

Table 2.10 shows how the calculations are performed for a small data set, with ties. Time 0 and the final interval are set in parentheses as these do not correspond to observation times, but the points are needed to specify the whole function. In between the points, the function is defined by being right continuous. This is also valid at time 7, but we cannot extend the value after 7. All we can say is that the estimate is $0 \leq S(t) \leq 0.267$, for $t > 7$.

As an alternative, the estimates can be found directly as the maximum likelihood estimate in an extended model. It is extended to allow for discrete components, and we first see that the probability will be positive exactly at the death times, which will be denoted $x_1, ..., x_m$. The probability of death at the jth death time is conditional on being alive immediately before it is denoted p_j, similar in approach to Equation (2.23), but now referring to a single time point rather than an interval. The probability of surviving the qth death time point for a person is $\prod_{j=1}^{q}(1 - p_j)$ and the probability of death at the qth death time point for a person is $p_j \prod_{j=1}^{q-1}(1 - p_j)$. To write this as a likelihood function, we first introduce extra notation, an indicator $D_{ij} = D_i 1\{T_i = x_j\}$ of the ith person dying at the jth death time. This is slightly different from above, where the same symbol was used in the jth interval. Similarly $R_{ij} = 1\{T_i \geq x_j\}$ describes whether the ith person is at risk at the jth death time. Then the likelihood can be written as

$$\prod_i \prod_j p_j^{D_{ij}}(1 - p_j)^{R_{ij} - D_{ij}}. \tag{2.26}$$

By reversing the order of making products, we have for each j a term that simply gives the maximum likelihood estimate $\hat{p}_j = D_{.j}/R_{.j}$, the Kaplan-Meier estimate.

Efron suggested a different procedure for obtaining the Kaplan-Meier estimate, the redistribution to the right algorithm. First each of the n individuals are assigned a mass of $1/n$, and the time points are ordered, into $T_1, ..., T_n$. Then they are considered in increasing order, and for each censoring the mass at that point is equally distributed over all later time points. This ends up giving the Kaplan-Meier estimate.

The variance can be evaluated by the so-called Greenwoods formula:

$$\text{Var}(\hat{S}(t)) = \hat{S}(t)^2 \sum_{r=1}^{q} \frac{N_r}{R(t_r)\{R(t_r) - N_r\}}.$$

This formula is based on the variance in the successive binomial distributions, combined by means of the variance formula for products. One consequence of this formula is that in an interval without deaths, not only is the estimated probability of death 0, but the estimated variance is also 0, suggesting that we are absolutely sure that deaths cannot occur in that interval. This is, of course, in conflict with common sense, and must be considered an inconvenience of the method used. For performing asymptotical evaluations, it is necessary to use the mathematical theory of counting processes.

In case of truncated data, the same method can be applied, by redefining the risk set to $R(t) = \sum_i 1\{T_i \geq t\}1\{V_i < t\}$, where V_i is defined as the

Truncation time (v)	Death time
0	1
0	2
3	4
3	5

Table 2.11. Problem data set for Kaplan-Meiers method with truncations giving an observation hole between time 2 and 3. No censoring.

time of start of observation. This still has a strong interpretation, as it describes the number of persons known to be alive and under observation, at time t. This extension to truncated data does create some problems, as there might be holes in the data, that is, periods where nobody are known to be at risk. The decrease in the survivor function during this period cannot be evaluated. Furthermore, if there is only one individual at risk, and this person dies, the estimate is zero, even though there might be later observations. As an example take the data in Table 2.11. This gives a survivor function estimate of 1/2 at time 1 and 0 at time 2, in conflict with there being survivors after time 3. To some extent this is a small-sample problem. With so few data as presented in the table, one should apply a parametric model instead. If the distribution of truncation times and censoring times are sufficiently rich, this problem will eventually disappear. This does require that some individuals are at risk at time 0. There is a problem, when, for example, we study the survival for individuals with a given disease using age as time scale. In this case, the risk set is empty at time 0 (birth), and then slowly builds up, as the persons develop the disease. Early deaths then have an enormous influence on the estimated survival function. An example of this is shown in Section 6.7.2.

Evaluation in SAS

The Kaplan-Meier estimate can be found by SAS using the following program:

```
data a;
  infile filename;
  input lifetime death;
proc lifetest plots=(s,ls) graphics;
  time lifetime*death(0);
```

The plots specification asks for a plot of the survivor function (s) and (minus) the log survival function (ls); that is, the integrated hazard function. This procedure only gives the values at the jump points (i.e., corresponding to the lower corners of the survivor function) as output, and therefore to get the step function drawn, one has to supplement with the left limits. All the corners are on the plot requested by the option graphics.

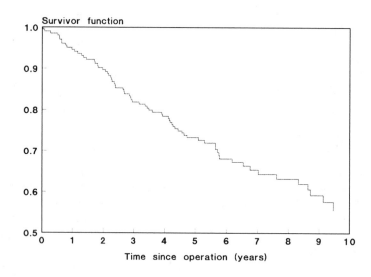

Figure 2.12. Kaplan-Meier estimate for the data on malignant melanoma.

Application

As an application take the malignant melanoma data of Section 1.10.2, where we study total mortality. The survival function is shown in Figure 2.12. It is easy to see the jumps at the death times. The size of the jumps increases owing to the censored observations. The overall picture shows a slight curvature. Whether this curvature is as expected for a model with constant hazard requires an examination on the hazard scale (see below).

2.3.2   The Nelson-Aalen estimate

This is an estimate of the integrated hazard function. Its derivation is similar to the Kaplan-Meier estimate. It can informally be derived as a limit estimate of a probability model based on Equation (2.1). The probability of observing a death is estimated as 0, when there are no deaths and as $1/R(t)$, if there is a death at time t. This corresponds to a Poisson model, so that in each infinitesimal interval (j), and for individual (i) under risk, there is a count variable D_{ij} with a Poisson distribution with mean λ_j, so that, in particular the probabilities of 0 or 1 events are

$$Pr(D_{ij} = 1) = \lambda_j \exp(-\lambda_j), \ Pr(D_{ij} = 0) = \exp(-\lambda_j), \qquad (2.27)$$

and thus this is slightly different from the Kaplan-Meier formulation, in Equation (2.23). Thus this model allows for $D_{ij} > 1$, even though it is impossible to die several times. When several individuals are combined, this

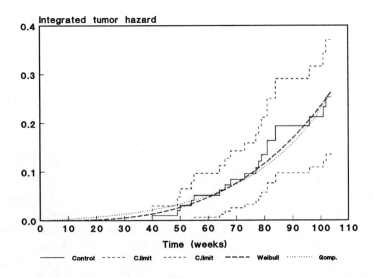

Figure 2.13. Integrated hazard function for the control rat tumorigenesis data, by the Nelson-Aalen method, and the Weibull and Gompertz models.

is no longer impossible; but ties, that is, multiple occurrences at the same time, happen with probability 0, as the assumed distribution is continuous. The total likelihood becomes

$$\prod_i \prod_j \{\lambda_j^{D_{ij}} \exp(-\lambda_j)\}^{R_{ij}}. \qquad (2.28)$$

By reversing the order of making products, we find the estimate $\hat{\lambda}_j = D_{.j}/R_{.j}$, utilizing that $D_{ij} = D_{ij}R_{ij}$. Thus, it is clear that there are only contributions at the death times, and therefore the integrated hazard function is then estimated as

$$\sum_{r=1}^{q} N_r/R(t_r), \qquad (2.29)$$

where the change of notation refers to N being evaluated at the times of events, where D could be defined at any time. Only the death times $t_1, ..., t_q$ before time t and including time t contribute. This function is a right continuous increasing step-function. If there are ties, the estimate is slightly below the value that would be obtained if the values occurred immediately after each other. This can be illustrated with the results when there are two simultaneous events. The Nelson-Aalen approach gives a contribution of $2/R(t)$, whereas if the second event occurred immediately after time t, the total contribution would be $1/R(t) + 1/\{R(t) - 1\}$.

The variance can similarly be evaluated as

$$\sum_{r=1}^{q} N_r / R(t_r)^2.$$
(2.30)

Also in this case, truncation can be handled by modifying the risk set definition as described for the Kaplan-Meier estimate. A formal derivation of the estimator and asymptotic evaluations is performed by means of the theory of counting processes.

The estimated integrated hazard is slightly lower than $-\log S(t)$ based on the Kaplan-Meier estimate, which can be explained by the (slight) difference between the models described in Equations (2.23) and (2.27).

Equation (2.28) is formally identical to Equation (2.14), when we substitute T_{ij} for R_{ij}. These are two different problems, as the piecewise constant hazards model is a continuous time model, whereas the Nelson-Aalen estimate is an extension to discrete time, but the identity of the likelihood functions implies that the Nelson-Aalen estimator can be found by piecewise constant hazards software, with the only restriction that the software should allow intervals with no events. A practical example using this identity is given later (Section 8.6).

Applications

As an application consider the tumorigenesis data. The integrated hazard function is shown in Figure 2.13, with pointwise 95 % confidence intervals. These are shown together with the estimates from the Weibull and Gompertz distributions. The Weibull hazard is slightly closer to the Nelson-Aalen estimate than the Gompertz hazard.

For the data on malignant melanoma of Section 1.10.2, Figure 2.14 shows the integrated hazard function. This seems to be very close to linear, suggesting a constant hazard function. This evaluation must be done on the integrated hazard scale; the Kaplan-Meier curves are bound to deviate from linearity, owing to the curvature of the exponential function.

2.4   Regression models

Above, independent identically distributed data have been considered exclusively. However, in most cases, a number of important explanatory variables, or risk factors, are known. These can be basic variables, like sex and age (if age is not used as time scale); they can be factors of particular interest, like treatment in a drug trial; or they can be nuisance variables, which are helpful to include in order to describe the risk of events as precisely as possible, but whose effect we are not directly interested in. In all cases, we will use terms like covariates, or explanatory variables for these variables. Such explanatory variables might be fixed variables, or they may

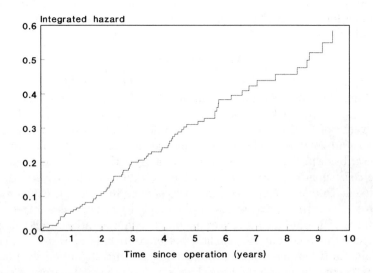

Figure 2.14. Nelson-Aalen estimate for the data on malignant melanoma.

change over time (time-dependent covariates). We will describe the relative risk parametrically, and the hazard function non-parametrically and therefore call the model semi-parametric. The standard model for such data is the so-called Cox model, or the proportional hazards model. However, to get the concepts right, it is an advantage to consider the whole procedure as two parts: the probability model (Section 2.4.1) and the estimation method (Section 2.4.2). The whole procedure is particularly designed to evaluate differences in risk related to the covariates. This means that the absolute risk is considered as less relevant. However, in many cases the absolute risk is indeed important (see Section 2.4.3). Truncation and time-dependent covariates are extremely important for handling the multivariate models considered later in this book (Section 2.4.4). Neglected covariates are considered in Section 2.4.6.

2.4.1 The proportional hazards probability model

In order to have a suitable notation for the most general models, we use a double notation for the regression variables, with one term, say, v, for the actual explanatory variables, and another, say, z, for the terms included in the model. In many cases, they are identical. In fact, we will only use different symbols for introducing the approach. Otherwise, we use z. Suppose we have a vector of explanatory variables, $v_1, ..., v_r$, for each individual and we are particularly interested in studying the effect of these variables on survival, and less interested in the actual lifetime distribution. One simple model for such an effect is the proportional hazards model, where the hazard is assumed to be of the form

$$\lambda(t; z) = \lambda_0(t) \exp(\beta_1 z_1 + \ldots + \beta_p z_p),$$

where $z_1, \ldots, z_p$ are known functions of $v_1, \ldots, v_r$. The term $\lambda_0(t)$ is a function describing the dependence of the hazard on the time t. This function is completely unspecified. The subscript 0 on it reflects that it is the hazard for a value of 0 of the covariates. For different values of z, the hazard functions are assumed to be proportional, so that the regression coefficient β_m describes the change in the hazard on a logarithmic scale for a change in the corresponding covariate z_m of 1 unit, while all other covariates are kept fixed. To take a simple example, let there be just a single explanatory variable v_1 describing sex, which is often coded so that males correspond to a value of 1 and females to a value of 2. Such a covariate could simply be included as it is, but it is slightly better to include $z_1 = v_1 - 1$. Thus the value is 0 for males and 1 for females. By this definition we obtain that $\lambda_0(t)$ corresponds to the hazard for a male. If the explanatory variable v_1 was included without modification, the model would essentially be the same, but $\lambda_0(t)$ would not be the hazard for an existing person. Whether we subtract 1 or not, the coefficient β_1 is the same, and $\exp(\beta_1)$ describes the relative risk, that is, the ratio of hazards between females and males.

The time scale can be any of the possibilities mentioned in Table 1.1. The advantage of selecting a given time scale is that it allows for an arbitrary dependence on that time scale, but the disadvantage is that it is much more difficult to evaluate the dependence of the hazard on that time scale, as we have to use the method of Section 2.4.3, supplemented with kernel function smoothing. In Section 2.4.4 the possibility of multiple time scales will be considered. If age, say a, is used as a covariate, that part of the relative risk is $\exp(\beta a)$, which corresponds to the Gompertz expression φ^a, using the parameter transformation $\beta = \log \varphi$.

If we assume that there is a linear effect, the value of v_j can be inserted, but often the variable might just describe one of several groups, for example, 1 for healthy individuals, 2 for type I (insulin-dependent) diabetics, and 3 for type II (non-insulin-dependent) diabetics. We must expect a large difference between the risk for the value 1 and the other values, whereas the risk for levels 2 and 3 might be similar. Such a variable is what SAS terms a class variable, and to include it into the model, it is necessary to define a set of dummy variables, for example, z_1 being an indicator function for $v_j = 2$ and z_2 an indicator function of $v_j = 3$. In that case, β_1 describes the difference between healthy and type I diabetics, whereas β_2 describes the difference between healthy and type II diabetics. This is one reason we chose to work with the double notation, v and z. One relevant hypothesis to test is whether the two types of diabetes lead to the same risk, i.e., $\beta_1 = \beta_2$. This can be tested by making a Wald test based on the difference

$\hat{\beta}_1 - \hat{\beta}_2$, and calculating the variability by means of the standard errors and the matrix of correlation's. A solution that is often computationally easier is to define a third dummy variable, say, z_3, being an indicator function of diabetes (i.e., 1 for both types); or in other words; $z_3 = z_1 + z_2$. If z_1 and z_3 are included instead, the coefficient β_1 gives the difference between type I and type II diabetics.

As in other regression models, we can also include interaction effects of some covariates, by defining new variables by the product of the relevant variables. Non-linear effects of a covariate can be modeled by a quadratic function ($z_1 = v$, $z_2 = v^2$), or as a piecewise constant function, ($z_q = 1\{x_{q-1} < v \le x_q\}$), where $x_1, ..., x_m$ are interval end points. This is done in practice by defining a set of covariates corresponding to the effect. That means, for example, as the square of the measured value, or as the product of two covariates, when an interaction is considered.

If we doubt that the hazards are proportional for a given covariate, it is possible to stratify according to that covariate. This means that for each value, say, w_s, $s = 1, ..., J$, of the covariate, there is a separate hazard function $\lambda_{0s}(t)$. The other covariates can be assumed to have the same effect in all stratas, or we may construct further variables, allowing the effect to be different in the different strata. By stratification we allow for non-proportional hazards, but the disadvantage is that it is much more difficult to describe the effect of that covariate. An example is considered in Section 2.4.8.

2.4.2 The partial likelihood estimation method

A major contribution of the paper by Cox (1972) was to suggest an estimation method for the proportional hazards model described above. The aim of this method was purely to estimate the regression coefficients (β), allowing for a general hazard function as a nuisance parameter. The method is based on successive conditioning, which is a repeated application of the conditioning principle introduced in Section 2.1.2 on the data. The idea is that there should be a likelihood contribution at each death time, corresponding to the conditional probability of observing the actual person experiencing an event given that there was an event at that time. First, we will assume that there is only one death at each such time. At the death time for individual i, the probability that the event is for person i is

$$\frac{\lambda_0(T_i) \exp(\beta' z_i)}{\sum_{j \in R(T_i)} \lambda_0(T_i) \exp(\beta' z_j)}, \qquad (2.31)$$

conditional on there being a death at this time. The important point here is that $\lambda_0(T_i)$ cancels out, meaning that only the β-parameters contribute to this term. The likelihood is then defined as the product over all death times. This could be brought in better correspondence to the parametric models by including factors of 1 at the censoring times using the trick of raising to the power of the death indicator. This would have the advantage that there would be one term per individual. However, we chose not to do so in order to emphasize that it is the death times that contribute to the likelihood. Then the total likelihood is

$$\prod_{i:deathtimes} \frac{\exp(\beta' z_i)}{\sum_{j \in R(T_i)} \exp(\beta' z_j)}. \tag{2.32}$$

In this way, the likelihood does not depend on the hazard function $(\lambda_0(t))$.

An alternative derivation of this likelihood is as a profile likelihood. That is, first the likelihood is set up as a function of both $\lambda_0(t)$ and β, as a parametric model, that is, as a generalization of Equation (2.2). This gives

$$\prod_i \lambda_0(T_i)^{D_i} \exp(D_i \beta' z_i) \exp\{-\int_0^{T_i} \lambda_0(u) \exp(\beta' z_i) du\}. \tag{2.33}$$

Using a discretization similar to the Nelson-Aalen estimate and observing that for known β, the estimate of λ_0 can be determined by an expression derived by the same principle as Equation (2.9). The expression at a death time t is then

$$\hat{\lambda}_0(t) = \frac{1}{\sum_{j \in R(t)} \exp(\beta' z_j)}. \tag{2.34}$$

If this expression is inserted in the full likelihood, the partial likelihood of Equation (2.32) is obtained.

The standard solution is to handle ties by an approximation suggested by Peto (1972), where the same denominator is used for all events at the time point t, including all terms with times greater than or equal to t. SAS denotes this the Breslow tie handling. In the case of two events at time t, say the ith and the mth, the Peto contribution is

$$\frac{\exp(\beta' z_i)}{\sum_{j \in R(t)} \exp(\beta' z_j)} \frac{\exp(\beta' z_m)}{\sum_{j \in R(t)} \exp(\beta' z_j)}. \tag{2.35}$$

If they occurred at distinct times, say, the ith person died slightly before the mth, the contribution ought to be

$$\frac{\exp(\beta' z_i)}{\sum_{j \in R(t)} \exp(\beta' z_j)} \frac{\exp(\beta' z_m)}{\sum_{j \in R(t) \setminus \{i\}} \exp(\beta' z_j)}, \tag{2.36}$$

the only difference being that the ith person is taken out of the second risk set. However, the order of persons i and m is unobservable, and to account for this, we add the probabilities corresponding to each of the possible orderings, as this is the probability of the observed quantity. This exact evaluation is possible in SAS, but computationally more complicated and markedly slower, if the number of ties is large.

The derivative of the log likelihood is

$$d\ell/d\beta_k = \sum_{i:deathtimes} \{ z_{ik} - \frac{\sum_{j \in R(T_i)} z_{jk} \exp(\beta' z_j)}{\sum_{j \in R(T_i)} \exp(\beta' z_j)} \}. \tag{2.37}$$

This has an interpretation of the sum of the z-values among the deaths should be the same as a weighted sum of the corresponding values for the survivors. We might define $\bar{z}_k(t)$ as that weighted average at time t, so that Equation (2.37) reads

$$d\ell/d\beta_k = \sum_{i:deathtimes} \{ z_{ik} - \bar{z}_k(T_i) \}. \tag{2.38}$$

As an alternative, the log likelihood can be written as a sum over all individuals, but with a zero term for the censored individuals, that is, as

$$d\ell/d\beta_k = \sum_i D_i \{ z_{ik} - \bar{z}_k(T_i) \}. \tag{2.39}$$

A second reformulation of Equation (2.37) is to reverse the order of summation over i and j, followed by reversing the symbols i and j in the second term. This gives

$$d\ell/d\beta_k = \sum_i z_{ik} \{ D_i - \exp(\beta' z_i) \sum_{j:T_j \leq T_i} \frac{1}{\sum_{q \in R(T_j)} \exp(\beta' z_q)} \}. \tag{2.40}$$

The sum over j equals $\hat{\Lambda}_0(T_i)$, so the advantage of this expression is an interpretation as a residual. In fact, if we substitute D_i by the time-dependent function $D_i 1\{T_i \leq t\}$ and only sum over times $T_j \leq t$, the function becomes a martingale, a fact that can be used for asymptotic evaluations.

The second derivative of the log likelihood is

$$d^2\ell/d\beta_k d\beta_m = - \sum_{i:deathtimes} \{ \frac{\sum_{j \in R(T_i)} z_{jk} z_{jm} \exp(\beta' z_j)}{\sum_{j \in R(T_i)} \exp(\beta' z_j)} - \bar{z}_k(T_i)\bar{z}_m(T_i) \}. \tag{2.41}$$

This is a reasonably well-behaved second derivative in the sense that minus the second derivative is always positive definite (or semi-definite), in contrast to general likelihoods, which are only known to satisfy this property locally around the estimate. If there are some zero eigenvalues, there is a linear restriction among the covariates. To be precise, this restriction can be detected at the first event time, but not necessarily among all observations, as there can be censorings before the first event time. Basically, this implies that checking for linear dependence between the covariates should be done immediately before the first event time. One can apply standard asymptotic arguments for the partial likelihood, giving, for example, asymptotic normality. It does not make sense to try to evaluate the mean of the second derivative, but as for parametric survival models, we use the second derivative directly in order to evaluate the asymptotic variance.

It is possible to get an infinite estimate of β. For example, if there are just two observations, a male and a female, and a single covariate z defined as the indicator of female sex, then $\hat{\beta} = -\infty$ if the male dies first, and $\hat{\beta} = +\infty$ if the female dies first. More generally, infinite estimates occur if there exists a linear function of the covariates so that the events happen in order of that function. This is a small sample problem, but one must be prepared to experience it, in particular, if one defines covariates, which are indicator functions for small subsets of the observations, for example, an indicator for a single person in a study of recurrent events, and this person either never experiences the event, or experiences the event early, and then is censored.

Hypothesis testing, for example for $H_0 : \beta_j = \beta_{0j}$, where β_{0j} is a specified value can be performed by a likelihood ratio test on the partial likelihood, acting as if it is an ordinary likelihood. An alternative test statistic is the Wald test, $(\hat{\beta}_j - \beta_{0j})/SE(\hat{\beta}_j)$, where the standard error used in the denominator is found from the inverse of (minus) the matrix of second derivatives, shown in Equation (2.41). This method generally works well in this model. A third possibility is a score test, where the model is evaluated under the hypothesis and the first and second derivatives with respect to β_j are found, say ℓ_1 and ℓ_2. Then the score test statistic is $S = \ell_1/\ell_2^{1/2}$. This is less used, because it is easy to handle the model including z_j as covariate.

The partial likelihood depends only on the ranked observations, that is, the order in which the events happen, and not the actual times. This means that it is a likelihood function for a set of discrete observations. This can be illustrated by a time observation which is allowed to vary, keeping the other fixed, in which case the estimate becomes a step function, and thus is not continuous. If the observation is only changed so the ranks are unchanged, there is no change in the estimate, but if the ranks are changed, the estimate is changed. In order to get the ranks right, we prefer observations in actual days rather than months or years. This is inconvenient in many cases, because there can be observation errors in some lifetimes, in particular in cancer studies, where the cancer may be developing over many years. Figure 2.15 illustrates the importance of this point. Two groups are compared. In group 1 the observations are $\log 3/2$ and $\log 3$. These numbers are chosen as the 1/3 and 2/3 fractiles in a unit exponential distribution. In group 2 there is a fixed observation at $\log 2$, the median in a unit exponential and an extra observation that will be varied, say with value t. This can be handled under the assumption of constant hazards in the two groups, in which case the estimated β (log relative risk) is $\log[\{\log(3/2) + \log 3\}/(\log 2 + t)]$, which is a decreasing and differentiable function of t. In the Cox partial likelihood the corresponding function is a step function. Using the exact method for handling ties, the estimate $(\hat{\beta})$ is also decreasing as function of t, but it is not a continuous function, meaning that a small change in t can

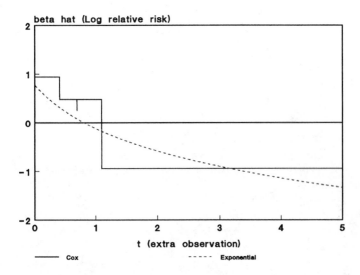

Figure 2.15. Illustration of the discontinuity of the partial likelihood as a function of the observations. Ties are handled by Breslows method.

lead to a large change in $\hat{\beta}$. The estimates in this illustration are also given in Table 2.12, where the ties are considered both in the way suggested by Breslow and the exact method. The tie handling method of Breslow implies that the function is not generally monotone. This can be seen at the time point $t = \log 2$. If the events happen simultaneously, the estimate (0.25) is lower than the estimate obtained if they happen immediately after each other (0.48), irrespective of the order. In order to avoid such problems, data should be recorded as detailed as possible; in practice, this is often in days. When there are ties, the exact method is preferable, unless there are so many that computing time becomes a problem. For data where the measurement error in the times is important, like cancer diagnosis, it might be preferable to use a parametric distribution for the hazard $\lambda_0(t)$ in order to avoid discontinuities in the likelihood function.

2.4.3 Estimation of absolute risk

The application of the Cox model has led to an almost exclusive consideration of relative risk. This is relevant in many models, but in equally many cases, the absolute risk is also of interest. In particular, this is the case, when the purpose is prediction, as introduced in Section 1.14. For example, for an insurance company, it is very interesting whether the risk of smokers and non-smokers is the same, which is a comparison of risks,

t	$\hat{\beta}(SE)$ Exact	$\hat{\beta}(SE)$ Breslow
Unknown	0.35 (1.44)	
$t < \log 3/2$	0.94 (1.24)	
$t = \log 3/2$	0.75 (1.27)	0.69 (1.22)
$\log 3/2 < t < \log 2$	0.48 (1.24)	
$t = \log 2$	0.48 (1.24)	0.25 (1.24)
$\log 2 < t < \log 3$	0.48 (1.24)	
$t = \log 3$	-0.35 (1.44)	-0.17 (1.01)
$t > \log 3$	-0.94 (1.24)	

Table 2.12. Illustration of the discontinuity of the partial likelihood estimate as a function of the observations. Artificial example. Blank space means that the two estimates coincide.

because it determines whether they should have different premiums for the two groups. However, the absolute risk is essential for calculating the actual premiums.

It is, in fact, easy to estimate the integrated hazard function. This is basically the terms described by Equation (2.34), except that in order to handle ties, the numerator should be exchanged by the number of deaths at the time considered (or sum over persons rather than over times). From these estimates the integrated hazard $\Lambda_0(t) = \int_0^t \lambda_0(u)du$ is estimated by summing the terms up to the actual time, giving

$$\hat{\Lambda}_0(t) = \sum_{i:deathtimes \leq t} \frac{N(T_i)}{\sum_{j \in R(T_i)} \exp(\hat{\beta}'z_j)}. \tag{2.42}$$

If there are no covariates, this corresponds to the Nelson-Aalen estimate. In that case, all the exponential terms are 1.

The full model can be analyzed as a Poisson multiplicative regression model, where for each patient, the number of events is evaluated at each death time. As there is at most one event for each person, most event counts are 0. This is done in the following way. Let x_q denote the death times. For each combination of i and q, for which the person is under observation, that is, $T_i \geq x_q$, a derived observation $D_{iq} = D_i 1\{T_i = x_q\}$ is considered to be Poisson distributed with mean $\exp(\beta'z_i)\lambda_q$. This is a log linear Poisson model and can be fitted by software for such models. The disadvantage of this approach is that the number of derived observations and the number of parameters increase very fast with the dimension of the data.

2.4.4 Truncation and time-dependent covariates

Truncation is mathematically simple to handle. Similar to the Kaplan-Meier and the Nelson-Aalen estimate, a person is only included in the risk set after the time of start of observation. Computationally, this is more complicated than the standard of starting at time 0, because, in the standard case, the risk set can be built up by sorting the observations in descending order according to the value of the time variable, and then evaluating cumulative sums. With truncation and time-dependent variables, it is necessary to make a new evaluation at each death time, adding and subtracting terms.

At the introduction of this model, Cox noted that the covariates could depend on time, the only requirement being that $z(t)$, the value of the covariate at time t, should be known at time t. This is not always satisfied, as will be demonstrated below. Time-dependent covariates are mathematically simple to handle, but conceptually difficult to understand fully, because they offer an extremely powerful modeling tool. The likelihood is the same as that shown in Equation (2.32), except that the values of z are replaced by the values of z evaluated at the death time. That gives the likelihood

$$\prod_{i:deathtimes} \frac{\exp\{\beta' z_i(T_i)\}}{\sum_{j \in R(T_i)} \exp\{\beta' z_j(T_i)\}}. \tag{2.43}$$

Computationally, this is more complicated than the truncation case, because all evaluations have to be done for each death time separately. One has to apply time-dependent covariates with care in order to get useful results. A key point in this regard is whether the covariates can be predicted. For example, if covariates monitoring the heart function, like pulse and blood pressure, are included, they will in many cases change immediately before death, and then explain the death, in the sense they have high predictive power. If we want to study the effect of a cardiovascular drug treatment, we might not directly see the effect, if the drug works by stabilizing pulse and blood pressure. This also makes it impossible to predict death well in advance, because we do not control how pulse and blood pressure change. To handle these problems pulse and blood pressure should be included as responses in the model. How to create such models is considered in Chapter 6. A similar extreme example is the menopausal model of Figure 1.3. Defining menopause at time B, the time when the woman has experienced a bleeding-free year, which makes sense from a survival analysis viewpoint, we can make a perfect description of the times, by including a time-dependent covariate, measuring time since latest menstruation. As long as this covariate is below 365 days, the incidence of menopause is 0, and when it gets to 365 days, there is a 100 % probability that menopause happens. Even though there are many other factors that influence time of menopause, this time-dependent covariate is completely capable of describing this event. It is impossible to make detailed predictions. All we can say if the value of the covariate is z is that if the woman does not have a bleeding within the next $365 - z$ days, she will obtain menopause at that time, and that if she bleeds, menopause will be more than a year away. This is exactly what can be deduced from the definition of menopause, and therefore it is not interesting. In other words, if we want to make a non-

Type	Application
Known linear, common slope	Multiple time scales
Known	Check of proportionality assumption
	Modeling non-proportionality
State-dependent	Multi-state models
Measured	Dependence examination

Table 2.13. Some types of time-dependent covariates.

trivial conclusion, we need to exclude such covariates. A similar example is that for studying births, the best predictor is a time-dependent variable describing pregnancy, but this is only good for a short-term prediction of births, i.e., up to 9 months. If we want to make a long-term prediction, or to examine the effect of age, race, partner, and number of previous births, we need to exclude pregnancy as a possible covariate for the evaluation. Another way to say this is that to choose a model, it is not only a matter of obtaining a good fit, but also the predictability of the time-dependent covariates must be taken into account. One more example is the risk of drunk driving. An insurance company might find out that drunk driving is related to an increased risk by a factor of c, say, by means of an analysis including a time-dependent indicator variable for whether the examined persons are drunk at any given time. However, to predict whether a new customer will have an accident owing to drunk driving, we cannot rely on whether the person is sober at the time of signing the contract. We must consider the probability of a person's changing status, that is, becoming drunk and driving at a later time.

We require the covariate function to be left continuous to exclude response dependent functions like $z(t) = 1\{T \leq t, D = 1\}$, which tells nothing, but has a perfect fit.

Here we will mention some key types of time-dependent covariates (see Table 2.13). It is possible that the covariate trajectory is known from the beginning, or it is possible that it changes in a more-or-less unpredictable way. Some possible applications can illustrate the points.

Multiple time scales

In a study of persons with a given disease, it is relevant to ask whether it is the age, say, a, or the duration of the disease, say, u, that determines the mortality. Both can be included when time-dependent covariates are allowed for. We can pick age as the time scale to make a model with hazard $\lambda_0(a) \exp(\beta u)$. Using that duration is time since age at diagnosis (a_0), this can be reformulated to

$$\lambda_0(a) \exp\{\beta(a - a_0)\} = \lambda_0(a) \exp(\beta a) \exp(-\beta a_0) = \tilde{\lambda}_0(a) \exp(\tilde{\beta} a_0).$$
$$(2.44)$$

Here we use the fact that the arbitrary function $\lambda_0(a)$ can absorb any function of a, simplifying the model to a fixed covariate model, with age at diagnosis as covariate, and $\tilde{\beta} = -\beta$ as regression coefficient. There will be truncation in this model. Alternatively, we can pick duration as the time scale to make a model with hazard $\mu_0(u)\exp(\kappa a)$. This model can similarly be transformed to a fixed covariate model with hazard $\tilde{\mu}_0(u)\exp(\kappa a_0)$. In this case, the regression coefficient is unchanged. Whether there is truncation is a matter of whether the patients are included from the time of diagnosis or later. This transfer of the time-dependent terms works for any set of linear functions with common slopes. Whether we should pick age or duration as the time scale is a matter of fit. We should choose the variable with the largest effect, or the most non-linear effect. A similar problem arises for fertility data; should we use age, or the time since the latest birth? This approach is illustrated by its application to the survival of diabetics.

Known functions

Known (pre-specified) functions can be used to make non-proportional hazards, for example, a non-proportional treatment effect (a treatment by time interaction) can be described by a fixed variable z_1 being the indicator function of treatment, and a time-dependent term $z_2(t) = tz_1$. This model implies that the hazard in the control group is $\lambda_0(t)$ and in the treatment group $\lambda_0(t)\exp(\beta_1 + \beta_2 t)$. This gives the same relative risk function as a Gompertz model with different values of φ in the two groups. In this model β_1 describes the initial treatment effect and β_2 the change in treatment effect over time. This is particularly relevant for checking the proportional hazards model, which is the hypothesis $\beta_2 = 0$, but less relevant for modeling non-proportional hazards, as the consequence of the assumption is that the treatment effect is reversed if β_1 and β_2 have opposite signs, and that the effect either increases to infinity or decreases to minus infinity with time. This problem can be reduced by taking $z_2(t) = z_1 \log t$, which gives the same relative risk function as a Weibull model with different values of γ in the two groups. The problem can be completely avoided by picking covariates that stay finite, for example, piecewise constant variables. This approach is illustrated by the application to malignant melanoma.

State-dependent covariates

The covariate can further be an indicator function of presence in a given state. This is a quite general approach and will be considered at length in Chapter 6. It can be used for modeling of the hazard of death by, for example, the presence of complications. What makes this type of variable special is that there are only a few possible states, and the transition between the states is included in the model and therefore, we are able to make probability statements about the future values of such a covariate. One example is the survival among the participants in the Stanford heart transplant program (Section 1.9.4), where the hazard of death differs before and after heart transplant.

Measured covariates

The final type of time-dependent covariates is the measured variables, which means that the covariate trajectory is external to the model, and thus by definition impossible to predict. These may be measured in a regular pattern, or at visits made with irregular intervals. If these intervals are long, and there is a clear development over time, which, for example, would be case for CD4 counts in AIDS and for albuminuria measurements in diabetes, it seems attractive to use interpolation to get the most precise evaluation of the variable at any given time. This, however, invalidates the principle that the value of $z(t)$ should be known at time t. It should, in fact, be clear that this is wrong, because it is not possible to use interpolation for those that die, and therefore the covariates are treated differently for the deaths and the survivors. If the simple approach of using the latest measurement is not satisfactory, it is possible to make an updating formula based on previous measurements. If there are many measurements, and a large person variation in development, we can use extrapolated values based on a fit of earlier measurements, but in other cases we can modify the latest measurement by some function of the time since the measurement. For the albuminuria example above, the concentration is known to increase by about 15 % per year as a mean over patients, and we can then use this number for extending past values.

Predictions

Evaluating the integrated hazard function is done in exactly the same way as for constant covariates, but it is more difficult to apply it for evaluating a prognosis in the case of time-dependent covariates, as it is necessary to know the future course of the covariates, either precisely, or the distribution of the covariates. This is not a problem for known covariates, where the course is fixed from the beginning. In the case of state-dependent covariates, the future development of it can be included as a random quantity in a multi-state model (see Chapter 6). The prediction is then found by the transition probabilities. In the case of measured covariates, we have to make an assumed development for the covariate process or to set up a stochastic process model for its future, which might be difficult or impossible.

The time-dependent covariates are very well suited to the successive conditioning in the partial likelihood estimation procedure. However, we could also have time-dependent covariates in parametric models. As mentioned, the treatment by time interaction model with known covariates, would in a Gompertz model just correspond to different φ values in the two treatment groups. The state dependent covariates correspond to a structure on the parametric functions in a multi-state model, see Chapter 6. The likelihood would still be of the form in Equation (2.2), but one should note that $\Lambda(t)$ should be substituted by the integral of the actual hazard experienced and this makes it much more complicated.

2.4.5 Residuals and robust variance estimates

In normal distribution models, residuals are commonly evaluated in order to check the assumptions of the models. Also residuals are computationally useful for evaluating the variance estimate. For survival data, it is more complicated. Residuals can still be evaluated, but their precision depend markedly on whether they originate from observed or censored observations. The variance estimate derived in this way will be different from that evaluated by the second derivative. The residuals are based on the univariate formulation of the likelihood in Equation (2.39). The terms needed are the influence diagnostics, describing for each individual the contributions to the log likelihood derivative from that individual. For the ith individual, and for covariate k, the quantity is

$$W_{ik} = D_i\{z_{ik} - \bar{z}_k(T_i)\} - \sum_q \frac{D_q R_i(T_q)\exp(\beta' z_{ik})}{\sum_r R_r(T_q)\exp(\beta' z_{rk})}\{z_{ik} - \bar{z}_k(T_q)\} \quad (2.45)$$

The kmth element of the estimated variance matrix V of the score vector of Equation (2.39) then is

$$v_{km} = \sum_i W_{ik}W_{im}. \quad (2.46)$$

The variance matrix of the regression coefficients then is the so-called sandwich estimator

$$B = A^{-1}VA^{-1}, \quad (2.47)$$

where A is the matrix of second derivatives of the log likelihood function, as defined in Equation (2.41). The standard derivation in a Cox model uses A as the variance of the score vector, leading to the variance of $\hat{\beta}$ being A^{-1}.

The theoretical basis for the sandwich estimator is the information evaluations for parametric working models. Instead of using the likelihood $\ell(\theta)$ in the correct model, one uses a likelihood $\tilde{\ell}(\theta)$ of another model (the so-called working model). The asymptotic variance of the estimate based on the working model, say, based on n independent identically distributed variables, is

$$\frac{1}{n}(Ed^2\tilde{\ell}/d\theta^2)^{-1}[E\{(d\tilde{\ell}/d\theta)(d\tilde{\ell}/d\theta)'\}](Ed^2\tilde{\ell}/d\theta^2)^{-1}, \quad (2.48)$$

where the expectations must be evaluated under the correct model. When $\tilde{\ell}$ is the likelihood of the correct model, the terms coincide, except for the sign, giving an asymptotic variance of $-(Ed^2\ell/d\theta^2)^{-1}/n$.

2.4.6   Neglected covariates

It is not possible in practice to include all relevant covariates. For example, we might know that some given factor is important, but if we do not know the value of the factor for each individual, we cannot include the variable in the analysis. For example it is known that excretion of small amounts of albumin (Section 1.9.1) in the urine is a diagnostic marker for increased mortality, not only for diabetic patients, but also for the general population. However, we are unable to include this variable, unless we actually obtain urine and analyze samples for each individual under study. It is furthermore possible that we are not aware that there exist variables that we ought to include. For example, this could be a genetic factor, as we do not know all possible genes having an influence on survival. This consideration is true for all regression models, not only survival models. If it is known that some factor is important, it makes sense to try to obtain the individual values, but if this is not possible, the standard is to ignore the presence of such variables. In general terms, we let the heterogeneity go into the error term. This will, of course, lead to an increase in the variability of the response compared to the case, when the variables are included. In the survival data case, however, the increased variability implies a change in the form of the hazard function, as will be illustrated by some more detailed calculations. We will assume that some covariates $z_1, ..., z_p$ are known and some further $w_1, ..., w_m$ are also important, but unknown. Suppose that theoretically both have an influence on the hazard in a proportional hazards model as

$$\lambda_0(t)\exp(\beta'z + \psi'w). \tag{2.49}$$

However, w is unknown, so this model cannot be used in practice. We then assume that the vector w is random. We have to make this assumption as we have no information on the individual values of w. For convenience it is assumed that w is independent of z. If this is not the case, the expected value of w given z should be subtracted from w, so the contribution of that part is moved over to z. Thus the hazard has the form

$$Y(w, \psi)\lambda_0(t)\exp(\beta'z), \tag{2.50}$$

with $Y(w, \psi) = \exp(\psi'w)$. This means that the hazard depends on the vector w only via the scalar function $Y(w, \psi)$, say Y. If w is assumed random, the multivariate distribution of the whole vector is not needed, all that matters is the distribution of the one-dimensional function Y. Here some of the distributions of Appendix A are considered and the calculations turn out much the same way as in Section 2.2.7 on mixture distributions. Inserting a gamma distribution gives a hazard function of $\delta\lambda_0(t)\exp(\beta'z)/\{\theta + \Lambda_0(t)\exp(\beta'z)\}$, after integrating Y out. As $\lambda_0(t)$ is arbitrary, it makes no further generality to include a scale parameter on Y, and therefore we assume that the mean is 1, which is obtained by $\delta = \theta$.

That gives a hazard function of the form

$$\lambda_0(t) \exp(\beta' z)/\{1 + \Lambda_0(t) \exp(\beta' z)/\theta\}. \tag{2.51}$$

These functions are no longer proportional for different values of z. In fact, the ratio of two such hazard functions, say, for z_1 and z_2 will start at the correct value $\exp\{\beta'(z_1 - z_2)\}$, but monotonically converge to 1, as $t \to \infty$ (or slightly more specific, as $\Lambda_0(t) \to \infty$). Here, the word *correct* refers to the value conditional on Y. The special case $\theta = 1$ gives the so-called proportional odds model, which has been suggested as an alternative regression model with non-proportional hazards. Instead of assuming a proportional odds model, it seems more sensible to consider the whole gamma frailty proportional hazards model in Equation (2.51). If instead an inverse Gaussian distribution is assumed, with $\theta > 0$ so the mean exists, we take $\delta = \theta^{1/2}$ to secure a mean value of 1, and the marginal hazard function becomes

$$\lambda_0(t) \exp(\beta' z)/\{1 + \Lambda_0(t) \exp(\beta' z)/\theta\}^{1/2}, \tag{2.52}$$

an expression that is very similar to Equation (2.51) for the gamma distribution, the only difference being a power of $1/2$ in the denominator. The ratio of two such hazard functions also starts at the value $\exp\{\beta'(z_1 - z_2)\}$, but, as $t \to \infty$, monotonically converges to $\exp\{\beta'(z_1 - z_2)/2\}$, the square root of the start value. This immediately generalizes to the PVF distributions with finite mean (again chosen to 1), and $\alpha > 0$, in which case we obtain the expression

$$\lambda_0(t) \exp(\beta' z)/\{1 + \Lambda_0(t) \exp(\beta' z)/\theta\}^{1-\alpha}, \tag{2.53}$$

which starts at the correct ratio and converges to $\exp\{\beta'(z_1 - z_2)\}^\alpha$. In fact, this expression is also valid for $\alpha < 0$, in which case the relative risk crosses the value 1, and the limiting value will be on the other side of 1. This is due to a proportion $(\exp(\theta/\alpha)$, the same proportion in both groups) having 0 risk of the event and they will eventually dominate the survivors, a domination that will occur faster in the high-risk group.

If instead a positive stable distribution is assumed, we cannot normalize by the mean, as it does not exist, but the scale can be fixed by choosing $\delta = \alpha$, and we obtain that the marginal hazard function is

$$\lambda_0(t) \exp(\alpha\beta' z)\alpha\Lambda_0(t)^{\alpha-1}, \tag{2.54}$$

which is a proportional hazards function of the form $\omega_0(t) \exp(\tilde{\beta}' z)$, with $\omega_0(t) = \alpha\lambda_0(t)\Lambda_0(t)^{\alpha-1}$ and $\tilde{\beta} = \alpha\beta$. This implies that when the distribution of the neglected covariates has a distribution corresponding to a positive stable distribution for Y, the model is consistent with there being neglected covariates, but the hazard function and the regression coefficients are not. The hazard function is changed corresponding to the increased variation. That is, the hazard function becomes decreasing or less increasing. Also the regression coefficients are changed owing to the increased variation, and they become numerically smaller. This can be interpreted as a bias. An alternative formulation is that the regression coefficients cannot be evaluated without consideration of the variability of neglected covariates. This is a serious drawback of relative risks models. The same problem is not present in accelerated failure times models, see Section 2.5.2.

In practice, fitting is typically done while ignoring this problem. The resulting estimated regression coefficient will be closer to 0 than the conditional regression coefficient β.

As the vector of unobserved covariates w only contributes via $\psi'w$, it is impossible to find out whether the number of components m is one or more. The largest flexibility is obtained if the distribution of $\psi'w$ (that is, $\log Y$) is infinitely divisible, as then any value of m is possible. The gamma and stable distributions are infinitely divisible on the logarithmic scale, whereas the general inverse Gaussian and PVF are not.

2.4.7 Computational aspects

The Cox model can be fitted by SAS, using proc phreg. A program for fitting the tumorigenesis data is

```
data a;
   infile filename';
   input treat tumtime death;
proc phreg;
   model tumtime*death(0)=treat/ties=exact;
```

This procedure cannot accept class variables, and thus it is necessary to code such variables. If the ties=exact option is omitted, the ties are handled by Breslows method. If one would stratify with respect to treatment, one can make a procedure call of

```
proc phreg;
   model tumtime*death(0)=/ties=exact;
   strata treat;
```

Time-dependent covariates are easily introduced by defining them in the procedure call. For example, the non-proportional treatment effect discussed in Section 2.4.4 is obtained by

```
proc phreg;
   model tumtime*death(0)=treat treattim/ties=exact;
   treattim=tumtime*treat;
```

It should be noted that to match this to Equation (2.43), tumtime should be indexed by i and treat by j. The survival function and the integrated hazard can be obtained by a call:

```
data covals;
  input treat;
cards;
  0
  1
;
proc phreg data=a;
  model tumtime*death(0)=treat/ties=exact;
  baseline out=res covariates=covals survival=surv logsurv=ls/nomean;
proc print data=res;
```

The default is to evaluate the survivor function (survival) or integrated hazard (logsurv) at the average value of the covariates. This is avoided by specifying the option nomean and giving a data set with the desired values of the covariates. The output is a data set that for each value in the covariate data set contains the values of the chosen quantities at all jump times. This means that in order to plot these as step functions, one should add points corresponding to the left limits at the jump times.

Truncation can be handled from release 6.10. If the variable start gives the start of observation, the procedure call could look like

```
proc phreg;
  model (start,tumtime)*death(0)=treat/ties=exact;
```

2.4.8 Applications

To illustrate the many interesting features of this model, a number of examples are considered. Further examples of time-dependent covariates of the state-dependent type are presented in Section 6.7.

Death after myocardial infarction

As this is a regression-type model, it has a lot of features common to other regression models. One such feature is that the regression coefficient describes the change in response (for survival models, the change in hazard), when the other variables are kept constant. It is easy, but incorrect, to interpret this as everything else being equal. It is only the variables in the model that are being kept equal. An illustration of this point can be the death hazard after myocardial infarction, a subset of the data of Section 1.9.3. Here the short-term survival (until 30 days) after infarction is studied in order to evaluate when the patients should be discharged from the hospital. There were 1140 such admissions to the hospital. Some patients contribute with several courses, but we will not account for this owing to the successive conditioning principle. The time scale used is time since onset of the infarction. If only sex is included in the model, the estimate is $\hat{\beta} = 0.36$, implying that the death risk for women is $1.44 = e^{0.36}$ times that for men. However, this is an unfair comparison, because typically women suffering an infarction are significantly older than men with the disease, and as age is not included in the model, this variable is not kept fixed. If both sex and age are included, the regression coefficients are -0.06 for sex and 0.054/year for age. This implies that the risk for women is lower (insignificantly) than for men *of the same age*, rather than increased as suggested by the estimate without age included. To make the comparison for fixed age, age must be included in the model. A further point is that the coefficient to age is lower than the Gompertz estimate obtained in Section 2.2.3 for the population, which was $\hat{\varphi} = 1.091$, corresponding to $\hat{\beta} = \log \hat{\varphi} = 0.087$/year. This difference is also expected, as age is less important for patients with a given disease, than for the population at large.

Tumorigenesis data

For the tumorigenesis data described in Section 1.5.3, neglecting dependence owing to litters, we obtain $\hat{\beta} = 0.905$ for the treatment effect, with standard error 0.318. The Wald test of no difference gives a χ^2 test statistic of 8.12, whereas the likelihood ratio test statistic is 7.98. The score test statistic is 8.68, illustrating the good agreement between the various test statistics. The p-value is of the order of 0.004.

Heart transplant data

The original analysis of the Stanford heart transplant data introduced in Section 1.9.4 used a covariate of 1 for the patients receiving a heart transplant and 0 for those who did not. The time used was time since acceptance in the program. This analysis is in conflict with the survival data principles, because the value of z was not known before actual transplantation, and survival data methods require it to be known at the start of follow-up, which was time of acceptance. This gives an implicit survival advantage to the transplanted group. In a model, also including age, the (invalid) estimated effect of transplantation was a coefficient of -1.80 (SE 0.27), corresponding to a relative risk of 0.17, suggesting a strongly significant improvement in survival with transplantation. The effect of age was 0.060 (SE 0.015). This problem can be handled correctly by a time-dependent covariate of the state-dependent type, and this is performed in Section 6.7.1.

Malignant melanoma

For the data on malignant melanoma of Section 1.10.2, we consider the deaths of the disease, i.e., treat the 14 deaths of other causes as censorings. Sex, age, and thickness are included as covariates. The estimated regression coefficients are, for sex -0.55 (SE 0.27), suggesting lower mortality for women than men, for age 0.012 (0.008) /year and for thickness 0.151 (0.033) /mm. Qualitatively, this is as expected. The sex effect suggests a higher risk for males, the age effect suggests a (non-significant) increase

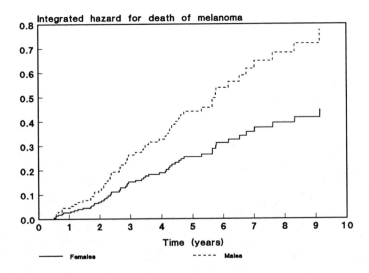

Figure 2.16. The estimated integrated hazard function for the melanoma data, for a male and a female patient of age 50 years and melanoma thickness 5 mm, based on an assumption of proportional hazards.

by age, with a coefficient that is much lower than known for the population, owing to the risk's being less dependent on age for people having a specific disease, and the thickness effect suggests a larger risk with increasing size of the melanoma. Figure 2.16 shows the estimated integrated hazard for two fictitious patients, a male and a female of age 50 years, and thickness 5 mm. This is based on the assumption of proportional hazards. To allow for and check the proportional hazards model, three methods are considered. The most general is stratification, where separate arbitrary hazards are assumed. The effect of the covariates is assumed to be the same in both stratas, and the estimates are, for age, 0.012 (0.009)/year and, for thickness, 0.151 (0.033)/mm. Regarding the sex effect, there is now no quantitative estimate, but the effect is illustrated in Figure 2.17, which shows the estimated integrated hazard functions. Thus the advantage of stratification is that we allow for non-proportional hazards, but at the price of being unable to quantify the effect, all we can do is to show the different curves in the figure. The covariate model gives a confidence interval of (1.03–2.91), for the relative risk for a male compared to a female, but a similar simple result cannot be obtained under stratification. A further disadvantage of the stratified approach is an increased variance on the integrated hazard estimate, which can be suggested just by observing that the sizes of the jumps are higher under stratification (Figure 2.17). A compromise, which

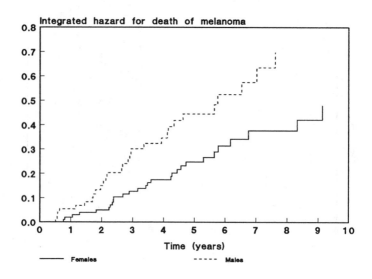

Figure 2.17. The estimated integrated hazard function for the melanoma data, for a male and a female patient of age 50 years and melanoma thickness 5 mm, based on stratification by sex.

is more effective at quantifying non-proportionality, is to include a time-dependent covariate, being 0 for males, and equal to the time for females. In that case, the sex effect is -1.06 (0.53), and the time-dependent covariate effect is 0.00041 (0.00037)/day. This effect is non-significant, but it suggests that there is a small relative risk of 0.35 at time 0, which increases with time since operation, and implies a reversal of the sex effect after an estimated 2584 days, or 7.1 years. We may or may not believe that the effect is really reversed after these 7.1 years, but this calculation is included to illustrate the point that although this approach is fine for testing the hypothesis of proportional hazards, it is less good as an actual model for non-proportionality, and should not be overinterpreted. This is an example of a model useful for model checking purposes, but unrealistic as a scientific model. The effect of age and thickness is the same as in the other models, to the accuracy the results are reported with.

Another model leading to non-proportional hazards is the neglected covariates model. For the melanoma data, using the same covariates and a gamma model for the neglected covariates, we obtain $\hat{\theta} = 0.207$ (0.091). The sex effect is -0.92 (0.51), the effect of age is 0.0073 (0.0147) / year, and the effect of thickness 0.512 (0.187) / mm. The log likelihood is significantly better than for the model without neglected covariates, corresponding to $-2 \log Q = 7.27$, where Q is the likelihood ratio. If we extend to the

PVF distribution for the neglected covariates, the likelihood is only non-significantly improved, giving an additional value of $-2 \log Q = 0.44$. The estimate of α is -0.13 (0.22). As the estimate is negative, it suggests that some patients are unable to die of this disease. This is possible, as we only study death owing to malignant melanoma and not total mortality. The estimated proportion with 0 risk is 11.6 %. A very resolute conclusion would be that this is the cure rate, but in practice, we should be careful not to overinterpret such a value. The estimated value of θ is 0.286 (0.159). The effect of sex is -0.91 (0.49), the effect of age is 0.0062 (0.0079), and the effect of thickness is 0.52 (1.40). The estimated integrated hazards for the same two fictitious patients as in the two previous figures are shown in Figure 2.18. These functions are the estimated marginal hazards, that is, after Y has been integrated out, as described in Equation (2.53). The difference between the estimates for the two sexes is initially as large as in the other model, but the two curves do not deviate further after about 5 years, suggesting that the hazards are comparable for the two sexes after this point. As there is a proportion with 0 risk, the hazards cross, and this is estimated to happen at 6.2 years after operation. Thus, this is comparable to the time-dependent covariate model, which said 7.1 years. However, the crossing of the hazards functions is not significant, because the PVF model is not significantly better than the gamma model, which does not imply crossing hazard functions.

Catheter infection data

A similar example is the catheter infection data of Section 1.7.3, if no account is taken of the pairing of data. The proportional hazards model including sex and age, leads to estimates of -0.82 (0.30) for sex and 0.0022 (0.0092) per year for age, suggesting that females have a significantly lower infection risk than men. In a gamma mixture model, the regression coefficients are -1.77 (0.61) and 0.0067 (0.0124) for age. These values are much larger, but the qualitative conclusion is the same. The numerical value of the regression coefficients is clearly increased compared to the proportional hazards model. The estimated value of θ is 1.51 (0.98).

Survival of diabetics

In the study of the survival among insulin-dependent diabetic patients in the county of Funen, Denmark, described in Section 1.2.2, all patients were followed from July 1, 1973. As age is more important for the mortality than duration and calendar time, it was decided to use age as the time scale, and thus the patients started observation at whatever age they were on July 1, 1973. The time-dependent variable duration could be included by using the fixed variable age at diagnosis as demonstrated in Section 2.4.4. This gave a coefficient of -0.014/year (SE 0.005), meaning that there was an increase with duration, of 0.014/year, for fixed age. Similarly calendar time could be

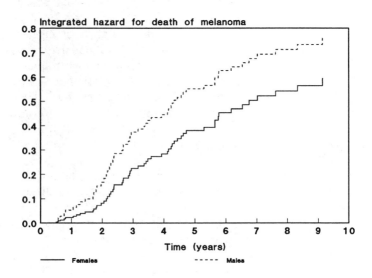

Figure 2.18. The estimated integrated hazard function for the melanoma data, for a male and a female patient of age 50 years and melanoma thickness 5 mm, based on the PVF frailty model and proportional conditional hazards.

included by means of the fixed covariate age on July 1, 1973. The effect of calendar time was -0.042/year (SE 0.026), suggesting a large change over time (4.2 % decrease per year). However, this is not statistically significant because the period of 7 years is short for such an analysis, and secondly, the effect might reflect selection. This corresponds to the mixture, where the high-risk patients die first in the period, leading to a change to low-risk patients. If the conditional distribution is exponential, the hazard function in the marginal distribution decreases over time. When a variable describing time is included, it is possible that the mixture effect is attributed to the calendar time.

2.4.9   Summary of the Cox model

Table 2.14 lists the major properties of the Cox model. It has become so popular because it is very good at describing relative risks. That is, it very effectively removes the effect of time. However, this is also a major disadvantage, because it suggests considering only the relative risk also in cases where it would be useful to evaluate the absolute risk. This, of course, is not a problem with the approach, but a problem regarding the way it has been applied in practice. Heterogeneity is a major problem. In the case where the distribution of the effect on the hazard of the neglected covariates

Advantages:
Extremely flexible regarding effect of covariates
No need for considering the absolute risk
Disadvantages:
Likelihood function not continuous as function of the observations
The assumption of proportional hazards influenced by heterogeneity
Hazard ratios influenced by heterogeneity
The absolute risk does not receive attention

Table 2.14. Major properties of the Cox proportional hazards model.

follows a positive stable distribution, the model still shows proportional hazards, but the regression coefficients are changed. This implies that it is difficult to interpret the value of a relative risk. Furthermore, if the effect of the neglected covariates follows any other distribution, the model is no longer correct. That is, the assumption of proportional hazards is violated. The influence of heterogeneity has been discussed in Section 2.4.6 and will be further considered in Section 2.5.2.

2.5 Accelerated failure times

Rather than having the hazard function's being described as a function of the explanatory variables, it is possible to let the explanatory variables act via a scale factor directly on the time. Thus there should be a basic survivor function $S_0(t)$, the survivor function for a person with covariate value 0, and then the survivor function for a person with covariates $z_1, ..., z_p$ is assumed to be $S_0\{t/\exp(\nu'z)\}$. The standard way to describe an accelerated failure time model is as

$$\log T_i = \nu'z_i + \epsilon_i, \tag{2.55}$$

where the ϵ_i are independent and identically distributed. Thus, this describes a linear model for the logarithm to the times.

If $S_0(t)$ corresponds to a Weibull distribution, of shape γ, this gives the same regression model as the proportional hazards model, but with a different parametrization. The relation between the parameters is

$$\nu = -\beta/\gamma. \tag{2.56}$$

There are no other models where the proportional hazards and the accelerated failure times are identical.

Typically, we make parametric assumptions regarding $S_0(t)$, because no expression like the Cox partial likelihood is available to remove the effect of the basic survival distribution.

2.5.1   Comparison of accelerated failure time models and proportional hazards models

The question is, of course, whether the accelerated failure time model makes more or less sense than the proportional hazards regression models. Accelerated failure times seem more sensible for wear related processes: for example, if a constant load differs between individuals. In some cases, this can be interpreted as a double time scale. The lifetime of a car might be measured in years but could maybe be better predicted by the mileage. Then the load could be the distance driven per year. Some cars are used only a little, and others a lot. The present model assumes that the mileage increases linearly for each single car (that is, constant use), but with different speeds. The distance is, however, typically not known and therefore the regression model is included in order to describe the distance as a function of the covariates. A hazard-based model, on the other hand, makes it easier to accommodate time-dependent covariates. It is also better for describing changes in risk corresponding to fixed points in the time scale, for example, the change in risk for boys when they attain the age to receive a drivers license.

On the graphical side, this can be understood on the integrated hazards scale. Suppose there are two groups. The proportional hazards model then says that $\Lambda_2(t) = c\Lambda_1(t)$ for some c, whereas the accelerated failure time model says that $\Lambda_2(t) = \Lambda_1(t/c)$ for some c. So the question is whether the integrated hazards are proportional on the time scale or the hazard scale.

This can be illustrated by considering the effect on a chosen hazard. Take the distribution for the Danish male population described in Section 1.2.1 and depicted in Figure 2.1. The mean lifetime is 72.5 years. If the hazard is multiplied by 5, the mean is reduced to 53.1 years. Multiplying on the time axis by 0.732, corresponding to an accelerated failure time model, leads to the same mean survival. Figure 2.19 shows the integrated hazard as suggested. The integrated hazards cross at a single point near the mean lifetime. The integrated hazard of the accelerated model is steeper suggesting a smaller variability in this case. The effect on the actual distribution is seen on Figure 2.20, which illustrates the density for the original distribution and the two modified distributions. The accelerated failure time approach leads to a decreased mean, with a constant relative variability and thus a decreased absolute variability, which is clearly seen by the higher peak density and the narrower peak. The proportional hazards approach similarly leads to a decreased mean, but except at low ages, it rather looks like a translation by about 20 years and the variability appears to be unchanged. For the infant mortality, there is a clear change for the proportional hazards model, but no big difference for the accelerated failure time approach.

This is further illustrated in Figure 2.21, where the baseline is a Gompertz distribution of mean 1 and standard deviation 1/2. Both the proportional hazards model and the accelerated failure time model lead to

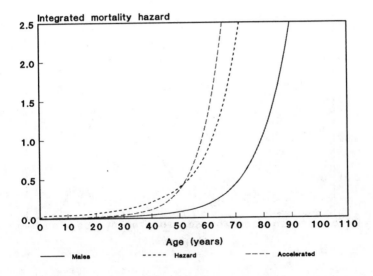

Figure 2.19. The integrated hazard for the mortality of Danish males, before and after modification by proportional hazards (factor 5) and accelerated failure time (factor 0.732).

Gompertz distributions. The figure shows the means and standard deviations obtainable in the two models. In the accelerated failure time model, the standard deviation is proportional to the mean as the modification acts like a scale factor on time. For the proportional hazards model, the standard deviation changes less than the mean value, similar to the results found for the population data.

A main advantage of the proportional hazards model is that an estimate can be found in this model allowing for an arbitrary hazard function, but this is more complicated in the accelerated failure time model and therefore, in practice, parametric models are applied.

Time-dependent covariates can also be introduced in accelerated failure time models, but this is more complicated than for proportional hazards models, as described by Hougaard (1999). This will not be further considered in this book.

2.5.2 Neglected covariates

In the case of neglected covariates in the model, we can use Equation (2.55) to show that this just leads to a distribution of ϵ with larger variability, but no change in the regression coefficients. The form of the distribution of ϵ may change. The simplest model, when there are no censorings, is the

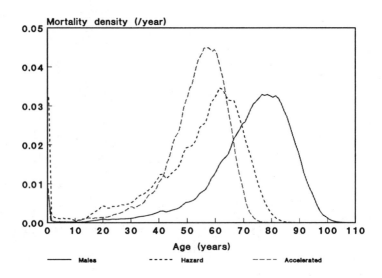

Figure 2.20. The density for the mortality of Danish males, before and after modification by proportional hazards (factor 5) and accelerated failure time (factor 0.732).

lognormal model, where both the neglected covariates and the error term (on the log scale) are assumed to follow normal distributions. It is well known that when the observed and neglected covariates are independent, the value of ν is unchanged, but the variance parameter is increased. Another interesting special case is the positive stable frailty model. Combining Equations (2.22) and (2.55) gives the model

$$\log T = \nu'z + \psi'W + \epsilon, \tag{2.57}$$

where z denotes the observed covariates and W the neglected covariates. If ϵ follows the distribution of the logarithm of a Weibull variable of shape γ and $\psi'W$ follows the distribution of the logarithm of a positive stable variable of index α, independently of the value of z, W can be integrated out giving

$$\log T = \nu'z + \tilde{\epsilon}, \tag{2.58}$$

where $\tilde{\epsilon}$ follows the logarithm of a Weibull variable, of shape $\alpha\gamma$. Most importantly, the regression term is unchanged showing the superiority of the parameter ν, which alternatively can be phrased as that ν is robust towards neglected covariates. Studying Equation (2.56) gives an explanation. Both β and γ are multiplied by α, so that their ratio is constant.

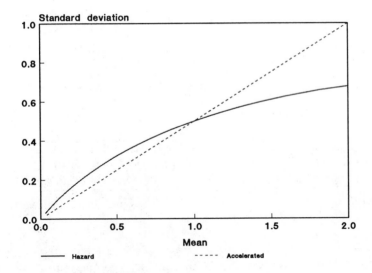

Figure 2.21. The relation between the mean and standard deviation in the proportional hazards and accelerated failure time model, based on a Gompertz distribution with mean 1 and standard deviation 1/2.

For other distributional assumptions in Equation (2.57), we still obtain the formula of Equation (2.58), so the only problem is that the distribution of $\tilde{\epsilon}$ typically is not in the same parametric family as used for ϵ.

2.5.3 Applications

The accelerated failure model can for Weibull times be analyzed by SAS, using the program described above in Section 2.2.2, but where the names of the variables in the model are inserted after the equality sign.

For the tumorigenesis data, an intercept (ν) of 5.222 (SE 0.160), and a treatment effect (ν_1) of -0.239 (SE 0.089) and a scale (σ) of 0.2638 (SE 0.0380) are obtained in the Weibull model. From this we derive that $\hat{\gamma} = 3.79$ and $\hat{\lambda} = 2.53 \cdot 10^{-9}$ in the control group, and $\hat{\lambda} = 6.25 \cdot 10^{-9}$ in the treatment group. Thus the log relative risk in the hazard function ($-\nu_1/\sigma$) is estimated to 0.904, agreeing very well with the semi-parametric proportional hazards model. This gives a relative risk of 2.47. The effect on the time scale is as a factor of e^ν, which is estimated as 0.79. Thus the alternative interpretations of the results of this model are that treatment increases the risk by 147 %, or it reduces the lifetime by 21 %. The reason for this large apparent discrepancy is that the hazard is increasing, in which case a large change in the hazard might lead to a more modest change in

	Males	Females
Year of onset	−0.0423 (0.0123)	−0.0322 (0.0113)
Age at onset	−0.035 (0.011)	0.216 (0.067)
Squared age at onset	0.0010 (0.0003)	−0.0081 (0.0022)
Worst age at onset	17.2 (1.5)	13.4 (1.2)

Table 2.15. Estimated hazard regression coefficients, for nephropathy data, with PVF frailty.

	Males	Females
Year of onset	0.0084 (0.0024)	0.0093 (0.0033)
Age at onset	0.175 (0.060)	−0.071 (0.021)
Squared age at onset	−0.0051 (0.0018)	0.0023 (0.0006)

Table 2.16. Estimated accelerated failure time regression coefficients, for nephropathy data, with PVF frailty.

lifetime. The Wald test for no treatment effect is a χ^2-statistic of 7.17, and a likelihood ratio test of 8.00, also in very good agreement with the proportional hazards model. To obtain the likelihood ratio test statistic by means of SAS, it is necessary to make a separate fit under the hypothesis.

If the treatment variable is not included in the model, the estimate of γ is reduced to 3.73, slightly lower than the first value of 3.79. This is an illustration of the increased variability, which in the survival data case is seen as a decreasing (or in this case less increasing) hazard.

For the data on diabetic nephropathy of Section 1.3.1, Hougaard, My-glegaard, and Borch-Johnsen (1994) applied various models combining Weibull distributions and heterogeneity. The calendar year of onset and the age of onset were included together with the square of the age of onset. This variable was included because the effect was known to be non-linear. The regression coefficients (β) are reported in Table 2.15. As it is difficult to evaluate the effect of a covariate entering both linearly and quadratically, the onset age with the highest risk is evaluated. This is a non-linear function of the two regression coefficients. Similarly, the accelerated failure time regression coefficients (ν) are reported in Table 2.16. The onset age with the highest risk is unchanged by this parameter transformation. The Wald test statistics are the similar for the two parametrizations, but the accelerated failure time parameters are less sensitive to possible assumptions regarding the frailty distribution.

2.6   Counting processes

The mathematical framework for considering univariate survival data is the theory of counting processes. A counting process is an increasing (right continuous) stochastic process with jumps of size 1, with an initial value

K(0)=0, giving later values of 0,1,.... In the simplest case, it counts, at time t, the number of times an individual has been observed to die before that time. Thus, it only attains values 0 or 1, and can be expressed as $K(t) = 1\{T \leq t\}D$. Processes for several individuals can be summed. In the one-individual case, the hazard of a jump at time t is $R(t)\lambda(t)$, where $R(t)$ is the indicator of the individual being under observation at time t. As in all other cases of survival data, this statement is conditional on the value of $R(t)$. The advantage of the counting process approach is that it accommodates for this conditioning. It generally conditions on everything that is known about the process during the period $[0, t)$. From a mathematical point of view, this is formulated as the process being measurable with respect to the σ-algebra created by the information until time t. As time grows this creates an increasing sequence of σ-algebras, which is called a filtration. The hazard formula immediately generalizes to the sum of the counting processes for several independent identically distributed individuals, in which case $R(t)$ becomes the size of the risk set. As the probability of a jump during a short period equals the mean of the indicator function for a jump, $R(t)\lambda(t)dt$ equals the mean of the increase in $K(t)$ during the infinitesimal time period from t to $t + dt$. We would like to sum this up over all infinitesimal time periods from time 0 to t, which gives $K(t)$ for the number of events, and $Q(t) = \int_0^t R(u)\lambda(u)du$ for the hazard. The term $Q(t)$ is an integral of conditional means and is denoted the compensator for $K(t)$. The consequence of this is that $K(t) - Q(t)$ is a martingale, a fact that opens up for a large mathematical theory on stochastic processes. In particular, this makes it easy to derive results on the asymptotic distributions of estimators. For example, for the Cox model, the expression in Equation (2.40) is directly suited for such an evaluation. The details will not be given here, but can be found in the books on counting processes.

2.7 Chapter summary

Censoring and truncation create technical problems special to survival data. A further special aspect is that at any time point, we will consider the conditional distribution of future occurrences given the present status, which in the simplest case is that the individual is alive, and in more general cases everything that has happened to the individual previously. This successive conditioning makes the hazard function, which describes the probability of an event's happening during a short interval, given that the individual is alive today (or more generally at risk for experiencing the event under study) the most relevant concept. Standard distributions available (normal, lognormal, gamma, inverse Gaussian, etc.) are either symmetric or right skewed, but survival distributions are in many cases left skewed positive variables. Furthermore, it is difficult to account for censoring and truncation. A few distributions satisfying these requirements are available, but often non-parametric methods are preferable, as they automatically account for these features, and, of course, give a better fit.

Univariate survival data is a rich statistical field, where we have only been able to refer to a few aspects, which are important for the later chapters. Classical parametric models include the exponential, the Weibull and the Gompertz distributions, where particularly the first two have nice mathematical properties. It is possible to extend these models to allow for more than two parameters, but it leads to mathematically more difficult models. The mixture models are of particular importance for the later chapters, because the model allows for several sources of variation, a feature that will be used to generate dependence. Non-parametric models can be evaluated simply and can adjust to any distribution, but does not allow for a theoretical interpretation and only the integrated hazard function is determined. The actual hazard function needs a smoothing technique, for example, a kernel function smoothing.

Including explanatory variables leads to a new field, where the proportional hazards models dominate, with a simple estimation procedure allowing for a completely general hazard function. It is, however, difficult to interpret the regression coefficients because they are sensitive toward neglected covariates. A great advantage that will be used later is the possibility of time-dependent covariates. An alternative model, which does not present the problem of neglected covariates, is the accelerated failure time model, but it is less good in allowing for time-dependent covariates and for arbitrary hazard functions.

2.8   Bibliographic comments

The Gompertz distribution has been used since it was introduced by Gompertz (1825). The Weibull distribution was essentially suggested by Fisher and Tippett (1928), who derived it as a minimum stable distribution, but it is named after Weibull (1939, 1951) who used it as a survival distribution in an engineering context. The idea of mixture distributions is old, dating back, at least, to Greenwood and Yule (1920). In the form applied here for survival data, it was introduced by Vaupel, Manton, and Stallard (1979) for the gamma case and by Hougaard (1986a) for the positive stable and PVF family. Hougaard (1984) demonstrated the importance of the Laplace transform for these calculations. Elbers and Ridder (1982) showed that a finite mean frailty model is identifiable with univariate data, when covariates are included.

The biostatistical non-parametric tradition was initiated by Kaplan and Meier (1958). Efron (1967) derives it by a re-distribution to the right algorithm. The introduction of regression models by Cox (1972) was a major breakthrough and has stimulated thousands of papers concerning statistical theory and not the least, application to medical problems. Practical experience on fitting time-dependent covariates of the measured type is described in Altman and de Stavola (1994). Robust inference in the Cox model was considered in Lin and Wei (1989) and the working model information evaluation can be found in Royall (1986). The effect of neglected covariates was considered by Hougaard (1986a) and Oakes and Jeong (1998). The proportional odds model was discussed by Bennett (1983) and Younes and Lachin (1997).

Using the theory of counting processes was suggested by Aalen (1978). Fleming and Harrington (1991) and Andersen et al. (1993) describe this theory in detail.

Table 2.1 and Figures 2.1, 2.20 and 2.21 first appeared in Hougaard (1999). Tables 2.5, 2.15, and 2.16 are transcripts from Hougaard, Myglegaard, and Borch-Johnsen (1994).

2.9 Exercises

Exercise 2.1 Transformation by the integrated hazard function

Let T be a random variable with integrated hazard function $\Lambda(t)$. Define $Y = \Lambda(T)$. Prove that Y has a unit exponential distribution. Similarly, show that $S(T)$ has a uniform distribution.

Exercise 2.2 Distribution of the minimum

Let T_1 and T_2 be independent with hazard functions $\lambda_1(t)$ and $\lambda_2(t)$, respectively. Define $T_{\min} = \min\{T_1, T_2\}$. Find the hazard function of $T_{\min}$.

Exercise 2.3 Distribution of the maximum

Let $T_1, ..., T_n$ be independent and identically distributed with survivor function $S(t)$. Define $T_{\max} = \max\{T_1, ..., T_n\}$. Find the survivor function of $T_{\max}$.

Exercise 2.4 Exact properties of exponential estimates

Find the exact distribution of $\hat{\lambda}$ based on n observations from the exponential distribution without censoring. Find the exact mean and variance of $\hat{\lambda}$.

Exercise 2.5 Comparison of exponential estimates

Consider independent, possibly censored, observations, of which n_1 have hazard λ_1 and n_2 have hazard λ_2. Derive explicitly the likelihood ratio test statistic for the hypothesis $\lambda_1 = \lambda_2$. What is the asymptotic distribution of this test statistic?

Exercise 2.6 Censored lifetime moments

Consider a lifetime random variable T censored at time c, with death indicator D. Show for $q = 1, 2, \ldots$ the following moment relations $ED^q = 1 - S(c)$, $ET^q = \int_0^c u^{q-1} S(u) du$ and $EDT = ET - cS(c)$.

Show that in the special case of the exponential distribution, $E(D - \lambda T) = 0$ and $Var(D - \lambda T) = 1 - \exp(-\lambda c)$.

How can the relations be used to find moments in the case of random censoring?

Exercise 2.7 Weibull moment estimate

Consider n independent observations from a Weibull distribution, without censoring. Use Equation (2.48) to derive the asymptotic variance of the moment estimate of the parameters (based on the mean and variance).

Exercise 2.8 Relation between the mean and hazard in the Weibull model

Study the parameters found for Danish males in the Weibull model. What is the mean lifetime according to these estimates? Now suppose the hazard is reduced to one half the previous. How much does that increase the expected lifetime?

Exercise 2.9 Gompertz median

Let T have a Gompertz distribution, with parameters λ and φ. Find the median lifetime.

Exercise 2.10 The relation between Weibull and Gompertz distributions

Let T be Weibull distributed with parameters λ and γ. Define $Y = \log T$. Truncate Y at 0, and prove that the resulting distribution is Gompertz.

Exercise 2.11 Gompertz profile likelihood

Evaluate the profile likelihood for φ and its first two derivatives for the Gompertz model of Section 2.2.3.

Exercise 2.12 Gompertz mixture

Let U have a Gompertz distribution in which λ is random, following a gamma distribution, with density $f(\lambda) = \lambda^{\delta-1} \theta^\delta \exp(-\theta\lambda)/\Gamma(\delta)$. Find the restriction on the parameters so that the marginal distribution is exponential. Show that with this case excluded, the parameters are identifiable.

Exercise 2.13 Gompertz marginals

Suppose the marginal hazard $(\omega(t))$ for a hazard based mixture model of Section 2.2.7 follows a Gompertz distribution and that the frailty Y

follows a gamma distribution. What is the conditional distribution ($\mu(t)$ in Equation (2.16))?

Exercise 2.14 Fisher information for piecewise constant hazards

Evaluate the Fisher information in an observation in a piecewise constant hazards model, without censoring.

Exercise 2.15 Binary mixture distributions

Consider a mixture distribution where Y can attain only two possible values, η_1 and η_2, with probabilities p and $1 - p$, respectively. What is the Laplace transform in this case? What is the hazard function if the conditional distribution is exponential? Secondly, consider a Cox model, and make an expression similar to Equation (2.53). What is the ratio between the marginal hazards for two groups, at time 0, and at time ∞? An illustration of this ratio can be found in Hougaard (1991).

Exercise 2.16 Moments in gamma frailty exponential models

Assume that T is exponential with hazard Y conditional on Y and that Y is gamma distributed. Prove that for a function h we can evaluate the moment $E_{\delta,\theta} \frac{h(T)}{(1+T/\delta)^q}$ as $\frac{\delta}{\delta+q} E_{\delta+q,\theta} h(T)$, where $E_{\delta,\theta}(\cdot)$ means that Y follows gamma(δ, θ). For the moment to exist, you can assume that $q > -\delta$ and that $E_{\delta+q,\theta} h(T) < \infty$. Use the result to show that $E_{\delta,\theta} \frac{1}{1+T/\delta} = \frac{\delta}{\delta+1}$, $E_{\delta,\theta} \frac{T}{1+T/\delta} = \frac{\delta}{\delta+1}$ and $E_{\delta,\theta} \frac{T\log(T)}{1+T/\delta} = \frac{\delta\{\psi(2)-\psi(\delta)+\log\delta\}}{\delta+1}$. The second expression can be derived in a different way directly from the first.

Exercise 2.17 Moments in gamma frailty Weibull models

Assume that T is Weibull with hazard $Y\gamma t^{\gamma-1}$ conditional on Y and that Y is distributed as gamma(δ, θ). For which q is $ET^q < \infty$? Evaluate the value when it exists. What is $E\log T$? Next, use the results of Exercise 2.16 to show that $E_{\delta,\theta} \frac{1}{1+T^\gamma/\delta} = \frac{\delta}{\delta+1}$ and $E_{\delta,\theta} \frac{T^\gamma \log(T)}{1+T^\gamma/\delta} = \frac{\delta\{\psi(2)-\psi(\delta)+\log\delta\}}{\gamma(\delta+1)}$.

Exercise 2.18 Likelihood in gamma frailty Weibull models

Assume that T is Weibull with hazard $Y\gamma t^{\gamma-1}$ conditional on Y and that Y is distributed as gamma(δ, θ). Suppose that we have a sample of n, possibly censored, observations from this distribution. Derive the likelihood and its first two derivatives.

Exercise 2.19 Gamma frailty Weibull regression model

Consider the gamma frailty regression model of Equation (2.51), assuming that $\lambda_0(t)$ is a Weibull hazard. Find the density of the distribution. Find explicitly the ratio of hazards (to an individual with $z = 0$). Show that this is an accelerated failure time model, both conditionally and unconditionally and derive the scale factor.

Exercise 2.20 Existence of moments in gamma frailty Gompertz models

Assume that T is Gompertz with hazard $Y\varphi^t$ conditional on Y and that Y is distributed as gamma(δ, θ). Show that for $\varphi > 1$ and $q > 0$, we have that $ET^q < \infty$.

Exercise 2.21 Constant + gamma frailty

Let the frailty be given as $Y = c + Z$, where c is a positive constant, and Z gamma distributed. What is the Laplace transform of Y? What is the mean and the variance of Y? Derive the survivor function. Choose the scale so that $EY = 1$. What is the distribution of Y among the survivors? How does the coefficient of variation change over time?

Exercise 2.22 Dependence between frailty and covariates

Consider a model of the form in Equation (2.49), but assume that for any z, the frailty $\exp(\psi'w)$ follows a positive stable distribution with parameters α and $\delta = \delta_0 \exp(\kappa'z)$. What is the distribution of the lifetime, when w is integrated out?

Exercise 2.23 Diabetic nephropathy data

Consider the estimates presented in Table 2.5. Make a figure of the survivor function up to duration 60 years. Discuss the differences between the gamma and PVF models.

Exercise 2.24 Melanoma data

Make a Weibull regression model for the melanoma data presented in Section 1.10.2 for the hazard of death of the disease, including suitable covariates. Is the hazard constant? Make a Kaplan-Meier estimate for these data. Make a Cox regression model for the data, including suitable covariates. Do you think the effect of tumor thickness is best explained by the untransformed variable or as the log thickness?

Exercise 2.25 Application to the tumorigenesis data

Study the female part of the data of Section 1.5.3, neglecting the dependence within litters. Analyze the data according to the methods above, including
1. Use the Weibull model for each treatment separately.
2. Calculate and draw the Kaplan-Meier estimate for each treatment separately.

3. Calculate and draw the Nelson-Aalen estimate for each treatment separately.

4. Find the hazard ratio of the drug treated to the control in the Weibull model.

5. Find the hazard ratio of the drug treated to the control in the Cox model.

Exercise 2.26 Catheter infection data

Consider the kidney catheter infection data of Section 1.7.3. Include time-dependent covariates in order to examine whether the hazards are proportional for males and females.

Exercise 2.27 First event among recurrent events

A standard approach to avoid problems with dependent observations among recurrent events is to consider only the time to the first event for each individual. Analyze the data of Section 1.7.1 by this approach using a proportional hazards model.

Exercise 2.28 Piecewise linear hazard

To avoid the discontinuity of the piecewise constant hazard, we suggest a piecewise linear hazard $\lambda(t) = \lambda_0 + \sum_{q=1}^{m}(t - x_{q-1})\lambda_q 1\{x_{q-1} < t\}$. Formally, it has one parameter more than the piecewise constant hazards model, but as the function is continuous, the number of intervals can sometimes be reduced. Derive the maximum likelihood equations for this model, when the data consist of n, possibly censored, independent observations from the same lifetime distribution.

Exercise 2.29 Frailty hidden cause of death model

Consider the hidden cause of death model in Section 2.2.7. Let the cause-specific frailties be independent, and let Y_j be gamma distributed with parameters δ_j and θ. What is the distribution of Y?

3
Dependence structures

The standard in ordinary multivariate analysis is to have a single parameter governing dependence. Such a parameter describes the degree of dependence. For many purposes, this might also be satisfactory for survival data, but for equally many cases it is useful to consider the dependence in more detail. In particular, with censored data, the assumed model for the dependence can have a major importance for the estimated degree of dependence, because the model for dependence for the period with data will extrapolate into the time period where all individuals are censored.

Before we consider the actual statistical models for dependence, we should reflect on how dependence between time variables appears. There are several possible probability mechanisms that can generate dependence in multivariate survival data. Three such mechanisms will be discussed in Section 3.1. One mechanism is common events, where, typically owing to accidents or natural disasters, several events happen simultaneously. Such models are handled by the multi-state models of Chapters 5. The second is common risks models, where the individuals are dependent owing to some common unobserved risk factors, corresponding to a random effects model. An obvious example of this is the common genes among twins or other family members. This model and its generalizations are considered in Chapters 7, 8, 10, and 11 for parallel data and Chapter 9 for longitudinal data on recurrent events. The third mechanism is the event-related mechanism, where it is the actual event that changes the risk. A simple example of this effect is infections. If a person obtains an infection, this implies that people close to him have an increased risk of becoming infected, because the first person transmits the disease. Models based on this mechanism are considered in Chapter 6. We emphasize here the mechanism as knowing this can create much more relevant models for the subject at hand, and allow for an interpretation regarding the subject matter. Some probability models do not have a known biologically plausible probability mechanism. Such models are judged as less relevant in the modeling of survival data and therefore are not considered in this book.

Furthermore, we go into much detail regarding the type of dependence. Correspondingly, in Section 3.2 we consider the various dependence time frames that the probability mechanisms can lead to. One consideration is whether the dependence is most important early or late. Another consideration is the duration of dependence, which we split into three time frames – instantaneous, short-term, and long-term dependence. Instantaneous dependence occurs when two events happen at the same time. Short-term dependence is when the dependence is most pronounced immediately after other individuals in the group have experienced an event, and long-term dependence is when an event implies that the risk among group members is increased forever. Most standard models give long-term dependence and a few give instantaneous dependence; but in practice, the dependence is often short-term. Section 3.3 gives some practical examples, both of dependence mechanisms and dependence time frames.

3.1 Probability mechanisms

By a probability mechanism we mean a way of generating the data by processes having a biological interpretation, avoiding specific distributional assumptions. Slightly more formally, a mechanism is a set of structural assumptions that specifies how a model with some feature, here dependence, is derived. By structural assumption we mean a qualitative assumption, like independence, or conditional independence. Assumptions on actual distributions (or more quantitative assumptions) are part of the model, and are not considered structural assumptions. The advantage of structural assumptions is that they allow for an interpretation, and it is biologically possible that the data are generated in this way. Here three mechanisms are considered, common events (Section 3.1.1), common risks (Section 3.1.2), and event-related dependence (Section 3.1.3). The relevance of each mechanism is considered in Section 3.1.4. Practical examples are discussed in Section 3.3. If one does not have a specific mechanism in mind, it is important to consider a model that is sufficiently general to catch the dependence.

Standard ways of deriving models for multivariate random variables are either as a random effects model, integrating out some third factor, corresponding to our common risks models, or by successive conditioning, building up a multivariate distribution by means of the univariate distribution of T_1, the conditional distribution of T_2 given T_1 and so on. For survival data, the second approach easily works for recurrent events, but for parallel data, the time aspect is not well recognized. However, including the time aspect leads to the event-related dependence.

3.1.1 Common events

The term *common events* refers to parallel data; for longitudinal data, we would prefer a term like *multiple simultaneous events*. In the parallel case common events are defined as a single cause leading to simultaneous failure for several individuals. For human lifetimes, the most relevant cases are natural disasters and accidents leading to the death of several persons at the same time. In the study of infectious diseases, two family members might together visit an infected person, and both become infected. There can be some discussion of whether this is a common event, or whether the persons share the environment, a model that will be discussed in Section 11.1. When we use the word *environment,* we refer to the short-term conditions, not to the common childhood environment considered by geneticists, and which may lead to a long-term effect. In industrial applications, an electrical shock might damage a number of components simultaneously.

A practical aspect is that the time scale must be chosen so that it corresponds to physical time for each group (i). For example, if we study the simultaneous death of a married couple, e.g., owing to traffic accidents, we must use a time scale corresponding to calendar time within each pair (which is most naturally done by choosing time since marriage), with some covariates describing the age of the persons. If we used individual age as the time scale, we would not be able to recognize that the accident took place at the same physical time, as it apparently took place at different time points (different ages) for them. This problem is not present when studying simultaneous death of twins, because they are born the same time, and thus the various time scales coincide within pairs. If a couple or a pair of twins does not die immediately in the accident, the exact time of death could vary between them, but we will might consider it a common event. This dependence structure is not relevant for matched pairs data in a drug trial, because it requires that the persons are physically together. It is similarly not relevant for repeated measurements, where the courses run at different physical times.

The classical example of such a model is the Marshall-Olkin model for bivariate data (see Section 5.5.4).

3.1.2 Common risks models

Conceptually, this corresponds to the variance components models for normally distributed data and thus is a random effects model. The idea is that

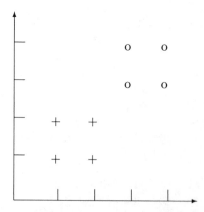

Figure 3.1. Example (fictitious data on eight pairs) illustrating conditional independence, + denotes high risk, o denotes low risk.

there are some unobserved risk factors that are common between the various courses for parallel data, and constant over time for longitudinal data. A key point for these models is the conditional independence when these common risks are known. The models are also termed latent risks models. From a statistical point of view, a common risks model is a mixture model, where the mixture term is common for several individuals or constant over time (for repeated events). For example, a pair of monozygotic twins have all their genes in common. It is expected that the genes have an influence on the lifetimes of the twins. For this model we will assume conditional independence, which means that the genes and other common risk factors are responsible for all the dependence seen between the members of a twin pair. It is assumed that, conditionally on the gene makeup and the other risk factors, the two twins have independent lifetimes. The problem with this approach is that we do not know the genes, and therefore we need to consider them as random and integrate the effect of the genes out, and this creates dependence between the lifetimes. The most common specific type of model is the frailty model based on a common factor in the hazard. The idea is illustrated in Figure 3.1, with artificial data on eight pairs, who are in two different risk groups. Within the high-risk group, each individual has a fifty-fifty chance of lifetimes of 1 and 2, and the lifetimes are independent. Within the low-risk group, each individual has a fifty-fifty chance of lifetimes of 3 and 4, and the lifetimes are independent. Thus when the two members of a pair are in the same known risk group, the lifetimes are independent, but if the group is unknown, there is dependence, because observing one lifetime will make it possible to find out which risk group the pair is in. Thus the dependence is created by their common risk. The example uses just two groups to illustrate the point, but generally we will prefer a continuous distribution because that is consistent with there being several risk factors behind the unknown risk. One consequence of this model for a data set on several individuals is that the death of one individual does not change the risk for the other individuals, but it changes the *knowledge* we have of the risk for the other individuals. It is essential in such a model to be able to account for known explanatory variables, because it makes sense to ask the question whether a given variable explains part or all of the dependence seen between the individuals. This means that we want to study whether the times are independent when the covariate is accounted for. Therefore, it becomes important whether a given explanatory variable is measurable, as it only makes sense to include it in the model if it is measurable.

From a calculation point of view, this model uses a multivariate version of the mixture results of Section 2.2.7.

An advantage of this model is that it offers an interpretation as a probability model; that is, the conditional independence implies that dependence is created by the common risk factors. This means that we can discuss concepts like variation within and between groups in the parallel case, and within and between individuals in the longitudinal case.

The common risk can be constant over a lifetime (see Chapter 7) or it can change over time, leading to markedly different dependence models (see Section 11.1), where an independent increments model leads to simultaneous events. The classical example of a common risks model is the negative binomial model for recurrent events, suggested by Greenwood and Yule (1920) (see Section 9.3.2).

3.1.3   Event-related dependence

In this case, it is the actual event that changes the risk for future events. A classical example is the risk after marital bereavement, where the death of a married person changes the risk of the spouse. This can be due to psychological effects, like sorrow, or to a changed environment, like housing, economy, or the missed help from the late person. Another example is kidneys, where the loss of one kidney implies that the other has to take over the load of both. The same happens for twin computers. If one breaks down, the other has to do twice the work that it used to do and this increases the risk that it will also break down. A person can have a heart attack while driving, leading to a traffic accident. An event-related dependence can both be positive and negative for the risk of future events. An airplane crash leads to changes in routines or maintenance policies, so that the risk of future events is reduced. A car accident can make the driver drive more carefully. A smoker might quit smoking after a myocardial infarction in order to reduce his risk of repeated events. Infectious diseases are tricky. An attack tends to reduce the risk for future events for the same person, because he obtains immunity toward the same or similar challenges, but to increased risk of infections for other people as he might infect them.

	Common events	Common risks	Event related
Individuals	+	++	++
Similar organs	++	++	+
Different events	+	+	++
Recurrent events	+	++	++
Repeated measurements	−	++	−
Competing risks	−	+	−

Table 3.1. The most relevant combinations of data types and dependence mechanisms. ++ means relevant, + means relevant in special cases and − means not relevant.

Event-related effects have to be considered in a longitudinal model and are best described by multi-state models (Chapter 6). The classical theoretical example of such models is the Freund model for bivariate survival (see Section 5.5.3).

3.1.4 Relevance of the mechanisms

Each of the suggested mechanisms of dependence has areas it is particularly relevant for. Table 3.1 shows this. For the study of individuals, both common risks and event-related effects are present. Common events are possible, but rare in practice. For similar organs, common events are more relevant owing to the organs' being physically and chemically close. For different events, the causal effect is typically event-related. For example, the dependence between heart disease and death is not that a person has a high risk of heart disease and death, but that the presence of heart disease leads to a high risk of death. The case of recurrent events is similar to several individuals. Owing to the different time scales used in repeated measurements, only common risks are applicable. For competing risks, we cannot estimate the effects, and therefore none of the models are really relevant. We have put common events and event-related effects as not relevant, a point that is discussed in Section 3.3.9. A number of examples are considered in Section 3.3.

3.2 Dependence time frame

For many purposes, we will just discuss dependence. This will be the standard. However, for other purposes, a more detailed evaluation is necessary. One aspect that will turn out to be important later is whether a given model leads to particularly high dependence early or late (Section 3.2.1). When there is dependence, for example, for bivariate parallel data, it will typically be a positive dependence, so that the time in between the events

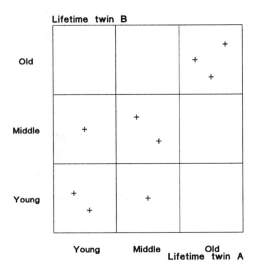

Figure 3.2. Artificial data for nine pairs, illustrating the joint distribution, when the dependence is high at old ages.

will be shorter than under independence. This timing will be considered in much more detail, and for this evaluation, one should not consider the time interval between events, but how the hazard function looks after an event. The general picture of the above mechanisms is that the common events leads to an instantaneous dependence, as failures happen at the same time (Section 3.2.2). The event-related dependence typically is on a short-term basis (Section 3.2.3), whereas the conditional independence typically leads to long-term dependence (Section 3.2.4). However, we will build up models of either type, both with short-term and long-term dependence, and therefore it makes sense to consider the time frame of dependence in detail.

Within the engineering reliability field, there are a number of classifications of dependence, based on multivariate generalizations of univariate concepts, like increasing failure rate (IFR) and new better than used (NBU). These are measures that originate for univariate data (corresponding to the marginal distributions) and extended to multivariate models. Such concepts will not be considered as they are not related to the dependence as such.

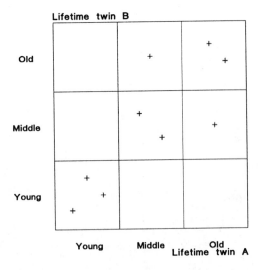

Figure 3.3. Artificial data for 9 pairs, illustrating the joint distribution, when the dependence is high at young ages.

3.2.1 Early/late dependence

One consideration is whether the dependence is most marked at early or late times. This concept will be needed in Chapter 7. An illustration of it is given in Figures 3.2, 3.3, and 3.4. The first two figures show the joint lifetimes of nine artificial pairs of twins. The time is split into three age groups, made so that the marginal distributions are uniform over the groups. Thus under independence of the times, there should be one pair in each of the nine cells. Figure 3.2 illustrates high dependence at old ages. If one twin dies old, we are sure the other will also die old, whereas if one twin dies young, we do not know the actual age class of death of the other one, only that it is either young or middle-aged. As an alternative, Figure 3.3 illustrates high dependence among young people. If one twin dies young, we are sure the other will also die young, whereas if one twin dies middle-aged or old, we do not know the actual age class of death of the other one, only that it is either middle-aged or old. An intermediate and more symmetric case cannot be illustrated with just nine pairs, but by overlaying the figures, we can make an example with 18 pairs (see Figure 3.4). Even though there is a clear dependence, we cannot, from the death age of one twin, say precisely, which age class the other twin will die in.

This concept will be discussed for multi-state models in Section 6.7, for frailty models in Section 7.8 and for non-parametric models in Section 14.9.2.

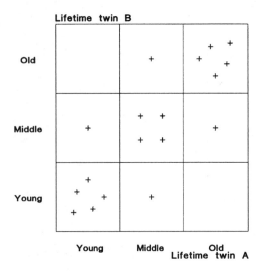

Figure 3.4. Artificial data for 18 pairs, illustrating the joint distribution, when the dependence is high at intermediate ages.

3.2.2   Instantaneous dependence

A more detailed evaluation is whether the dependence time frame is instantaneous, short-term, or long-term. By instantaneous dependence we mean that there are multiple events happening at exactly the same time. This is the case for the common events described in Section 3.1.1. In a multi-state model (see Chapter 6), we can make this a single event, by redefining the states and/or transitions. This is a solution that from a technical point of view removes the problem, but it should still be remembered for the interpretation. Therefore, this problem is most intrinsic for parallel data, where several individuals die simultaneously. From a technical statistical point of view, this implies that the multivariate distribution is not continuous, as there is a positive probability that the bivariate observation is on the diagonal, which only has zero Lebesgue measure. The most well-known model for such data is the Marshall-Olkin model of Section 5.5.4. Another model is the independent increments frailty model of Section 11.1.

3.2.3   Short-term dependence

In some cases, the risk of an event is particularly high shortly after a previous event, whereas the increase in risk fades away over time. This will be called short-term dependence. In this section, the term is introduced in a vague fashion, but in Section 3.2.4 it will be defined more explicitly. The concept can be illustrated by twins. Suppose we study a twin alive by the age of 70 years, and we want to predict his residual lifetime. If we know the twin partner is dead, this must influence our prediction in a negative sense. Now first consider the case, where the twin partner died of heart disease by the age of 69. Is this important for our prediction? It must be, because the survivor is expected to have an increased risk of heart disease. Now suppose instead that the partner died of poliomyelitis, by the age of 30 years. This suggests that the twin couple is susceptible to infectious diseases, a common risk factor explanation. However, given the time passed, we might as well judge the surviving twin as having the same risk as a twin with a surviving partner. The information on the partner would have been very relevant immediately after the death of the partner, both because the twin couple could have been infected by the same infection path, a common events explanation, or because the first infected person infects the other one, an event-related dependence.

It is easy to construct such models for multi-state models, as exemplified by twin data in Section 6.7.2. Frailty models for short-term dependence are derived in Section 11.3 and 11.5.

3.2.4 Long-term dependence

In this time frame, the whole history is important. Long-term dependence seems particularly relevant to the study of genetic effects as a number of other effects will only lead to short-term dependence, because the risk factors might change over time. It will be argued later that the observed dependence is often of short-term nature, but the models considered, including Markov models (Section 5.6), and shared frailty models (Chapter 7), do show a long-term dependence.

In order to make such a consideration we need to define what is short-term and what is long-term dependence. The following will be an informal definition. Consider first a bivariate parallel data set. This can be exemplified by a pair of twins with lifetimes (T_1, T_2). As long as twin member 1 is alive, the hazard of death of member 2 at time t is $\lambda_2(t)$. If member 1 has died at time t_1, (where we only consider $t_1 < t$ to make it relevant from a survival data point of view), the hazard of death of member 2 is $\mu_2(t, t_1)$, conditionally on the history, that is, that member 1 is dead at time t_1, and automatically also that member 2 is alive at time t. The actual expressions for λ and μ depend on the model considered. If T_1 and T_2 are independent, we will have $\mu_2(t, t_1) = \lambda_2(t)$, for all values of t_1. Under dependence, we will expect positive dependence, which means that $\mu_2(t, t_1) > \lambda_2(t)$. The most famous example is a Markov model, where $\mu_2(t, t_1)$ is independent of t_1. We will say that the dependence is of short-term nature when $\mu_2(t, t_1)$ is increasing as function of t_1 for any fixed value of t, and of long-term nature, when $\mu_2(t, t_1)$ is constant or decreasing as function of t_1 for any fixed t. Thus the Markov models have long-term dependence. Stated in words, it can be formulated as the following. Consider a twin of age t. If the recent death of his partner leads to a markedly increased risk, whereas if the partner died a long time ago leads to a slight increase, the dependence is short-term. On the other hand, if the recent death leads to a smaller increase than the distant death, the dependence is long-term. In case the dependence is negative, the inequalities have to be reversed. The comparison hazard $\lambda_2(t)$ is only used to evaluate whether the dependence is negative or positive. For longitudinal data sets, we can use the same definition if we exchange the comparison hazard. For example, for recurrent events, it makes no sense to consider the hazard of event number 2 given number 1 has not occurred. In that case the comparison hazard should be the hazard of a (first) event at time t.

These considerations are naturally formulated in Markov extension models, which is a subclass of the multi-state models and defined in Section 5.7, and is difficult to generalize to general models, where the hazards can depend on the previous events in an arbitrary fashion.

3.3 Examples

In practice, it might well be so that several or all of these aspects are relevant. Some examples are considered here.

3.3.1 Birth histories

Suppose we study the birth histories for a group of women: that is, for each woman, the ages at which she gives birth to her children. This is longitudinal recurrent events data. If the woman has a twin birth, this is a multiple event (Section 3.1.1), leading to instantaneous dependence for the birth times (Section 3.2.2). There are large differences in fertility between women, with a fraction of 5–10 % who cannot conceive children. This is described by conditional independence, or common risk models (Section 3.1.2), and leads to a long-term dependence, Section 3.2.4. After a birth, there is a period of about 9 months, where the mother cannot give birth again, and a period after that when the birth intensity is reduced. This is an event-related dependence (Section 3.1.3). Furthermore, many women have some sort of stopping rule, meaning, for example, no more than two children. This is also an example of event-related dependence. The presence of a partner and contraceptive use leads to a common risk model of short-term dependence as these factors may change over time (Section 3.2.3).

3.3.2 Married couples

The lifetimes of married couples are parallel data of the type referred to as *several individuals*. A married couple does not have common risks owing to genetics, but they might have them owing to selection of the partner; for example, a non-smoker might prefer a non-smoker, leading to smoking concordance within pairs, but it might also be due to shared risks or lifestyle. The latter could be the case even though a non-smoker choses a smoker, as they will both have the risk from the smoke, one as an active smoker, one as a passive smoker. Furthermore, they share diet and the local environment. We have previously mentioned the event-related dependence seen after the death of one partner. Probably short-term dependence is more important than long-term dependence in this case. If a widow survives a couple of years after the loss of her husband, her risk is approximately back to normal risk. There is also a risk of common events, as couples are physically together and can die simultaneously in accidents. However, this accounts for only a small part of the events.

3.3.3 Twin dependence

The lifetimes of twins are also parallel data of the several individuals type. Compared to married couples, the common events are not so relevant for adult twins because they are not physically together to the same degree. They have common risks owing to their common genetic basis and their common environment during fetal life and childhood. This is the most important dependence structure for twins. There have been cases of one twin committing suicide after the death of the partner, which is an extreme type of short-term event-related dependence.

Models to examine whether the dependence is short-term or long-term are considered in Section 6.7.2. Probably the dependence is closer to long-term than for married couples.

3.3.4 Adoptive children

The lifetimes of adoptive children compared with their biological and adoptive parents make up parallel data of the several individuals type. The dependence between the biological parents and the adoptive child would be a long-term common risk owing to their common genes. The dependence between the adoptive parents and the child could be of all types, but is probably of a short-term time frame.

3.3.5 Traffic deaths

If one describes the traffic deaths in a country over time (say, each day) or in various areas at the same time, this is longitudinal data for recurrent events. There will be an overdispersion compared to a Poisson model, that is, dependence. There can be common events owing to single accidents leading to multiple deaths. Traffic accidents can be event-related, as it is well known that if there is an accident on a motorway, it often leads to accidents in the other direction owing to the drivers' being distracted by the first accident. There can be variations owing to season, weather, and time of day. Obviously, season and time of day are explanatory factors it would make sense to include in the model, whereas weather is more difficult to measure, can only be predicted a few days ahead, and varies with geography. Thus weather is a short-term common risk for the drivers in an area.

3.3.6   Epileptic seizures

Seizures for epileptic patients are also recurrent events. It is well known that there are marked differences in rates between patients. This is a common risk dependence, for longitudinal data. But there are also more short-term fluctuations. The common events make no sense in this case, as we will never say that a patient has two seizures simultaneously. However, it is suggested that the electric disturbances present during a seizure can pave the way for another seizure, arriving shortly after the first, an event-related dependence. This will appear as a cluster of events, a short-term dependence. Another event-related effect is that a large number of seizures will lead to changes in medication in order to reduce the seizure frequency.

3.3.7   Bleeding patterns

First, we consider menstrual bleeding patterns. This is longitudinal recurrent events data, with times of start of menstruation. The standard time scale for the initiation of menstruation is time since start of the last menstruation. Clearly, there is a common risk effect, corresponding to some women having short intervals, and others long intervals. So in terms of intervals between menstruations, there is a positive dependence. In this book, we prefer to keep track of events by means of running time, typically age; but as the times of previous events may influence the hazard, it is not a problem that the main determinant is time since latest menstruation. In particular, this can be handled by the current state models (Section 5.7). This will appear as an event-related effect. Shortly after an event, the risk is extremely low; later it increases, and eventually it decreases again, owing to the possibility that the woman will experience pregnancy or menopause. This dependence is unclassifiable using age as the time scale, that is, neither positive nor negative and neither short-term nor long-term.

Slightly different considerations are relevant for post-menopausal bleedings. A woman who has stopped bleeding might start again if she receives hormone replacement therapy (estrogen treatment). Some treatments are designed to lead to regular bleedings but bleeding is also experienced with drugs that are not supposed to stimulate bleeding. The frequency depends on the drug and its formulation, but generally, this problem is different from menstrual bleeding in the sense that the timing to the previous events is less important and the variability is larger.

3.3.8 Amalgam fillings

The times until breakdown of amalgam fillings is parallel data for similar organs, when the number of fillings is fixed. The breakdown is probably related to wear of the teeth, and to the chemical and physical environment in the mouth. Common events are possible, but not frequent. Event-related mechanisms do not seem relevant. Common risks seem sensible, but the environment may change over time, leading to short-term dependence. The analysis referred to in Section 1.6.2 uses time since filling as the time scale. This, in fact, makes it impossible to consider common events and event-related mechanisms. The original analysis was based on a common risks model.

3.3.9 Competing risks

For cause of death data, the concept of dependence is not relevant, owing to there being at most one event. And therefore, the dependence time frame is not relevant either. But in order to understand such data, dependence must be discussed in detail. A key aspect for considering competing risks is the definition of the cause of death. Definitions have changed over time. The present definition of cause is the immediate cause of death. For example, say a person gets insulin-dependent diabetes, this leads untreated to diabetic ketoacidosis, which then leads to death. The cause of death in this case is ketoacidosis, even though one could alternatively say it was diabetes.

Diabetes should be quoted as a pre-existing condition. The reason for this definition is probably that the diabetic disease could be treated with insulin, and thus ketoacidosis and death were preventable. Reading the above description, one immediately thinks of an event-related dependence, with diabetes as a state leading to an increased risk of ketoacidosis. If one wants to follow this line of reasoning, however, one should notice that diabetes develops before death, and therefore the whole process should be treated as a life history model, and thus not as a cause of death model.

3.4 Chapter summary

This chapter has been a general and non-mathematical description of how dependence is created in multivariate survival data. Three mechanisms are defined that are the natural ways to obtain dependence. Common events mean that several events happen simultaneously. The other two mechanisms are completely opposite. Event-related dependence implies that the actual occurrence of an event changes the risk of later events, whereas for common risks (random effects) dependence, the occurrence of an event does not change the risk of later events, but gives information on the risk of a later event. This is typically the point for genetic factors. They are constant throughout life, but we update our knowledge on them through observing the individual.

Furthermore, the time frame of dependence is considered. The typical course is that the common events create instantaneous dependence. The common risks (random effects) model and event-related dependence, where the occurrence of one event implies a changed risk for future events, lead in the simple cases to a long-term dependence. It can be argued that short-term dependence is more common in practice, but to model this, the common risks models and the multi-state models used for event-related dependence need to be generalized.

3.5   Bibliographic comments

The various probability mechanisms have been discussed separately in the papers introducing specific distributions. An overview was published by Hougaard (1987). The material on dependence time frame is new, although that some of it is discussed in Hougaard (1995).

Figures 3.2, 3.3, and 3.4 are reproduced from Hougaard (1995), with kind permission from Kluwer Academic Publishers.

3.6   Exercises

Exercise 3.1 Early/late dependence and censoring

Consider the data illustrated in Figures 3.2 and 3.3. Suppose censoring is introduced when passing from young to middle age. Which of the data sets suggests the highest dependence in that case? Use the figures to discuss what bias you may make if the true distribution shows early dependence and you apply a late dependence model to censored data. What bias do you make if the true distribution shows late dependence and you apply an early dependence model?

Exercise 3.2 Early/late dependence and truncation

Consider the data illustrated in Figures 3.2 and 3.3. Suppose truncation applies so that only pairs where both have survived the young period are included. Which of the data sets suggests the highest dependence in that case? Do you think this is reasonable in light of the original distributions?

Exercise 3.3 Myocardial infarctions

Suppose the events studied are recurrent instances of myocardial infarctions (heart attack). Which probability mechanism do you find relevant in this case? What is the dependence time frame?

Exercise 3.4 Diabetic retinopathy

Consider data of the type described in Section 1.6.1. Which probability mechanism do you find relevant in this case? What is the dependence time frame?

4

Bivariate dependence measures

The previous chapter has considered how dependence is generated. The next problem is to assess or quantify the dependence in a sensible way. In normal distribution models, we are familiar with using the ordinary product moment correlation (Pearson correlation) for measuring the dependence between the various coordinates. This quantity, however, measures only linear dependence, but for survival data, the marginal distributions are not normal and the dependence structure is nonlinear and therefore we need more general measures of dependence. In a parametric model, we may quote some parameter values as expressing dependence, but for more general discussion and for comparing different models, it makes more sense to have a measure not related to a particular model. That is, a measure that is defined on the bivariate distribution rather than tied up to a specific parametrization of a model.

In this chapter only bivariate time data are considered. The reason is that these measures are designed to measure dependence in a bivariate response. In the case of considering the dependence between a covariate and a univariate response, it is typically more relevant with some other measure of dependence. Further, they are designed for measuring dependence among parallel data. Whether they are relevant for longitudinal data is unclear.

We start by discussing the product moment correlation coefficient (Section 4.1), and then move on to some more general rank based measures of dependence, specifically Kendall's coefficient of concordance τ (Section 4.2), Spearman's correlation coefficient ρ (Section 4.3), and the median concordance (Section 4.4). These are all standard measures of overall dependence and have a number of simple properties (Table 4.1). They are normal-

Property	Requirement
Range	[-1;1]
Identity	$m(T,T) = 1$
Oddity	$m(T_1, -T_2) = -m(T_1, T_2)$
Symmetry	$m(T_1, T_2) = m(T_2, T_1)$
Independence	$m(T_1, T_2) = 0$
Translation invariance	$m(\alpha_1 + T_1, \alpha_2 + T_2) = m(T_1, T_2)$
Scale invariance ($\beta_1 > 0, \beta_2 > 0$)	$m(\beta_1 T_1, \beta_2 T_2) = m(T_1, T_2)$
Continuity ($X_n \to X, Y_n \to Y$)	$m(X_n, Y_n) \to m(X, Y)$

Table 4.1. Basic properties of dependence measures considered. $m(X, Y)$ is the measure of dependence between X and Y.

ized so that they do not depend on the unit of measurement, are 0 under independence, and 1 with complete agreement between the coordinates. Furthermore, we consider the correlation after transformation to marginal exponential distributions (Section 4.5).

Instead of assessing the overall dependence, one can consider more local measures of dependence, related to the hazards of events. One such measure is the cross-ratio function (Section 4.6), which compares the hazard given the time of death of the other person in the pair to the hazard when the other person is known to be alive.

The suggested measures are defined theoretically for distributions with continuous marginal distributions, but, of course, we would also like to estimate them, without having to specify a parametric or semi-parametric model. They all have empirical counterparts. The Pearson correlation can be estimated in the usual way by the product moment expression, for complete data. Similarly, the Spearman correlation can be estimated by means of the ranks for complete data. The median concordance and Kendall's coefficient of concordance can be estimated non-parametrically, both for complete and for censored data.

Generally, Spearman's correlation, Kendall's τ and the median concordance agree as to whether there is dependence. The Spearman correlation has an interpretation more like that of the Pearson correlation but avoids its inconveniences. Kendall's τ and the median concordance agree rather closely numerically and give values lower than Spearman's correlation in the cases studied in this book.

4.1   Correlation coefficients

The traditional way of evaluating dependence in a bivariate distribution is by means of the correlation coefficient (Pearson correlation), defined as

$$\rho(T_1, T_2) = \frac{E\{(T_1 - ET_1)(T_2 - ET_2)\}}{\{E(T_1 - ET_1)^2\}^{1/2}\{E(T_2 - ET_2)^2\}^{1/2}} \tag{4.1}$$

or alternatively, the possibly more familiar formulation

$$\rho(T_1, T_2) = \frac{Cov(T_1, T_2)}{\{Var(T_1)Var(T_2)\}^{1/2}}.$$

The correlation is undefined when the variances in the denominator are 0 or infinite. An alternative expression based on the bivariate survivor function, $S(t_1, t_2) = Pr(T_1 > t_1, T_2 > t_2)$, is

$$Cov(T_1, T_2) = \int_0^\infty \int_0^\infty \{S(t_1, t_2) - S_1(t_1)S_2(t_2)\} dt_1 dt_2,$$

where $S_1(t_1) = S(t_1, 0)$ and $S_2(t_2) = S(0, t_2)$ are the marginal survivor functions. Similarly, the denominator can be found from the expression

$$Var(T_1) = 2 \int_0^\infty t S_1(t) dt - \{\int_0^\infty S_1(t) dt\}^2.$$

The properties of this measure are that the range is $[-1, 1]$, with the values ± 1, if and only if $T_2 = \alpha + \beta T_1$, in which case $\rho = 1$ for $\beta > 0$, and -1 for $\beta < 0$. Under independence $\rho = 0$. It is not possible in general to reverse this statement; that is, to go from $\rho = 0$ to independence requires some further conditions. It is symmetric, $\rho(T_1, T_2) = \rho(T_2, T_1)$, and unchanged by linear transformations; that is $\rho(T_1, f(T_2)) = \rho(T_1, T_2)$, when $f(t) = \alpha + \beta t$, $(\beta > 0)$. The continuity condition in Table 4.1 requires that the convergence of X_n to X and Y_n to Y is in L_2 norm. The correlation coefficient is, for normally distributed random variables, intimately related to the conditional distributions. The conditional mean is linear $E(T_2 \mid T_1) = E(T_2) + \rho\{Var(T_2)/Var(T_1)\}^{1/2}\{T_1 - E(T_1)\}$. More interesting is the important formula for the variances in the conditional and unconditional distributions,

$$Var(T_2 \mid T_1) = (1 - \rho^2)Var(T_2). \tag{4.2}$$

This equation has the interpretation that knowledge of T_1 explains the proportion ρ^2 of the total variance. The correlation is very well suited for measuring the linear dependence seen in the bivariate normal distribution, but for general bivariate distributions, it is typically not a good measure. The problem is that a marginal transformation of the observations changes the correlation. In mathematical terms, $\rho(f(T_1), f(T_2))$ is generally different from $\rho(T_1, T_2)$, when $f(t)$ is a nonlinear function. For a bivariate normal, a marginal transformation always makes the correlation lower, in absolute value. The consequence of this is that the correlation coefficient can be low if the dependence is nonlinear, even with a high degree of dependence. This is illustrated in an exercise in Section 4.9. If one wants to evaluate the correlation coefficient, one must first consider the right scale to measure the correlation on. An example of how this can be done is presented in Section 7.4.3. An alternative is to use a non-parametric correlation type measure, like Kendall's τ or the median concordance, which is unchanged by transformation of the marginal.

Estimation with complete data is simple, we just substitute the empirical moments into the defining equation. That is, defining $\bar{T}_j = \sum_i T_{ij}/n$ and $SPD_{jm} = \sum_i (T_{ij} - \bar{T}_j)(T_{im} - \bar{T}_m)$, the expression is

$$\hat{\rho} = \frac{SPD_{12}}{(SPD_{11}SPD_{22})^{1/2}}.$$

The properties of this estimate are well known, when the distribution is the bivariate normal, but without this assumption, we do not know much about its properties.

4.2   Kendall's coefficient of concordance

This measure of dependence is designed as a rank-based correlation-type measure. It was introduced as a simple measure of dependence, which did not require the assumption of normality. For a set of bivariate parallel data T_{ij}, $i = 1, ..., n, j = 1, 2$, which for the different values of i are assumed independent and identically distributed, it is defined as

$$\tau = E\text{sign}\{(T_{11} - T_{21})(T_{12} - T_{22})\}, \qquad (4.3)$$

where $\text{sign}(x)$ is the sign of x, -1 for $x < 0$, 0 for $x = 0$, and 1 for $x > 0$. A somewhat more transparent formulation, valid for continuous distributions, is $\tau = 2p - 1$, where p is the probability that the order of the coordinate 1 observations is the same as the order of the coordinate 2 observations

$$p = Pr[\{(T_{11} - T_{21})(T_{12} - T_{22})\} > 0].$$

In plain words this can be formulated by an example. Suppose we want to study the dependence within married couples, and observe that Mr. Smith dies before Mr. Peterson. Then p expresses the probability that Mrs. Smith dies before Mrs. Peterson. This approach accepts that males and females have differential mortality, and thus the lifetime of a male is never compared to that of a female. But we can compare persons of the same sex, studying whether the early deaths happen in the same families. Under independence within couples, and assuming a continuous distribution, $p = 1/2$ and $\tau = 0$. For τ the same nice properties as for the correlation coefficient are satisfied, with the extension that τ is unchanged by both linear and nonlinear increasing transformations. A conceptual drawback is that the interpretation of τ requires two pairs, in contrast to the correlation coefficient, which can be interpreted with only one pair, as demonstrated in Equation (4.2).

Alternatively, the measure can be evaluated by integration of the bivariate survivor function,

$$\tau = 4 \int_0^1 \int_0^1 f(t_1, t_2) S(t_1, t_2) dt_1 dt_2 - 1 \tag{4.4}$$

when the marginal distributions are uniform. When the marginals are not uniform, the same formula applies if the integration range covers the full distribution.

The value of the coefficient can be found in various models (see Equation (7.23)).

It can be estimated non-parametrically for complete data, by considering each combination of two pairs, scoring each concordant set as 1, and each discordant set as −1. In case of a tie, a score of 0 is used. This is then normalized in a similar way as a standard correlation. To make this precise, suppose we have bivariate parallel data, in the standard setup, $T_{ij}, i = 1, ..., n, j = 1, 2$. For each set of two pairs, indexed by i and m, we define for coordinate 1 a term a_{im} as

$$a_{im} = \begin{cases} 1 & \text{if } T_{i1} > T_{m1} \\ 0 & \text{if } T_{i1} = T_{m1} \\ -1 & \text{if } T_{i1} < T_{m1} \end{cases} \tag{4.5}$$

and similarly for coordinate 2 a term b_{im} as

$$b_{im} = \begin{cases} 1 & \text{if } T_{i2} > T_{m2} \\ 0 & \text{if } T_{i2} = T_{m2} \\ -1 & \text{if } T_{i2} < T_{m2} \end{cases}. \tag{4.6}$$

The expression for the coefficient of concordance is, in the case of complete data without ties

$$\hat{\tau} = \frac{\sum_{i,m} a_{im} b_{im}}{n(n-1)}. \tag{4.7}$$

If τ is zero, the variance is $2(2n+5)/\{9n(n-1)\}$.

In the case of ties or censored data, the formula is generalized to

$$\tau = \frac{\sum_{i,m} a_{im} b_{im}}{\{(\sum_{i,m} a_{im}^2)(\sum_{i,m} b_{im}^2)\}^{1/2}}. \tag{4.8}$$

The first suggestion is to use a score (a, b) of 0 in all cases, when the death order is not certain, owing to censoring. This gives the so-called simple estimate. However, this will typically underestimate the dependence, and we do not account for the fact that as censoring happens at different times, there is a higher probability of early death for the person censored first. This can be accounted for by using a score based on the marginal Kaplan-Meier estimate. This is called the adjusted estimate. The scores are as described in Equations (4.5) and (4.6) when both observations are complete. More generally, the scores for a are described in Table 4.2. The values for the

(D_{i1}, D_{m1})	$T_{i1} > T_{m1}$	$T_{i1} = T_{m1}$	$T_{i1} < T_{m1}$
(1,1)	1	0	-1
(0,1)	1	1	$2\{\hat{S}(T_{m1})/\hat{S}(T_{i1})\} - 1$
(1,0)	$1 - 2\hat{S}(T_{i1})/\hat{S}(T_{m1})$	-1	-1
(0,0)	$1 - \hat{S}(T_{i1})/\hat{S}(T_{m1})$	0	$\{\hat{S}(T_{m1})/\hat{S}(T_{i1})\} - 1$

Table 4.2. Kaplan-Meier adjusted scores for coordinate 1, for evaluating Kendall's τ. $\hat{S}(t)$ denotes the Kaplan-Meier estimate of the survivor function.

b-scores are similar, just changing the second subscript on T and D from 1 to 2. The variability of this estimate can be evaluated under an assumption of independence, by considering each set of three pairs, by the formula

$$\frac{4(\sum_{imr} a_{im} a_{ir} - \sum_{im} a_{im}^2)(\sum_{imr} b_{im} b_{ir} - \sum_{im} b_{im}^2)}{n(n-1)(n-2)}$$

$$+\frac{2\sum_{im} a_{im}^2 \sum_{im} b_{im}^2}{n(n-1)}. \tag{4.9}$$

However, this formula can be reduced to be expressed as a two-dimensional sum:

$$\frac{4(\sum_i(\sum_m a_{im})^2 - \sum_{im} a_{im}^2)(\sum_i(\sum_m b_{im})^2 - \sum_{im} b_{im}^2)}{n(n-1)(n-2)}$$

$$+\frac{2\sum_{im} a_{im}^2 \sum_{im} b_{im}^2}{n(n-1)},$$

making it less computationally cumbersome for large data sets.

It is useful to have an expression that is also valid for regression models, but in that case, formulas are only available in specific models. It is, however, possible to stratify and thus one can add the various sums for each stratum.

To put it into perspective, the value for a bivariate normal distribution is $\tau = 2\sin^{-1}(\rho)/\pi$, where ρ is the correlation coefficient.

4.2.1 Applications

For the Danish twin data of Section 1.5.1, the values found are given in Table 4.3. The dependence is higher for monozygotic twins than for dizygotic twins. The adjusted estimates are higher than the simple estimates, and they are more satisfying. As the largest data set contains 2756 pairs, this leads to about 3.8 million sets of two pairs, clearly demonstrating that this evaluation is designed for small data sets.

For the leukemia data of Freireich (Section 1.5.4), the simple estimate is -0.11 (SE 0.17), and the Kaplan-Meier adjusted value is -0.09 (0.18). Thus the estimates suggest a non-significant negative dependence. In particular,

Sex	Data set	Simple	Adjusted
Males	MZ	0.127 (0.019)	0.173 (0.023)
	DZ	0.079 (0.015)	0.091 (0.017)
	UZ	0.185 (0.037)	0.228 (0.042)
Females	MZ	0.106 (0.019)	0.147 (0.023)
	DZ	0.080 (0.014)	0.104 (0.017)
	UZ	0.154 (0.032)	0.175 (0.037)

Table 4.3. Non-parametric estimates of Kendall's τ for Danish twin data. With standard errors in parentheses.

this shows that the pairing is not important and a simpler study design could have been used.

For the data on kidney catheter infections, of Section 1.7.3, we obtain that the scores in the simple case are 166 for the product and 1126 and 798 for the sums of a and b. This gives a value of 0.175. For the males alone, the scores are 20, 90, and 56, giving an estimate of 0.282. For the females alone, the scores are -30, 534 and 384, giving an estimate of -0.066. Thus the pooled value is based on scores -10, 624 and 440, which gives a τ-value of -0.02, suggesting that the dependence seen in the total material is due to differences between the two sexes.

4.3   Spearman's correlation coefficient

An alternative measure is Spearman's correlation coefficient, say ρ, or ρ_S, when it can be confused with the Pearson correlation. This is a particularly interesting measure, because it is a non-parametric measure, which is independent of marginal transformations and is conceptually more like an ordinary correlation, in the sense that it accounts for the values, and not just the order of the observations. If the marginals are uniform on [0,1], the value is defined as

$$\rho_S = 12 \int_0^1 \int_0^1 S(u,v)dudv - 3. \tag{4.10}$$

This corresponds to the correlation coefficient, when the marginals are uniform, and thus

$$\rho_S = 12 \int_0^1 \int_0^1 uvf(u,v)dudv - 3.$$

Equation (4.10) can be generalized to arbitrary continuous marginal distributions by the formula

$$\rho_S = 12 \int_0^1 \int_0^1 S(S_1^{-1}(u), S_2^{-1}(v))dudv - 3. \tag{4.11}$$

Unfortunately, these expressions are not simple to integrate in the models considered, but Equation (4.10) is simple to handle by numerical integration. This approach does not work for marginal distributions that are not continuous as they cannot be transformed to marginal uniformity. This is a particular problem in survival data, where it is not certain that the event will happen, because in that case, there is a point mass at ∞, and then Spearman's measure cannot be evaluated.

In the normal distribution, it can be simply found from the correlation coefficient by $\rho_S = 6 \sin^{-1}(\rho/2)/\pi$. There is an approximate relation, with $\rho_S = 3\tau/2$, valid near 0 for most distributions.

The standard estimate with complete data is based on the marginal ranks, (R_{i1}, R_{i2}), and equals

$$\hat{\rho}_S = \frac{\sum_i \{R_{i1} - (n+1)/2\}\{R_{i2} - (n+1)/2\}}{n(n^2 - 1)/12}.$$

It is understood in this formula that the two coordinates are ordered separately, that is, R_{ij} is the rank of T_{ij} among $T_{1j}, ..., T_{nj}$. In fact, this empirical formula was the original suggestion of Spearman, and Equation (4.10) is the corresponding population value.

4.4 Median concordance

To avoid the conceptual difficulties with the Kendall's τ, that is, that the interpretation requires two pairs, we will also study other measures of dependence. Instead of comparing with a second pair, we might evaluate the concordance of a single observation (T_1, T_2) in relation to a fixed (bivariate) point (t_{01}, t_{02}), by defining

$$\kappa_{t_0} = E \text{sign}\{(T_1 - t_{01})(T_2 - t_{02})\}. \tag{4.12}$$

The problem with this definition is that there is a high dependence on the value of (t_{01}, t_{02}). If both values are very high, or very low, κ_{t_0} is far from 0, even when the observations are independent. If there are covariates, the value will generally depend on the value of the covariates, even in simple models. To avoid these problems, we can choose t_{01} as the median of T_1, and t_{02} as the median of T_2, giving the median concordance. Thus, the definition is

$$\kappa = E \text{sign}\{(T_1 - \text{median}(T_1))(T_2 - \text{median}(T_2))\}. \tag{4.13}$$

It can be easily derived from the probability of being on the same side of the median; that is, if $p = Pr\{0 < (T_1 - \text{median}(T_1))(T_2 - \text{median}(T_2))\}$, then $\kappa = 2p - 1$. It might be simpler to interpret the value of p than that of κ, but the use of κ is motivated by the fact that κ is standardized and satisfies the same simple properties as the Kendall's τ and Spearman's ρ. It lies between -1 and 1, is 0 under independence, and does not change under increasing transformations of the time. Similarly as for ρ and τ, a zero value of κ does not imply independence. In particular for κ it is easy to suggest bivariate dependent distributions with zero values, using that κ is zero, just when the probability of the four quadrants created by splitting at the medians, each have probability $1/4$. Thus the probability can have any pattern within each quadrant.

Actually to derive the value the bivariate survival function $S(t_1, t_2)$ is needed. The medians are found by solving the equations $S(t_{01}, 0) = 1/2$, $S(0, t_{02}) = 1/2$, and then the value is $\kappa = 4S(t_{01}, t_{02}) - 1$. An even shorter way of defining it, is as

$$\kappa = 4S(S_1^{-1}(1/2), S_2^{-1}(1/2)) - 1. \tag{4.14}$$

Thus it can easily be derived in a parametric model, and some semi-parametric models. In the normal distribution $\kappa = 2\sin^{-1}(\rho)/\pi$, and thus is identical to τ. To derive it non-parametrically, requires an estimate of the bivariate survival function. This is done in Chapter 14.

4.5   Integrated hazard correlation

Where Spearman's ρ is the correlation coefficient after a transformation to uniform marginals, one could alternatively use a transformation to exponential marginal distributions. This, however, implies that it does not satisfy the requirement on odd random variables in Table 4.1. Rather than expressing this using such a marginal, we express it, when the marginals are uniform, which gives the expression

$$\rho_H = \int_0^1 \int_0^1 (\log u)(\log v) f(u, v) du dv - 1. \tag{4.15}$$

Typically, this measures requires numerical integration, like Spearman's ρ.

4.6   Local dependence measures

All the suggestions above are global measures of dependence, and thus they do not address the concepts of early/late dependence and short-term and long-term dependence described in Section 3.2. For discussing such concepts, we need more local measures. The measure suggested in this section will not describe the type of dependence, but the degree of dependence evaluated at a single time point. It is defined as

$$\rho(t) = \frac{S(t) D_1 D_2 S(t)}{\{D_1 S(t)\}\{D_2 S(t)\}}, \tag{4.16}$$

where D_j is the derivative operator for coordinate j and $t = (t_1, t_2)$. It can be given an alternative formula as a ratio of hazard functions, for a pair,

Property	Pearson	Spearman	τ	κ
Invariant under time transf.	No	Yes	Yes	Yes
Non.-par. est., censored data	No	No	Yes	See Ch. 14
Simple exp. for frailty models	No	No	Yes	Yes

Table 4.4. Some properties of bivariate dependence measures. τ is Kendall's coefficient of concordance. κ is the median concordance.

where individual 1 is alive at time t_1 and individual 2 at time t_2:

$$\rho(t) = \lim_{\Delta t \searrow 0} \frac{Pr(t_1 < T_1 < t_1 + \Delta, t_2 < T_2 < t_2 + \Delta \mid t_1 < T_1, t_2 < T_2)}{\prod_{j=1}^{2} Pr(t_j < T_j < t_j + \Delta \mid t_1 < T_1, t_2 < T_2)}.$$

4.7 Chapter summary

It is a major problem to estimate the dependence between multivariate responses in a sensible way that is not too model dependent. Various possibilities are available, the ordinary Kendall's coefficient of concordance, Spearman's correlation, and the median concordance. Some basic properties of the various measures are summarized in Table 4.4. The ordinary correlation coefficient is not relevant as it is sensitive to the marginal distribution. From a theoretical point of view, Spearman's measure seems to be the most interesting, but it is difficult to examine theoretically. It seems, however, to be the simplest for numerical integration. Kendall's coefficient is simple to evaluate in many models and can be simply estimated based on censored data. The median concordance depends only on the bivariate survivor function, and can therefore be evaluated in many cases.

For more detailed evaluations, local measures of dependence are necessary.

4.8 Bibliographic comments

The Spearman correlation coefficient was suggested by Spearman (1904), and the coefficient of concordance by Fechner (1897) and later discovered independently by Kendall (1938), who also examined it more completely. Brown, Hollander, and Korwar (1974) suggested the Kaplan-Meier adjustment and the variance estimate of Equation (4.9). This was studied further by Weier and Basu (1980). Oakes (1982a) made a more refined variance estimate, but did not adjust. The median concordance was first suggested by Blomqvist (1950). The correlation of the integrated hazards was suggested by Prentice and Cai (1992) and advocated by Hsu and Prentice (1996). The local measure of dependence was suggested by Clayton (1978), who used it to derive the gamma frailty model of Section 7.3. It has been further studied by Oakes (1989).

Only the most classical measures are discussed above. Many other measures of dependence are possible. Several other measures are considered by Fan, Prentice, and Hsu (2000).

Table 4.3 is taken from Hougaard, Harvald, and Holm (1992a).

4.9 Exercises

Exercise 4.1 Correlation in a gamma distribution

To illustrate that the correlation coefficient can be lower than 1, even when the dependence is perfect (that is, differentiable, monotone, and one-to-one), evaluate the correlation between X, and $Y = X^2$, when $X > 0$ follows a gamma distribution, of parameters (δ, θ), defined in the Appendix. Show that ρ is independent of θ, and that it is an increasing function of δ starting from a value of $\sqrt{2/3}$ at $\delta = 0$ to a value of 1, for $\delta = \infty$. What is Spearman's ρ in this case?

Exercise 4.2 Correlation in the additive gamma distribution

Let Y_0, Y_1, and Y_2 be independent and gamma distributed, with parameters (δ_0, θ), (δ_1, θ), and (δ_1, θ), respectively. What is the Pearson correlation between $Y_0 + Y_1$ and $Y_0 + Y_2$?

Exercise 4.3 Application of Kendall's τ

Based on the data of Table 1.12, calculate the estimate of τ for OI3 and OP3, with and without adjustment. Does this give information relevant to the purpose of the study?

Exercise 4.4 Comparison of Kendall's τ and Spearman's ρ

Based on the data of Table 1.12, calculate the estimate of τ and ρ_S for OP0 and OP1, where data are complete. Calculate also the Pearson correlation for the times as well as for the log times. Discuss the differences.

5
Probability aspects of multi-state models

Multi-state models are the most commonly used models for describing the development for longitudinal data. A multi-state model is defined as a model for a stochastic process, which at any time point occupies one of a set of discrete states. In medicine, the states can describe conditions like healthy, diseased, diseased with complications, and dead. A change of state is called a transition. This then corresponds to outbreak of disease, occurrence of complications and death. The state structure specifies the states and which transitions from state to state are possible. It is possible to make a figure of the state structure. Some examples of state structures have already been shown in Figures 1.4–1.7. The full statistical model specifies the state structure and the form of the hazard function for each possible transition. This chapter is a description of how multi-state models can be used to model multivariate and multiple survival data. In principle, all kinds of such data can be formulated as multi-state models and this is often convenient for considering predictions. The approach is particularly well suited to event-related dependence. But the approach does have some shortcomings for recurrent events, because it considers states, rather than events (see below). Furthermore, multi-state models consider all data as longitudinal, which make them less useful for repeated measurements and require the censoring pattern for parallel data to be homogeneous.

The state structure is not unique. By choosing the best structure, we can, first of all, make the assumptions in the model much more transparent, we can simplify some calculations and possibly make the process a Markov process. Six special cases stand out as standard state structures. These are illustrated in Figure 5.1 as small figures, and more detailed figures

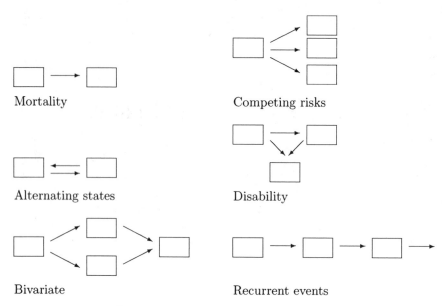

Figure 5.1. Standard multi-state models.

Name	Illustration	References
Mortality	Figure 1.1	Chapter 2
Competing risks	Figure 1.7	Section 5.4.1, Chapter 12
Alternating (two state)	Figure 2.2	Section 10.5.6
Disability	Figure 1.5	Section 5.3.2
Bivariate	Figure 5.12	Sections 5.3.3, 5.5.3
Recurrent events	Figure 1.4	Section 5.4.4, Chapter 9

Table 5.1. Standard multi-state models.

are referenced in Table 5.1, which also includes references to where the models are considered in detail. The mortality model (with states alive and dead) is the simplest possible multi-state model, in fact, so simple that there is no advantage in putting it into the multi-state framework. The competing risks model (with states alive and dead of cause j, $j = 1, ..., k$) is particularly relevant for cause of death data, and considered as such in Chapter 12. However, the mathematics behind it is relevant for multi-state models in general, as it covers the case when we only consider the first event in a process. Therefore, it is considered in Section 5.4.1. The alternating state model is relevant for reversible diseases, where the individuals move back and forth between being healthy and ill. In this case, we will often prefer a common risks model. The disability model (with states healthy, ill, and dead) is relevant for irreversible diseases, in particular when the disease increases the risk of death. The bivariate model is the multi-state model for bivariate parallel data, with states both alive, individual 1 dead, individual 2 dead and both dead. This case can alternatively be modeled in a common risks model. Similarly, recurrent events can both be described by multi-state models (with states describing the cumulative number of events) and common risks models.

One more consideration in terms of the state structure is that the graphical layout is important. In particular, for more complicated models, it is important to think about how to depict the model to show the key aspects in the best way. For example, one rule followed here, except for one figure, is that one-way transitions are shown either right or down, so that if there is a natural direction with time, it follows the reading direction.

When necessary, the states will be numbered $1, ..., S$. In the present framework, we can accept an infinite number of states, in which case the numbers are $1, ...$ In some cases, like recurrent events, it is more convenient to denote the states $0, ...$ We will require that there be only a finite number of possible transitions from each state. If all processes start in the same state, it is sometimes convenient to define this as state 1. Censoring can be considered as an artificial state, numbered 0 (or -1), a convention that can simplify computer storage of the life histories. More details on how to record the process development are in Section 5.2. In some cases, numbering of the states is inconvenient, and below we will only introduce numbering when necessary for writing the expressions for the transition probabilities. A state can be *absorbing*; that is, there are no transitions going out from the state. Thus after entry into the state the process stays in it forever. From a practical viewpoint, we may see two cases. There are states that are absorbing by their nature, the main example being dead (in cases where several individuals are studied jointly, this means that all individuals are dead) and there are states that are absorbing owing to the design of the study. For example we may decide that if some specific event happens, we will not consider the process further. To be concrete, if we are studying the natural history of heart disease, transplantation of the heart may be considered an event after which the study aim makes no sense (in other studies, this could be the interesting point, as we demonstrate in an application in Section 6.7.1).

The stochastic process X_t describing the course of the multi-state model is defined as ℓ, if the process is in state ℓ at time t. It is a piecewise constant process and it has to be right continuous, with limits from the left.

By the word *history* (or the past) at time t, we mean the information contained in the development of the process over time $[0, t]$. That is, $X_s, 0 \leq s \leq t$. This can be made mathematically precise, as a σ-algebra, indexed by t, say, F_t, covering the information over $[0, t]$, which, as time increases, makes up an increasing sequence of σ-algebras, a so-called filtration. However, we do not need the mathematical definition for setting up the models.

The hazard functions consider the hazard of the next transition. There is one hazard function for each possible transition. They are defined by a generalization to Equation (2.1),

$$\lambda_\ell(t \mid F_{t-}) = \lim_{\Delta t \searrow 0} \frac{Pr\{X_{t+\Delta t} = \ell \mid F_{t-}\}}{\Delta t}, \tag{5.1}$$

in the case $X_{t-} \neq \ell$. In the case $X_{t-} = \ell$ a transition to state ℓ is impossible, and the hazard is not defined. This is then conditional on the whole history up to, but not including, the actual time point. We need to use F_{t-} rather than F_t in order to make the risk set continuous from the left. This formulation makes the model very dynamic, meaning that the course of the process is allowed to depend on everything that has happened.

From the hazard function, it is directly possible to evaluate the probability of no events during an interval. But in order to look several transitions ahead, the transition probabilities must be considered, that is, the probability of being in a given state at a given time, possibly conditional on what has happened until some time point. Therefore, the transition probabilities are the keys to make long-term predictions. These probabilities are defined in Section 5.1.

From the state structure, it is possible to see, whether a process is progressive, that is, each state has only a single possible transition into it, and the initial state has no entries. This implies that it is possible from knowing the state at time t to determine, which states have been visited previously and in which order. The advantage of this is that some calculations are simplified (Section 5.4).

For more detailed considerations, we classify the various state models, based on the states, the possible transitions, and the functional form of the transition hazard functions. This has enormous importance for the probability calculations, that is, on how easy it is to express and evaluate transition probabilities; but for setting up a statistical model and for estimation of transition hazards, this will turn out to be less important. For estimation purposes, it is more important how the transition hazards are related. Typically, the transition hazards are simple for common events models (Section 3.1.1) and event-related models (Section 3.1.3), and complicated for common risks models (Section 3.1.2). Often they can be evaluated in a Cox proportional hazards model with time-dependent covariates and/or strata.

The subset of models that are the most studied from a probability point of view is the Markov models. In simple terms, the Markov assumption implies that the past and the future are conditionally independent given the present. This means that the development of the process after time t, given the whole history at time t only depends on the state at time t. In other words, for making a prediction at time t, the relevant part of the memory is the state at time t; that is, no further information on how the process developed before time t is needed. Mathematically, this can be described as that $\lambda_\ell(t)$ in Equation (5.1) depends on F_{t-} only via X_{t-}.

When the hazard functions do not depend on t (that is, constant hazards), the Markov process is called homogeneous, and the transition probabilities depend on v and t, only via $t - v$. The Markov assumption generally allows for a separate hazard function for each transition (whether there is a structure, like proportional hazards or common parameters, between the various possible transitions is not relevant for the Markov assumption), and it can depend on time t, but it does not depend on any other aspect of the history, like states visited on the way, and the times of previous transitions (except to the extent that this information is reflected by the present state). This is often forgotten, but non-homogeneous Markov models is a rich and important class of models. The Markov assumption can be interpreted as that the present state contains all the memory, and this is the reason why the graphical approach is particularly relevant for Markov models, you can directly see what the relevant memory contains. Extension to the general models is somewhat counterintuitive, because the graphical depiction of separate states suggests that it is irrelevant how the process arrived to the actual state. In a Markov model, the hazard functions are, inter alia, independent of the time spent in the current state. We consider such an extension, Markov extension models, which is intermediate between Markov models and general models, by allowing the transition hazards to depend on the time of transition into the present state, besides depending on the current time value. We will thus consider three sets of models for the hazard. Besides the Markov models (Section 5.6), and the general models (Section 5.8) that allow for an arbitrary dependence on all previous transitions and the times of previous transitions, we study Markov extension models (Section 5.7). The multi-state framework is designed to handle Markov models, but conceptually easily extended to the Markov extension models.

These models are literally state models, rather than event models. This is a major shortcoming of multi-state models for recurrent events, where we are more interested in the events than in defining sensible states. The problem will be exemplified below for the fertility model, Section 5.3.1.

This chapter starts with basic definitions for the transition probabilities, Section 5.1. How to record the observations is described in Section 5.2. A discussion then follows on how to select the state structure for the model, and which properties that can be obtained in this way (Section 5.3). Then the probability calculations will be discussed for various models. Section 5.4 specifically describes the transition probabilities for progressive models, where they can be expressed by integrals. The simplest case is the homogeneous Markov models (Section 5.5), where all probabilities can be found explicitly. In Section 5.6, the general Markov models are considered, to illustrate how much the Markov assumption implies, without the homogeneity assumption. The transition probabilities are solutions to a differential equation. Markov extension models are considered in Section 5.7. Furthermore, there are the general models (Section 5.8), where we cannot simplify the calculations. Then Section 5.9 studies conditional processes, to show one way of handling more general models. The final model concept to consider is hidden states, which is an extension to the standard state structure, where some states cannot be discriminated (Section 5.10). Statistical inference for multi-state models is described in Chapter 6.

5.1   Transition probabilities

The transition probabilities are in the simplest cases defined as

$$P_\ell(t) = Pr(X_t = \ell), \tag{5.2}$$

the probability of the process X being in state ℓ at time t. The transition probabilities can be found from the specified transition hazards, as they are expressed by differential equations or integral formulas. The transition probability is conditional on the initial state; that is, it is understood that all processes start in the same state at time 0. If they do not, the expression (5.2) should depend on the initial state, also. Where the transition hazards only look one event ahead of the current time, the transition probabilities consider the distributions at a fixed time point, and thus look possibly several events ahead. Therefore, the transition probabilities are the keys to making long-term predictions. Transition probabilities are most simple for Markov processes, but can also be used for non-Markov processes. To make this clear, we will also need the transition probabilities evaluated at time v. These are defined as

$$P_\ell(v, t) = Pr(X_t = \ell \mid X_u, u \in [0, v]), \tag{5.3}$$

which are conditional on the whole development up to time v. This expression is only considered for $t \geq v$, as it is trivial otherwise. In formula terms, the Markov condition can be written as

$$Pr(X_t = \ell \mid X_u, u \in [0, v]) = Pr(X_t = \ell \mid X_v), \tag{5.4}$$

for $v \leq t$. This has the interpretation that for prediction purposes at time t, the course from 0 to t is completely summarized by the state at time t. The notation becomes more clear when we let the state occupied at time v be specified directly in the expression. Thus we define Markov transition probabilities as

$$P_{m\ell}(v, t) = Pr(X_t = \ell \mid X_v = m), \tag{5.5}$$

where $v \leq t$. This is equal to Equation (5.3), when $X_v = m$.

5.2   Observations and censoring patterns

The standard observation plan considered here is to observe a set of n processes over time periods, as described in Section 1.4.2. When needed, the process will be indexed by i, when not needed, the index will be neglected. We typically start at time 0 in state 1, and observe until some time C that may differ between processes. In case of processes with an absorbing state, there is no information to gain from observing the process after the entry into that state. When an absorbing state is not reached, the end of observation is a censoring time. For each process we observe a number of events, say, E. The observed process can be recorded as the times of transition $T_1, ..., T_E$ and the states entered $S_1, ..., S_E$, but to avoid special formulas to describe the period from T_E until C, we introduce a further time, when $T_E < C$, namely, $T_{E+1} = C$, with state variable $S_{E+1} = 0$. Thus, if there is an event at time C, the number of times K equals E, when there is not an event, the last time is a censoring and $K = E+1$. The times of transitions are denoted $T_1, ..., T_K$, and the states that the transitions lead into are denoted $S_1, ..., S_K$. In the case of censoring $S_K = 0$. In order to simplify some formulas, we define S_0 as the initial state.

When this observation pattern should be interpreted for parallel data, this means that the censoring is homogeneous; that is, when censoring happens for one individual, it should apply to all individuals in the group. An alternative formulation is that it is necessary to have precise information on the state from time 0 to C, but if one individual is censored and the other is not, we do not have this information.

5.3   Selection of state structure

By choosing the right way to define the states, and the transitions, we can obtain various advantages. The most important features are that we can simplify some probability calculations and we can turn some non-Markov models into Markov models. Owing to the intuitive graphical understanding of a multi-state Markov model, it is a clear advantage if it is possible to formulate the model as a Markov model. This makes the model more transparent.

We have to consider what the possible events are. The minimal model is one where there is one transition for each type of event. When we study the outbreak of disease, complications, and deaths, this has to be considered as, at least, three types of events. The type of event is a concept, which is not necessarily well defined. For example, for recurrent events, we typically consider the events as a single type, but for some purposes, it might be preferable to discriminate between them.

An important property that can be seen in the state structure is whether the process is progressive. This is defined as there being at most one possible transition into each state, and none into the initial state. It has the consequence that at any time, the events experienced earlier and the order they happened in and the states visited earlier, are known by knowing which state the individual is in presently. Among the standard models, the mortality model, the competing risks model, and the recurrent events model are progressive. The disability model and the bivariate model are not progressive, but can easily be extended to become progressive, by adding an extra state, as will be demonstrated below. Finally, the alternating state model is not progressive, as there is an entry into the initial state. This means that when the process is in the initial state, we cannot deduce the number of previous transitions, only that the number is even. It is possible to make this process progressive, but it requires a large number of states.

Examples considered below are the fertility model for recurrent events, the disability model, and the bivariate data model. Most of the discussion is related to the state structure, but some other aspects are also considered.

5.3.1 The fertility model

The fertility model depicted earlier, in Figure 1.4, is a standard recurrent events type of model. Here, we discuss the reproductive history for a set of women. In this section, it will be shown how the model can be reformulated and extended to allow for various features. It will also clarify the shortcomings of the multi-state models. Some of these considerations are general to recurrent events, some of them specific to fertility models. The natural numbering of states is as 0,1,..., corresponding to the present number of children and thus possible censoring must be denoted like a state of -1. The natural time scale is the age of the woman. A Markov model suggests that the probability of getting a child depends only on how many children the woman already has, and her age. Thus it does not account for the pregnancy period; that is, that birth intervals below nine months are not relevant. In a Markov extension model the transition hazards are allowed also to depend on the time since the latest birth, and thus can account for the pregnancy period. This is a clear advantage of Markov extension models.

In this model, the state is defined by the previous number of events. That is a shortcoming of multi-state models for recurrent events, because in some cases, we are not interested in the actual state (i.e., the accumulated number of events), but only in the transitions. For example, if we want to decide on the size of a school to be built, or a birth clinic, we would prefer to use a simple method rather than go into a detailed scientific analysis. Thus one would apply a Poisson model (that is, a Markov model with the extra assumption that the transition hazards do not depend on the previous number of children). Thus the hazard of giving birth is assumed

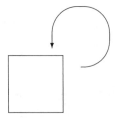

Figure 5.2. General model for recurrent events. Not acceptable as a multi-state model.

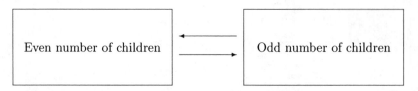

Figure 5.3. Alternating birth model.

to be of the form $\lambda(t)$, where t denotes the age. It is simple and operational to get public data on the age distribution of women in the area, and the number of births in each maternal age class. From this we can calculate birth rates in a piecewise constant hazard model, by the number of births divided by the observation time, within each age class. This can then be applied to predict the number of births in the area over the coming years, based on the development in the number of women in the age classes. This procedure does not account for the previous number of children. In other words, even though it is scientifically interesting to examine the influence on the current number of children, it is not worth the effort in this example. When we do not have the information on the current family size, it seems irrelevant to illustrate the model by Figure 1.4. Furthermore, the simple birth rate approach easily accommodates left truncated data, where we do not know the previous number of children. The general Markov multi-state approach requires us to know the state at entry into the study period. A further, minor, disadvantage is that the total number of possible states is not known. In summary, we would prefer a depiction like that shown in Figure 5.2. Even though it is clear what this model describes, it is illegal as a multi-state model, because in such models the transitions are defined as a change of state, and there is no change of state. The model illustrated is an event model, rather than a state model. To make a non-trivial state model requires at least two states. If we consider the fertility model as an alternating state model (Figure 5.3), we can keep it down to two states, but still the model is illogical, and requires knowledge on the parity, the previous number of children. In conclusion, we have to stick with the model of Figure 1.4 together with an assumption of the same hazard in all cases.

Another, more biological, model is shown in Figure 5.4. This model does

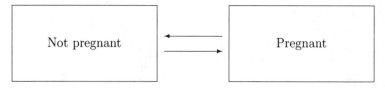

Figure 5.4. Pregnancy-birth model.

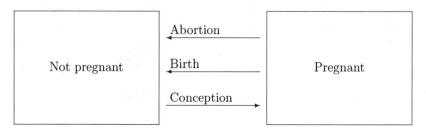

Figure 5.5. Pregnancy-birth model, with birth and abortion. Not acceptable as a multi-state model.

have some advantages: for example, all births correspond to the same transition and it is more transparent that the interval between successive births is at least nine months. The major disadvantage of that model is that application of it requires knowledge of pregnancy status. For the school planning problem above, the first many years are based on children already born, where prediction is precise, after which the fertility model comes in, with less precise estimates. Including the pregnancy period would add six to nine months to the period where we can make a precise estimate, but otherwise not help. It would require more detailed data, and therefore not be worth the effort. A further problem with this model is that, even if we were able to get the necessary information, it is not all transitions from pregnancy to the state of not pregnant that correspond to the birth of a healthy child. The transition could also correspond to an abortion, either provoked or spontaneous. We will not consider the provoked abortions here, as the decisions for performing such follow a different pattern. To include spontaneous abortions, we would prefer to extend the model to that of Figure 5.5. This model is also illegal as a multi-state model, because there are two different transitions from the state pregnant to the state of not pregnant. Transitions are defined implicitly as a change of state. To turn it into an acceptable model, we need to change it to that of Figure 5.6. There is one state corresponding to each event (abortion, birth, conception); that is, the arrival state recalls the type of the latest event. This model has the further advantage that it makes it transparent that the model allows for the hazard function for a new pregnancy's being higher when the last pregnancy led to abortion than when it led to birth of a child.

We will expect that the hazard function for pregnancy also depends on the number of children. To make this visible in the figure, a model of

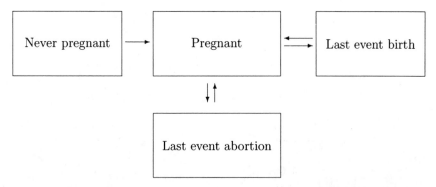

Figure 5.6. Fertility model accounting for outcome of last pregnancy.

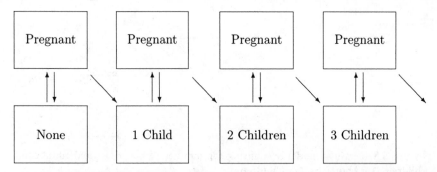

Figure 5.7. Fertility model accounting for pregnancies and number of children.

the form shown in Figure 5.7 is suggested. Such a model is interesting under the assumption that couples continue until they have the desired number of children. This type of hazard function dependence on the state corresponds to an event-related type of dependence. To test the validity of such an assumption requires a larger model, which might also be relevant for studying the occurrence of multiple abortions for a woman. This gives a much more complicated structure, and to simplify it, we do not show the pregnancy states. They could be put in as intermediate states. That gives the model shown in Figure 5.8.

A further point worth illustrating is how to account for twin births (Figure 5.9). A transition directly from 0 to 2 children is possible in this model. Thus, similar to the bivariate case below, this state structure means that simultaneous events are turned into single transitions, between distant states. A consequence of this is that the model is no longer progressive, in contrast to the original model (Figure 1.4).

The conclusion to be drawn from these illustrations is that by choosing the right state structure, we can obtain various effects, in particular making an intuitive graphical depiction of the model leading to the assumptions

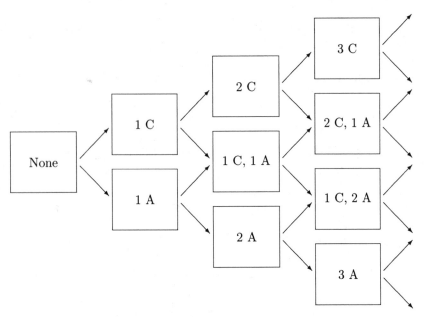

Figure 5.8. Fertility model accounting for number of abortions and number of children. A=Abortions; C=Children.

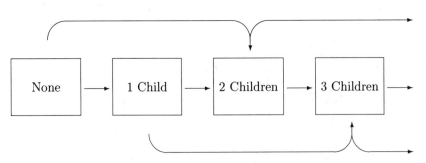

Figure 5.9. Fertility model for a woman, allowing for twin births.

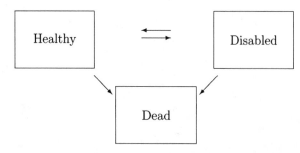

Figure 5.10. Disability model with reactivation.

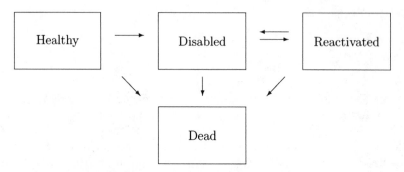

Figure 5.11. Disability model with reactivation as a separate state.

being more transparent. Therefore, it is useful to consider the model in detail before doing actual calculations.

5.3.2 The disability model

As another example, consider the disability model depicted in Figure 1.5. A person starts in state healthy, and then can die, or can become disabled and then die. It is thus a model with different events. It also goes under the name illness-death model. In this model it is impossible to become reactivated, i.e., return from the state disabled to the state healthy. Such a feature could be introduced by including a transition arrow back to the healthy state (see Figure 5.10). The question is, of course, whether persons who previously have been disabled have the same risk of death (and recurrent disability) as persons who have been healthy all their life. This can be modeled by letting the hazard of death (respectively, disability) depend on whether their history includes disability. In Figure 5.10 this is not transparent, and therefore it is advantageous to illustrate the model as in Figure 5.11. In this model it is clear that the death hazard for a previously disabled person is possibly different from the death hazard for a person who has never been disabled. Indeed, this feature can be obtained under the assumption that the model in Figure 5.11 is a Markov model, whereas a Markov model in

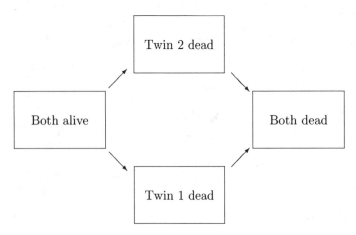

Figure 5.12. Twin survival model.

Figure 5.10 implies that a previously disabled person has exactly the same risk of future events as a person who has never been disabled.

The same model (Figure 5.11) can give some insight into menstrual bleeding patterns, epilepsy, psychiatric hospital admissions, and cancer. A classical example in demography is marriage status, considered as never married, married, divorced, widowed, and dead. In this model one could join never married, divorced, and widowed into a category not married (like Figure 5.10), but demographic experience says that it is more relevant to consider those that are never married as separate from those who have previously been married, either divorced or widowed. In all cases, we would use a completely different set of parameters for the first event than for later events. For example, the model for the first menstruation is determined by the age, whereas future menstruations are determined by the time since the last event. For epilepsy, the first seizure marks the onset of the disease, and thus the hazard measures the incidence of epilepsy, whereas the hazard for later events measures the seizure frequency among people with the disease. In both these cases, the distinction between the first and later events is so large that one would, in fact, prefer to consider two different data sets to evaluate the two transition hazards. Also for studying the effect of smoking, it is relevant to consider never-smokers and ex-smokers separately.

The disability model is applied to the heart transplant data in Section 6.7.1. An extension to two complications is used for modeling complications and survival after a myocardial infarction in Section 6.7.3.

5.3.3 Bivariate parallel data

Any continuous multivariate distribution can be described by a multi-state model, with one major limitation, the censoring pattern. This will be exemplified for bivariate data. The limitation is that the multi-state model requires homogeneous censoring (Section 1.11), so that if any individual is censored, the other individual in the pair must be censored at the same time. Basically, the consideration is whether a pair should be considered as two dependent individuals (the parallel case) or as a single process for the pair (the longitudinal case). Multi-state models make a longitudinal approach. To make the points concrete, we will discuss the model as describing the lifetimes of a pair of twins. Consider a continuous bivariate parallel random variable (W_1, W_2), so that W_1 is the survival time of twin 1 and W_2 the survival time of twin 2. This notation makes it possible to see, when we use the parallel formulation (W) or the longitudinal formulation (T). The bivariate survivor function is $S(w_1, w_2)$. We can implement this in the multi-state model shown in Figure 5.12. The process is in state 1 at time t, when both are alive, that is the set $\{W_1 > t, W_2 > t\}$, which occurs with probability $S(t, t)$. The process is in state 2, twin 1 dead, for the set $\{W_1 \leq t, W_2 > t\}$, which occurs with probability $S(0, t) - S(t, t)$. The process is in state 3, twin 2 dead, for the set $\{W_1 > t, W_2 \leq t\}$, which occurs with probability $S(t, 0) - S(t, t)$. It is in state 4, both dead, for the set $\{W_1 \leq t, W_2 \leq t\}$, which occurs with probability

$$1 - S(0, t) - S(t, 0) + S(t, t). \tag{5.6}$$

This shows that the multi-state transition probabilities are well defined by the survivor function. The hazard function of death of twin 1 when both twins are alive is

$$\lambda_1(t) = -\{D_1 \log S(t_1, t_2)\}(t, t), \tag{5.7}$$

where D_1 denotes differentiation with respect to the first coordinate. The hazard of death of twin 1 at time t, when twin 2 is known to have died at time t_2 is

$$\mu(t, t_2) = -\{D_1 \log -D_2 S(t_1, t_2)\}(t, t_2). \tag{5.8}$$

This is well defined and correct in the bivariate distribution for any combination of t and t_2, but from a dynamic point of view (that is, in the multi-state model), it only makes sense when twin 2 has already died, that is, for $t > t_2$. The corresponding expression for death of twin 2 is analogous.

The model can be extended to allow for simultaneous events, as discussed in Section 3.1.1; that is, death of both twins at the same time. This implies that $Pr(W_1 = W_2) > 0$. In that case, the bivariate distribution is no longer continuous, but has a discrete component on the diagonal (the identity line). In that case, the model should look like Figure 5.13. Thus the parallel model considers it as two events, where the stochastic process considers it as a single transition, but between more distant states. The evaluations above on the sets and the survival function are still correct, but the hazard functions are different. The hazard function of death of any twin is $d \log S(t, t)/dt$. The total hazard of death of twin 1 is as described in Equation (5.7). So to find the hazard of death of twin 1 alone, when

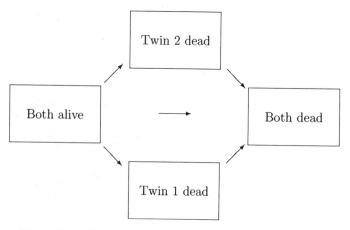

Figure 5.13. Twin survival model with simultaneous events.

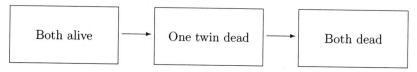

Figure 5.14. Twin survival model based on the ordered observations.

both are alive, we use the total hazard minus the hazard of death of twin 2; that is,

$$\lambda_1(t) = -d \log S(t, t)/dt + \{D_2 \log S(t_1, t_2)\}(t, t).$$

The hazard of simultaneous event is

$$\lambda_0(t) = -d \log S(t, t)/dt + \lambda_1(t) + \lambda_2(t).$$

For death of twin 1 when twin 2 is known to have died previously at time t_2 the expression is like that without the possibility of simultaneous death (Equation (5.8)).

Another way to change the model of Figure 5.12 is shown in Figure 5.14. In that formulation it is not recorded which twin dies first. From a statistical point of view, this corresponds to a reduction of the data to the ordered observations within pairs. This reduction is sufficient under the assumption of symmetry, but not sufficient if the distribution is not symmetric. This figure makes the model look like a recurrent events problem, for example, like the fertility model of Figure 1.4. There are, however, two major differences, because under the assumption of independence, the hazard of the first transition equals twice the hazard of the second transition. In the recurrent events problem, the hypothesis of events happening independently of each other corresponds to the two hazard functions's being identical. Secondly, the maximum number of events in the twin model is two, whereas there is no limit for recurrent data. In other words, there is

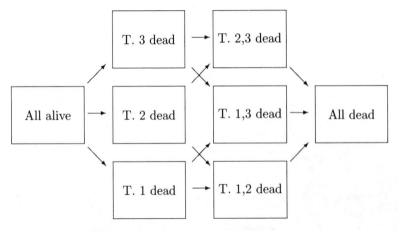

Figure 5.15. Trivariate survival model. T, triplet number.

an absorbing state in the twin model, corresponding to both twins being dead. A further difference is that in the twin case, we know we have two separate objects.

These calculations can be done in all bivariate models, and thus also in repeated measurements models. However, as the physical times are not identical, it makes no sense from a prediction point of view, and event-related dependence is impossible. This is why we say that multi-state models should not be considered for repeated measurements data.

The same model can be generalized to dimensions higher than two, but the structure becomes much more complicated, as illustrated in Figure 5.15 for the trivariate case.

The bivariate model is applied to data on twins in Section 6.7.2.

5.4 Progressive models

The simplest definition of a progressive model is that all states, except the initial state, should only have one possible transition into the state. The initial state should have no possible transitions into the state. We have already seen such models, for example, Figure 1.4 for the fertility histories for women and Figure 1.7 for competing risks. Figure 5.12 is not progressive, because the both dead state has two possible entries into the state, but by a simple modification it can become progressive (see Figure 5.16). The interpretation is that the current state includes the information on how many and which states have been visited previously, and the order, they have been visited in, but not the times of the transitions. An alternative formulation is that from the present state, we know what has happened until now, but not when it happened. The advantage of a model's being progressive is that the differential equations for the transition probabilities

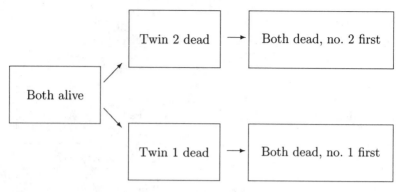

Figure 5.16. The continuous twin survival model as a progressive model.

can be simplified to integrals, which are much easier to handle even though they might be multiple integrals. In the twin case the solution for the original model can be found by combining the states again, as discussed in Section 5.10. A further advantage of studying progressive models is that the likelihood for general models will be based on expressions for progressive models.

5.4.1 Competing risks

The simplest progressive model is the competing risks model shown in Figure 1.7. Only the alive state is not absorbing. In other words, all transitions are from the state alive, and therefore we only need to index the hazard functions with the type of event. This also means that all models are trivially Markov models. Let $\lambda_m(t)$ be the hazard of death of cause m, $m = 1, ..., k$. The hazard corresponding to the total mortality is $\lambda(t) = \sum_m \lambda_m(t)$. Thus the survivor function can be given the usual representation

$$S(t) = \exp\{-\Lambda(t)\} = \exp\{-\int_0^t \lambda(u)du\}. \tag{5.9}$$

The contribution to the likelihood of a censoring at time t will thus be $S(t)$. The contribution of a death of cause m at time t is the corresponding density $\lambda_m(t)S(t)$. Thus the transition probability for cause m is

$$P_m(t) = \int_0^t \lambda_m(u)S(u)du = \int_0^t \lambda_m(u)\exp\{-\int_0^u \sum_\ell \lambda_\ell(v)dv\}du. \tag{5.10}$$

In this formula, the term $\sum_\ell \lambda_\ell(v)$ could be shortened to $\lambda(v)$. The reason it is not done here is that the present expression makes it clearer how the various causes of death contribute. For each cause of death, there is a hazard term, depending only on the actual cause, and an exponential term depending on the integrated hazard for all causes together.

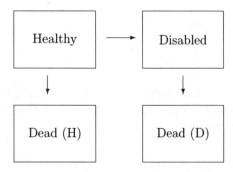

Figure 5.17. The disability model as a progressive model.

5.4.2 Bivariate parallel data

The progressive calculations can be further illustrated for the twin model. In the symmetric case, we consider the model of Figure 5.14, to simplify the notation. The hazard for death of one twin will be called $\psi(t)$, not accounting for which twin dies first. As shown previously, it equals $2\lambda(t)$, where $\lambda(t)$ is the hazard of death of a chosen individual given both are alive. The hazard of death of the second twin, when one has died is denoted $\mu(t, t_1)$, where t_1 is the time of death of the first. The probability of both being alive at time t, that is, no transitions before t, is

$$P_0(t) = \exp\{-\int_0^t \psi(u)du\}, \tag{5.11}$$

in particular, it is independent of the assumptions for $\mu(.)$. The probability of being in the one twin dead state is calculated by integrating over u, which denotes the time of the first transition.

$$P_1(t) = \int_0^t \psi(u)\exp\{-\int_0^u \psi(v)dv\}\exp\{-\int_u^t \mu(v, u)dv\}du. \tag{5.12}$$

This expression has a strong interpretation. There is one term for survival of both twins from time 0 to u, then a hazard of an event at time u, and then a term for survival of the other from time u to time t. The probability of both being dead can be found as $1 - P_0(t) - P_1(t)$.

5.4.3 The disability model

Now we consider a more complicated model, for example, the progressive version of the disability model, shown in Figure 5.17. The hazard of death for a healthy person is denoted $\lambda(t)$. The hazard of becoming disabled is denoted $\psi(t)$. The hazard of death for a disabled person is denoted $\mu(t, t_1)$, where t_1 is the time of disablement. The probability of staying in the healthy state is then

$$P_1(t) = \exp\{-\int_0^t \lambda(u) + \psi(u)du\},$$

in complete analogy with Equation (5.9). The probability of having died without ever being disabled, that is, the probability of being in the state denoted dead (H), is

$$P_3(t) = \int_0^t \lambda(u) \exp[-\int_0^u \{\lambda(v) + \psi(v)\}dv]du,$$

mathematically identical to the probabilities in the competing risks case (5.10), and independent of the expression for $\mu(t, t_1)$. The probability of being in the disabled state is

$$P_2(t) = \int_0^t \psi(u) \exp[-\int_0^u \{\lambda(v) + \psi(v)\}dv] \exp\{-\int_u^t \mu(v, u)dv\}du.$$
(5.13)

This has a similar strong interpretation as the expression for the twin model. There is a term for no events in the period 0 to time u, then a hazard term at u, and a term for staying in the state from time u to time t. This then needs to be integrated over u. The probability, say, $P_4(t)$, of being in the final state is most easily evaluated by 1 minus the sum of the probabilities of all other states. An alternative evaluation is

$$\int_0^t \int_u^t \psi(u) \exp[-\int_0^u \{\lambda(v) + \psi(v)\}dv]\mu(w, u) \exp\{-\int_u^w \mu(v, u)dv\}dwdu.$$
(5.14)

This also has a strong interpretation: first there is a term corresponding to no events before time u, then a hazard term at time u, then a term for no events from time u to time w, then a hazard term at time w, and then there ought to be a term corresponding to no events from time w to time t, but as the state is absorbing, this probability is 1 and therefore omitted in the expression. In the case of Markov hazard functions, the argument u is removed from $\mu(\cdot, u)$ and the equation can be reduced to

$$\int_0^t \int_u^t P_{11}(0, u)\psi(u)P_{22}(u, w)\mu(w)P_{44}(w, t)dwdu. \qquad (5.15)$$

That is, there are terms for the hazard functions at the times of events, and the probability functions for no events in between. The terms are rearranged so that they correspond to the order things happen in, that first you stay in state 1 from time 0 to u, then you change to state 2, then you stay in state 2 until time w, then you change to state 4, and finally you stay there for the rest of the time. The term P_{44} is technically redundant as it is 1, but it is included to make the point more clear.

5.4.4 Recurrent events

The standard recurrent events model, which is illustrated in Figure 1.4, is a progressive model. These models to some extent also cover models, with only a single time path; for example, Equations (5.11) and (5.12) are still correct. Further transition probabilities can be found by the same approach.

Semi-Markov models are technically simple to handle, but the necessary assumptions are rarely satisfied. In this case, the total waiting time can be described as a convolution of independent waiting times for the intermediate states. Among the examples considered in this work, menstrual bleeding is the closest example.

5.4.5 General progressive models

The general expression will follow the same line, but the problem is that all terms depend on the whole history, and therefore are more complicated. First we need some notation. The hazard of transition from state m to state ℓ is generally defined as $\lambda_{m\ell}(t \mid X_u, u \in [0, t))$. As it is a progressive model, the state m implicitly specifies how many states have been visited up to that time, say, k, and also which, so the state arrived at for all previous transitions; that is, s_j is known for $j = 0, 1, ..., k$, where $s_k = m$. So the hazard of transition above can be reduced to $\lambda_{m\ell}(t \mid T_1, ..., T_k)$. It might not appear obvious that this is also conditional on $X_t = m$, or in other words that $T_{k+1} \geq t$, but this is implicit in the subscript m that specifies that the process must be in this state immediately before t. To simplify the equation, we will define $\tilde{u}_j = (u_1, ..., u_j)$. Thus this vector describes all times up to the jth. Then the general expression for $P_m(t)$ is

$$\int_0^t \int_{t_1}^t \cdots \int_{t_{k-1}}^t [\prod_{j=1}^k \lambda_{s_{j-1}s_j}(u_j \mid \tilde{u}_{j-1}) \exp\{-\int_{u_{j-1}}^{u_j} \lambda_{s_{j-1}}(v \mid \tilde{u}_{j-1}) dv\}]$$

$$\exp\{-\int_{u_k}^t \lambda_{s_k}(v \mid \tilde{u}_k)\} du_1 ... du_k. \tag{5.16}$$

5.5 Homogeneous Markov processes

This is, in many ways, the simplest possible case. It is a well-known class of models. All transition hazards are assumed to be constant as functions of time. The actual values of the transition hazards can, of course, be different, i.e. depend on the states that the transition goes from and to, and it is possible to include fixed and known covariates. Time-dependent covariates are not acceptable. There may, or may not be, a parametric model relating some of the transitions. The transition hazard from state m to state ℓ is denoted $\lambda_{m\ell}$. The total hazard for a state is defined as $\lambda_m = \sum_{\ell \neq m} \lambda_{m\ell}$.

In this model, the transition probabilities can be evaluated by means of exponential functions. The transition probabilities can be described by a set of differential equations with constant coefficients. The form of these equations is, for a finite number of states, in vector language

$$dP(t)/dt = P(t)'G. \qquad (5.17)$$

The vector formulation says that for any fixed initial state m, the vector of transition probabilities from m, $(P_{m1}(t), ..., P_{mS}(t))$ satisfies the equation. The matrix G has off diagonal elements $G_{m\ell} = \lambda_{m\ell}$, and the diagonal elements are $G_{mm} = -\lambda_m = -\sum_{\ell \neq m} \lambda_{m\ell}$. In coordinates (5.17) is $dP_{m\ell}(t)/dt = \sum_k P_{mk}(t)G_{k\ell}$, the forward recurrence equations. In general, we can show that

$$P_{m\ell}(v, t) = P_{m\ell}(0, t - v). \qquad (5.18)$$

The solution can be elegantly described by means of the matrix exponential function, where the matrix of transition probabilities satisfy

$$P(v, t) = \exp\{G(t - v)\} = \sum_{r=0}^{\infty} \frac{G^r(t - v)^r}{r!}.$$

In practice, one needs to decompose G to have fast convergence of the sum. In most cases, the eigenvalues of G are distinct and the solutions for the transition probabilities are sums of exponential functions, where the rate constants are the eigenvalues of G. If some eigenvalues have multiplicities higher than 1, the solutions contain combined polynomials and exponential functions. With the simpler models, it might be most convenient to evaluate them explicitly knowing that the transition probabilities are of the form

$$P_{m\ell}(v, t) = \sum_r \alpha_{m\ell r} \exp\{-\beta_r(t - v)\}, \qquad (5.19)$$

where $-\beta_r$, $r = 1, ..., S$ are the eigenvalues of G. The eigenvalues are generally negative, and therefore, we change sign, so that β_r values are positive. The solution is only valid, when the eigenvalues are distinct. The eigenvalues are found as the solutions to the general matrix determinant equation

$$| G + \beta I | = 0, \qquad (5.20)$$

where I is the identity matrix. The set of constants $\alpha_{m\ell r}$ are found from the corresponding eigenvectors, or alternatively by knowing that they are required to satisfy a set of boundary conditions and a set of balance equations. These equations are all linear and therefore easy to solve. The boundary conditions are that

$$P_{mm}(t, t) = 1, P_{m\ell}(t, t) = 0, \text{ for } m \neq \ell, \qquad (5.21)$$

which can be expressed as

$$\sum_r \alpha_{mmr} = 1, \sum_r \alpha_{m\ell r} = 0, m \neq \ell. \tag{5.22}$$

The balance equations specify that the solutions have to satisfy Equation (5.17). This can generally be written as

$$-\alpha_{m\ell r}\beta_r = \sum_k \alpha_{mkr}\lambda_{k\ell}, \tag{5.23}$$

for each r.

Classical analysis of homogeneous Markov models emphasizes that stationary distributions exist and that these are (under certain conditions) obtained under the limit of time going to infinity. Survival analysis considers the transition probabilities at finite times, and thus the limiting behavior is a too simple concept. Therefore, this is not considered further.

First, we will consider a disability model in order to show how to simplify the calculations. This is also done for recurrent events. Two classical models for bivariate data are the Freund and Marshall-Olkin models. The two models can be combined to a larger model. Finally, the alternating state model is considered.

5.5.1   The disability model

The derivation can be illustrated for the disability model, with reactivation (Figure 5.10). To simplify the expressions, the standard notation is not used. The death hazard for healthy individuals is simply denoted λ. The death hazard for disabled individuals is denoted μ. The transition hazard of becoming disabled is ψ. The transition hazard of becoming reactivated is ϕ. The states are numbered as healthy (1), disabled (2), and dead (3). Then the matrix G is

$$\begin{pmatrix} -(\lambda + \psi) & \psi & \lambda \\ \phi & -(\phi + \mu) & \mu \\ 0 & 0 & 0 \end{pmatrix}.$$

In this model the sign-changed eigenvalues are $\beta = (B \pm \sqrt{B^2 - 4C})/2$ and 0, where $B = \lambda + \psi + \phi + \mu$ and $C = \lambda\phi + \lambda\mu + \psi\mu$. Thus the transition probabilities are of the form (5.19), which combined with the boundary conditions (5.21) and the balance equation (5.23) give the solutions. We will, however, not do this, because it is possible to simplify the problem a little, first. Equations (5.19) and (5.20) are still valid for a defective Markov model. This implies that we can delete the absorbing state dead, giving the reduced matrix

$$\tilde{G} = \begin{pmatrix} -(\lambda + \psi) & \psi \\ \phi & -(\phi + \mu) \end{pmatrix}.$$

This model is defective, because the rows do not sum to 0, so there is a flow out of the two states considered. The sign-changed eigenvalues are $\beta = (B \pm \sqrt{B^2 - 4C})/2$, where B and C are as above. Thus, these eigenvalues are the same as before, and the 0 eigenvalue is lost. The advantage of this approach is that Equation (5.19) is reduced from three dimensions to two dimensions, and it can still be used to derive P_{11}, P_{12}, P_{22}, and P_{21}. The boundary conditions tell us that $\alpha_{111} + \alpha_{112} = 1$, that $\alpha_{121} + \alpha_{122} = 0$, that $\alpha_{211} + \alpha_{212} = 0$, and that $\alpha_{221} + \alpha_{222} = 1$. The balance equation for P_{11} says that the flow out of state 1 at time t is $-(\lambda + \psi)P_{11}(0, t)$ and the flow into it is $\phi P_{12}(0, t)$. According to Equation (5.19), the net flow is $\sum_r \alpha_{11r}\beta_r \exp\{-\beta_r t\}$. These functions have to agree for all t, and thus have to agree term by term, giving equations

$$-(\lambda + \psi)\alpha_{11r} + \phi\alpha_{12r} = -\beta_r\alpha_{11r}, r = 1, 2,$$

which are special cases of Equation (5.23). These two equations give together with the boundary conditions for P_{11} and P_{12}, four linear equations to determine $\alpha_{1\ell r}$. Similarly, the balance equations for P_{22},

$$-(\phi + \mu)\alpha_{22r} + \psi\alpha_{21r} = -\beta_r\alpha_{22r}, r = 1, 2,$$

give, together with the boundary conditions for P_{21} and P_{22}, four linear equations to determine $\alpha_{2\ell r}$. The balance equations for P_{12} and P_{21} are not necessary. If they are included, we end up with the determinant equation (Equation (5.20)).

To return to the full three-state problem, the last transition probabilities are easily determined by means of formulas $P_{m3} = 1 - P_{m1} - P_{m2}$, $m = 1, 2$. The term 1 is the term corresponding to the zero eigenvalue. The transition probabilities starting in state three are trivial as the state is absorbing.

5.5.2 Recurrent events

This will be formulated in terms of the fertility model of Figure 1.4, even though we know fertility is not a Markov process. State j is defined as the state where the woman has j children, $j = 0, 1, \dots$. This is the most natural, but the expressions below become slightly more complicated compared to numbering them $1, 2, \dots$. We do not need to specify a maximal value of j, because the model is progressive. The hazard of getting child number j is denoted as ϕ_j, when the woman has $j - 1$ children. The transition matrix G is upper triangular, implying that the eigenvalues are $-\phi_1, -\phi_2, \dots$. In the general case, when no two values of ϕ's are equal, the solution to Equation (5.19) is of the form $P_{m\ell}(v, t) = \sum_r \alpha_{m\ell r}\exp\{-\phi_r(t-v)\}$, for $m \le \ell$. When $m > \ell$, the value is 0. However, by repeated applications of the defective Markov model method described above, we can see that the solution does not depend on $\phi_{\ell+2}, \phi_{\ell+3}, \dots$. Also it does not depend on $\phi_1, \dots, \phi_m$ as these refer to previous transitions. Thus the solution is of the form $P_{m\ell}(v, t) = \sum_{r:m<r\le\ell+1}\alpha_{m\ell r}\exp\{-\phi_r(t-v)\}$. Solutions for different values of m have

the same structure, so we only consider $m = 0$. We then build up the transition probabilities sequentially. First $P_{00}(v,t) = \exp\{-\phi_1(t-v)\}$, that is $\alpha_{001} = 1$. The balance equation for the P_{01} coefficient to $\exp\{-\phi_1(t-u)\}$ implies

$$\phi_1\alpha_{001} - \phi_2\alpha_{011} = -\phi_1\alpha_{011}, \qquad (5.24)$$

from which we derive $\alpha_{011} = \phi_1\alpha_{001}/(\phi_2 - \phi_1)$. The other balance equation is empty, but the boundary condition $P_{01}(t,t) = 0$ implies that $\alpha_{012} = -\alpha_{011}$. This can be generalized so that $\alpha_{0\ell r} = \phi_r\alpha_{0,\ell-1,r}/(\phi_{\ell+1} - \phi_r)$, for $r \leq \ell$ and $\alpha_{0\ell,\ell+1} = -\sum_{r=1}^{\ell} \alpha_{0,\ell,r}$. This gives the full solution.

In the classical case, where all ϕ's are equal there are repeated eigenvalues, found in Equation (5.20), and polynomial terms are included. In this case, the solution becomes

$$P_{0\ell}(v,t) = \{\phi(t-v)\}^\ell \exp\{-\phi(t-v)\}/\ell! \qquad (5.25)$$

corresponding to the number of children being Poisson distributed with mean $\phi(t - v)$. These solutions can be built up in the same way.

The moments are easily found, because each waiting time is independent of what has happened previously, and thus they can be summed. Letting T_ℓ denote the time of birth of child number ℓ, we directly notice that $ET_\ell = \sum_{r=1}^{\ell} 1/\phi_r$. Also the variances are immediately derived to be $\mathrm{Var}(T_\ell) = \sum_{r=1}^{\ell} 1/\phi_r^2$. The covariances are similarly $\mathrm{Cov}(T_\ell, T_m) = \sum_{r=1}^{\min\{\ell,m\}} 1/\phi_r^2$.

5.5.3   The Freund model

The Freund model is the homogeneous Markov model with state structure illustrated in Figure 5.12. Thus the hazard of death of twin 1 is λ_1, when both are alive, and μ_1, when the partner is dead. Similarly, for twin 2 the hazards are λ_2 and μ_2. These are also the transition hazards. In the symmetric case, the indices can be dropped. In that case, λ is the hazard of death of any single individual, when both are alive, and μ the hazard of death of the last survivor. This model was originally developed for event-related dependence in industrial applications, where a two-unit system has a risk of failure λ for any given component, but where the failure rate increases to μ for a single component, when one component fails, due to the increased workload. A standard example is a twin computer, where if a computer breaks down, the other can take over. However, the other computer has to work harder, which increases its risk of breaking down also. The model is also valid for $\mu < \lambda$. This could be the case where the two components compete for resources. The marginal distributions are not exponential, unless $\mu = \lambda$, in which case, W_1 and W_2 are independent. The distribution of the time to the first event (T_1) is exponential with hazard $\lambda_1 + \lambda_2$.

The transition probabilities, using the state numbering from Section 5.3.3, are

$$P_{11}(v,t) = \exp\{-(\lambda_1 + \lambda_2)(t - v)\}$$

for survival of both until time t. For individual 1 dead, we obtain

$$P_{12}(v,t) = \frac{-\lambda_1}{\delta} \exp\{-(\lambda_1 + \lambda_2)(t - v)\} + \frac{\lambda_1}{\delta} \exp\{-\mu_2(t - v)\},$$

where $\delta = \lambda_1 + \lambda_2 - \mu_2$. There is a similar expression for twin 2 dead. The last value is most easily found from the relation $P_{14}(v,t) = 1 - \{P_{11}(v,t) + P_{12}(v,t) + P_{13}(v,t)\}$. The other transition probabilities are easily found, for example,

$$P_{22}(v,t) = \exp\{-\mu_2(t - v)\},$$

and $P_{24}(v,t) = 1 - P_{22}(v,t)$ and $P_{44}(v,t) = 1$. The expressions above are only correct when the denominators are different from 0. When they are 0, there are repeated eigenvalues and a different solution (not shown) applies.

The marginal survival distribution for component 2 is

$$S_2(w) = \frac{\lambda_2 - \mu_2}{\lambda_1 + \lambda_2 - \mu_2} \exp\{-(\lambda_1 + \lambda_2)w\} + \frac{\lambda_1}{\lambda_1 + \lambda_2 - \mu_2} \exp\{-\mu_2 w\},$$

with a similar expression for $S_1(w)$. The bivariate density is

$$f(w_1, w_2) = \lambda_1 \mu_2 \exp\{-\mu_2 w_2 - (\lambda_1 + \lambda_2 - \mu_2)w_1\}$$

when $w_1 < w_2$, with an expression with the coordinates reversed for $w_1 > w_2$. The survivor function $S(w_1, w_2)$ is

$$\frac{\lambda_1}{\lambda_1 + \lambda_2 - \mu_2} \exp\{-(\lambda_1 + \lambda_2 - \mu_2)w_1 - \mu_2 w_2\} + \frac{\lambda_2 - \mu_2}{\lambda_1 + \lambda_2 - \mu_2} \exp\{-(\lambda_1 + \lambda_2)w_2\}$$

when $w_1 < w_2$, with an expression with the coordinates reversed for $w_1 > w_2$. It has previously been stated that multi-state models require homogeneous censoring, even though we can evaluate any quantity we need from the bivariate survivor function, also for general censoring, but the problem is that the terms are completely different from the terms found under homogeneous censoring (where the terms corresponding to censoring and the terms corresponding to events are easily combined), and therefore we prefer to consider only homogeneous censoring.

An alternative description of the time is as $W_1 = T_1 + H_2 U_1$, where $T_1 = \min\{W_1, W_2\}$, $H_2 = 1\{W_2 = T_1\}$ and $U_1 = W_1 - T_1$, corresponding to the interpretation of first experiencing the first event in each pair, and then, if component 1 does not fail at this time, we experience a further time. The distribution of T_1 is exponential with hazard $\lambda_1 + \lambda_2$, the distribution of H_2 is independent of T_1 and is Bernoulli, with probability $\lambda_2/(\lambda_1 + \lambda_2)$. Conditional on $H_2 = 1$, the distribution of U_1 is exponential with hazard μ_1. On the set $H_2 = 0$, the value of U_1 is zero by definition, but as it is multiplied by 0, we are allowed to fill in other definitions. This relation suggests a way of simulating such data. Let U_0, U_1, U_2, and H_2 be independent. The U's should be exponential, with hazards $\lambda_1 + \lambda_2$, μ_1 and μ_2, respectively, and let H_2 be Bernoulli, with probability $\lambda_2/(\lambda_1 + \lambda_2)$. Now define $H_1 = 1 - H_2$, and $W_1 = U_0 + H_2 U_1$, $W_2 = U_0 + H_1 U_2$. This is an alternative way of deriving the Freund distribution. This approach could be called successive conditioning, as we move one event forward by each term. One of the advantages of this approach is that we can immediately calculate the mean value as

$$EW_1 = \frac{1}{\lambda_1 + \lambda_2} + \frac{\lambda_2}{\lambda_1 + \lambda_2} \frac{1}{\mu_1},$$

which can be reduced to $(\mu_1 + \lambda_2)/\{\mu_1(\lambda_1 + \lambda_2)\}$. By extension of this approach, we calculate the variance of W_1 to be $(\mu_1^2 + 2\lambda_1\lambda_2 + \lambda_2^2)/\{\mu_1^2(\lambda_1 + \lambda_2)^2\}$ and the correlation coefficient between W_1 and W_2 is found as

$$\frac{\mu_1\mu_2 - \lambda_1\lambda_2}{\sqrt{(\mu_1^2 + 2\lambda_1\lambda_2 + \lambda_2^2)(\mu_2^2 + 2\lambda_1\lambda_2 + \lambda_1^2)}},$$

which spans the range of $(-1/3, 1)$.

5.5.4   The Marshall-Olkin model

This is a model for bivariate data, allowing for simultaneous events: that is, corresponding to Figure 5.13. According to this figure, the hazard of simultaneous death is φ_0, and the hazard of death of individual 1 alone is φ_1, when the partner is alive, and $\varphi_0 + \varphi_1$, when the partner is dead. The classical derivation of this model is as a shock model, where shocks arrive according to Poisson processes, and which may be fatal to one or both individuals. Alternatively, it can be given a parallel data derivation by means of three independent exponentially distributed variables U_0, U_1, U_2, with hazards $\varphi_0, \varphi_1, \varphi_2$, respectively. Then $W_1 = \min(U_0, U_1)$ and $W_2 = \min(U_0, U_2)$. This means that U_0 corresponds to an event that hits both individuals giving simultaneous events, if the individuals both are alive at that point in time. Furthermore, U_1 is an event hitting only individual 1 and U_2 is an event hitting only individual 2. This distribution has exponential marginal distributions with hazards $\varphi_0 + \varphi_1$ and $\varphi_0 + \varphi_2$, respectively. Also the distribution of the time to the first event $T_1 = \min(W_1, W_2)$ is exponential, with hazard $\varphi_0 + \varphi_1 + \varphi_2$. The probability of simultaneous events is $\varphi_0/(\varphi_0 + \varphi_1 + \varphi_2)$. This is true, both stated alone, and conditionally upon T_1. In popular terms, this implies that all the dependence is placed at the diagonal. To illustrate this point, consider the total hazard of death of individual 1, total meaning containing both the case of death of the individual alone, and simultaneous with the other individual. When both are alive, this hazard is $\varphi_0 + \varphi_1$. When only individual 1 is alive, the hazard is also $\varphi_0 + \varphi_1$. This appears like independence, but that is because the evaluation does not catch the possibility of simultaneous events. Consistent with the previous use of the word *long-term*, this type of dependence can be called long-term independence.

The transition probabilities, using the state numbering of Section 5.3.3, are

$$P_{11}(v,t) = \exp\{-(\varphi_0 + \varphi_1 + \varphi_2)(t - v)\}$$

for survival of both until time t. For individual 1 dead, we obtain

$$P_{12}(v,t) = -\exp\{-(\varphi_0 + \varphi_1 + \varphi_2)(t - v)\} + \exp\{-(\varphi_0 + \varphi_2)(t - v)\},$$

which is derived by means of an expression very close to Equation (5.24). There is a similar expression for twin 2 dead. The last value is most easily found from the relation $P_{14}(v,t) = 1 - \{P_{11}(v,t) + P_{12}(v,t) + P_{13}(v,t)\}$.

The means are $EW_1 = 1/(\varphi_0 + \varphi_1)$ and $EW_2 = 1/(\varphi_0 + \varphi_2)$, easily derived, as the marginal distributions are exponential. The correlation of (W_1, W_2) equals Kendall's τ and is simply $\varphi_0/(\varphi_0 + \varphi_1 + \varphi_2)$, which spans a range of $(0,1)$. The distributions satisfy a bivariate lack of memory property so that conditional on both individuals alive at age v, the distribution of $(W_1 - v, W_2 - v)$ is the same as the original distribution of (W_1, W_2). The survivor function is $S(w_1, w_2) = \exp\{-\varphi_1 w_1 - \varphi_2 w_2 - \varphi_0 \max(w_1, w_2)\}$. This equation, together with (4.14), gives that the dependence measure based on the median concordance equals

$$\kappa = 2^{\varphi_0/\{\varphi_0 + \max(\varphi_1, \varphi_2)\}} - 1.$$

It is further possible to evaluate the bivariate Laplace transform, which is

$$L(s_1, s_2) = E \exp(-s_1 W_1 - s_2 W_2) =$$

$$\frac{(\varphi_0 + \varphi_1 + \varphi_2 + s_1 + s_2)(\varphi_0 + \varphi_1)(\varphi_0 + \varphi_2) + \varphi_0 s_1 s_2}{\varphi_0 + \varphi_1 + \varphi_2 + s_1 + s_2)(\varphi_0 + \varphi_1 + s_1)(\varphi_0 + \varphi_2 + s_2)}. \qquad (5.26)$$

From a technical point of view, the Marshall-Olkin model is a three parameter submodel of the full five parameter homogeneous Markov model for the state structure of Figure 5.13, which is the reason for it's being difficult to estimate in this model.

5.5.5   The combined model

This is the model of Figure 5.13, where there is a separate parameter for each transition. Thus it is an extension of the Freund model, in that simultaneous death is possible, and it is an extension of the Marshall-Olkin model, by allowing a freely varying parameter for the hazard of a second event. Besides being an extension, the model has the advantage compared to the Marshall-Olkin model that it allows for explicit estimation. Despite its simplicity, it has not been considered as much as the Marshall-Olkin model.

5.5.6   The alternating state model

The alternating state model is not progressive, implying that the approach of Section 5.4 cannot be used to evaluate the transition probabilities. Therefore the assumption of a homogeneous Markov model is particularly attractive in this case. If the two hazards are ψ and ϕ, the eigenvalues are 0 and $\psi + \phi$ and the transition probabilities are

$$P_{00}(v, t) = \frac{\phi}{\psi + \phi} + \frac{\psi}{\psi + \phi} \exp\{-(t - v)(\psi + \phi)\}. \qquad (5.27)$$

The value of P_{01} is found as $1 - P_{00}$, and P_{11} and P_{10} are found similarly.

5.6   General Markov processes

Another formulation of the Markov property is that the relevant summary of the history at time t is the state at that time. The word *relevant* refers to being relevant for predicting the future course of the process. This is the main point in the intuitive understanding of the graphical part of the model. The future course depends on where you are at the current time, but not on how you got there. Also in this case, the transition probabilities are given by a set of differential equations, which are

$$dP(t)/dt = P(t)'G(t). \qquad (5.28)$$

Similar to the homogeneous case, this is a vector equation. In coordinates this is

$$dP_{m\ell}(t)/dt = \sum_r P_{mr}(t)G_{r\ell}(t) \qquad (5.29)$$

Unfortunately, this equation cannot be solved in general, as in the homogeneous case, because the coefficients $G(t)$ do not make up a constant matrix. Thus Equations (5.18) and (5.19) no longer hold.

As demonstrated above in the disability model, we can, by splitting up the states, make the state contain more information, which then allows for the model's being a Markov model. In some cases, we have a choice between a non-Markov model with a simple state structure or a Markov model in a complicated state structure. It is also possible to make the state contain information on the times of the transitions, although it is much more complicated. For example, the model of Figure 5.14 can be modified to that shown in Figure 5.18. The first transition hazards are such that at any time point one of them is positive, and the two other 0. At times 25 and 50 years, another transition becomes positive. The advantage of a process's being Markov is not big enough to make it an advantage to perform this trick. It is better to keep with the original model, and describe it as a Markov extension model.

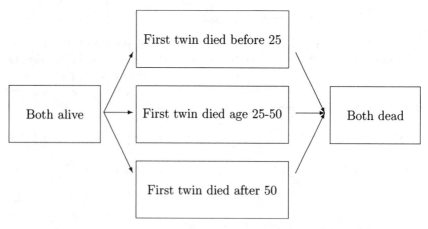

Figure 5.18. Twin survival model based on the ordered observations, with a partial memory of the time of first transition.

In Markov models, there is a relation (the Chapman-Kolmogorov equation) between the transition probabilities

$$P_{m\ell}(v, t) = \sum_r P_{mr}(v, u)P_{r\ell}(u, t), \tag{5.30}$$

whenever $v \leq u \leq t$. This equation has a strong interpretation that we can split according to intermediate times and states.

The case of piecewise constant hazard functions can be treated with help from these formulas, by considering each interval separately. To be precise, when both v and t are in the same interval, the solution is as described in the homogeneous case (Equation (5.19)). When v and t are in different intervals, we need to use the Chapman-Kolmogorov equation (Equation (5.30)), repeatedly, choosing for u all interval end points between v and t.

Markov models lead to long-term dependence, because the times of earlier transitions are irrelevant for future events. All that matters is the fact that they have happened.

5.7 Markov extension models

This is a slight extension of the Markov models. The hazard functions are also allowed to depend on the time of the latest transition. As the hazard functions are allowed to depend on the current time, it can alternatively be formulated as that the hazard might depend on the current duration in the state. Therefore, these models are sometimes called models with duration dependence. The graphical version of the model is still very relevant. Equation (5.30) no longer holds.

The Markov extension models make up a necessary tool in order to discuss whether dependence is of short-term or long-term time frame.

The semi-Markov processes make up an important special case, where the hazards do not depend on the current time, but only the current duration in the state.

If we study only the first two transitions in a process, all models are Markov extension models. Thus, for example, the bivariate model (Figure 5.12) is a Markov extension model for any assumptions on the hazard functions.

It has already been shown that fertility data cannot be described by a Markov model, but it seems sensible to use a Markov extension model. The simplest possibility is just to assume that the hazard of birth is 0, the first nine months after a previous delivery. This is, in fact, very simple to accommodate in the estimation. More refined models could call for a slow return to a normal fertility level, either as a piecewise constant model, or a nonlinear differentiable model.

Similarly, data on menstrual patterns could be studied in this way. In that case, it might be most convenient to let the time since the latest menstruation have a non-parametric effect and the age have a parametric effect.

5.8 General models

In general models we allow for the hazard showing an arbitrary dependence on the history. This is easily accommodated in a progressive model, as described in Section 5.4. There is not much to say about this case, when the model is not progressive, because basically, this makes it impossible to write general formulas for the transition probabilities. Typically, however, we cannot conceptualize such an arbitrary dependence; in particular, when the hazard functions are complicated, we will automatically consider it as a progressive model. For example, in the alternating state model of Figure 2.2, a general model will allow for an arbitrary dependence on the number and times of all previous transitions. To be specific in the example of the alternating state model, we will, after one event, have one explanatory variable, corresponding to the time T_1, but after j events, we have j explanatory variables, $T_1, ..., T_j$. This is difficult to accommodate, and therefore, we would turn it into a progressive model, because then it would be known from the state how many previous events there are. The model would then be as shown in Figure 5.19. The structure is much like the recurrent events model, but there are two different events involved.

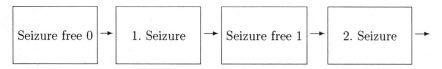

Figure 5.19. The alternating state model for epileptic seizures as a progressive model.

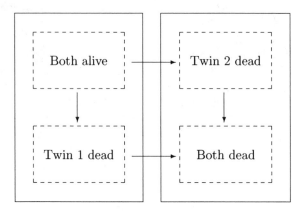

Figure 5.20. Twin survival model. Hidden state model showing the marginal distribution of the lifetime of twin 2.

5.9   Conditionally simple processes

Some models can be described simply, conditional on some random variable. Such models will be considered in detail in Chapter 9. The idea is to calculate the transition probabilities conditional on the random variable and then integrate out the variable to give the unconditional transition probabilities. For example, it is possible that the process is Markov conditionally, but not unconditionally. Similarly, it could have constant hazards conditionally, but not unconditionally. One advantage that might be obtainable in this case is that left truncation could be acceptable, because it is acceptable conditionally.

5.10   Hidden states

The term *hidden states* refers to the case when it is impossible to observe each single state, but only some superstates, which are combinations of the original states. This is thus an extension of the state structure. The topic is only relevant in special cases, and therefore this section can be omitted. A very simple example is shown in Figure 5.12, which can be modified to that of Figure 5.20. There is one superstate corresponding to twin 2 alive, and one superstate corresponding to twin 2 begin dead. Combining the states

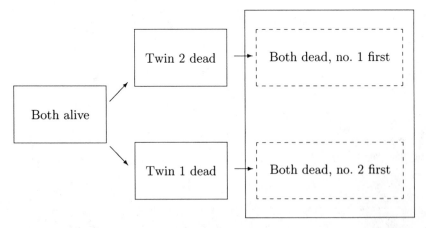

Figure 5.21. The continuous twin survival model as a hidden state model.

as shown in the figure corresponds to consider the marginal lifetime of twin 2 alone, as we collapse the states connected by transitions for twin 1.

Hidden states also make the clue for getting back from the progressive models to the original model. For example, the model in Figure 5.16 is really a hidden state version of Figure 5.12, as demonstrated in Figure 5.21. The consequence is that the transition probabilities should be added over the two both-dead states. In fact, in the case where we combine some absorbing states, there is not much to be gained from considering the model as a hidden state model, because typically the transition probability corresponding to the absorbing state can be calculated as 1 minus all other probabilities. Therefore, the interesting cases are hidden non-absorbing states.

Such an example is the albuminuria model of Figure 1.6. Before the invention of the precise assay to measure the albuminuria content, it was not possible to discriminate between normo- and microalbuminuria, and thus the model corresponded to the solid boxes shown in Figure 5.22. The same model can be applied to screening for cancer or other diseases, where we ordinarily cannot see whether the person has a tumor; that is, we can only observe the superstates, except that by some screening procedure, we can observe the true state.

A further example is the survival-sacrifice approach to cancer data. The model is depicted in Figure 5.23. In such an experiment, a number of animals, typically mice or rats, are exposed to some possible carcinogen, and one wants to know whether more tumors develop compared to a control group. The problem is that one does not know whether a living animal has a tumor. To find out, one can at one or more time points sacrifice some animals, that is, kill them to examine them for presence of tumors. Without doing so it is impossible to estimate the tumor incidence. When an animal dies, it is examined for presence of tumors, and thus it is known whether it dies from the healthy or the tumor state. That is, it is possible to observe

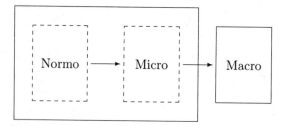

Figure 5.22. Hidden state model illustrating albuminuria before invention of the precise assay.

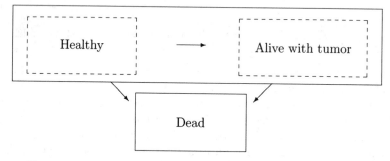

Figure 5.23. The survival-sacrifice model as a hidden state model.

whether the deaths originate in one or the other hidden state. Tumors are classified according to whether they are fatal or non-fatal. Fatal means that the death hazard with tumor is very high, and thus the death hazard with tumor reflects the tumor incidence. The other extreme is that the death hazard is unrelated to presence of tumors. To do the actual calculations in a statistical model, we need to add the terms for the transition probabilities, corresponding to the states that are combined.

A requirement for handling such models is that the initial state is known precisely. In the twin model, this assumption implies that initially both twins should be alive, which is clearly satisfied. In the albuminuria model, all start with normoalbuminuria, and thus this model is also acceptable. In the survival-sacrifice model, all animals start being healthy.

Phase-type distributions are defined as possible distributions of the time to reach an absorbing state in a homogeneous Markov model, and thus corresponds to a multi-state model with hidden states. That approach might consider an unspecified state structure. This book emphasizes the case, where the states and the state structure are precisely defined and have a sensible interpretation.

5.11   Chapter summary

The multi-state models provide an extremely flexible approach that can model almost any kind of longitudinal data. In particular this is relevant to different events and when the probability mechanism that creates dependence is an event-related dependence. For parallel data sets, this approach requires homogeneous censoring. It might not be useful for recurrent events, because it focuses too much on the accumulated number of events.

Before one applies a multi-state model, one should choose the state structure in the best way for the problem at hand. The Markov models stand out as much simpler from a probability point of view, in particular for evaluating transition probabilities, but this also simplifies the likelihood evaluation. However, in many cases, the Markov models do not fit satisfactorily, and happily, it is reasonably simple to study non-Markov models, in particular when the state structure is progressive or the model is a Markov extension model. This also makes it possible to consider whether the dependence is of short-term or long-term nature.

5.12   Bibliographic comments

The Markov models, in particular the homogeneous models, make up a classical probability model. Early important papers on homogeneous Markov models are Fix and Neyman (1951) and Sverdrup (1965). Review papers are Hoem (1976) and Andersen and Borgan (1984). Cox and Miller (1965) have a chapter on multi-state models. The Freund model was suggested by Freund (1961), and the Marshall-Olkin model by Marshall and Olkin (1967) and put into a common framework by Proschan and Sullo (1974) and independently developed by Platz (1984). The animal carcinogenicity model has a large literature (see, for example, Omar, Stallard, and Whitehead, (1995).

The multi-state models for twin survival were considered by Hougaard, Harvald, and Holm (1992b).

5.13   Exercises

Exercise 5.1 Transition probabilities in disability model

Find explicitly the transition probabilities in the homogeneous Markov disability model without reactivation (Figure 1.5).

Exercise 5.2 Fertility model with mortality

Consider the combined fertility-mortality model in Figure 5.24. Suppose that the death hazard is $\lambda(t)$, independent of the present number of chil-

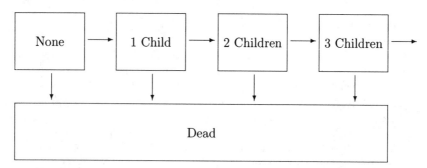

Figure 5.24. Fertility model for a woman, with mortality.

dren. For simplicity, assume that the model is a Markov model. Prove that the transition probabilities $P_{m\ell}(u,t)$, between two alive states can be described by the formula $Q_{m\ell}(u,t)\exp\{-\int_u^t \lambda(v)dv\}$, where $Q_{m\ell}(u,t)$ is the solution to the fertility model, where the dead state, and all death hazards are neglected.

Exercise 5.3 Twin birth model

Consider the fertility model of Figure 5.9, where there are separate transitions for twin birth and births of singletons. Let the hazard of birth be 0 during a period of length Δ after birth. At other times, let the hazard of giving birth to a singleton be $\varphi(t)$, where t denotes the age of the woman. Correspondingly, let the hazard of a twin birth be $\psi(t)$. In particular, these are assumed independent of the current number of children.

Evaluate the probability of having exactly one child at age t. Evaluate the probability of having exactly two children at age t. Is this a Markov model?

Hint: Make this model a progressive model and combine the probability of having two singletons and that of having one set of twins.

Exercise 5.4 Recurrent events with separate first hazard

As mentioned in Section 5.3.2, the hazard of the first event may differ from that of later events. This exercise studies this idea in a recurrent events frame (Figure 1.4). Suppose the hazard of the first event is ψ and that the hazard of a later event is λ, not depending on the actual number of events. Find first $P_{00}(v,t)$ and $P_{m\ell}(v,t)$, when $m \geq 1$. Then write $P_{0m}(v,t)$ as an integral split according to the time of the first event. Finally, evaluate this integral explicitly.

Exercise 5.5 Constant hazard models with periods without events

A model that has been used for Geiger counters of radioactive particles describes that in a period of known length Δ after an event, one cannot measure a new particle, for technical reasons. This model for the observed events can be formulated as a recurrent events model with the hazard being 0 during the period after each event and ϕ at other times. Does this make a homogeneous Markov, inhomogeneous Markov, Markov extension, or general model? The aim of this exercise is to evaluate the transition probabilities regarding recorded events from a starting point of no events, with the system able to observe an event immediately from start. What is the distribution of T_1? What is the distribution of $T_2 - T_1$? From this you should be able to derive the distribution of T_j. How is the set $\{X_t = j\}$ related to the sets $\{T_j \geq t\}$ and $\{T_{j+1} \geq t\}$? Use this and Equation (A.29) to derive an explicit expression for the probability $Pr\{X_t = j\}$.

Exercise 5.6 Freund model with multiple eigenvalues

Find out for which parameter values there are multiple eigenvalues in the model of Section 5.5.3. Find the transition probabilities in this case.

Exercise 5.7 Maximum in the Marshall-Olkin model

In industrial reliability, having two identical components for the same function is one way of extending the lifetime of the whole system. The success of this approach is judged by the distribution of $W_{\max} = \max\{W_1, W_2\}$. Find the distribution of $W_{\max}$ in the symmetric Marshall-Olkin model. Evaluate the ratio $\rho = E(W_{\max})/E(W_1)$. What is the maximum obtainable value of ρ and for which parameter value is this obtained?

Exercise 5.8 Marshall-Olkin Weibull extension

An extension of the Marshall-Olkin model is defined by the distribution of (W_1, W_2), when (W_1^γ, W_2^γ) follows the Marshall-Olkin model of Section 5.5.4, where $\gamma > 0$ is a parameter. Show that W_1, W_2 and $T_1 = \min\{W_1, W_2\}$ follow Weibull distributions and that the distribution can be defined by means of Weibull distributed U_0, U_1, U_2 as $W_1 = \min\{U_0, U_1\}$ and $W_2 = \min\{U_0, U_2\}$. What are the transition hazards, when considered as a multi-state model? Is it a Markov model? What are the values of the dependence measures τ and κ?

Exercise 5.9 Alternating state models

Consider an alternating state Markov model of Figure 2.2. What is the expected number of seizures during a time period from v to t, given that the person is seizure free at time v? Make an explicit evaluation in the homogeneous case (using Equation (5.27)). What is the expected time to the jth event in the homogeneous case?

Exercise 5.10 Purged models

A purged model is one studied conditional on survival to some time, say t_0. A typical example is the disability model of Figure 5.17. We assume that the model is homogeneous Markov and use the notation of Section 5.4.3, that is, ψ, λ, and μ. To simplify the data collection, we only gather data on persons alive at age t_0. What is the probability of being disabled at time t ($t < t_0$), given that the person is healthy at age 0 and disabled and alive at age t_0? What is the transition hazard, say, $\tilde{\psi}(t)$, in this conditional model? Which two-parameter function can be identified in this case? What is $\tilde{\psi}(t)$ in the special case $\lambda(t) = \mu(t)$?

Exercise 5.11 Bivariate data survivor function

Consider the bivariate model in Figure 5.12. How can you express the bivariate survivor function $S(w_1, w_2)$ as function of the transition probabilities in the multi-state model?

Exercise 5.12 Freund model conditional distribution

Consider the Freund model assuming $\mu_1 = \lambda_1$, but $\mu_2 \neq \lambda_2$. Show that in the dynamic frame, failure of individual 2 does not influence the hazard of death of individual 1. What is the marginal distribution of W_1? Show, however, that the ordinary conditional distribution of W_1 given W_2 depends on W_2.

Exercise 5.13 Gumbel model

A classical bivariate distribution due to Gumbel (1960) has survivor function $S(w_1, w_2) = \exp(-\omega_1 w_1 - \omega_2 w_2 - \rho w_1 w_2)$, where $\omega_j > 0$ and $\rho \geq 0$. Show that it has exponential marginals. Let (W_1, W_2) be a random variable from this distribution. Which parameter values make W_1 and W_2 independent? Show that the distribution of W_1 given $W_2 > t_2$ is exponential for any t_2. Derive the transition hazards in the bivariate multi-state model.

6

Statistical inference for multi-state models

Where the previous chapter has discussed choosing the state structure for multi-state models and the probabilistic consequences (like evaluation of transition probabilities) of assumptions like the Markov assumption, the present chapter goes more deeply into the statistical modeling and analysis of the transition hazards.

Overall, there is a wide range of statistical models that are easily fitted by the modern non-parametric methods, including proportional hazards models. The ability to handle time-dependent covariates and left truncation are important tools to manage this flexibility. Of course, the classical modeling of such processes by homogeneous Markov models (constant hazards) is still possible, but there is no need to be restricted by either the assumption of constant hazards or the Markov assumption. The key feature for obtaining a likelihood allowing for simple estimation is the extent to which different transitions share parameters. If the transitions do not share parameters, each possible transition can be studied separately. If two transition hazards are assumed to be proportional, they can be considered simultaneously by means of proportional hazards models with left-truncation (or in some cases, with time-dependent covariates). Difficulties can, for example, arise when there are specific relations between the hazards, as in the Marshall-Olkin model. Asymptotic properties are well understood and make few requirements. Where the estimation of transition hazards is simple in these models, the transition probabilities are not necessarily easy to evaluate. However, evaluation is possible in quite a few models.

Examples of statistical models are discussed in Section 6.1. They differ by the influence the history of the process can have on the hazard functions.

Model for the hazard $\mu(t, u)$	Name
$\lambda(t)$	Independence
$c\lambda(t)$	Proportional hazards Markov
$\mu(t)$	Markov
$\mu(t - u)$	Semi-Markov
$\exp(\beta u)\mu(t)$	Proportional hazards Markov extension
$\mu(t, u)$	General (Markov extension)

Table 6.1. Classification of mortality models for a disable person according to the disability model, where $\lambda(t)$ is the hazard of death when the person is healthy, t the current time, and u the time of disablement.

The likelihood function is derived in Section 6.2. Computational aspects regarding estimation of transition hazards are considered in Section 6.3. Estimation of transition probabilities in non-parametric models is considered in Section 6.4. Asymptotic properties are discussed in Section 6.5. Model checking is considered in Section 6.6. The most immediate way of checking a multi-state model is to consider a more detailed (extended) multi-state model in which the relevant assumption is relaxed. Applications are considered in Section 6.7. Key points illustrated in these applications are the possibility of non- or semi-parametric models for the hazards, the flexibility of the multi-state approach and the simplicity of fitting non-Markov models. Also, the choice of time scale is considered. The applications presented here are all based on the standard sampling plan of observing the exact times of all transitions. In some models, however, it is possible to estimate the hazard functions even with reduced sampling plans, like knowing the state only at some discrete time points, or observing only individuals with specified histories, like case-control studies. A few such examples are referenced in Section 6.7.5.

6.1   Statistical models

Above, we have considered how to go from the hazard functions to the transition probabilities. In this section, we consider various models and how to derive the likelihood function, in order to estimate the parameters. We first consider four of the standard state structures as special cases, and then give general results. The mortality model is covered by Chapter 2 and therefore not treated here. For the competing risks model, it will follow from the results below that each cause of death can be considered separately.

Model for second transition	Name
$\lambda(t)$	Independence
$c\lambda(t)$	Proportional hazards Markov
$\mu(t)$	Markov
$\mu(t - t_1)$	Semi-Markov
$\exp(\beta t_1)\mu(t)$	Proportional hazards Markov extension
$\mu(t, t_1)$	General (Markov extension)

Table 6.2. Classification of symmetric models for twin hazards, where $\lambda(t)$ is the hazard of death when the partner is alive, t the current time and t_1 the time of the first event.

6.1.1   The disability model

In the disability model of Figure 1.5, there are just three hazard functions. It generally makes little sense to model the relation between the disability hazard and the mortality hazard and therefore this is not considered here. What we can do is to make a model relating the death hazard for a healthy person, say, $\lambda(t)$, and the death hazard for a disabled person, say, $\mu(t, u)$, where u is the time of becoming disabled. Some possible models are illustrated in Table 6.1. The semi-Markov model is only relevant when the model describes a disease with a major impact on the death hazard. The proportional hazards Markov extension model is mostly relevant for checking the Markov model.

6.1.2   Bivariate parallel data

Table 6.2 shows some possible models for the hazard functions of the twin model of Figure 5.12. The semi-Markov model is less relevant for parallel lifetimes, because the hypothesis of independence is not present in this model. Another side of this problem is that the age of the individual is not part of the model. This is unsatisfactory in mortality models covering longer periods of time, as age is an important predictor of mortality, possibly with the exception of some short-term conditions. The proportional hazards Markov model is the simplest model with dependence and could also be called the extension of Freunds model to proportional hazards. As there is a maximum of two transitions in the bivariate model, the general model is the same as the Markov extension model. The model specified as Markov is the most general Markov model in this state structure. The model described as proportional hazards Markov extension is a model, where it is simple to check the Markov assumption. This assumption is obtained for $\beta = 0$. For the application to twins in Section 6.7.2, we assume a parametric relation between $\lambda(t)$ and $\mu(t, t_1)$ as this makes it much more easy to discuss the dependence. This is a quite flexible approach, but apart from the proportional hazards Markov model, they are not yet given names.

Table 6.2 looks very similar to Table 6.1 for the disability model, except for the change of u to t_1. This reflects the fact that they both describe the mortality hazard from a starting state and from a single later state. In fact, the most important difference in this respect is that the disability model also operates with the disability hazard, which should be modeled separately. In fact, the reason for choosing different symbols (u respectively t_1) was that we wanted to emphasize the different types of events involved.

Covariates can easily be introduced in this case in the usual proportional hazards model. The standard assumption is that the effect of a covariate is the same for the first and the second transition.

6.1.3   Recurrent events

For the recurrent events model of Figure 1.4, the most general model will have hazard $\lambda_1(t)$ for the first transition, $\lambda_2(t, t_1)$ for the second event, where t_1 is the time of the first transition, $\lambda_3(t, t_1, t_2)$ for the third event, etc. Generally, this is of the form $\lambda_j(t, t_1, ..., t_{j-1})$ for the jth event. The function only makes sense when $0 < t_1 < t_2 < ... < t_{j-1} < t$. The model, where the hazard depends only on t, that is, $\lambda(t)$ is a Poisson model, which is further described in Section 9.2. The Markov model is obtained when the hazard depends only on j and t, that is $\lambda_j(t)$. A further relevant model is the proportional hazards Markov model, where $\lambda_j(t) = \phi_j \lambda(t)$.

When covariates are available, a standard model is the stratified model of Prentice, Williams, and Peterson (1981), where $\lambda_j(t, z) = \exp(\beta' z)\lambda_j(t)$, where the various transition hazards are allowed to vary freely, but the effect of the covariate is the same at all stages of the process.

6.1.4   Alternating states

The alternating state model is not progressive and therefore it is most sensible to include the history only in a rather limited fashion. In practice, this suggests a Markov, semi-Markov, or Markov extension model. The principal difference between the two possible transitions implies that it is typically not relevant to let the two transitions share parameters. Therefore, there is no point in making tables like Tables 6.1 and 6.2.

6.1.5   General models

General models can be handled much the same way as the above examples. First, one should consider (as already done for choosing the state structure) whether the various transitions correspond to comparable events are not. As a general principle, different event types should not share parameters. Transitions corresponding to similar events may share parameters. Inspiration as to how models can be set up in that case can be obtained from Tables 6.1 and 6.2.

6.2   Likelihood evaluation

For evaluating the likelihood function, the Markov models are considered first (Section 6.2.1). In that case, it is possible to simplify the expressions. In the general case (Section 6.2.2), such simplification is not possible. This section does not attempt to evaluate the estimate. This topic is postponed to the following section (Section 6.3).

6.2.1   Markov likelihood functions

For deriving the likelihood function, we will neglect the index corresponding to process number (i), because multiplication over processes is simple. Before we derive the likelihood in the general case, we start with the Markov model. Suppose there are S states, numbered 1,...,S. If the model includes an infinite number of states, we can reduce the model to a finite state model, because we consider a given process outcome. The derivation will be very much like the progressive model. The reason is that for considering a single process result, we know the actual number of transitions and the order of the transitions. The hazard from state m to state ℓ is denoted $\lambda_{m\ell}(t)$. According to the state structure, some of these terms will be known to be identically 0. This is not a problem, because the formulas are still valid. The total hazard from a state m is $\sum_{\ell \neq m} \lambda_{m\ell}(t)$ and is simply denoted $\lambda_m(t)$. A given observation then covers a time period from 0 to C, in which there are E events. The process starts in state s_0, at time $T_0 = 0$. The jth event is a transition into state $s_j, j = 1, ..., E$. Then the likelihood is

$$[\prod_{j=1}^{E} \lambda_{s_{j-1}s_j}(T_j) \exp\{-\int_{T_{j-1}}^{T_j} \lambda_{s_{j-1}}(u)du\}] \exp\{-\int_{T_E}^{C} \lambda_{s_E}(u)du\}. \quad (6.1)$$

It is inconvenient to have the two exponential terms, which are quite similar, so by introducing notation $K = E + 1$, $T_K = C, s_K = 0$, in the case of censoring (and $K = E$ in the case of an event at time C), we can reformulate the likelihood to

$$\prod_{j=1}^{K} \lambda_{s_{j-1}s_j}(T_j)^{1\{s_j \neq 0\}} \exp\{-\int_{T_{j-1}}^{T_j} \lambda_{s_{j-1}}(u)du\}. \quad (6.2)$$

This likelihood says that for each transition there is a contribution corresponding to the hazard at that time and that for the periods without transitions there are exponential terms with the integral of the hazard experienced by the process, that is, the hazard in the state, where the process is. In the Markov model, the likelihood can be reformulated along this line. The advantage of this is that we can collect terms from different patients and repeated occurrences of the same transition for single patients. To do so, we introduce indicators $D_{m\ell j} = 1\{s_{j-1} = m, s_j = \ell\}$ which are 1, precisely when the jth transition goes from state m to state ℓ and risk set functions $R_m(t)$, which are 1 when the process is in state m at time t^-. The formula for this function is

$$R_m(t) = \sum_{j=1}^{K} 1\{s_{j-1} = m, T_{j-1} < t \le T_j\}.$$

Then the likelihood can be formulated as

$$\prod_m \prod_\ell [\{\prod_{j=1}^{K} \lambda_{m\ell}(T_j)^{D_{m\ell j}}\} \exp\{-\int_0^C R_m(u)\lambda_{m\ell}(u)du\}]. \qquad (6.3)$$

This describes the likelihood as a product over all possible transitions and each term involves only the hazard function for that particular transition.

6.2.2   General likelihood functions

In the general case, we can extend Equation (6.1) by exchanging the hazard function argument t with the general expression, where the times of earlier transitions also enter. The general expression will look very much like Equation (5.16), showing the transition probability for a progressive model, except that we do no longer integrate over the times of transitions. For a progressive model for a process experiencing transitions to states $s_1, ..., s_E$ at times $T_1, ..., T_E$, the likelihood is

$$\{\prod_{j=1}^{E} \lambda_{s_{j-1},j}(T_j \mid \tilde{T}_{j-1}) \exp\{-\int_{T_{j-1}}^{T_j} \lambda_{s_{j-1}}(v \mid \tilde{T}_{j-1})dv\}\} \exp\{-\int_{T_E}^{C} \lambda_{s_E}(v \mid \tilde{T}_E)\},$$

$$(6.4)$$

where $\tilde{T}_j = (T_1, ..., T_j)$. For Markov extension models, the same formula applies by removing the tilde over t in the conditioning arguments. We cannot quite reduce this to a formula like Equation (6.3), but we can still collect terms corresponding to the various transitions. That is, instead of considering the data as a process from time 0 to time C, we may list each time period as an observation in state s_{j-1}, with left truncation at time T_{j-1} until time T_j, where there is a transition into state s_j. The last interval can be included by using an event indicator. Thus the likelihood is

$$\prod_m \prod_\ell \prod_{j=1}^{K} [\lambda_{m\ell}(T_j \mid T_{j-1})^{D_{m\ell j}} \exp\{-1\{s_{j-1} = m\} \int_{T_{j-1}}^{T_j} \lambda_{m\ell}(t \mid T_{j-1})dt\}].$$

$$(6.5)$$

The consequence of this formula is that each transition can be considered separately, if it has its own set of parameters. If there are some parameters common to several transitions, they have to be considered together.

6.3   Estimation of transition hazards

This section discusses the theoretical and computational problems in estimating the parameters based on the likelihood functions described above. We consider here n processes, followed over time periods from time 0 until some time C_i for the ith process. First, constant hazards models are considered, which allow for explicit estimation, using generalizations of univariate exponential distribution formulas, when the various hazards are either common or varying freely (Section 6.3.1). Then parametric models are considered (Section 6.3.2). Non-parametric models can in many cases be handled by Nelson-Aalen estimates with truncation or proportional hazards models with truncation and time-dependent covariates. Such models are not described in general, but two examples are described, the disability model in Section 6.3.3 and the bivariate model in Section 6.3.4. Based on these examples, it should be possible to handle other multi-state models. It should be clear from these examples that the problem is not whether the model is Markov or not, but rather the way in which parameters are shared between different transitions.

6.3.1   Separate and common constant hazards

The classical way to handle multi-state models is to consider homogeneous Markov models, that is, assuming constant hazard functions. In this case, it is easy to estimate the parameters and all formulas are explicit, finding hazard functions as occurrence/exposure rates in the case, where there is one parameter for each possible transition. That is, each transition hazard is denoted $\lambda_{m\ell}$ and varies freely independently of all other parameters. When there is a relation between the transition hazards, as in the Marshall-Olkin model (Section 5.5.4), estimation might require iteration (see Section 6.3.2).

Constant hazards models make up a simple case. If a transition hazard is known to be 0, we may neglect that term, but it turns out that we can as well include it, because as there are no events, it will be estimated to be 0 anyway. The likelihood in Equation (6.3) is a product of terms with separate parameters and each term has the same form as Equation (2.4). For giving the final formula for the parameters, process number (i) is included as index. The sufficient statistics are the total number of transitions from m to ℓ, $D_{.m\ell.} = \sum_{i,j} D_{im\ell j}$ and the total time spent in state m, $Q_m = \sum_i \int_0^C R_{im}(u)du$, which alternatively can be found as $\sum_{i,j} 1\{s_{i,j-1} = m\}(T_{i,j} - T_{i,j-1})$. The likelihood estimate becomes

$$\hat{\lambda}_{m\ell} = \frac{D_{.m\ell.}}{Q_m}. \tag{6.6}$$

This expression, which has a strong interpretation as the observed number of relevant events divided by the total time under observation in the relevant state generalizes the univariate exponential distribution formula.

For evaluating variances, we note that the product structure of the likelihood implies that all the mixed second derivatives are 0. This again implies that also in this sense, each transition can be considered separately. Again, for each transition, this is just the same evaluation as in Section 2.2.1. This means that the variance is estimated as $D_{.m\ell}/Q_m^2$.

If the hazards for several transitions are assumed to be common, the estimate can be found similarly by adding the number of events for the numerator and adding the observation times for the denominator. A classical example of this is the Poisson model for recurrent events (Section 5.5.2), where the estimated hazard is the total number of events divided by the total time under observation, irrespective of the state. Another classical example is the symmetric Freund model of Section 5.5.3, where the common first hazard is estimated as $(D_{12} + D_{13})/(2Q_1)$. This example shows that an observation time may appear several times in the denominator, because there are equal transition rates out from the state.

6.3.2 Parametric models

The standard case is when the parameters for each possible transition hazard vary freely. Then each hazard function can be considered separately by the methods of Chapter 2, with truncation at entry into the relevant state. The hazard can then be modeled, e.g., by a Weibull model. The time scale for these evaluations can be time since the beginning or time since entry into the state.

Piecewise constant hazards can be considered in exactly the same way as constant hazards models, the only difference being that Equation (6.6) should be used for each interval separately, that is, counting only events and time at risk within the interval. This is the classical approach used in demography, epidemiology, and other fields and also leads to an occurrence/exposure rate.

In the general case, where parameters are shared for several transitions, we must include all the transitions with shared parameters. For example, the Marshall-Olkin model has three parameters for the five possible transitions and they need to be considered simultaneously. In this case, there is an eight-dimensional sufficient statistic, which is the same as for the model, where all hazards are constant and vary freely. The sufficient statistic consists of the number of observed transitions for each of the five possible transitions $(D_{12}, D_{13}, D_{14}, D_{24}, D_{34}$, using the notation of Equation (6.6) without the dots and the state numbering of Section 5.3.3) and the total time (Q_1, Q_2, Q_3) experienced in each of the three non-absorbing states. As this is a Markov model, the likelihood of Equation (6.3) can still be used, but we need to insert the expressions for the hazards. This gives a log likelihood of

$$D_{12} \log \varphi_1 + D_{13} \log \varphi_2 + D_{14} \log \varphi_0 + D_{24} \log(\varphi_0 + \varphi_2) + D_{34} \log(\varphi_0 + \varphi_1)$$

$$-Q_1(\varphi_0 + \varphi_1 + \varphi_2) - Q_2(\varphi_0 + \varphi_2) - Q_3(\varphi_0 + \varphi_1).$$

For doing a standard iterative estimation, we evaluate the derivatives,

$$\frac{d\ell}{d\varphi_0} = \frac{D_{14}}{\varphi_0} + \frac{D_{24}}{\varphi_0 + \varphi_2} + \frac{D_{34}}{\varphi_0 + \varphi_1} - Q_1 - Q_2 - Q_3,$$

$$\frac{d\ell}{d\varphi_1} = \frac{D_{12}}{\varphi_1} + \frac{D_{34}}{\varphi_0 + \varphi_1} - Q_1 - Q_3,$$

with a similar expression for $\frac{d\ell}{d\varphi_2}$. Although it is possible that an explicit solution can be found, a Newton-Raphson approach can be applied in order to use a general approach. The second derivatives can be found directly. The mixed second derivative for φ_1 and φ_2 is 0, because there are no transitions depending on both of these parameters. The conclusion to draw from this is that it is the relation between the hazards for different transitions that makes it necessary to apply an iterative procedure.

6.3.3 Non-parametric models for the disability model

This case is considered in order to illustrate the approach. For the evaluation, it is assumed that there are no common parameters for the hazard of disablement and the mortality hazards. According to the standard observation plan, there are at most two times. If censoring takes place in the healthy state, we have $T_1 = C$, $S_1 = 0$. If censoring takes place in the disable state, we have observations T_1 (time of disablement), $S_1 = 2$, $T_2 = C$, and $S_2 = 0$. If the person dies without being disabled, the observations are the death time T_1 and $S_1 = 3$. If the person dies disabled, the observations are time of disability T_1 and time of death T_2 and $S_1 = 2$ and $S_2 = 3$.

For studying the disability hazard, we extract the observation time in the healthy state, $U = T_1$, and indicator of the event's being disability, $1\{S_1 = 2\}$. This can then be analyzed in the usual way, by a Nelson-Aalen estimate or a proportional hazards model.

For studying the mortality hazard, we can have separate or common parameters, as described in Table 6.1. Because Section 6.3.4 will present a more detailed example, this section will just describe the simple case of separate non-parametric estimates, without covariates. The mortality from the healthy state can be analyzed by a Nelson-Aalen estimate, the observation starts at 0 and the observation time is T_1 and the indicator of death is $1\{S_1 = 3\}$. The mortality from the disabled state depends both on the current time t and the time of disablement, T_1. In the Markov case, the hazard only generally depends on the current time and the estimated integrated mortality hazard is found from individuals that have positive observation periods in the disabled state, a condition that can be specified as $S_1 = 2$. These individuals contribute with observations T_2, with left truncation at T_1 and the event indicator is $1\{S_2 = 3\}$. When the model applied is the proportional hazards Markov extension model, the observations are the same, but they must be analyzed by the proportional hazards model, including T_1 as covariate.

6.3.4 Non-parametric models for bivariate parallel data

Constant hazard functions are generally not satisfying and therefore we do need more general estimation routines. Depending on the assumptions, many of the more advanced models can be estimated by means of Nelson-Aalen estimates with truncation, or Cox models with time-dependent variables and possibly with truncation. This will be illustrated in the symmetric twin model of Figure 5.12, using the expressions of Table 6.2. The approaches are sometimes formulated by the standard observation plan for multi-state models and sometimes as bivariate time observations. We have bivariate observations (W_1, W_2), with corresponding death indicators (F_1, F_2). The symbols W and F rather than T and D as defined in Section 1.4.1 are used in order to make it clear when the data are considered as bivariate parallel data and as longitudinal data. The homogeneous censoring implies that if $F_1 = F_2 = 0$, it follows that $W_1 = W_2$ and that if $F_1 = 1, F_2 = 0$, it must be so that $W_1 \leq W_2$, with a corresponding expression for $F_1 = 0, F_2 = 1$. The time of the first event is $T_1 = \min\{W_1, W_2\}$, with a censoring indicator $D_1 = \max\{F_1, F_2\}$. If $D_1 = 1$, we further observe a second time $T_2 = \max\{W_1, W_2\}$, with corresponding death indicator $D_2 = \min(F_1, F_2)$. This time is left truncated at time T_1. One could also include pairs with $D_1 = 0$ for the second transition, noting that they contribute with no information (a censored observation after an empty observation period). The number of pairs contributing real information regarding the second transition is n_1, which is found by summing $D_1 1\{T_2 > T_1\}$.

An interesting case is the most general Markov model. In this case, $\lambda(t)$ is estimated by means of only the first transition in each pair. This brings it down to using the procedures described in Chapter 2. In the general case, this can be performed by a Nelson-Aalen estimate of the integrated hazard function $\Lambda(t)$. One way of finding this estimate is to include an observation time for each individual, with death if the twin is observed to die before the other one and censoring at the time of death of the partner, if the twin partner dies first. Thus there are $2n$ times. An alternative is to reduce the data to the first event, T_1, with censoring indicator D_1. This gives only n times, but with hazard $2\lambda(t)$ and the same number of observed events. In this model, we evaluate the Nelson-Aalen estimate of the integrated hazard and divide by 2 to estimate $\Lambda(t)$. If we do not make the assumption of symmetry, we have to consider the two coordinates separately. For the second hazard function $\mu(t)$, we have left truncated data. There is a single time observation for the pair with at least one observed death and no times for pairs, with censoring before the first death. With an arbitrary function $\mu(t)$, this can be evaluated by a Nelson-Aalen estimate with left truncation, using observation times of T_2, truncation times T_1 and death indicators D_2.

In the case of the semi-Markov model, evaluation is easier, because all pairs with a second time start observation at time 0. The observation times are then $T_2 - T_1$ and death indicators D_2. The semi-Markov model is the most simple to handle, because the restarting of time implies that no truncation is necessary. These observation times can then be analyzed by the standard Nelson-Aalen estimate or a proportional hazards model, and in this model, it is acceptable to include T_1 as a covariate, which turns out to be a constant covariate since it is considered only for $t > T_1$.

The extension to Markov extension models, called the proportional hazards Markov extension, refers only to the second transition and thus can be fitted based only on the second spell in the pairs. This is a Cox model, of the time T_2, with left truncation at time T_1, censoring indicator D_2 and covariate T_1. This covariate is constant in this frame.

The proportional hazards Markov model can be fitted in various ways by a Cox proportional hazards model with time-dependent covariates or truncation. The relative risk owing to experiencing death of the partner is c. This corresponds to the time-dependent covariate's being of the state-dependent type, being 0 when both are alive and 1 when the pair has experienced a death. There are, at least, four possibilities on how the calculations can be performed in practice. One possibility is the individual approach. For twin number 1, the observation time is W_1, with death indicator F_1 and a time-dependent covariate describing the status of the partner $z(t) = 1\{t > W_2\}$. Then $c = \exp\beta$. There is a similar observation for twin number 2. This gives $2n$ observations, one for each twin. The second approach is the split process approach. Individual 1 contributes time until T_1, with a death indicator of $F_1 1\{W_1 = T_1\}$ and similarly for twin 2. The covariate is 0 for this interval. The survivor (if there is a survivor) contributes an observation time to T_2, with death indicator D_2, left truncation at T_1 and constant covariate 1. This model has left truncation and a single constant covariate. The total number of observations is $2n + n_1$. Then $c = \exp\beta$. The third approach is the stochastic process approach, which completely corresponds to the ordered observations T_1 and, when relevant, T_2. This requires two covariates (z_1, z_2), for which one regression coefficient is known, $\beta_2 = \log 2$. The reason for having z_2 is the factor 2 present in the hazard of the first event. In SAS, this can be obtained by an OFFSET option. For the first observation T_1, the death indicator is D_1 and $z_1 = 0, z_2 = 1$. The second observation, if present, is T_2 with death indicator D_2 and covariates $z_1 = 1, z_2 = 0$. Then $c = \exp\beta_1$. This gives a data set with $n + n_1$ observations, left truncation and two constant covariates, satisfying $z_1 + z_2 = 1$. The fourth approach utilizes this relation to reduce

Name	Truncation	Observations	Covariate	Covariate
Parallel	0	W_1	$1\{t > W_2\}$	
	0	W_2	$1\{t > W_1\}$	
Split process	0	W_1 (until T_1)	0	
	0	W_2 (until T_1)	0	
	T_1	T_2	1	
Stochastic process	0	T_1	0	1 (*)
(Figure 5.12)	T_1	T_2	1	0
Stochastic process	0	T_1	0	
(Figure 5.14)	T_1	T_2	1	

Table 6.3. Four ways to code times and covariates in order to estimate in the proportional hazards Markov model for bivariate data. The * means that the corresponding coefficient is fixed.

the number of covariates to 1. We can fit the model without z_2, in which case $c = 2\exp(\beta_1)$. This data set has $n + n_1$ observations, left truncation and a single constant covariate, where the hypothesis of independence of lifetimes is $\beta_1 = -\log 2$. The four methods are summarized in Table 6.3.

The conclusion from these evaluations is that quite complicated Markov models relating the various transition hazards to each other can be fitted by ordinary survival data methods by means of methods for truncated data. So, even though there are time-dependent covariates of the state-dependent type, it is not important whether the software can actually handle time-dependent covariates. This is because each stay in a state can be handled separately by means of multiple truncated times.

6.4   Estimation of transition probabilities

Above, we have shown how to estimate the transition hazards, the building blocks of the models. This is generally straightforward. However, it only gives an incomplete picture, as the hazards just look one event ahead. This means that the transition hazards immediately tell the probability of there being no events during an interval and in the case of one or more events in the interval, it describes the distribution of the time to the first event. In order to look further ahead, we need the transition probabilities.

For parametric models we might very well have an analytical expression for the transition probabilities. This is, for example, the case for constant hazards and piecewise constant hazards. In that case, one can just insert the estimated parameters in the expressions.

For non-parametric Markov models without covariates, one can use the Aalen-Johansen estimator. This generalizes the Kaplan-Meier estimate of the simple mortality model. At each time point with events, the local transition probabilities (that is, the transition probabilities over the interval from just before to just after the time) are estimated as the observed probabilities. At times without events, the transition probabilities are given by the identity matrix and cancel out of calculations. For evaluating the transition probability for an interval, the local matrices are combined by using Equation (5.30). For the derivation, we consider a non-homogeneous Markov model, where all hazards are varying freely and independently of each other. Suppose, the observed times of events are $x_1, ..., x_m$. At time point x_q there are $D_{m\ell q}$ transitions from state m to state ℓ. Normally, for each q only a single $D_{m\ell q}$ is 1 and the rest is 0, but the general formulation allows for ties. The risk set in state m is $R_m(x_q) = R_{mq}$. The local observed transition matrix $\hat{G}_q$ then has (m, m) element $-D_{m.q}/R_{mq}$ and (m, ℓ) element $D_{m\ell q}/R_{mq}$ for $m \neq \ell$. The matrix of transition probabilities $P(v, t)$ with (m, ℓ) element $P_{m\ell}(v, t)$ is then estimated by

$$\hat{P}(v, t) = \prod_{q:v < x_q \leq t} (I + \hat{G}_q). \tag{6.7}$$

This is quite a nice estimator. When there is no censoring, it agrees with the empirical estimate,

$$P_{m\ell}(v, t) = \frac{\sum_i 1\{X_{iv} = m, X_{it} = \ell\}}{\sum_i 1\{X_{iv} = m\}}.$$

In the simple mortality model (Figure 1.1), it gives the Kaplan-Meier estimate. Keiding and Andersen (1989) illustrate this method by an alternating-state Markov model with non-parametric hazards.

This idea can be generalized also to more general Markov models, for example, the proportional hazards Markov models. This means that the local matrix $\hat{G}$ at time t will have contributions for all transitions included in the model involving observed events at time t. To be specific, the symmetric bivariate proportional hazards model gives estimates $\hat{\beta}$ and $\hat{\Lambda}_0(t)$, which are then inserted in the transition matrix. At death times this gives off diagonal elements of $\hat{\Lambda}_0(dt)$ and $\exp(\hat{\beta})\hat{\Lambda}_0(dt)$ for the first and second transition, respectively. The diagonal elements for the non-absorbing states are the same, but modified by factors of -2 and -1.

Transition probabilities can also be estimated in non-Markov models, by inserting the estimates into expressions like Equation (5.12), in the symmetric bivariate case. For example, if we assume the proportional hazards Markov extension model, we obtain an estimate of $\Psi(t) = \int_0^t \psi(u)du$, as a step function with masses $\Delta\hat{\psi}(u)$ whenever u is a time of an observed event. For the second transition, we obtain an estimate $\hat{\beta}$ for the regression coefficient and $\hat{M}(t)$ for the integrated hazard. For finding the probability of no events before time t, we insert in Equation (5.11) and obtain $\hat{P}_0(t) = \exp\{-\hat{\Psi}(t)\}$, which is completely like ordinary univariate expressions. Inserting this into Equation (5.12) gives

$$\hat{P}_1(t) = \sum_{0 < u \le t} \Delta\hat{\psi}(u)\exp\{-\hat{\Psi}(u)\}\exp[-\exp(\hat{\beta}u)\{\hat{M}(t) - \hat{M}(u)\}],$$

where the sum over u is over all event times for the first transition. This approach works for progressive models.

6.5   Censoring patterns and asymptotics

Applying these models, one often does not consider whether the asymptotic distributions really apply. However, nice asymptotic distributions are not automatic. Just consider the bivariate models listed in Table 6.2. Even under the assumption of independence $\lambda(t)$ can only be estimated and the asymptotic distribution applies only for time points that have positive information; that is, there should be a positive risk set at all times considered. Therefore the censoring pattern has to be considered. This is similar to the univariate case, where the hazard can only be identified up to the upper limit in the censoring distribution.

Process-dependent censoring is generally acceptable; that is, an individual can be censored based on the history of the individual. For example, it is acceptable to censor an individual after three transitions. This includes censoring times' being defined as stopping times in stochastic processes. The problem of doing so is not the asymptotic validity of the approach, but that process-dependent censoring can lead to some hazard functions's not being estimable at certain times. As an extreme case one can have a censoring pattern that censors the process, when there is an event. This corresponds to making all states, except the starting state, absorbing. This makes it impossible to identify anything but the hazard of the first event. In a bivariate model this means that we can only estimate the marginal lifetimes in a model assuming independence and that the degree of dependence cannot be estimated. This is precisely the problem of the competing risks model, for which the identifiability problems are further discussed in Chapter 12. Common sense will immediately detect such problems.

As a further example, it is acceptable to censor an individual after a certain period without events, for example, if we study repeated cases of myocardial infarctions for patients who have already had one, it is acceptable to censor the individual if he has not had an attack for five years. From a practical point of view, such a patient could be considered as cured. In some general models for the hazards, this will show up as an empty risk set and consequently some aspects will not be estimable. In other models, for example, if the time scale is age and there is a parametric dependence on time since last infarction, one might not notice the problem. In that case, it is not a problem from an asymptotic point of view, but it is impossible to check whether the model applied is correct. Therefore, one should consider possible problems before using such a design.

A deeper problem is that in the Markov model for bivariate parallel data, the risk set for the second hazard ($\mu(t)$) starts at 0 at the time of birth. Therefore, the integrated hazard $M(t)$ cannot be estimated well in the non-parametric case, but for any fixed $v > 0$, we can estimate $M(t) - M(v)$, asymptotically, without problems. This problem is illustrated in practice in the application to twins (Section 6.7.2). The standard way to avoid this problem is to require that there be a positive probability of a non-empty risk set at all times, including time 0. However, as illustrated by the bivariate survival model, this cannot always be satisfied in practice and therefore we have to live with the problem or make a parametric component so that data from other times are used to give information on the transition hazards. To be specific, for the models listed in Table 6.2, the problem is avoided for the proportional hazards Markov model, the semi-Markov model, and, of course, under the independence assumption.

Subject to regularity conditions (like those following as consequences of the discussion above), the estimates will be consistent and asymptotically normally distributed.

6.5.1 Estimation of variance

For estimation of the variance the standard approach is to use (minus) the inverse of the matrix of second derivatives of the log likelihood function: that is, the inverse of the observed information matrix.

An alternative is to use the expected (or Fisher) information based on the mean of the second derivatives. There are two reasons for not using the expected information. First, for the evaluation, it is necessary to make assumptions on the general censoring pattern (that is, on what time censoring is done in the case of fixed censoring, respectively, on the censoring distribution in case of random censoring), whereas the observed information is based only on the actual observed censoring times. Consequently, the evaluation is only valid under precisely that censoring pattern. Second, for censored data, the expected information is more complicated to evaluate than the observed information because integration is necessary. This is in contrast to many other models, like nonlinear regression and exponential families, where taking the expectation makes some terms vanish. Happily, we may justify the choice by the fact that the observed information better reflects the precision realized in the actual sample. This is a deeper discussion, and here the reader is referred to Efron and Hinkley (1978). Some people may argue that this is the reason for using the observed information, but I believe this is a subsequent rationalization.

This implies that the Fisher information is not important for the analysis of actual data. It may, however, be relevant at the planning stage and for discussing efficiency of various procedures. Therefore, a series of exercises has been made to illustrate when the Fisher information is simple to evaluate (see Section 6.10).

6.6   Model checking

Checking a multi-state model is most naturally done by considering a more flexible multi-state model, but it can also be done by other means. First, we may extend the state structure to allow for checking. The most obvious example of this above is the extension of Figure 5.10 to Figure 5.11. Second, the transition hazard functions may be given a more general form. For example, for the recurrent events case with common constant hazard function considered in Equation (5.25), we may allow completely different constant hazards, as described in the same section (Section 5.5.2). As a compromise between these models, one may let the hazard of the first event deviate from the other, as considered in an exercise in Section 5.13. A homogeneous Markov model may be extended by using a Weibull hazard instead or a non-parametric hazard giving an inhomogeneous Markov model. An inhomogeneous Markov model may be extended to a Markov extension model. More examples of how to extend models may be derived from Tables 6.1 and 6.2. Further examples will be considered in the application in Section 6.7.2. If a variable is suspected to influence the hazard, it can be included in the model as a covariate giving proportional hazards. If the proportionality assumption needs checking, one may suggest a stratified model or construct time-dependent covariates to include in the model. If the log linearity of the effect of a given covariate is suspected, one may suggest quadratic, piecewise constant, or piecewise linear models. Overall, for just about any multi-state model, one can suggest more general multi-state models to check any of the assumptions. Most important is the simplicity by which this is done at the hazard function level. If transition probabilities are needed, it may be more complicated.

As the methods of analysis for multi-state models are simple extensions of univariate methods, any univariate model checking procedure may be applied. The only problem with such a procedure is that multi-state models often lead to truncated times, and some univariate methods are not able to handle truncated observations.

6.7   Applications

Applications include Danish twins as parallel data for several individuals, where the interesting aspect is the dependence and there is only a single covariate, year of birth. The Stanford heart transplant data are structurally like the disability model. A more complicated data set is the data on my-

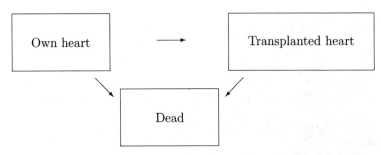

Figure 6.1. Heart transplant model.

ocardial infarctions, where there are three main types of events. Finally, we have data on albuminuria progression.

6.7.1   Heart transplant data

The heart transplant data of Section 1.9.4 can be analyzed by the state structure of Figure 6.1, which is the same structure as the disability model of Figure 1.5. We are particularly interested in studying whether transplantation of a new heart changes the mortality. Let the death hazard while untransplanted be $\lambda(t)$, where t is the time since acceptance in the heart transplant program. The transplantation hazard is denoted $\psi(t)$. The time of transplant is denoted u and, of course, only defined for those patients that were actually transplanted. After transplantation, the death hazard is denoted $\mu(t, u)$. It is a Markov model, when it does not depend on u, i.e., is of the form $\mu(t)$. Within the Cox model, the most natural model is the proportional hazards Markov model, where $\mu(t) = c\lambda(t)$. This can be fitted as a Cox model with a time-dependent variable, which is 0 when the patient is not transplanted and 1 after transplantation. From a computational point of view this is most easily done by defining $u = \infty$ (or a very large number) when a transplant is not performed and letting $z(t) = 1\{t > u\}$. We may include further covariates in the model, the most natural being the age at entry into the program. In that case, we obtain estimated regression coefficients of 0.031 (SE 0.015) for the age and -0.004 (SE 0.312) for transplantation. This value corresponds to $c = 0.996$, that is, a slight and non-significant decrease in mortality owing to transplantation.

Transplantation might lead to increased mortality in the immediate period after the operation owing to complications, and therefore it is interesting to include also the time since operation as covariate. Such an effect would give short-term dependence. This is done as a model with a hazard of $\exp(\beta_1 a)\lambda_0(t)$ without transplantation, where a denotes the age and $\exp\{\beta_1 a + \beta_2 + \beta_3(t - u)\}\lambda_0(t)$ after transplantation. This is no longer a Markov model, but only a Markov extension model. The estimates are given in Table 6.4. There is no effect of time since operation and thus there

Parameter	Variable	$\hat{\beta}(\text{SE})$	p
β_1	Age (years)	0.031 (0.015)	< 0.05
β_2	Indicator	-0.015 (0.336)	0.96
β_3	Time since transplant (days)	0.00014 (0.00158)	0.93

Table 6.4. Estimates for mortality based on heart transplant data.

is no initial increase in the hazard. In other words, the Markov model is satisfactory.

The possibility of ties creates a special problem in this case. It is a possibility (although no patients in the data set experience this) that a person might die on the same day he obtains a new heart. In light of this, the covariate should rather be defined as $z(t) = 1\{t \geq u\}$, in which case, it would be right continuous instead of left continuous as is generally required for time-dependent covariates, as described in Section 2.4.4. This definition would lead to a different estimate, because there are ties between death times for some persons and transplantation times for other patients. If this aspect is important, one should record times with greater precision, or be very careful in the handling of the estimates.

To complete the model, we can estimate the transition hazard corresponding to receiving a new heart. In this model, the age can be included, and, of course, other relevant covariates known at the entry into the study. As the event transplantation can only take place from the initial state, state-dependent covariates are not relevant. The coefficient to age is estimated to be 0.031 (SE 0.014) and thus the chance of obtaining a new heart increases significantly with age. It does not make sense to compare this estimate to the coefficient to age in Table 6.4 because the transitions are of very different types.

6.7.2 Danish twins

The Danish twin data of Section 1.5.1 are evaluated by the bivariate model of Figure 5.12 or Figure 5.14 (as all models used are symmetric). There are just a couple of pairs that appear to die the same day, but these are individuals where only the year of death was known and these have been assumed to die July 1. Therefore, the model with simultaneous events will not be considered.

Markov model

The most general symmetric Markov model with hazard $\lambda(t)$ for the first death and $\mu(t)$ for the second death is considered first. Figure 6.2 shows the integrated hazards for these transitions, for monozygotic males, evaluated by a standard Nelson-Aalen estimate and a left-truncated Nelson-Aalen estimate. It is seen that $M(t)$ is larger than $\Lambda(t)$, and from looking at the derivative, we also conclude that $\mu(t)$ is larger than $\lambda(t)$, corresponding to

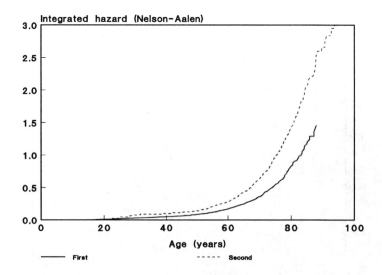

Figure 6.2. Integrated hazard functions for first and second transition in the bivariate symmetric Markov model, for male monozygotic twins.

a positive dependence. Similarly, Figure 6.3 shows the integrated hazard functions for monozygotic females. This case illustrates a general problem with this approach. The risk set in the one-twin-dead state starts at 0 and that means that an early death in the one-dead state can give a very large contribution to the integrated hazard, but, of course, subject to a large variability. Owing to the integrated hazard being considered, this contribution influences the integrated hazard function for all later age classes. It would be more satisfying to evaluate the hazard function by means of kernel function smoothing, or apply a model that would weight this observation corresponding to the variability present. An even simpler approach is to start the integrated hazard at a later time, for example, 20 years.

If we apply the proportional hazards Markov model, the estimates of the regression coefficients $(\hat{\beta})$ and relative risks $(\exp \hat{\beta})$ are given in Table 6.5. The relative risks are included, because they are intuitively easier to understand and the regression coefficients are included in order to compare to later models. The relative risks are significantly above 1 and they thus demonstrate a positive dependence between the lifetimes of twins.

General models

The most specific test of the Markov property is made considering only the second transition, the so-called proportional hazards Markov extension model. We can include a covariate describing the time of the transition

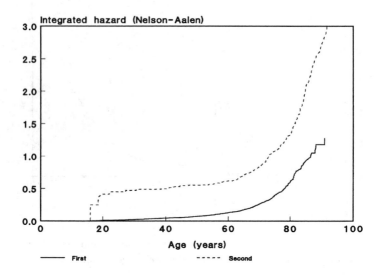

Figure 6.3. Integrated hazard functions for first and second transition in the bivariate symmetric Markov model, for female monozygotic twins.

	$\hat{\beta}$ (SE)	Relative risk (SE)
Males		
MZ	0.57 (0.07)	1.76 (0.13)
DZ	0.25 (0.06)	1.29 (0.07)
UZ	0.71 (0.13)	2.04 (0.27)
Females		
MZ	0.52 (0.08)	1.68 (0.14)
DZ	0.36 (0.06)	1.43 (0.09)
UZ	0.48 (0.12)	1.62 (0.19)

Table 6.5. Estimates of regression coefficients and the relative risk ($\exp(\hat{\beta})$) in the proportional hazards Markov model applied to Danish twin data.

	$\hat{\beta}$ (SE) %/year
Males	
MZ	0.47 (0.37)
DZ	0.05 (0.26)
UZ	0.08 (0.74)
Females	
MZ	0.77 (0.41)
DZ	0.36 (0.27)
UZ	0.69 (0.56)

Table 6.6. Estimates of the coefficient to age at partner's death in the Cox proportional hazards Markov extension model for the second transition for the Danish twin data.

Covariates	c	c, t	$c, t - t_1$	c, t_1	$c, t_1, t - t_1$
Males					
MZ	29.20	29.23	30.13	30.09	30.18
DZ	10.15	12.69	10.21	10.45	12.71
UZ	13.87	14.58	13.88	14.07	14.58
Females					
MZ	19.65	19.65	21.69	21.19	21.69
DZ	17.91	18.35	18.95	18.25	19.30
UZ	8.13	9.40	9.12	8.17	10.27
Sum	98.90	103.89	103.99	102.22	108.73

Table 6.7. Log likelihood values for five models applied to Danish twin data, compared to independence.

into the second state. This is mathematically identical to include the duration in the state, as was demonstrated in Equation (2.44). The estimates are described in Table 6.6 separately for each sex and zygosity group (MZ, monozygotic; DZ, dizygotic; and UZ, unknown zygosity). All estimates are positive, suggesting short-term dependence, but none of them are significantly differently from 0.

In order to evaluate how the relative risk develops over time, we have examined more detailed models for the relation between the first and the second transition. In our terminology, we want to find out whether the risk is of short-term or long-term time frame, under a parametric relation between $\lambda(t)$ and $\mu(t, t_1)$. Table 6.7 gives the maximized log likelihood values for various models. These are normalized, compared to independence, so that no effects of the covariates correspond to a 0 value of the log likelihood. The first two columns are Markov models. The three-parameter model in the last column includes all the two-parameter models, owing to the linear relation between age, age at death of partner death, and time since death

	Indicator $\hat{\beta}(\text{SE})$	t_1 $\hat{\beta}(\text{SE})$ %/year	$t - t_1$ $\hat{\beta}(\text{SE})$ %/year
Males			
MZ	0.52 (0.44)	−0.19 (0.64)	−0.31 (0.73)
DZ	0.94 (0.30)	−1.02 (0.44)	−1.07 (0.49)
UZ	1.39 (0.57)	−1.03 (0.85)	−1.12 (1.11)
Females			
MZ	0.63 (0.48)	0.02 (0.67)	−0.78 (0.77)
DZ	0.69 (0.32)	−0.39 (0.46)	−0.76 (0.52)
UZ	1.35 (0.49)	−1.14 (0.73)	−1.86 (0.89)

Table 6.8. Estimates of regression coefficients in a three-parameter model for the relative risk after death of partner applied to Danish twin data.

of partner. This model does not fit better than the other models, evaluated by a likelihood ratio test for the sum over the six data sets. The estimates in the most general model are given in Table 6.8. One way to illustrate these numbers is as a life history model. That is, the ratio of the hazard when the partner is dead to that when the partner is alive, $\mu(t, t_1)/\lambda(t)$ is evaluated for various values of t_1 and considered for $t > t_1$. This has the interpretation that the person stays on the baseline as long as the partner is alive and then follows his curve after death of the partner. This is shown in Figure 6.4. The values are above 1, corresponding to a positive dependence between the lifetimes. An alternative consideration is needed in order to discuss whether the dependence is of short or long-term time frame. Then we need curves for each value of t, as a function of age at partner's death t_1. This is done in Figure 6.5. The estimates suggest that the dependence is of a short-term nature, because each curve increases as a function of the age at the time of death of the partner. But as shown above, the model is not significantly better than the Markov model, which by definition shows long-term dependence.

Whether the model has the highest dependence early or late, as discussed in Section 3.2.1, is considered in the Markov model, that is, the model including the indicator describing status of the partner and current age t as covariates after the death of the partner. This gives a hazard model of $\lambda(t)$, when the partner is alive, and $\mu(t) = \lambda(t)\exp(\beta_1 + \beta_2 t)$, when the partner has died before time t. The estimates are given in Table 6.9. For the monozygotic twins of both sexes, the coefficients to t are so close to 0 that we conclude that the relative risk is constant. For the other groups, negative coefficients are obtained, leading to decreasing relative risk by age, that is, a high early dependence.

It is also possible to include other covariates, the most natural in this case being the birth year. If this is included together with the indicator for death of partner, the results of Table 6.10 are obtained. By comparison to

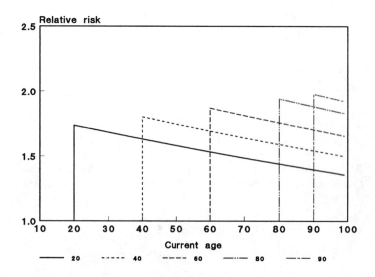

Figure 6.4. Relative hazards $\mu(t, t_1)/\lambda(t)$ as function of t, for various values (20, 40, 60, 80 and 90 years) of age at partners death t_1. Based on Danish twins data.

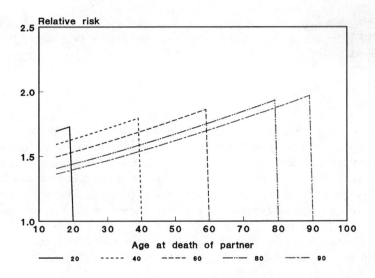

Figure 6.5. Relative hazards $\mu(t, t_1)/\lambda(t)$ as function of age at partners death t_1, for various values (20, 40, 60, 80 and 90 years) of current age t. Based on Danish twins data.

	Indicator $\hat{\beta}$(SE)	t $\hat{\beta}$(SE) (%/year)
Males		
MZ	0.47 (0.44)	0.15 (0.64)
DZ	0.93 (0.30)	−1.03 (0.44)
UZ	1.38 (0.56)	−1.04(0.85)
Females		
MZ	0.55 (0.48)	−0.04 (0.68)
DZ	0.66 (0.32)	−0.43 (0.46)
UZ	1.28 (0.49)	−1.21 (0.73)

Table 6.9. Estimates of regression coefficients in a two-parameter Markov model for the relative risk after death of a partner applied to Danish twin data.

	Indicator $\hat{\beta}$(SE)	Birth year $\hat{\beta}$(SE) (% /year)
Males		
MZ	0.54 (0.07)	−1.56 (0.31)
DZ	0.23 (0.06)	−1.58 (0.22)
UZ	0.70 (0.13)	0.64 (0.50)
Females		
MZ	0.48 (0.08)	−2.48 (0.33)
DZ	0.31 (0.06)	−2.49 (0.23)
UZ	0.48 (0.12)	−0.34 (0.42)

Table 6.10. Estimates of regression coefficients in a two-parameter model, including a relative risk after death of a partner and the birth year applied to Danish twin data.

Table 6.5, it is seen that the influence of the death of a partner is slightly reduced. This is because the relative risk of a partner's death measures dependence and one cause for dependence is the birth year, as mortality decreases with calendar time. Such an analysis is much more suited for a frailty model, see Section 8.12.5. The mortality decreases with year of birth, as seen in the general population. The rate of decrease seems to depend on sex and not on zygosity.

In conclusion, we have found dependence between the lifetimes of twins, which can be described by means of the proportional hazards Markov model. The dependence is higher for monozygotic twins than for dizygotic twins. Regarding year of birth, we find that there is a decreasing mortality trend over time and that when this factor is accounted for, the dependence within pairs is reduced but is still significant.

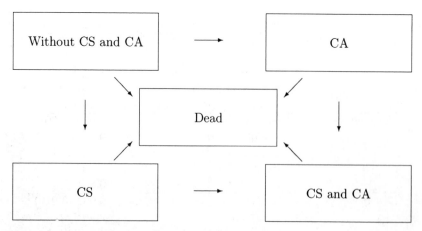

Figure 6.6. Myocardial infarction complication model. CS=cardiogenic shock, CA=cardiac arrest.

6.7.3 Myocardial infarctions

For the data on patients with myocardial infarction (Section 1.9.3), the purpose was to evaluate the risk of death or severe complications (cardiac arrest and cardiogenic shock), in order to discharge low-risk patients early. In our terminology of purposes, this is prediction. This was done by means of the model of the form shown in Figure 6.6. The estimates are described in Table 6.11. The risk of death after cardiogenic shock was so high (more than 90 % within 44 days) that early discharge should not be considered and therefore mortality after cardiogenic shock was not considered further. The age effect for the hazard of death is similar to the effect for people in general. For cardiac arrest and cardiogenic shock, the age effect is much lower. Heart failure is a complication diagnosed within the first five days, leading to a markedly increased risk. Asystole is a subtype of cardiac arrest, leading to a higher risk than for ventricular fibrillation, the other subtype. The coding of this complication for death means that a ventricular fibrillation leads to an increase by a factor of $e^{2.7} = 15$, whereas an asystole (with or without simultaneous presence of ventricular fibrillation) leads to an increase by a factor of $e^{2.7+0.7} = 30$. Supraventricular tachycardia, extension of MI, ventricular premature beats, and nodal rhythm are time-dependent variables not controlled by the state structure.

The desired discharge criterion used for considering whether the patient could be discharged is that the probability of death, cardiogenic shock, or cardiac arrest within 14 days from the current day should be below some given threshold. Thresholds examined were 2 % and 5 %. A problem was that only the time of the first cardiogenic shock and the first cardiac arrest was recorded. Patients having experienced a cardiac arrest are known to have a high risk of future cardiac arrests. For these patients, it was necessary to make some assumptions and the assumption was made in the

Endpoint	Variable	$\hat{\beta}$ (SE)
Cardiac arrest	Age (years)	0.010 (0.007)
	Heart failure	2.2 (0.4)
	Supraventricular tachycardia	1.0 (0.3)
	Extension of MI	1.0 (0.5)
	Ventricular premature beats	0.9 (0.2)
Cardiogenic shock	Age (years)	0.028 (0.007)
	No. of Previous MI	0.22 (0.07)
	Cardiac arrest	1.22 (0.17)
	Heart failure	3.3 (1.0)
	Nodal rhythm	0.8 (0.3)
Death	Age (years)	0.082 (0.010)
	Heart failure	2.3 (0.6)
	Cardiac arrest	2.7 (0.2)
	Asystole	0.7 (0.3)

Table 6.11. Estimates for myocardial infarction data. Age is measured in years, whereas all other variables are time-dependent 0-1 variables describing whether the complication has happened before the current time.

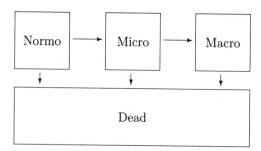

Figure 6.7. Albuminuria model with mortality.

prediction phase that the hazard of a future cardiac arrest was unchanged by experiencing an arrest. Typically, such patients would have a risk above the threshold, owing to their increased risk of cardiogenic shock and death. For patients experiencing a cardiogenic shock, we had, in principle, the same problem, but this factor was so important for future death that it was unnecessary to perform the calculation; their risk was clearly above the threshold. Reporting the effect of the prediction-based discharge is outside the scope of this book, so the reader is referred to Hougaard and Madsen (1985).

6.7.4 Albuminuria progression

This is an example of a state structure that is not among the six standard structures. We want to analyze the data set of Section 1.9.1 both regard-

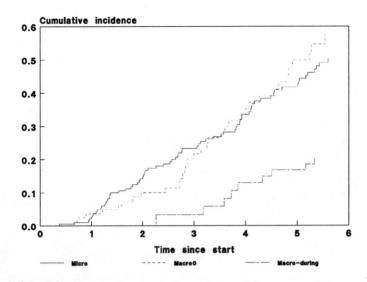

Figure 6.8. Estimate of integrated albuminuria progression hazards, based on Nelson-Aalen estimates, solid: microalbuminuria, dashed: macroalbuminuria (patients with microalbuminuria at baseline), dot-dashed: macroalbuminuria (patients turning microalbuminuric during the study).

ing mortality and albuminuria progression as illustrated by the model of Figure 1.6. That gives the model of Figure 6.7, which can alternatively be considered an extension of the disability model, with two progressive degrees of disability. First, we study the albuminuria progression using the time scale of time since the baseline measurement. As this does not involve the hazard of death, this analysis is identical to an analysis in the model of Figure 1.6, letting death lead to censoring. This is an application of the principle that when a model only involves a subset of the transitions, other transitions can be neglected in the likelihood function. In particular, when the other transitions are to an absorbing state, the observations can be regarded as censorings. Without covariates, we can model the transition hazard from normoalbuminuria to microalbuminuria as $\psi(t)$. The transition hazard from microalbuminuria to macroalbuminuria, say, $\mu(t)$, can be modeled as a Markov model or as a non-Markov model. As the data are really interval censored, it is difficult to make a detailed model and, therefore, only a simple non-Markov model is studied here. For model checking we may use the fact that it is possible to estimate this hazard, based on the patients being in the microalbuminuria state at baseline and based on the patients entering microalbuminuria during the follow-up period. The latter presents left truncated data. In a Markov model these are just two esti-

Variable	$\hat{\beta}$ (SE)	p
Age (years)	0.033 (0.015)	< 0.05
Diabetic retinopathy	0.62 (0.25)	< 0.02
Albumin (log base 10)	1.47 (0.40)	< 0.001

Table 6.12. Estimates of regression coefficients for progression from normoalbuminuria to microalbuminuria.

Variable	$\hat{\beta}$ (SE)	p
Age (years)	0.083 (0.022)	< 0.001
Micro	0.77 (0.35)	< 0.05
Macro	1.54 (0.34)	< 0.0001

Table 6.13. Estimates of regression coefficients for death according to time on study, using albuminuria state at baseline.

mates of the same quantity, based on different patients and therefore they should agree. All three hazards are shown in Figure 6.8. The two macroalbuminuria hazard functions can quantitatively be compared by a proportional hazards model including left truncation. The regression coefficient for those that become microalbuminuric during the study is -0.94 (0.39), which implies a relative risk of 0.39 compared to those that were microalbuminuric at the start of the study. The conclusion is that the process is not Markov. It makes no sense to compare the hazard of microalbuminuria with that of macroalbuminuria, as the events are different.

Covariates can be included in these models in the usual way. If we include age, presence of diabetic retinopathy and the log (base 10) of albumin, in all cases using the value at start, the results described in Table 6.12 are obtained. The high effect of albumin also illustrates that the multi-state model is not Markov. This is, in fact, not surprising, because albumin is a continuous variable and modeling it as a multi-state model implies grouping the value. If the process of albumin as a continuous variable is Markov, we cannot expect that the process obtained by grouping will be Markov.

Similarly, the mortality can be studied. The typical medical application would consider the mortality according to time since the baseline examination and with (constant) covariates describing the albuminuria state at baseline. The estimates are described in Table 6.13. However, in the multi-state model, it makes more sense to use time-dependent covariates, describing the current albuminuria state. This, in fact, corresponds to assuming proportional hazards for the three death hazards in Figure 6.7. The estimates are described in Table 6.14. The estimates are roughly comparable to the previous, although there is no longer a significant difference between normo- and microalbuminuria.

It is debatable whether time since baseline is such an important variable that it deserves non-parametric modeling, in particular, when the covariate is updated according to the albuminuria development. Alternatively, we

Variable	$\hat{\beta}$ (SE)	p
Age (years)	0.080 (0.022)	< 0.001
Micro	0.50 (0.39)	0.20
Macro	1.41 (0.36)	< 0.0001

Table 6.14. Estimates of regression coefficients for death according to time since baseline, using time-dependent covariates describing the current albuminuria state.

Variable	$\hat{\beta}$ (SE)	p
Micro	0.80 (0.35)	< 0.05
Macro	1.66 (0.35)	< 0.0001

Table 6.15. Estimates of regression coefficients for death according to age, using time-dependent covariates describing the current albuminuria state.

can let age be the variable given a non-parametric hazard model, again assuming proportional hazards for the albuminuria state. This is again analyzed by time-dependent covariates. The estimates are given in Table 6.15. It is no longer possible simply to quote the effect of age. In order to examine this effect, one must consider the integrated hazard function. This is a simpler model in the sense that time on study is no longer influential. To examine whether it is acceptable to exclude this variable, one could include it as a time-dependent covariate, or alternatively include age at the start of the study as a constant covariate, following Equation (2.44). This works as a check of the model. In that case, the estimates are given in Table 6.16. The effect of age at baseline is not significant and, therefore, the model of Table 6.15 can be used instead.

This example also serves to illustrate that it is possible and often relevant to have different time scales for the different transitions. For the albuminuria progression hazards, it seems most relevant to use the time the baseline, or the duration as the time with a non-parametric effect on the hazard, and for mortality it seems most relevant to use the age as the time with a non-parametric effect on the hazard.

Variable	$\hat{\beta}$ (SE)	p
Age (at baseline)	-0.01 (0.09)	0.89
Micro	0.54 (0.39)	0.16
Macro	1.52 (0.36)	< 0.0001

Table 6.16. Estimates of regression coefficients for death according to age, using time-dependent covariates describing the current albuminuria state.

6.7.5   Other applications

This section is by no means complete. It lists a few examples, which can serve as further inspiration. Some of these examples do not have full information on all times of transitions.

Kay (1986) is a nice application of cancer markers and shows how far we can get using homogeneous Markov models in a non-progressive state structure.

Hoem (1977) uses an non-homogeneous Markov model for the movement to and from the work force, corresponding to the disability model with reactivation (Figure 5.10).

Klein and Keiding (1989) use a proportional hazards extension of the Marshall and Olkin model for breast cancer metastasis at multiple sites.

Klein, Keiding, and Copelan (1994) calculate various transition probabilities in a non-homogeneous Markov model with four different types of events.

Therneau and Hamilton (1997) study various approaches to recurrent events data.

Aalen *et al.* (1997) study back-calculation. This is a sort of truncated data. In a Markov model for the development of HIV infection and outbreak of AIDS, there is only information on persons getting AIDS. For these persons the time of HIV infection is obtained (and, of course, the time of getting AIDS). By the use of the Markov assumption and various extra assumptions, it is possible to obtain an estimate of the incidence of HIV infection.

Andersen and Green (1985) study the incidence of diabetes among males by the disability model with data describing the status at the conscript examination about age 18-19 years. This is potentially biased due to emigration and differential mortality in the two states. They found that the bias was small in this application.

6.8   Chapter summary

It is generally simple to perform statistical inference in multi-state models. The likelihood function can be evaluated as the hazard evaluated at the times of transition multiplied by the exponential of the integrated hazard experienced during the risk periods. The likelihood can be described as a product over the possible transitions, implying that when there are separate parameters, each transition can be considered separately. Many of the commonly applied models can be fitted simply. In the constant hazards case the estimates are ratios of number of events and times under risk. In the non-parametric case when the hazard functions are either identical or varying separately, this might be done as a Nelson-Aalen estimate with left truncation. In the case where the various transition hazards are assumed to be proportional, this is done by means of the proportional hazards model with time-dependent covariates.

Transition probabilities are somewhat more difficult, but with Markov models with hazard functions varying separately, there is an explicit formula, which seems to be generalizable also to progressive models.

Asymptotic theory is well understood and also allows for process-dependent censoring.

6.9   Bibliographic comments

Hoem (1977) considered the statistical inference in piecewise constant hazards for Markov models. Aalen and Johansen (1978) derived the non-parametric estimate of the transition probabilities in a non-homogeneous Markov model. Andersen et al. (1993) is a key reference to the multi-state models and to the statistical inference and, in particular, the asymptotic evaluations for such models.

Kalbfleisch and Lawless (1985) describe the statistical inference in Markov models, where the state is only known at selected time points.

Tables 6.5, 6.7 and 6.8 first appeared in Hougaard et al. (1992b). A couple of corrections have been made to the tables. Table 6.11 is reproduced from Hougaard and Madsen (1985) with permission.

6.10   Exercises

Exercise 6.1 Competing risks as an exponential family

Consider the competing risks model with k causes of death, constant hazards and without censoring. How can you formulate this model as an exponential family?

Exercise 6.2 Random left truncation

The multi-state model of Figure 5.16 can also be used to evaluate the effect of left truncation in ordinary univariate survival data. Let the bivariate observation (V, T) follow a multi-state Markov model with hazard functions $\lambda_v(t)$, $\lambda_t(t)$, $\mu_v(t)$ and $\mu_t(t)$. Let V and T have the same support. What is the marginal distribution of T? Which of the hazard functions does not contribute to this distribution?

Suppose that if $V > T$ we observe nothing (that is, we do not even know the number of such pairs). If $V < T$, we observe (V, T). Formulate this observation pattern in the multi-state frame.

Describe the likelihood of the observations as $Pr\{V = v, V < T\}Pr\{T = t \mid V = v, V < T\}$. Which hazard functions contribute to which of these terms? Consider $\lambda_v(t)$ and $\mu_v(t)$ as arbitrary nuisance parameters. Is it possible to estimate $\lambda_t(t)$? Is it possible to estimate $\mu_t(t)$?

Now assume that V and T are independent. How can you estimate the marginal distribution of T?

Exercise 6.3 Marshall-Olkin first event

To avoid the iterative estimation procedure, we can restrict our attention to only the time to the first event, with data (T_1, H_1, H_2) for each of n pairs. Here H_1 is defined as $F_1 1\{W_1 = T_1\}$ and similarly for H_2. Find the maximum likelihood estimate of the parameters? What is the asymptotic distribution of the estimate?

Derive the likelihood ratio test for symmetry ($\varphi_1 = \varphi_2$).

Exercise 6.4 Disability model with duration effect

Consider the simple disability model, of Figure 1.5, with Gompertz-like transition hazards. Let t denote the age and v the duration of disability, that is, $v = t - T_1$ in the notation of the text, which, of course, is only considered for $v \geq 0$. Let the hazard of disability be $\beta \varphi^t$, the hazard of death of healthy persons be $\lambda(t) = \psi \gamma^t$, and the hazard of death for a disabled person be $\mu(t, v) = \delta \kappa^t \rho^v$. The observations consist of life histories for n independent individuals, followed from birth to death or to an individual and independent censoring time C_i, where i denotes the individual.

Introduce suitable notation and derive the likelihood function. Find the derivatives of the log likelihood function for all seven parameters and describe how the estimates of ψ, β, and δ can be found, when γ, φ, κ, and ρ are known. Split the parameter vector into the asymptotically independent parameter subsets.

Which restriction makes the model be of Markov type? Describe a test of this hypothesis. Which subset of the persons has an influence on this test?

Another special case of the original model is $\kappa = 1$. What does this hypothesis mean for the underlying disease process? What is the computational simplification in this case?

Consider only the transition from disabled to dead. In order to find initial estimates for the parameters, we first calculate estimates $\hat{\mu}_{jk}$ in age class j and duration class k based on a bivariate piecewise constant hazard model, that is, of the form $D_{.jk}/T_{.jk}$. What is the asymptotic distribution of $\hat{\mu}_{jk}$? What is the asymptotic distribution of $\log \hat{\mu}_{jk}$? How can you use this to find an initial estimate of δ, κ, and ρ? What is the advantage of using the log-scale rather than the original scale?

What would you do in order to evaluate the transition probabilities?

Exercise 6.5 The fertility model with pregnancy periods

Consider first the fertility model, depicted in Figure 1.4, where the hazard of getting a child is $\phi_j(t)$ in age t, when the woman already has $j - 1$ children. Suppose the data consists of independent life histories for n women, followed from birth to age 50. To simplify the notation, consider the process only for $j \leq 5$; that is, a woman is censored when she has the fifth child. Death leads to censoring. Twins are not accounted for. We assume that we do not have knowledge on pregnancy status. Is this model a Markov model, a Markov extension model, or a general model? Introduce suitable notation and describe the likelihood function, under the assumption of identical distributions for all women.

Secondly, we will account for the pregnancy period of about nine months. For mathematical simplicity, let the period length Δ be common and known. The consequence of this is that during a period of length Δ after a birth, the fertility is 0, after which it is as in the first case, that is, $\phi_j(t)$ in age t, when the woman already has $j - 1$ children. Is this model a Markov model, a Markov extension model or a general model? Calculate the transition probability, corresponding to having exactly one child at age t. Describe the likelihood function, under the assumption of identical distributions for all women.

To reduce the number of parameters and to make a powerful test of the hypothesis of the hazard being independent of the parity, we assume proportional hazards $\phi_j(t) = \psi_j\phi(t)$. How would you solve the unidentifiability problem? How would you fit this model by means of a Cox model with time-dependent covariates? What difference does it make for the complexity of the estimation approach whether you do or do not account for the pregnancy period?

Exercise 6.6 Survival of widows and widowers

The aim is to construct a multi-state model to discuss whether a person has increased risk of death after marital bereavement, as discussed in Section 3.3.2. For this exercise, we neglect problems owing to divorces and remarriages. We also neglect the possibility of simultaneous events. To put it into the multi-state framework, we use the state structure of Figure 5.12, measuring time by time since marriage, say, t. Denote the ages of the persons at the time of marriage as a_1 for the husband and a_2 for the wife. First, we assume that the four hazard functions depend only on the current age of the relevant person and vary independently of each other. Does this make a Markov model? Observations are denoted as W_1 (time since marriage for the husband) with death indicator F_1 and similar W_2 and F_2 for the wife. How would you estimate the hazard functions non-parametrically? Which problem is there regarding asymptotic distributions in this case?

Now, assume proportional hazards before and after death of the partner, still allowing for an arbitrary dependence on sex and age. How would you estimate the proportionality factors? Which of the possibilities of Table 6.3 can be modified to handle this model and how should these be modified?

How would you turn this model into one where the risk is more increased immediately after death of the partner than in the long term (there are several possibilities, so you may make a few suggestions)?

Exercise 6.7 Recurrent events with separate first hazard

This describes the statistical analysis of the model described in Exercise 5.4. Suppose all individuals are followed from time 0 to C (common). For each individual, the total number of events K_i is known, and when there are events, the times T_{ij} of events are known. Describe precisely the estimates of ψ and λ by means of T_{ij}, K_i, and C.

Exercise 6.8 Constant hazards models with periods without events

This describes the statistical analysis of the model described in Exercise 5.5. Suppose all individuals are followed from time 0 to C (common). For each individual, the total number of events K_i is known, and when there are events, the times T_{ij} of events are known. Describe precisely the estimate of ϕ by means of T_{ij}, K_i, and C.

Exercise 6.9 Alternating state model

Consider the homogeneous Markov model for alternating states with parameters ψ and ϕ, as described in Section 5.5.6. Suppose we only observe the state at time 1 for n_1 persons starting in state 1 at time 0. Show that it is not possible to identify both parameters from such data.

Suppose then that there are similar observations for n_2 persons starting in state 2. Show that it is possible to identify both parameters from such data. Describe the equations to solve in order to obtain the estimates. Are there data patterns that do not lead to valid estimates of the parameters?

Exercise 6.10 Transition probabilities in the bivariate model

Consider the most general symmetric Markov model for the bivariate multi-state model of Figure 5.12. How can you estimate the transition probabilities by means of the Aalen-Johansen approach, modified to account for the symmetry? How can you estimate the marginal survivor function of a single lifetime in this frame?

Exercise 6.11 The effect of screening

The aim is to study a simple screening model, for example, applicable to cancer screening (see Figure 6.9). Whether a person is in the healthy state or the subclinical state can only be detected by screening, performed by, for example, a blood sample or X-ray. The subclinical state is assumed not

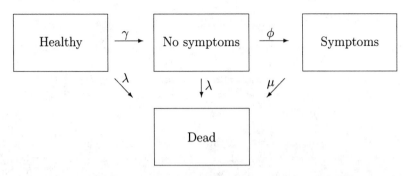

Figure 6.9. Screening model. Symptoms mean clinical disease. No symptoms mean subclinical disease detectable by screening.

to influence the mortality. To study the screening itself, we do not assume that treatment can change the mortality.

Show that the following transition probabilities are correct:

$$P_{11}(v,t) = \exp\{-(\gamma + \lambda)(t - v)\}$$

$$P_{12}(v,t) = \frac{\gamma}{\phi - \gamma}[\exp\{-(\gamma + \lambda)(t - v)\} - \exp\{-(\phi + \lambda)(t - v)\}]$$

$$P_{23}(v,t) = \frac{\phi}{\mu - (\phi + \lambda)}[\exp\{-(\phi + \lambda)(t - v)\} - \exp\{-\mu(t - v)\}].$$

How would you estimate the four parameters based on complete data for n persons starting in the healthy state followed until death or individual censoring times C_i? What is the asymptotic distribution? How would you estimate the asymptotic variance?

Before screening is implemented, this is a hidden state model, meaning that transitions healthy to no symptoms are completely unknown, and possible deaths from the healthy and no symptoms states cannot be discriminated. It is still assumed that all persons start in the healthy state. Is this a Markov model? Derive the transition hazards for the superstates. Derive the likelihood function. How would you estimate λ and μ based on such data? What is the asymptotic distribution, and how would you estimate the asymptotic variance? To which extent can γ and ϕ be identified? Describe a method for estimating the parameter function that can be identified. There is no explicit solution to this problem.

What is the expected residual lifetime for a person entering the state with symptoms? What is the expected residual lifetime for a person whose disease is detected by screening? Compare these two values and discuss what faulty conclusions they can lead to.

Exercise 6.12 Fisher information for some competing risks models

Consider the k-cause constant hazards model for competing risks data. That is, with hazards $\lambda_1, ..., \lambda_k$, respectively. Find the Fisher information of the parameters for an individual without censoring. Find the Fisher information of the parameters for an individual with fixed censoring at time c. Consider now random censoring at time C, which is assumed to follow an exponential distribution with hazard λ_0. Show that the Fisher information in this case can be found by considering the $(k + 1)$-cause competing risks model obtained by considering censoring as an artificial cause of death, but where only the k-dimensional parameter $(\lambda_1, ..., \lambda_k)$ is estimated.

Exercise 6.13 Exact moments for a competing risks model

Consider the two-cause constant hazards model for competing risks data without censoring. That is, with hazards λ_1 and λ_2, respectively. Find the exact mean and variance of $\hat{\lambda}_1$ and $\hat{\lambda}_2$, and the exact covariance in the case of n independent individuals. Show that the two estimates are asymptotically uncorrelated. Hint: Use the independence of T and (D_1, D_2).

Consider now random censoring at time C assumed to follow an exponential distribution with hazard λ_0. Find the exact mean and variance of $\hat{\lambda}_1$ and $\hat{\lambda}_2$, and the exact covariance in the case of n independent individuals, treating censoring as an artificial cause of death like in Exercise 6.12.

Exercise 6.14 Fisher information for a Weibull competing risks model

Consider the k-cause model for competing risks Weibull data without censoring: that is, with hazards $\lambda_1 t^{\gamma_1 - 1}, ..., \lambda_k t^{\gamma_k - 1}$, respectively. Find the Fisher information of the parameters for an individual without censoring and assuming common shape parameters $\gamma_1 = ... = \gamma_k$.

Do you think the assumption of common shape parameters makes sense for cause of death data? Can the Fisher information be evaluated simply without the restriction?

It is tempting to introduce random censoring in the common shape parameter case using a Weibull censoring distribution of the same shape. Why is this unacceptable? Hint: See Section 2.2.

Exercise 6.15 Fisher information for the Freund model

Consider the Freund model of Section 5.5.3 with hazards $\lambda_1, \lambda_2, \mu_1, \mu_2$. Derive the Fisher information about the parameters in the case of no censoring. What is the Fisher information under the hypothesis $\mu_1 = \mu_2$?

Now allow for random process-dependent censoring so that there is hazard ψ of censoring while both are alive and κ, when one individual is alive. Derive the Fisher information about the parameters $(\lambda_1, \lambda_2, \mu_1, \mu_2)$ in this case.

Now, instead assume fixed censoring at time c. For this case, you are allowed to simplify the problem by assuming symmetry, $(\lambda_1 = \lambda_2, \mu_1 = \mu_2)$. Derive the Fisher information.

Building upon the results for fixed censoring, you may derive the Fisher information for random censoring, when you consider a censoring distribution having Laplace transform $L(s)$.

Exercise 6.16 Fisher information for a Weibull extension of the Freund model

Consider the bivariate multi-state semi-Markov Weibull model of Figure 5.12 with hazard $\lambda_j t^{\gamma_j - 1}$ for death of individual j, when both are alive and $\mu_j(t - t_1)^{\kappa_j - 1}$, when individual j is alive $(j = 1, 2)$, but the other individual died at time t_1. Derive the Fisher information about the parameters in the case of no censoring and assuming $\gamma_1 = \gamma_2$.

Exercise 6.17 Exact distributions for the Freund model

Consider the Freund model of Section 5.5.3 with hazards $\lambda_1, \lambda_2, \mu_1, \mu_2$. Assume first that $\mu_1 = \mu_2$. Derive the exact distributions of the parameters in the case of n independent pairs without censoring.

Now, allow for freely varying μ_1, μ_2. Find the exact distribution of $\hat{\mu}_1$, $\hat{\mu}_2$ conditional on $D_{.12}$. There is positive probability that some risk sets are empty and thus μ_1 or μ_2 are undefined. When you have realized this problem, you do not need to account for it in the formulas. Use the result to write the exact density of all estimated parameters as a finite sum.

Now allow for random process-dependent censoring so that there is hazard ψ of censoring while both are alive and κ when one individual is alive. What is the exact density of all estimated parameters in this case?

Exercise 6.18 Fisher information for a piecewise constant hazards extension of the Freund model

The Fisher information can also be evaluated in this case. To illustrate the point without needing a complicated notation, consider the following very simple example. Use the symmetric bivariate multi-state model of Figure 5.12 with first hazard λ. The second hazard is assumed to be piecewise constant, with value μ_1 from time 0 to x_1 and μ_2 after x_1. Derive the Fisher information about the parameters in the case of no censoring.

Exercise 6.19 Bivariate parallel data software

Write SAS programs to fit symmetric bivariate parallel data, with the proportional hazards Markov model, by each of the four approaches described in Section 6.3, from data of the form (W_1, W_2, F_1, F_2).

Exercise 6.20 Disability model

Describe two different approaches to fit mortality data in the proportional hazards Markov model for the disability model, based on time-dependent covariates for data starting at time 0, respectively, as constant covariates for left-truncated data.

Exercise 6.21 Weibull proportional hazards Markov model

Describe how you can fit the bivariate proportional hazards Markov model with $\lambda(t)$ of Weibull form, by means of a procedure that can handle two groups with different λ and common γ in a Weibull model, allowing for truncation. Make such a program.

Exercise 6.22 Gompertz proportional hazards Markov model

Describe how you can fit the bivariate proportional hazards Markov model with $\lambda(t)$ of Gompertz form, using the method developed in Exercise 6.21. Hint: Use Exercise 2.10.

Exercise 6.23 Gompertz Markov model

Describe how you can fit the bivariate Markov model with $\mu(t) = \exp(\beta_1 + \beta_2 t)\lambda(t)$ and $\lambda(t)$ of Gompertz form using a program that can handle a single Gompertz sample, but allowing for left truncation.

Exercise 6.24 Tie handling

Download the twin data and study them in the proportional hazards Markov model using the parallel approach of Table 6.3 and all the options for tie handling that your software allows.

Try recoding the covariate from $1\{t > W_2\}$ to $1\{t \geq W_2\}$. Why does the estimate change, even for datasets, where no pairs with events have $W_1 = W_2$?

Exercise 6.25 Recurrent events model

Describe precisely how you in standard statistical software can fit the recurrent events model of Prentice et al. (1981) described in Section 6.1.3 having a single covariate z_i and observed times $T_{i1}, ..., T_{iK_i}$ within an observation period $(0, C_i)$ for a set of independent individuals $i = 1, ..., n$.

Exercise 6.26 Plotting transition probabilities

Consider the heart transplant data of Section 1.9.4 using the disability model without covariates. Estimate the transition probabilities for a patient being enrolled in the program, in the most general Markov model by means of the Aalen-Johansen estimator, Equation (6.7). Make a figure of the estimate.

7
Shared frailty models

The shared frailty model is a specific kind of the common risks model described in Section 3.1.2. The frailty is the term that describes the common risks, acting as a factor on the hazard function. The approach makes sense both for parallel data and recurrent events data. In this chapter, only parallel data are considered. The results are presented in terms of individuals, which have the same risk in some groups. Recurrent events data will be separately considered in Chapter 9. The shared frailty model is relevant to lifetimes of several individuals, similar organs and repeated measurements. It is not generally relevant for the case of different events. It is a mixture model, because in most cases the common risks are assumed random. The mixture term is the frailty and for this the notation Y will be used. The model assumes that all time observations are independent given the values of the frailties. In other words, it is a conditional independence model. The value of Y is constant over time and common to the individuals in the group and thus is responsible for creating dependence. This is the reason for the word *shared*, although it would be more correct to call the models of this chapter constant shared frailty models. The interpretation of this model is that the between-groups variability (the random variation in Y) leads to different risks for the groups, which then show up as dependence within groups. The approach is a multivariate version of the mixture calculations of Sections 2.2.7 and 2.4.6.

A shared frailty model can be considered as a random effects model with two sources of variation. There is the group variation, described by the random variable Y (the frailty). Secondly, there is the simple (or individual) random variation described by the hazard function, which will be called

$\mu(t)$. It is more difficult to understand this model than normal distribution random effects models, because such models allow for a more symmetric handling of the various sources of variation, that is, both can be described by random variables. Technically, it would be possible to write the lifetime in a frailty model as a function of several random variables, but the formulas can be difficult to interpret. In the special case that the conditional distribution is of Weibull form, the formula becomes reasonably simple.

It is assumed that there is independence between groups (different values of i), and, as described above, dependence between the times for the same value of i, owing to the common value Y_i of Y. Thus Y's having no variation implies independence between the time observations. If Y is not degenerate, there is positive dependence between the times. The number of times (k) in a group is assumed to be known, but as censoring is possible, the actual number of events might be lower than k. This chapter covers both the case where the dependence is the interesting aspect, and the case, where some regression coefficients are the interesting parameters and the dependence is a nuisance. We may not be interested in the dependence by itself, but want to use the approach as a variance reduction technique by making a paired analysis. The typical example of this is a repeated measurements data set. Finally, the approach can be used to evaluate probabilities for certain events, possibly conditional on what has been observed for the group. This is what we call prediction.

The shared frailty model leads to absolutely continuous distributions (when the frailty is strictly positive) and thus cannot describe dependence owing to common events. It is not relevant for event-related dependence, because an event has no influence on the frailty and the other individuals, it only changes the information available on the frailty.

First we consider to which extent Y can be completely unspecified (Section 7.1). This corresponds to letting each group have a parameter giving the risk level for that group. That is, we do not model the random variation. For many purposes, the group parameter will be a nuisance parameter, that is, the parameter is included in order to describe different risk levels for the groups, but we are not particularly interested in the value of the parameter for each single group. This approach corresponds to the paired t-test for normally distributed data. However, the approach does not work for survival data, because we cannot make exact inferences as in the normal distribution model and the asymptotical statistical inference is only correct when the number of observations within the groups (k) tends to infinity. As we consider a fixed k, we cannot base inference on such asymptotic results. In some cases, the problem can be solved by stratification, that is, by not assuming proportional hazards between groups. Another solution to this problem is to assign a distribution to the frailty, that is, to consider the group levels random, the main approach of this chapter. Assuming a random frailty means that we can integrate the frailty out of the expressions and thus evaluate the multivariate distribution of the times. Conceptually, this corresponds to the variance components models for the normal distribution. The dependence structure is conceptually similar to the compound symmetry models for normally distributed data, with one random component besides the random error. General evaluations for such models are considered in Section 7.2. Almost all calculations can be done based on the Laplace transform. The standard assumption about the frailty is that it follows a gamma distribution (Section 7.3). However, the gamma family has some theoretical shortcomings for regression models, which can be avoided by studying positive stable distributions (Section 7.4). Furthermore, by taking a larger family we obtain a better fit (Section 7.5). A main point recommended here is that we should allow for the larger family of distributions, rather than be restricted by the gamma distributions. For heavily censored data, we might not be able to observe a difference in the fit, but the gamma model has the property that the dependence later is estimable from the observed early values. This might be seen as an advantage, but the fact is that we have no information on whether the dependence follows the projected pattern, that is, no information on whether the dependence is early or late, as described in Section 3.2.1. Using a larger family leads to an increased variance for the projected dependence, that is, a variance estimate that better reflects the variability in the basic quantities. The calculations are, of course, more difficult in the larger family, but one purpose of this chapter is to make it easier to perform the necessary calculations. The specific family considered here is the PVF (power variance function) family, which has an extra parameter compared to the gamma family. Some results for these mixture distributions are described in Appendix A. This family includes the gamma, the inverse Gaussian, and the positive stable distributions. The lognormal distribution (Section 7.6), does not allow similar explicit probability results, but has other advantages owing to the simplicity of the normal distributions. Other distributions are considered in Section 7.7. A comparison of the theoretical properties is performed in Section 7.8. Statistical inference is described in Chapter 8.

It is assumed that the frailty term is common to the individuals in a group and constant over time. Various extensions to this will be considered in Chapters 10 and 11. In the bivariate case, the main disadvantage of this model is that it describes long-term dependence. The problem can be illustrated by an extreme example. Suppose in a twin pair, one child is choked in the umbilical cord. In terms of the common risks model, this is the worst that can happen, as it is an event happening immediately after birth. However, in practice, this event is irrelevant for the future risk of the surviving twin. Instead, it appears more sensible to assume that there is a separate dependence for each possible cause of death, leading to short-term dependence. Extensions that create short-term dependence are considered in Chapter 11. Chapter 10 considers multivariate extensions, where different degrees of dependence are present. In particular, Section 10.1 also considers the specific question of comparing the degree of dependence in two bivariate samples.

The parallel data are given in the standard design of Section 1.4.1, that is, time responses of the form $T_{ij}, i = 1, ..., n, j = 1, ..., k$, where i denotes group, and j denotes individual within the group, with a corresponding set of individual failure indicators, $D_{ij}, i = 1, ..., n, j = 1, ..., k$. The number of individuals may vary between the groups, but as most formulas are given for single groups, there is no need to include this feature in the notation. Censoring is arbitrary, that is, not restricted to be homogeneous. The simplest case is when censoring times are independent of the failure times, but some cases of process-dependent censoring are also acceptable.

7.1   Unspecified frailty

The aim of the analysis described in this section is to estimate the effect of covariates, allowing for group differences in survival, but requiring as few assumptions as possible on the group differences. This approach is relevant when the problem is to examine the effect of covariates that vary between the individuals in a group, like the matched pairs covariates. The most natural example is a repeated measurements study or a drug trial with matched pairs. The latter is a trial where sets of two individuals are created on the basis of common values of some explanatory variables, and then the members of the pair are assigned one to each of the two treatments to compare. A major purpose of this design is to create balance regarding risk factors and to reduce response variability by making a paired analysis. Pairing is done by their values of key factors, in particular risk factors that are not easy to assign relevant numeric values, for example, geography or families. One such example is the tumorigenesis experiment of Section 1.5.3, which was, in fact, not based on pairs but included three members from each litter, of which one was given the experimental treatment and the two other served as controls. When risk factors are more easily quantifiable, like age, or there are just a few well-known groups, like sex, or center in a multi-center drug trial, it makes more sense not to match the individuals, but instead model the dependence on these explanatory factors, for example, by means of a proportional hazards model.

A standard approach used for the normal distribution linear models for matched pairs is to include the groups as a factor in the model, and then analyze the treatment effect in a two-way additive model, which in the paired case corresponds to perform the paired t-test of the treatment effect. The same approach is technically easy to do in the survival data proportional hazards model. The immediate suggestion is to include the group factor as a regression variable, that is, define $z_2, ..., z_n$ as indicator functions for the $n - 1$ last groups, and include them in the model, together with z_1, the indicator of treatment. Group 1 has been excluded as a covariate, because the corresponding parameter acts as a scale parameter and there already is a hazard scale parameter in the model owing to the completely general hazard function. This is then studied as a standard Cox model. As the covariates are 0 in most cases, we explicitly describe the assumed hazard in each. The hazard for an individual with treatment variable z_1 is $\lambda_0(t) \exp(\beta_1 z_1)$ in group 1, and

$$\lambda_0(t) \exp(\beta_1 z_1 + \xi_i) \tag{7.1}$$

in group $i, i = 2, ..., n$. The parameters ξ could also have been denoted as β, but a different symbol is used in order to avoid confusion between the interesting parameter β and the nuisance parameters $\xi_2, ..., \xi_n$. It was found by Holt and Prentice (1974) that this should not be done by including the group factor as regression variables as in Equation (7.1), but as stratas. Thus, the model should say

$$\lambda_{0i}(t) \exp(\beta_1 z_1)$$

for $i = 1, ..., n$. The argument for using stratification was based on invariance, but another argument could be asymptotics. In order for the asymptotic calculations to be correct in the regression case (Equation (7.1)), the number of individuals in each group (k) must tend to ∞. This problem is also present in the normal distribution case, but there we can make exact calculations (using the right sums of squared deviations and the degrees of freedom) rather than make use of the asymptotic calculations, for precisely this reason. In the survival case, we do not have corresponding exact calculations. If, stratification is used instead, the contribution from each pair reduces to a term depending on whether the treated individual dies first or last, which is a more drastic reduction than the difference within pairs done in the paired linear case, but it serves the same purpose, to avoid the problem of the asymptotics.

Some pairs contain no information on the treatment effect, namely, if the first observed time corresponds to a censoring.

When there are just a few groups, which could be the case in a multi-center drug trials with just a few centers, it can be possible to justify the use of asymptotic results for $k \to \infty$.

The disadvantages of this approach are first that it is designed to examine the effect of variables that vary within pairs, and very often, it is also interesting to examine the effect of variables common within the pairs. It may be difficult or impossible to examine such effects. This includes that it is impossible to quantify the strata differences (the dependence within strata) and it is impossible to make predictions. The second disadvantage is that the stratified approach implies a loss of resources, making it more difficult to obtain a large number of individuals. For example, in the litter-matched study of Section 1.5.3, litters of only one and two rats cannot be used for the experiments, and for litters of more than three, only three of them can be used. Or for the leukemia data of Section 1.5.4, the pairs are matched according to the hospital they are treated at and whether their remission is partial or complete. If a hospital has an odd number of patients in a given remission group, they cannot all participate in the trial. The third disadvantage is that there is a loss of information. If one individual is censored very early, the pair is considered uninformative, whereas if there were a model for the influence of the variables used for the matching, it would have contained some information. Similarly, the information on whether there is short time or long time in between the events in pairs with two events cannot be used, because the short time could be due to a steeply increasing hazard in that stratum. In the case where the matching was done on simple explanatory variables, like sex, age, or remission status, we could instead have included all the covariates in a proportional hazards model and in the case of complicated variables, like hospitals or litters, we could make a model for the random variability between groups as will be done next.

Only a few of the data sets considered here allow for making a stratified model because the approach only works for covariates that vary within groups. The tumorigenesis data of Section 1.5.3 are considered in Section 8.12.1, the exercise test times of Section 1.8.2 are considered in Section 8.12.2, and the leukemia data of Section 1.5.4 are considered in Section 8.12.6.

7.2   General probability results

The general shared frailty model can be considered as a modification of the model of the previous section. Instead of having a parameter ξ_i for the ith group, this quantity is considered as a random variable. This implies a different interpretation. With a random group level, we are not interested in each group as such, but we consider the groups as representing a population, for example, a population of litters. This is a typical common risks model. The parameters of the distribution of ξ_i are then the interesting parameters as they describe the general variation between litters. For making the formulas more readable, it is an advantage to exponentiate the quantity and to emphasize that it is a random variable; we denote the quantity by an upper case letter, Y. Thus, the relation is $Y_i = \exp(\xi_i)$. It is then assumed that conditionally on the value of the frailty Y_i, the individuals in the ith group have independent lifetimes, as in the unspecified frailty case. The main difference from the preceding section is the conceptual exchange of the parameter ξ_i by a random variable. In particular, it becomes easier to quantify the differences between groups, which is almost impossible in the stratified analysis and it becomes possible to predict the responses for other individuals (both in the groups in the study and in future groups).

The second difference is that more general regression covariates can be included, as we can now (besides the matched pairs covariates) study common covariates and examine whether they are the underlying causes of the group differences. That is, testing the hypothesis that the responses are independent when these covariates are accounted for. A third, more technical, difference is that it is necessary to solve the unidentifiability problem in a different way. In the unspecified frailty case, we measure all relative risks in relation to a chosen group. Above, group number 1 was the chosen group, which was done by defining $\xi_1 = 0$, or in practice by not having a covariate corresponding to that group. We cannot do that in a random model, because we require the groups to be independent. Instead, the scale parameter of the distribution of Y must be fixed in some way. The problem is that we cannot identify the parameters if there is a scale factor in the hazard function and one in the distribution of relative risks, Y_i. One possibility is to consider a hazard function without a scale parameter, but this is only possible in some cases. This was the approach used in Section 2.2.7. A second possibility is to start by fixing the scale parameter in the distribution of Y, and this solution is the most common in the literature. Here the standard solution is an extension of this approach, first to make the probability evaluations with scale parameters in both terms, and, when necessary for statistical estimation, to fix the scale in some way. The reason for doing so is that some probability calculations become more transparent, in particular when considering truncation, successive conditioning over time and updating. The disadvantage of this approach is that we will need more components in the parameter vector and sometimes several sets of parameters. When the mean exists, we will choose the restriction that $EY = 1$, but we will also consider models with infinite mean. As far as possible, the group index i is neglected in the formulas to simplify the expressions.

7.2.1   The conditional parametrization

This model is a common risks model and is derived conditionally on the shared frailty Y. Only a single group is considered and thus the group index i is omitted. In this section we derive the quantities based on this conditional formulation. Conditionally on Y, the hazard function for individual j is assumed to be of the form

$$Y\mu_j(t). \tag{7.2}$$

This is similar to the calculations of Section 2.2.7, except that here we will also allow arbitrary (non-parametric) expressions for the conditional hazard $\mu_j(t)$, and that the value of Y is common to several individuals in a group. Independence of the lifetimes corresponds to no variability in the distribution of Y, that is, when Y has a degenerate distribution. When the distribution is not degenerate, the dependence is positive. In a few cases, the model can be extended to allow for negative dependence (see for example, Section 7.3.3). The value of Y can be considered as just some value applicable to the group, or as generated from unknown values of some explanatory variables (see Section 2.4.6). Then, by an argument similar to Equation (2.18), we can find the multivariate survival function, $S(t_1, t_2) = P(T_1 > t_1, T_2 > t_2)$. For simplicity of the formula, we first make the bivariate derivation. Conditional on Y, the bivariate survival function is

$$S(t_1, t_2 \mid Y) = \exp[-Y\{M_1(t_1) + M_2(t_2)\}], \qquad (7.3)$$

where $M_j(t) = \int_0^t \mu_j(u)du$, $j = 1, 2$ are the integrated conditional hazards. From this, we immediately derive the bivariate survival function by integrating Y out

$$S(t_1, t_2) = E\exp[-Y\{M_1(t_1) + M_2(t_2)\}] = L(M_1(t_1) + M_2(t_2)), \quad (7.4)$$

where $L(s)$ is the Laplace transform of the distribution of Y. Thus, the bivariate survivor function is easily expressed by means of the Laplace transform of the frailty distribution, evaluated at the total integrated conditional hazard. Letting $M.(t_1, ..., t_k) = \sum_{j=1}^{k} M_j(t_j)$, the multivariate expression for k observations is

$$S(t_1, ..., t_k) = L(M.(t_1, ..., t_k)). \qquad (7.5)$$

From this, the density is immediately derived by differentiation with respect to $t_1, ..., t_k$, giving

$$(-1)^k \{\prod_{j=1}^{k} \mu_j(t_j)\} L^{(k)}(M.(t_1, ..., t_k)).$$

For handling the likelihood of actual observations, we will also need combinations corresponding to observing some exact times T_j with event indicator $D_j = 1$, and some censorings T_j with event indicator $D_j = 0$. For this to be valid, it is necessary to assume that censoring takes place independent of Y. To derive this expression we should find the derivatives only with respect to the times for the coordinates showing exact observations, and change sign $D. = \sum D_j$ times, to give

$$(-1)^{D.} \{\prod_{j=1}^{k} \mu_j(t_j)^{D_j}\} L^{(D.)}(M.(t_1, ..., t_k)). \qquad (7.6)$$

This expression goes directly into the likelihood and has a very strong interpretation; it includes the hazard function for the actual events and the Laplace transform evaluated at the total integrated conditional hazard and differentiated as many times as there are events. In particular, the censored individuals contribute only to the $M.$-term.

Regarding the hazard functions $\mu_j(t)$, various choices will be considered. The simplest is symmetry $\mu_j(t) = \mu(t)$; that is, all hazards are equal. Another is that they are unrelated; that is, each $\mu_j(t)$ has a separate set of parameters, or is arbitrary, independently of the other. Finally, there is a proportional hazards compromise, $\mu_j(t) = \rho_j\mu_0(t)$, where the $\rho_j, j = 1, ..., k$ are a set of parameters. It might be convenient to let $\rho_1 = 1$, to resolve the identifiability issue. This model corresponds to the matched pairs covariates, discussed below in Section 7.2.7. Finally, it can be a proportional hazards regression model, with $\mu_j(t) = \exp(\beta'z_j)\mu_0(t)$.

The various choices of frailty distributions give us some freedom as to what the multivariate distribution looks like. This will be illustrated and discussed later in Section 7.8 and in Chapter 10.

7.2.2 The marginal parametrization

As an alternative, all formulas can be expressed by means of the marginal distributions. It will, in some cases, be convenient to parametrize in this way. A major advantage is that there is an approximate orthogonality between the parameters, so it is easier to estimate the quantities. Furthermore, the standard error found by not accounting for the variability of the estimate of the marginal distribution is a good approximation to the correct standard error.

This can be done by means of the marginal survivor functions $S_j(t) = Pr(T_j > t)$, defined by $S_1(t) = S(t, 0)$ and $S_2(t) = S(0, t)$, or the model may be based on the marginal hazard function, that is, the hazard in the marginal distribution. These are denoted $\omega_j(t)$, with integrated hazard $\Omega_j(t)$, and, of course, satisfying the usual expression $S_j(t) = \exp\{-\Omega_j(t)\}$. From the relation

$$S_j(t) = L(M_j(t)), \tag{7.7}$$

it is found that $M_j(t) = L^{-1}(S_j(t))$. The bivariate survival function corresponding to Equation (7.4) is

$$S(t_1, t_2) = L(L^{-1}(S_1(t_1)) + L^{-1}(S_2(t_2))). \tag{7.8}$$

The multivariate version of this formula is

$$S(t_1, ..., t_k) = L[\sum_j L^{-1}(S_j(t_j))].$$

The same expression formulated by the marginal integrated hazard functions is, in the multivariate case,

$$S(t_1, ..., t_k) = L[\sum_j L^{-1}(\exp\{-\Omega_j(t_j)\})]. \tag{7.9}$$

This expression can be differentiated to give the multivariate density, utilizing that for a function $df^{-1}(x)/dx = 1/(df/dy)|_{y=f^{-1}(x)}$; that is, the derivative of an inverse function is the reciprocal of the derivative of the function, evaluated at the corresponding point. For ease of notation, the expression above is written as $(f^{-1})'(x) = 1/f'(f^{-1}(x))$. This gives a multivariate density of

$$f(t_1, ..., t_k) =$$

$$\{\prod_j [\omega_j(t_j)S_j(t_j)/L'(L^{-1}(S_j(t_j)))]\}L^{(k)}[\sum_j L^{-1}(S_j(t_j))]. \qquad (7.10)$$

If there is a scale parameter for the distribution of Y, it will disappear by this operation, that is, cancel out of the calculations in Equations (7.8), (7.9), and (7.10). This can be considered as an automatic solution to the scale unidentifiability problem. The censored version of Equation (7.10) is a likelihood contribution, which apart from a constant factor is

$$(\prod_j [\omega_j(T_j)S_j(T_j)/L'(L^{-1}(S_j(T_j)))]^{D_j})L^{(D.)}[\sum_j L^{-1}(S_j(T_j))]. \qquad (7.11)$$

A related result, which will be useful for the derivation of the estimate in practice, is that if the times are transformed by an increasing differentiable function, say, U=g(T), the expression in Equation (7.6) and (7.11) is only modified by multiplication with $\prod\{g'(T_j)\}^{-D_j}$. In particular, the Laplace transform term is unchanged. This implies that it is acceptable to make a time transformation before estimating the parameters of the frailty distribution. One of the estimation methods is based on this approach, using a transformation based on the integrated marginal hazard function.

7.2.3   Updating

After having observed some events and some time periods without events, we know more about Y. This is due to high-risk group's probably having experienced some events, whereas low-risk groups have experienced no or a few events. Then, it is possible to evaluate the conditional distribution of Y given the observed quantities. That is, we can update the distribution, based on the information accumulated since start of the study. In fact, this can have several purposes. As in the univariate case, it can be used to consider the effect of truncation. If we use some specific family of the distributions at the time of birth, is the same family applicable if data are truncated? It can be used for evaluating conditional distributions; so it is the relevant theory if the purpose is to make individual predictions. Finally, some estimation methods (like that of Section 8.3) will make use of these formulas in order to find the expected value of the frailty for each group giving everything that is observed for that group.

In a bivariate model, the conditional distributions are interesting to study. Owing to the conditional independence in a frailty model, there is no direct dependence between the times, or in other words, in order to evaluate the conditional distribution of T_2 given T_1, we can, instead of considering the bivariate distribution of (T_1, T_2), evaluate the conditional distribution of Y given T_1, and then use this distribution as frailty distribution for T_2. This can be done both when T_1 is known precisely, but it can also be done at each time point, that is, knowing that $T_1 > t_1$. This can be studied in a dynamic fashion, and therefore, we denote this as updating, describing that the conditional distribution of T_2 is updated according to the available information regarding T_1. One point to emphasize is that the frailty value for a group is unchanged over time; the only quantity that changes is the information we have on the value.

First, the case of no observed events is considered. This corresponds to the distribution of Y after multivariate truncation, but it will also be denoted selection. The latter term reflects that the high-risk groups are more probable to have events, and thus be removed from the set of groups we consider. So, conditioning on no events is a procedure that selects the low-risk groups. The survivor function given Y is $\exp[-Y\{\sum_j M_j(t_j)\}]$. This should be multiplied with the density of Y at a given point y, say, $g(y)$, and divided by the multivariate version of the marginal expression for the survival function for the times, Equation (7.5), to give the conditional density of Y given survival to time $(t_1, ..., t_k)$

$$\exp\{-y \sum_j M_j(t_j)\}g(y)/L(\sum_j M_j(t_j)).$$

By defining $\theta = \sum_j M_j(t_j)$, this is seen to be of the form

$$\exp(-\theta y)g(y)/ \int_0^\infty \exp(-\theta s)g(s)ds, \tag{7.12}$$

which is a member of the natural exponential family generated by $g(y)$ (see Appendix A). In other words, if the family of distributions for Y is a natural exponential family, the frailty distribution among the survivors is another member of the family. The canonical parameter is changed by the total integrated hazards experienced for the family. An alternative expression for the denominator in Equation (7.12) is $L(\theta)$. The updating formula is particularly relevant for truncation, because it implies that if the frailty distribution at birth is a member of a given natural exponential family, it is acceptable to truncate, that is, condition on all members of the group being alive at certain time point, and the frailty distribution will still be a member of the same exponential family. In fact, the same is true if the conditioning is done at different time points for the members. The only problem there could be with different conditioning times is whether the parameters of the frailty distribution are the same for all groups. That is, if each group has different times of updating or different covariates, the parameters of the truncated distributions will generally be different.

In the general case, updating with both events and censorings, we need the conditional density of the observations given Y. At time t, the information available is $D_j(t) = D_j 1\{T_j < t\}$ and letting $t_j = \min(t, T_j)$, the density for Y at y is

$$(-1)^{D.(t)} y^{D.(t)} \{ \prod_{j=1}^{k} \mu_j(t_j)^{D_j(t)} \} \exp\{-y M.(t_1, ..., t_k)\}.$$

This should be multiplied by $g(y)$, and divided by the expression in Equation (7.6), which gives

$$\exp(-\theta y) g(y) y^{D.(t)} / \int_0^\infty \exp(-\theta s) g(s) s^{D.(t)} ds.$$

By defining $\zeta = D.(t)$, this can be given the alternative formulation

$$\exp(-\theta y + \zeta \log y) g(y) / \int_0^\infty \exp(-\theta u + \zeta \log u) g(u) du, \qquad (7.13)$$

which shows that this distribution is a member of the exponential family with canonical statistics y and $\log y$ generated from the distribution of Y. In other words, if the family of distributions for Y is a natural exponential family with canonical statistics y and $\log y$, this is another member of the family, with θ increased by the integrated hazard and ζ increased by the observed number of events. An alternative version of the denominator of Equation (7.13) is the Laplace transform derivative $(-1)^\zeta L^{(\zeta)}(\theta)$. The Laplace transform of the updated distribution is

$$L^{(\zeta)}(\theta + s) / L^{(\zeta)}(\theta). \qquad (7.14)$$

An alternative approach is the dynamic evaluation, where the hazard at each instant is calculated on the basis of all the information known at that time, like Equation (5.1). Under this approach, the hazard of death for the jth individual given he is alive at time t is

$$\lambda_j(t \mid F_t) = \mu_j(t) E(Y \mid F_t). \qquad (7.15)$$

This is a generalization of Equation (2.21). This mean value can be calculated on the basis of the Laplace transform. When there are ζ events before time t, the function reads

$$-\mu_j(t) L^{(\zeta+1)}(\sum_q M_q(t_q)) / L^{(\zeta)}(\sum_q M_q(t_q)). \qquad (7.16)$$

Measures of dependence, like Kendall's τ, will generally change by truncation. That is, if we consider only groups with all members surviving at a given age, it is possible that the dependence in the residual lifetimes is different from that of the full lifetimes evaluated at birth. The updating formulas can be used to quantify this change. Specifically, the local measure defined in Equation (4.16) equals 1 plus the coefficient of variation (standard deviation divided by the mean) in the conditional distribution giving survival to (t_1, t_2), that is,

$$\rho(t_1, t_2) = 1 + \frac{Var(Y \mid T_1 > t_1, T_2 > t_2)^{1/2}}{E(Y \mid T_1 > t_1, T_2 > t_2)}. \qquad (7.17)$$

7.2.4   Weibull conditional distributions

The most natural parametric distribution to consider is the Weibull model, because it allows for both the proportional hazards model and the accelerated failure time model. We assume that the conditional hazard for the jth individual is $Y\lambda_j\gamma t^{\gamma-1}$. If we restrict attention to such models for the conditional hazards, the model can also be formulated as an accelerated failure time distribution, as described in Section 2.2.7, and elaborated on in Section 2.5.2, giving, inter alia, the advantage that we can evaluate moments and correlations of the lifetimes. To do this in the symmetric bivariate case, we assume that W_1, W_2 are independent, and distributed as Weibull(1,γ). Then, following Equation (2.7), the times are given by

$$T_j = Y^{-1/\gamma}W_j, j = 1, 2. \tag{7.18}$$

As a general result, we can evaluate that conditionally on Y, the mean is $Y^{-1/\gamma}\Gamma(1 + 1/\gamma)$, say, $c_1(\gamma)Y^{-1/\gamma}$. From this it is immediate that the unconditional mean is $c_1(\gamma)E(Y^{-1/\gamma})$. The conditional variance is $Y^{-2/\gamma}\{\Gamma(1+2/\gamma) - \Gamma(1+1/\gamma)^2\}$, say $c_2(\gamma)Y^{-2/\gamma}$, giving an unconditional variance of

$$Var(T) = c_1(\gamma)^2 Var(Y^{-1/\gamma}) + c_2(\gamma)E(Y^{-2/\gamma}) \tag{7.19}$$

and a correlation of

$$\text{corr}(T_1, T_2) = \{c_1(\gamma)^2 Var(Y^{-1/\gamma})\}/Var(T) \tag{7.20}$$

between two individuals with common Y. This shows that for this evaluation, the inverse moments of Y are more relevant than the ordinary positive power moments. It is undesirable that the expressions are so dependent on the powers. Simpler formulas are obtained for the logarithm of the times, because the expression in Equation (7.18) becomes additive. The conditional mean of $\log T$ is $\{\psi(1) - \log Y\}/\gamma$ and the conditional variance is $\pi^2/(6\gamma^2)$, independently of Y, giving an unconditional variance of

$$Var(\log T) = \{Var(\log Y) + \pi^2/6\}/\gamma^2, \tag{7.21}$$

and a correlation, which is

$$\text{corr}(\log T_1, \log T_2) = Var(\log Y)/\{Var(\log Y) + \pi^2/6\}. \tag{7.22}$$

This value is then independent of the value of γ and of any scale parameter in Y. The moments and correlations are, however, markedly changed by time transformations. This can be seen because a power transformation can lead to any value of γ in Equation (7.20). This makes it an advantage to consider the value of other measures of dependence than the Pearson product moment correlation, for example, the Kendall coefficient of concordance (Section 4.2), Spearman's correlation (Section 4.3), or the median concordance (Section 4.4).

7.2.5   Quantification of dependence

A major problem is to quantify the degree of dependence. The reason is that it is not simple quantitatively to compare the degree of dependence for two different frailty distributions. The first measure considered for the gamma model was the variance in the frailty distribution, but this measure is useless in a stable frailty model, because it is always infinite. We need some measures that are relevant in a more general frame.

On the general level, we have three ways of expressing dependence in a frailty model. Some measure of variability of the frailty can be used. In the normal distribution case, this corresponds to reporting the actual variance components. This approach is specific to common risks models, as it directly involves the common risk (frailty) term. The second possibility is to evaluate dependence by a correlation type measure. This approach can be used generally for continuous bivariate data, and therefore was discussed generally, in Chapter 4. The third possibility is to evaluate the conditional distributions. In the normal distribution models, this corresponds to evaluating the regression function, which in that case is a simple linear function. In the multi-state models of Chapter 6, a dynamic version of this relation was the key object. In frailty models, this is more complicated but can be handled by the updating formulas. Owing to the complicated dependence on t and t_1, such measures will not be discussed further from a theoretical point of view, but they will be considered in the applications. The approach will be illustrated by Equation (7.40).

As an example of the first suggestion, it is common in applications based on the gamma frailty distribution to quote the variance of the frailty distribution, assuming a mean value of 1. This quantity will be called the squared coefficient of variation in this work. This is basically the same, but the term recognizes that the scale parameter is unidentifiable. Such measures are typically not comparable for the different families of distributions, and therefore not recommended. In other words, this measure is not robust toward the choice of model. If we want to evaluate the dependence by means of some measure of variability of the frailty distribution, it is better to use the variance of $\log Y$. The disadvantages of this quantity are that it requires the frailty distribution to be concentrated on the positive numbers, and for non-fatal events this is a true restriction, and second that it may require numerical integration to evaluate. For example, in the PVF family, we have explicit formulas for $\alpha = 0$ and $1/2$ and $\theta = 0$, and the moment does not exist for $\alpha < 0$.

The second suggestion of evaluating some measure of bivariate dependence makes more sense, and was the approach introduced in Chapter 4. A standard choice of this kind is the correlation coefficient, but as this is dependent on the time scale, it has been common in the literature to calculate it after the data have been transformed to a scale, where the conditional hazard $\mu(t)$ is constant. This is done by choosing $\gamma = 1$ in Equation (7.20).

This is quite inconvenient, because $\mu(t)$ cannot be estimated without the model, and this means that this measure is incomparable between models. A better choice is to transform so that the marginal distributions are exponential, that is, $\omega(t)$ is constant (Section 4.5). The marginal distributions can be estimated without assuming a specific model, but it is more complicated to study the theoretical properties. We will prefer to use a measure that is independent of marginal time transformations, Kendall's τ, Spearman's ρ, and the median concordance. All of these measures depend only on the frailty distribution, and thus are not changed by a transformation of the time scale. Kendall's coefficient of concordance can be found by means of the formula

$$\tau = 4 \int_0^\infty sL(s)L''(s)ds - 1. \tag{7.23}$$

This is derived by studying Equation (4.3) conditional on the frailties. Suppose there are two pairs. The first (T_{11}, T_{12}) has frailty Y_1 and the second (T_{21}, T_{22}) has frailty Y_2. The conditional probability that $T_{1j} < T_{2j}$ equals $Y_1/(Y_1+Y_2)$ using the proportional hazards assumption, from which we find

$$E\{sign(T_{1j} - T_{2j}) \mid Y_1, Y_2\} = \frac{Y_2 - Y_1}{Y_1 + Y_2}.$$

Thus, using that the lifetimes are independent given the frailties, we find

$$\tau = E\left(\frac{Y_2 - Y_1}{Y_1 + Y_2}\right)^2.$$

Using the expression $a^{-2} = \int_0^\infty u \exp(-ua)du$ and reversing the order of integration, we obtain

$$\tau = \int \int \int u \exp\{-u(y_1 + y_2)\}(y_2 - y_1)^2 f(y_1)f(y_2)dy_1 dy_2 du.$$

Integrating over first y_2 and then y_1 using Equation (A.3) gives

$$2 \int_0^\infty sL(s)L''(s)ds - 2 \int_0^\infty sL'(s)^2 ds,$$

from which Equation (7.23) follows by partial integration. An alternative expression is given by means of the inverse of the Laplace transform,

$$\tau = 4 \int_0^\infty \frac{q(v)}{q'(v)}dv + 1,$$

where $q(v) = L^{-1}(v)$.

The median concordance can be found by combining Equations (4.14) and (7.8) to be

$$\kappa = 4L(L^{-1}(1/2) + L^{-1}(1/2)) - 1. \tag{7.24}$$

There are no known simplifications for Spearman's ρ, so it is necessary to perform numerical integration in Equation (4.10) to evaluate this measure.

The third approach of calculating some predicted distribution has the problem that it does not give a single number, but a whole curve, like that expressed in Equation (7.40). Therefore, it is not good as a summary measure, but it will be used in the application to illustrate the conditional hazard functions. This is done by considering the ratio of the hazards under various patterns of previous observation and events. The cross ratio function of Equation (4.16) is an example of such a ratio.

In conclusion, it makes more sense to evaluate some measure of dependence for the bivariate time distribution (see Chapter 4). For Weibull models, we will evaluate the correlation coefficients of the times, and discuss the relevance of this. For the various models considered, we will compare the measures in Section 7.8.3.

7.2.6 Derived quantities

It is useful to have a range of probability results in order to evaluate various moments and distributions. A few such results will be formulated here for a frailty model with conditional hazard $Y\mu_j(t)$ for the jth individual. The simplest result is that as the marginal survivor function is $S(t) = L(M_j(t))$, we immediately know that $L(M_j(T_j))$ follows a uniform distribution on the unit interval. This result can be extended to the bivariate case in the following way. We consider the statistics $V = M_1(T_1) + M_2(T_2)$ and $W = M_1(T_1)/V$. The range of W is (0,1) and for V, it is $(0, \infty)$. In that case, W is independent of V and

$$Pr(W > w) = 1 - w, \quad Pr(V > v) = L(v) - vL'(v). \qquad (7.25)$$

This is not difficult to prove. Conditional on Y, it is known that $M_j(T_j)$, $j = 1, 2$ are independent and exponentially distributed with a common scale $(1/Y)$. That the distribution W is uniform and independent of both the sum V and the scale $(1/Y)$ is a classic result (it is a special case of the beta distribution version of the test statistic in an analysis of variance). The distribution of V follows by first finding the distribution conditional on Y, using Equation (A.29) and then integrating Y out. This is a useful result for simulating according to the distribution. It is easy to simulate W and it may be easy to simulate V as we have an explicit expression for its distribution function. Then, the times can be found from the expressions $M_1(T_1) = WV$ and $M_2(T_2) = (1 - W)V$.

Another type of distributional result is that if T_1 is observed, the conditional distribution of Y has Laplace transform as stated in Equation (7.14). This directly gives the conditional survivor function of T_2 given T_1 as

$$Pr(T_2 > t_2 \mid T_1) = \frac{L'(M_1(T_1))}{L'(M_1(T_1) + M_2(t_2))}, \qquad (7.26)$$

in terms of the original Laplace transform of Y. Thus, if we insert T_2 instead of t_2, we obtain a random variable that is uniformly distributed for all values of T_1 and correspondingly is independent of T_1.

7.2.7 Regression models

In a frailty model, it is absolutely necessary to be able to include explanatory variables. The reason is that the frailty describes the influence of common unknown factors. If some common covariate is included in the model, the variation owing to unknown covariates should be reduced. Thus we assume that there are, for each individual, p observed covariates z_{ijm}, $i = 1, ..., n$, $j = 1, ..., k$, $m = 1, ..., p$. Typically, this will be written in vector form z_{ij}. In general, these covariates are individual, that is, depend in an arbitrary way on i and j. Two important special cases stand out, the common covariates, and the matched pairs covariates (Section 1.13).

Common covariates are common for all members of the group, that is, depend on i only. For monozygotic twins, examples are sex and any other genetically based covariate. Both monozygotic and dizygotic twins share year of birth and the common pre-birth environment. By measuring some potentially important covariates, we can examine the influence of the covariates, and we can examine, whether they explain the dependence, that is, whether the frailty has no effect (or more correctly, no variation), when the covariate is included in the model.

Risk factors that are not common can also be included, but for a different reason, because they have no influence on the dependence as such. *Matched pairs covariates* is a term for covariates that only depend on j. The typical example is treatment in a repeated measurements study or a drug trial, where individuals are paired and then one in each pair receives each treatment. For matched pairs covariates, the testing of a hypothesis is done using the variation within pairs, whereas common covariates should be evaluated by means of the larger variation between pairs, that is, the frailty variation. The effect of covariates varying within the group can be estimated with better precision than with independent observations; that is, they can be based on the within-group variability rather than the total variability. This problem could be studied by stratification (Section 7.1).

The model applied is the usual proportional hazards model, but in the conditional distribution of Y. In fact, the frailty model can be given a common unobserved risk factor interpretation, generalizing the univariate Equation (2.49). The conditional hazard of the (i, j)-th individual is assumed of the form

$$\mu_j(t) \exp(\beta' z_{ij} + \psi' w_i), \qquad (7.27)$$

where w_i is the vector of common unobserved covariates and the hazard term $\mu_j(t)$ may or may not depend on j. Defining $Y_i = \exp(\psi' w_i)$, a conditional hazard of

$$\exp(\beta' z_{ij}) Y_i \mu_j(t) \tag{7.28}$$

is obtained, and this will be the standard formulation of the model. As shown in Section 2.4.6, we can take one individual, and integrate Y out to get the marginal dependence on the covariates. Whenever $EY < \infty$, the hazards for different values of the covariates will be non-proportional. Unfortunately, this non-proportionality makes it possible to identify all parameters. This is a disadvantage, because it implies that in the finite mean frailty case, the regression parameters and the dependence structure are confounded. Thus it is possible to identify the degree of dependence based on only a single individual from each pair. To take an extreme example, suppose we want to examine the dependence in lifetimes of fathers and daughters. If there are important covariates, for example, smoking, it is sufficient to examine the lifetimes of the fathers, which apparently is convenient because they die first, and we can therefore obtain results earlier. The reason for the identifiability is that the frailty term leads to non-proportionality between the marginal hazards for smokers and non-smokers, and this non-proportionality makes it possible to identify the dependence within pairs. Common sense suggests that this is an undesirable property. We have made some wrong assumptions that mix the regression structure and the dependence structure. A further illustration of this problem is that as this is based only on the data for the fathers, the same results are obtained when we study their relation to daughters, grand-daughters, wives, or persons with any other relation; and obviously this is incorrect. There are various ways to fix, or reduce, this problem. A positive stable frailty distribution (Section 7.4), which has an infinite mean, may be applied. In this case, the proportional conditional hazards leads to proportional marginal hazards. A second solution is that the assumption of proportional hazards in the conditional distribution may be changed to proportional hazards in the marginal distribution, which is in conflict with the original thoughts, but allows for various more simple estimation procedures (see Chapter 13). If there are just a few values of the covariates, we might stratify according to the covariates, to avoid the proportionality assumption. In the example above, that would correspond to assuming that there was one hazard, say $\mu_1(t)$, for smokers and another, say, $\mu_2(t)$, for non-smokers. In that case, it would be impossible to identify the dependence from data on fathers only. In the application to twins, stratification is done for sex, as we make a separate analysis for each sex. Finally, the shared frailty assumption can be extended to a bivariate frailty (Chapter 10). The solutions mentioned are listed in Table 7.1.

Solution	Reference
Positive stable shared frailty	Section 7.4
Marginal model instead of conditional	Section 13.6
Stratified hazard function	This section
Bivariate frailty	Chapter 10

Table 7.1. Some solutions to the problem of the regression and the dependence parameters' being confounded.

7.3   Gamma frailty models

Gamma distributions have been used for many years to generate mixtures in exponential and Poisson models. From a computational point of view, they fit very well to survival models, because it is easy to derive the formulas for any number of events. This is due to the simplicity of the derivatives of the Laplace transform. This is also the reason why this distribution has been applied in most of the applications published until now. We use the parametrization of the gamma distribution, gamma(δ, θ), described in Appendix A.3.1, with a parameter δ and an (inverse) scale parameter θ. For many calculations, it makes sense to restrict the scale parameter, and the standard restriction is $\theta = \delta$, as this implies a mean of 1 for Y. However, some other formulas become less transparent using the restriction, and therefore we will make the restriction at a late stage, only. Independence of the lifetimes is obtained when the distribution becomes degenerate, which happens under the limit $\delta \to \infty$. Alternatively, one could parametrize by means of the variance of Y, which is $1/\delta$. In the literature, this model is sometimes called the Clayton or Clayton-Oakes model. In this book, it is called the gamma frailty model.

The bivariate survivor function can be written as

$$S(t_1, t_2) = \theta^\delta / \{\theta + M_1(t_1) + M_2(t_2)\}^\delta, \tag{7.29}$$

following Equation (7.4). From this, we can derive the inverse relation

$$M_1(t_1) = \theta\{S_1(t_1)^{-1/\delta} - 1\}, \tag{7.30}$$

where $S_1(t_1) = S(t_1, 0)$ is the marginal survivor function. This gives the alternative expression based on the marginals, following Equation (7.8),

$$S(t_1, t_2) = \{S_1(t_1)^{-1/\delta} + S_2(t_2)^{-1/\delta} - 1\}^{-\delta}. \tag{7.31}$$

In this equation, the scale parameter has disappeared, and thus only δ enters, automatically solving the scale identifiability problem. The multivariate generalization of this equation is

$$S(t_1, ..., t_k) = \{\sum_j S_j(t_j)^{-1/\delta} - (k-1)\}^{-\delta}. \tag{7.32}$$

In the bivariate case, the density of the lifetimes is

$$\mu_1(t_1)\mu_2(t_2)\{\theta + M_1(t_1) + M_2(t_2)\}^{-\delta-2}\theta^\delta(\delta + 1)\delta. \qquad (7.33)$$

For general calculations, we need the contribution to the likelihood of arbitrary censored data. The version of Equation (7.6) in this case is

$$\{\prod_{j=1}^{k} \mu_j(T_j)^{D_j}\}\theta^\delta(\theta + M.)^{-\delta-D.}\Gamma(\delta + d.)/\Gamma(\delta), \qquad (7.34)$$

where $M. = M.(T_1, ..., T_k)$. This expression is generally simple to handle. An alternative formulation is by the derivative of Equation (7.32), that is,

$$\{\prod_{j=1}^{k} \omega_j(t_j)^{D_j} S_j(T_j)^{-D_j/\delta}\}S(T_1, ..., T_k)^{(\delta+D.)/\delta}\delta^{-D.}\Gamma(\delta+D.)/\Gamma(\delta), \qquad (7.35)$$

where $\omega_j(t)$ is the hazard in the marginal distribution.

Kendall's τ can be evaluated to $1/(1 + 2\delta)$. The median concordance is

$$\kappa = 4(2^{1+1/\delta} - 1)^{-\delta} - 1. \qquad (7.36)$$

Spearman's ρ can be evaluated by numerical integration or by the formula

$$\rho = \frac{12\delta(\delta + 1)}{(1 + 2\delta)^2} \, {}_3F_2(\delta + 1, 1, 1, 2(\delta + 1), 2(\delta + 1), 1), \qquad (7.37)$$

where the hypergeometric function ${}_3F_2$ is defined in Equation (A.33). The power series converges slowly for large dependence.

7.3.1 Updating

The distribution of Y among the survivors at time t is also gamma with the parameter δ unchanged, and θ changed to $\theta + \sum_j M_j(t)$. This is the original distribution modified by a scale parameter, or more precisely by a factor of $\theta/\{\theta + \sum_j M_j(t)\}$. Thus the relative distribution of the frailty is unchanged by selection. This is a very nice property, and unique to the gamma distributions. This result is also a major reason for initially not restricting the frailty distribution to a mean of 1 in the probability calculations. If the parameters were restricted, it would be more difficult to communicate this result. One consequence is that τ and other measures of dependence are unchanged by truncation. In the general case, when we have observed some deaths and some censorings, the distribution of Y conditional on the observations is still gamma, of parameters $\delta + \sum_j D_j(t)$ and $\theta + \sum_j M_j(\min(t, T_j))$. Thus the ζ parameter in the general case, Equation (7.13), combines with δ for the gamma model. This is because the gamma model is an exponential family with Y and $\log Y$ as canonical statistics. The dynamic approach is easily handled in this distribution, we immediately obtain

$$\lambda(t \mid F_t) = \mu(t)E(Y \mid F_t) = \mu(t)\frac{\delta + \sum_j D_j(t)}{\theta + \sum_j M_j(\min(t, T_j))}, \qquad (7.38)$$

where $D_j(t)$ is an indicator of the jth individual's being observed to die before time t; that is, $D_j(t) = D_j 1\{T_j \le t\}$. The hazard for death of individual 2 at time t, conditional on individual 1's being alive at time t_1, that is, conditional on the event $\{T_1 > t_1\}$, is $\mu_2(t)\delta\{\theta + M_1(t_1) + M_2(t)\}^{-1}$. Conditional on death at time t_1, the hazard is $\mu_2(t)(\delta + 1)\{\theta + M_1(t_1) + M_2(t)\}^{-1}$. This implies that the ratio (which equals the cross-ratio of Equation (4.16)) is simply

$$\frac{\lambda(t \mid T_1 = t_1)}{\lambda(t \mid T_1 > t_1)} = 1 + \delta^{-1}. \qquad (7.39)$$

This is a very nice formula, and was the basis for some of the early derivations of the model, but for making a prognosis for a surviving individual (number 2) at some time t given the status of the other, it seems more relevant to use a denominator of the partner's being currently alive, that is, at time t. This gives the expression

$$\frac{\lambda(t \mid T_1 = t_1)}{\lambda(t \mid T_1 > t)} = (1 + \delta^{-1})\frac{\theta + M_1(t) + M_2(t)}{\theta + M_1(t_1) + M_2(t)}, \qquad (7.40)$$

which is less nice. However, it makes more sense, because it can be interpreted in the multi-state model of Figure 5.12 as the ratio of the hazard $\mu(t, t_1)$, when the partner is dead, to the hazard $\lambda(t)$, when the partner is alive.

In the proportional hazards regression models, the marginal hazards will be non-proportional, as derived in Section 2.4.6. In this case, it is possible to identify all parameters, even when $k = 1$. This is an inconvenience of the model. A practical example is given in Section 8.12.3.

7.3.2   Weibull models

In the case where the conditional hazard is of Weibull form, that is, of the form $Y\lambda_j\gamma t^{\gamma-1}$ for the jth individual and Y is gamma(δ, δ), the bivariate survivor function becomes

$$S(t_1, t_2) = 1/\{1 + (\lambda_1 t_1^\gamma + \lambda_2 t_2^\gamma)/\delta\}^\delta. \qquad (7.41)$$

This is called a bivariate Burr distribution, generalizing the Pareto power distribution.

The correlation can be found by combining Equations (7.19), (7.20), and (A.9). It is independent of λ_1 and λ_2. It exists for $\delta > 2/\gamma$. For $\delta < 2/\gamma$, the variance of T is infinite and the correlation is undefined. The correlation of the logarithms depends only on δ and equals

$$corr(\log T_1, \log T_2) = \psi'(\delta)/\{\psi'(\delta) + \pi^2/6\}. \qquad (7.42)$$

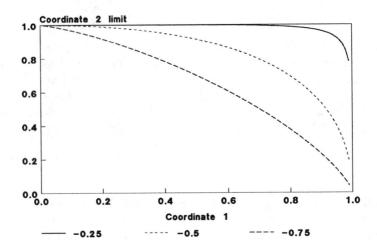

Figure 7.1. Upper limit of the support of the extension of the gamma frailty bivariate distribution with uniform marginals to negative dependence, for $\varphi = -0.25$, -0.5, and -0.75.

7.3.3 Extension to negative dependence

The model can be extended to allow for negative dependence. To do this, we need to make a reparametrization, because the hypothesis of independence of lifetimes $\delta = \infty$ needs to be an interior point in the parameter set. We insert $\varphi = 1/\delta$ in Equation (7.31), so that the hypothesis of independence corresponds to $\varphi = 0$. Simple insertion allows for $\varphi < 0$, but sometimes gives a negative expression for the survivor function in a neighborhood of (∞, ∞). Then, the expression should be changed to 0, so that it reads

$$S(t_1, t_2) = [\max\{S_1(t_1)^{-\varphi} + S_2(t_2)^{-\varphi} - 1, 0\}]^{-1/\varphi}. \qquad (7.43)$$

This is a valid bivariate survivor function. When $\varphi < 0$, this model shows negative dependence, and there is no frailty interpretation. There is a subset of $(0, \infty)^2$ which has probability 0. The subset for various choices of φ are shown in Figure 7.1. When φ is below -0.5, the distribution is no longer continuous, but has a discrete component along the line given by the first term in the maximum's being equal to 0.

An alternative formulation is to rewrite Equation (7.38) to

$$\mu(t)\frac{1 + \varphi \sum_j D_j(t)}{1 + \varphi \sum_j M_j(\min(t, T_j))},$$

which is valid for both positive and negative φ.

7.4 Positive stable frailty distributions

The family of positive stable distributions make up an interesting alternative, which shows nicer results concerning the marginal distributions, but the derivatives of the Laplace transform are more complicated, which makes some calculations more difficult. In this case, we will not include a scale parameter, because the formulas where this parameter is useful are covered by Section 7.5, which describes a generalization of the positive stable distributions. Background information on the positive stable distributions is described in the Appendix, Section A.3.3. The Laplace transform is $L(s) = \exp(-s^\alpha)$, from which we derive the bivariate survival function

$$S(t_1, t_2) = \exp[-\{M_1(t_1) + M_2(t_2)\}^\alpha] \tag{7.44}$$

The general expression for the likelihood is obtained by insertion in Equation (7.6), using the Laplace transform of Equation (A.18) with $\delta = \alpha$ and $\theta = 0$.

$$[\prod_j \mu_j(t_j)^{D_j}]Q \exp(-M.^\alpha), \tag{7.45}$$

where $Q = \sum_{m=1}^{D.} c_{D.,m}\alpha^m M.^{m\alpha - D.}$. The coefficients c_{dm} depend on α and are described in Equation (A.19).

Expressed in terms of the marginal survivor functions, the expression is

$$S(t_1, t_2) = \exp(-[\{-\log S_1(t_1)\}^{1/\alpha} + \{-\log S_2(t_2)\}^{1/\alpha}]^\alpha). \tag{7.46}$$

In terms of the integrated marginal hazards $\Omega_j(t)$, the expression is simplified to

$$S(t_1, t_2) = \exp[-\{\Omega_1(t_1)^{1/\alpha} + \Omega_2(t_2)^{1/\alpha}\}^\alpha]. \tag{7.47}$$

Formulated by means of the marginal distributions, the multivariate density is

$$[\prod_j \{\omega_j(t_j)\Omega(t_j)^{\varphi-1}\}^{d_j}]Q \exp(-M.^\alpha), \tag{7.48}$$

where $\varphi = 1/\alpha$, $M. = \sum \Omega_j(t_j)^\varphi$ and Q is as defined above.

Kendall's τ is simply $1 - \alpha$. The median concordance is $\kappa = 2^{2-2^\alpha} - 1$. No simple formula is known for Spearman's ρ.

This distribution cannot be extended to negative dependence, because in that case, the density should be negative near (0,0). However, the likelihood function is well defined in a neighborhood of $\alpha = 1$.

To apply the distributional result in Equation (7.25), we evaluate that V has survivor function $(1 + \alpha v^\alpha) \exp(-v^\alpha)$, from which we can derive that $S = V^\alpha$ has the density $(1 - \alpha + \alpha s) \exp(-s)$. This distribution has an interpretation as a mixture of gamma distributions.

7.4.1 Updating

The conditional distribution of Y given survival of the individuals until some time t is a member of the PVF family. The precise result is a special case of the results for that family (see Section 7.5.2). These results can also be used to evaluate dependence measures like τ for survivors at a given age. Generally, these measures decrease with truncation time.

The hazard for death of individual 2 at time t, conditional on individual 1, is easily calculated by means of Equation (7.16). Conditional on individual 1's being alive at time t_1, that is, the event $\{T_1 > t_1\}$, the hazard of death of individual 2 is

$$\mu_2(t)\alpha\{M_1(t_1) + M_2(t)\}^{\alpha-1}.$$

Conditional on death at time t_1, the hazard is

$$\mu_2(t)[(1 - \alpha)\{M_1(t_1) + M_2(t)\}^{-1} + \alpha\{M_1(t_1) + M_2(t)\}^{\alpha-1}].$$

The ratio of these hazards, similar to that of Equation (7.40), is

$$\frac{\lambda(t \mid T_1 = t_1)}{\lambda(t \mid T_1 > t)} = \frac{(1 - \alpha)\{M.(t_1, t)\}^{-1} + \alpha\{M.(t_1, t)\}^{\alpha-1}}{\alpha\{M.(t, t)\}^{\alpha-1}}. \tag{7.49}$$

This ratio will be considered in the example in Section 8.12.5.

7.4.2 Regression models

In the case of a proportional hazards model as shown in Equation (7.28), the marginal hazards also show proportional hazards, but with the regression coefficient changed from β to $\alpha\beta$, as demonstrated in Section 2.4.6. This means that the dependence parameter and the regression coefficients cannot be estimated by means of univariate data ($k = 1$); that is, it is necessary to have multiple observations in the same group. This is an advantage of the positive stable frailty distribution. An alternative phrasing is that the model is consistent with the possibility that a part of the variation originates from unobserved covariates. However, it becomes important whether relative risks are evaluated in the conditional or the marginal distribution. Generally, the regression coefficients have larger absolute values in the conditional distribution than in the marginal distribution. This is a complication for the interpretation of a relative risk regression coefficient, as it is very important under which circumstances it is evaluated. Also the integrated hazard is different, being steeper in the conditional distribution than in the marginal distribution.

7.4.3 The stable-Weibull model

The Weibull distribution is particularly well suited to the positive stable frailty model. The bivariate Weibull model is obtained by assuming

$\mu_j(t) = \epsilon_j\gamma t^{\gamma-1}$. This means that conditionally on Y, the distribution of T_j is Weibull$(\epsilon_j Y, \gamma)$. The bivariate survivor function is

$$S(t_1, t_2) = \exp\{-(\epsilon_1 t_1^\gamma + \epsilon_2 t_2^\gamma)^\alpha\}. \tag{7.50}$$

The advantage of this model is that also the marginal distributions are of Weibull form. The marginal distribution is Weibull$(\epsilon_j^\alpha, \alpha\gamma)$, which we parametrize as Weibull(ω_j, ρ). For expressing the bivariate distribution by means of the marginal distributions, we use the parametrization $(\omega_1, \omega_2, \rho)$. The change of the shape parameter from γ to $\rho = \alpha\gamma$ corresponds to the increased variation in the marginal distribution compared to the conditional distribution.

Also, the time to the first event $T_{\min} = \min(T_1, T_2)$ is Weibull distributed, Weibull$((\sum_j \epsilon_j)^\alpha, \alpha\gamma)$. This fact can be seen in two ways, either in the conditional distribution, where the hazard of the minimum generally is the sum of the component hazards, followed by integrating Y out, or by studying $S(t, t)$ in the bivariate survivor function of Equation (7.44). The probability that $T_j = T_{\min}$ is $\epsilon_j/(\epsilon_1 + \epsilon_2)$, independently of $T_{\min}$. The family allows for scale and power transformations, so that if the distribution of (T_1, T_2) has parameters $(\epsilon_1, \epsilon_2, \gamma, \alpha)$, the distribution of $(c_1 T_1^q, c_2 T_2^q)$ has parameters $(\epsilon_1 c_1^{-\gamma/q}, \epsilon_2 c_2^{-\gamma/q}, \gamma/q, \alpha)$. In particular, the dependence parameter is unchanged.

The density $f(t_1, t_2)$ for the bivariate distribution is

$$\rho^2 \omega_1^\varphi \omega_2^\varphi t_1^{\rho\varphi-1} t_2^{\rho\varphi-1} [M.^{2(\alpha-1)} + (\varphi - 1)M.^{(\alpha-2)}] \exp(-M.^\alpha) \tag{7.51}$$

where $M. = \sum \omega_j^\varphi t_j^{\rho\varphi}$. The density for the symmetric bivariate distribution with exponential marginals $(\rho = 1)$ is

$$\omega^2 t_1^{\varphi-1} t_2^{\varphi-1} (t_1^\varphi + t_2^\varphi)^{2(\alpha-1)} \{1 + \omega^{-1}(\varphi - 1)(t_1^\varphi + t_2^\varphi)^{-\alpha}\} \exp\{-\omega(t_1^\varphi + t_2^\varphi)^\alpha\}. \tag{7.52}$$

The Weibull model can also be given an accelerated failure time interpretation, as shown in Section 7.2.4. The moments are easily found, using that the marginals are Weibull (Section 2.2.2). The correlation is

$$\mathrm{corr}(T_1, T_2) = 1 - h(1/\gamma)/h(\alpha/\gamma), \tag{7.53}$$

where $h(x) = 1 - \Gamma(1 + x)^2/\Gamma(1 + 2x)$, which depends on γ, but not on (ϵ_1, ϵ_2). A simpler formula is obtained on the logarithmic scale

$$\mathrm{corr}(\log T_1, \log T_2) = 1 - \alpha^2.$$

This formula is particularly interesting, because it does not depend on the shape parameter γ. The correlation is illustrated in Figure 7.2 for various values of the marginal shape parameter ρ. The distributions can be transformed to any other distribution with the same value of α by a monotone time transformation (a power transformation as described above). Therefore the low correlations for $\rho = 0.02$ do not reflect low dependence, but high variance, and that the correlation is evaluated on a wrong time scale.

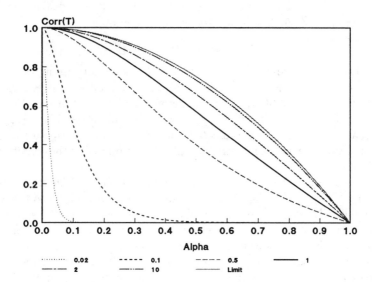

Figure 7.2. Correlation in the bivariate stable frailty Weibull distribution, for various marginal shape parameters (ρ), from 0.02 to 10. The limit for $\rho \to \infty$ equals the correlation for the log times.

It appears that the value for the log transform is the highest obtainable. Inserting $\gamma = 1/\alpha$ gives the integrated hazard correlation of Section 4.5 and this is seen on the figure as $\rho = 1$.

The distribution is a multivariate minimum stable distribution. With observations T_{ij}, $i = 1, ..., n$, $j = 1, ..., k$, where there is independence over i, and $(T_{i1}, ...T_{ik})$ follows a stable-Weibull model, with parameters $(\epsilon_1, ..., \epsilon_k, \gamma, \alpha)$, the vector minimum over groups, $(T_{\min,1}, ...T_{\min,k})$, defined coordinate-wise by $T_{\min,j} = \min(T_{1j}, ..., T_{nj})$ follows a stable-Weibull model with parameters $(n\epsilon_1, ..., n\epsilon_k, \gamma, \alpha)$, which is the same distribution as that of $n^{-\gamma}(T_{11}, ..., T_{1k})$.

The Fisher information for complete data in this model is described in Section 8.11.2.

7.4.4   Weibull regression models

A particularly interesting model is obtained by combining the regression model of Section 7.4.2 with the Weibull hazard assumption of Section 7.4.3, so that $\epsilon_j = \exp(\beta' z_j)$, or in the marginal distribution formulation $\omega_j = \exp(\kappa' z_j)$. In this case, there are three possible parametrizations of the regression coefficients. One is the conditional proportional hazards parameter β, corresponding to Equation (7.28). The second is the marginal proportional hazards version, where the regression coefficients are $\alpha\beta$, say, κ. Finally, there is the accelerated failure time parameters, as in Equation (2.57), denoted ν. The latter has the advantage that it applies as an accelerated failure time coefficient both in the conditional and the marginal distribution. The relation between the parameters is

$$\nu = -\beta/\gamma = -\kappa/\rho.$$

The κ parameters have the advantage that they are comparable to the hazard regression parameters obtained under an assumption of independence, whereas the β parameters will be numerically larger than those obtained under independence. In conclusion, it appears that the ν-parameters seem preferable.

7.5   PVF frailty distributions

The PVF family of distributions is a natural exponential family, where the variance is a power function of the mean. This is the reason for the name PVF or power variance function. It includes as special cases the gamma distributions and the positive stable distributions, and furthermore, the inverse Gaussian distributions. Thus it generalizes the models of Sections 7.3 and 7.4. The family is further described in Appendix A.3.4. It has three parameters, α, δ, and θ. In the case of $0 < \alpha \le 1$, it can be obtained as the distribution of Y in a stable frailty model, after truncation. This is a consequence of this distribution family's being the natural exponential family generated from the positive stable distributions, combined with the updating expression in the case of no events corresponding to a change of parameter value in the exponential family generated by the original distribution. The special case of $\delta = \alpha$, $\theta = 0$ gives the positive stable model of Section 7.4. For $\alpha = 0$, we obtain the gamma distributions, with the same parametrization as used for that distribution. Some formulas will be valid in this case, some will not. For $\alpha = 1/2$, the mixture distribution is an inverse Gaussian distribution and a few formulas can be simplified. For $\alpha < 0$, we obtain distributions with a point mass at zero, implying that some groups have 0 risk. In the case of lifetimes, this is impossible, because it would correspond to the persons' being immortal, but for other times, it is quite possible that some groups have 0 risk. This would then correspond to the actual group's being unable to experience the event considered. One of the three parameters is essentially a scale parameter. When we need to restrict the parameters, we will assume a mean of 1. As the mean in the PVF family is $EY = \delta\theta^{\alpha-1}$, this is obtained by restricting $\delta = \theta^{1-\alpha}$. To make it clear when this restriction is performed, we introduce a new parameter, say, η, so that when this parameter is used it covers the distribution with $\delta = \eta^{1-\alpha}$ and $\theta = \eta$. This standard distribution has a mean of 1 and the variance is $(1-\alpha)/\eta$. For a given value of (α, δ, θ), we can find a standardized distribution as a scale transform of the original distribution by defining

$$\eta = \delta\theta^\alpha. \tag{7.54}$$

This means that when Y follows $\mathrm{PVF}(\alpha, \delta, \theta)$, the distribution of Y/EY follows $\mathrm{PVF}(\alpha, (\delta\theta^\alpha)^{1-\alpha}, \delta\theta^\alpha)$, that is, $\mathrm{PVF}(\alpha, \eta^{1-\alpha}, \eta)$. The distributions with infinite mean (the stable distributions, $\theta = 0$) are excluded. For calculations in this case, please see Section 7.4.

This model extends both the stable and the gamma models and thus is useful for testing either of the models. It can also be used as a flexible way to describe dependence. However, it makes less sense for testing the hypothesis of independence, because there are two parameters to describe the dependence. In particular, when the dependence is slight, it is difficult to identify both parameters, and only the degree of dependence, as measured by Kendall's τ or Spearman's ρ can be determined with reasonable precision.

The bivariate survival function is

$$S(t_1, t_2) = \exp[-\delta\{\theta + M_1(t_1) + M_2(t_2)\}^\alpha/\alpha + \delta\theta^\alpha/\alpha]. \tag{7.55}$$

The integrated hazard is found from the marginal distribution functions by means of the formula

$$M_j(t) = [\theta^\alpha - \alpha\{\log S_j(t)\}/\delta]^{1/\alpha} - \theta.$$

Expressed by the marginal distributions, the bivariate survivor function is

$$\exp(-[\{\eta/\alpha - \log S_1(t)\}^{1/\alpha} + \{\eta/\alpha - \log S_2(t)\}^{1/\alpha} - (\eta/\alpha)^{1/\alpha}]^\alpha + \eta/\alpha). \tag{7.56}$$

In this way, the scale parameter has disappeared from the equation. This formula is slightly simplified, when expressed by the marginal hazard function

$$S(t_1, t_2) =$$

$$\exp(-[\{\eta/\alpha + \Omega_1(t_1)\}^{1/\alpha} + \{\eta/\alpha + \Omega_2(t_2)\}^{1/\alpha} - (\eta/\alpha)^{1/\alpha}]^\alpha + \eta/\alpha). \tag{7.57}$$

The multivariate version of this formula is

$$S(t_1, ..., t_k) = \exp\{-[\sum_j \{\eta/\alpha + \Omega_j(t_j)\}^{1/\alpha} - (k-1)(\eta/\alpha)^{1/\alpha}]^\alpha + \eta/\alpha)\}.$$

The likelihood follows by insertion in Equation (7.6). The actual formula is postponed to Section 8.6.2.

Measures of dependence can be evaluated when the model is continuous, that is, $\alpha \geq 0$. When $\alpha > 0$, Kendall's τ is given by the expression

$$\tau = (1 - \alpha) - 2\eta + (4\eta^2/\alpha)\exp(2\eta/\alpha)E_{(1/\alpha)-1}(2\eta/\alpha), \tag{7.58}$$

where $E_m(x)$ is the generalized exponential integral (see Appendix A.4.1). In the case of $\alpha = 1/2$, it is the ordinary exponential integral. The median concordance is

$$\kappa = 4\exp[-\{2(\eta/\alpha + \log 2)^{1/\alpha} - (\eta/\alpha)^{1/\alpha}\}^\alpha + \eta/\alpha] - 1. \tag{7.59}$$

No specific formula is available for Spearman's ρ. When α is fixed, there is an upper limit to the dependence, obtained corresponding to the positive stable boundary at $\theta = 0$. This can be illustrated by, for example, $\tau \leq 1-\alpha$. Thus, if one wants to have a model allowing any degree of dependence, α must vary freely.

7.5.1 Weibull and regression models

Following the general approach of Section 7.2.4, the conditional hazard can be assumed of Weibull form. In general, the formulas do not seem to simplify and they are therefore omitted.

In the case of $\alpha = 1/2$, the correlation of $\log T_1$ and $\log T_2$ can be found by combining Equations (A.15) and (7.22). In the general case, numerical integration must be used.

Similarly, covariates can be included in a proportional hazards regression model as described in Section 7.2.7. The marginal distributions are described in Equation (2.53). Owing to the finite mean, the marginal distributions also identify the dependence parameter.

7.5.2 Updating

Conditioning on survival until some time t gives a different distribution of Y. It is still a distribution in the power variance family, as this family is a natural exponential family, and the parameters α and δ are unchanged. The parameter θ is changed to $\theta + \sum_j M_j(t)$. This result also covers the positive stable frailty distribution, by setting $\delta = \alpha$ and $\theta = 0$. A consequence of this truncation result is that for $\alpha > 0$, the relative variance decreases toward 0, as the coefficient of variation after truncation is $(1-\alpha)\{\theta+\sum_j M_j(t)\}^{-\alpha}/\delta$. This implies that the surviving population turns more homogeneous over time, or, in other words that the group differences decrease by time. That is, if truncation is applied, the degree of dependence is smaller than it was in the full distribution. This can be illustrated by Kendall's τ, by combining Equations (7.54) and (7.58), inserting the modification of θ by truncation.

If the conditioning also involves some actual events, the updated distribution is no longer in the family. In the case of $\alpha = 1/2$, corresponding to an inverse Gaussian frailty distribution, the conditional distribution is a generalized inverse Gaussian distribution, with parameters GIG($1/2 + \sum D_j(t), \delta, \theta + \sum M_j(\min(t, T_j))$). In the general case, the distributions have not been considered previously.

The hazard for death of individual 2 at time t, conditional on individual 1's being alive at time t_1, that is, the event $\{T_1 > t_1\}$, is

$$\lambda_2(t)\delta\{\theta + M_1(t_1) + M_2(t)\}^{\alpha-1}.$$

Conditional on death of individual 1 at time t_1, the hazard for individual 2 is

$$\lambda_2(t)\delta[(1-\alpha)\{\theta + M_1(t_1) + M_2(t)\}^{-1} + \alpha\{\theta + M_1(t_1) + M_2(t)\}^{\alpha-1}].$$

The ratio of these hazards, similar to that of Equation (7.40) is

$$\frac{\lambda(t \mid T_1 = t_1)}{\lambda(t \mid T_1 > t)} = \frac{(1-\alpha)\{\theta + M.(t_1, t)\}^{-1} + \alpha\{\theta + M.(t_1, t)\}^{\alpha-1}}{\delta\{\theta + M.(t_1, t)\}^{\alpha-1}}. \tag{7.60}$$

Similarly, these expressions can be used to derive the cross-ratio function of Section 4.6 as a measure of local dependence. Using Equation (7.17), this is $\rho(t) = 1 + (1-\alpha)\{\theta + M_1(t_1) + M_2(t_2)\}^{-\alpha}/\delta$, which decreases to 1 with age.

7.6 Lognormal frailty distributions

The lognormal distributions have also been used as frailty distributions. In this case, the Laplace transforms are theoretically intractable and therefore probability results have to be evaluated by means of an approximation or numerical integration. Simple explicit results for dependence measures like τ and Spearman's ρ are not known. The Laplace transform and its derivatives can, however, be approximated (see Section A.3.5), and this makes it possible to do probability evaluations and to evaluate τ by means of one-dimensional numerical integration, using Equation (7.23). This approximation seems to work very well and will be used when necessary. Alternatively, it is possible to evaluate results by simulation. The need for approximations places some restrictions on the available estimation procedures.

Furthermore, we know some moments. With ξ and σ^2, the mean and variance on the log scale, the mean of Y is $\exp(\xi + \sigma^2/2)$ and the variance is $\exp(2\xi + \sigma^2)\{\exp(\sigma^2) - 1\}$, from which we derive the coefficient of variation as $\{\exp(\sigma^2) - 1\}^{1/2}$. The natural restriction to obtain scale identifiability is $\xi = 0$, in this case being simpler than the restriction $EY = 1$.

As the variance of Y on the log scale is σ^2, we can derive from Equation (7.22) that the correlation of log times in a Weibull model is

$$\text{corr}(\log T_1, \log T_2) = \sigma^2/(\sigma^2 + \pi^2/6), \tag{7.61}$$

which is independent of λ_1, λ_2 and γ. In fact, the Weibull model of Equation (7.18) can be simplified to

$$T_j = \tilde{Y} W_j, \tag{7.62}$$

where $\tilde{Y} = Y^{-1/\gamma}$. Also $\tilde{Y}$ follows a log normal distribution, with parameter $\tilde{\sigma}^2 = \sigma^2/\gamma^2$. The advantage of this reformulation is that we avoid the strange relation between the parameters of the distributions of Y and W_j, making it much easier to argue in favor of (7.62) as an accelerated failure time model. Also moments are immediately found by means of this equation, in fact, they are so simple that we do not need to apply the restriction on ξ. The q'th moment exists when $q > -\gamma$, in which case

$$ET^q = \exp\{-q\xi/\gamma + q^2\sigma^2/(2\gamma^2)\}\lambda^{-q/\gamma}\Gamma(1+q/\gamma).$$

As the mean frailty is finite, all parameters can be identified from univariate data, when covariates are available. How the marginal hazards deviate from proportionality is unknown. The lognormal distributions are in practice very close to the inverse Gaussian distributions. Thus, these models should behave approximately similarly. But there are some advantages to using the lognormal. The distribution of the unobserved covariates, w_i, in Equation (7.27) can be multivariate normal with an arbitrary variance matrix, which is much simpler than the standard case, where the distributions considered have a relation with the corresponding regression coefficient so that it is the distribution of the combined effect of covariates and regression coefficients ($\psi'w_i$) that must be within a given family.

It follows from the general results that truncation leads to an updated distribution in the exponential family generated from the lognormal distribution, as defined in Section A.3.5. Thus, we can directly describe that the distribution is $\text{LNEF}(\sum_j M_j(t), \xi, \sigma^2)$. Furthermore, as the exponential family also has $\log Y$ as canonical statistic, we can directly describe the general updated distribution as $\text{LNEF}(\sum_j M_j(t_j), \xi + \sigma^2 \sum D_j(t), \sigma^2)$. Based on the experience from other models, we expect that truncation implies a reduction in dependence, but the extent to which this happens requires further study.

Another advantage of relying on the normal distribution is that alternative estimation methods are available, for example, based on the REML approach. In the general frailty models of Chapter 10, it is easy to make more detailed dependence models by means of the multivariate normal distributions and this makes them relevant in that case. Furthermore, in the normal case, there are more possible estimation procedures.

7.7   Other distributions

In principle, any other distribution on the positive numbers can be applied as frailty distribution. The point that matters the most for theoretical evaluations is the simplicity of the Laplace transform.

The so-called Franks distributions also make a frailty model, but the actual frailty distribution has not been derived. The Laplace transform when $0 < \varphi < 1$ is

$$L(s) = \log\{1 - (1 - \varphi)e^{-s}\}/\log\varphi,$$

giving a bivariate distribution, corresponding to Equation (7.8):

$$S(u,v) = \log\{1 + \frac{(\varphi^u - 1)(\varphi^v - 1)}{\varphi - 1}\}/\log\varphi.$$

An alternative family that also includes the gamma and the inverse Gaussian distributions is the generalized inverse Gaussian distributions (see the Appendix). In this case, the Laplace transform is given by means of the Bessel function. The generalized inverse Gaussian distribution is an exponential family with $(Y, \log Y, 1/Y)$ as canonical statistics. The presence of Y and $\log Y$ implies that arbitrary updating is simple. The conditional distribution of Y given some events and some censorings is still within the family. This means that if the distribution of Y initially is $\text{GIG}(\gamma, \delta, \theta)$, the distribution conditional on the information at time t is $\text{GIG}(\gamma + \sum_j D_j(t), \delta, \theta + \sum M_j(\min(t, T_j)))$.

An extension, different from the PVF model, but including both the gamma and stable model is considered in an exercise.

7.8 Comparison of frailty distributions

Having suggested several frailty distributions, it makes sense to compare them in order to find out whether any of them is preferable to the other. Before that, we should discuss the relevance of having several distribution families. That is, would it be simpler just to pick a single one-parameter family of frailty distributions and use that as a general model. This idea, which, of course, is motivated by the normal distribution models seems attractive. For frailty models (and, more generally, for random effects models for other distributions than the normal) there is no single family having all desirable properties. Therefore, choosing a model requires a more detailed study of the model properties of each distribution family and of which properties are relevant to the actual problem considered. This, of course, also implies that the choice of family depends on the problem considered. This can be seen as a complication of the model, but I would certainly prefer to see it as a challenge. Finding the right tools for a given problem is more exciting than using a single tool for all problems.

The comparison will be done along three directions. First we make a theoretical comparison describing which nice properties these models have. Second we make a comparison of fit, that is, what the various models look like. Third, the various measures of dependence are compared for the various models.

7.8.1   Theoretical comparison

As described above, the various families of distributions have some theoretical advantages. If the frailty distribution is a natural exponential family, selection, that is, truncation (updating when no events have happened), implies that the conditional distribution of the frailty is still within the same family. The gamma model has the advantage that selection is only a change of scale of the frailty distribution, implying that the hazard ratio in Equation (7.39) is independent of time, and the measures of dependence are unchanged by truncation. The positive stable model has the advantage that it fits proportional hazards models and Weibull models. The statement that it fits proportional hazards means that if the conditional model has proportional hazards, so does the marginal distribution. This is an advantage, when considering the model as a random effects model. The PVF model has the advantage that it includes both the gamma and the positive stable model, and thus can be used to judge whether the fit of these models is satisfactory. The inverse Gaussian model stands out as a simple special case, where the density is known, and updating gives a distribution that has been described previously. However, these two points are only minor advantages compared to the full PVF family. Table 7.2 shows key differences between the various frailty distributions. The gamma and positive stable distributions are extreme cases, which show nice probability results, and the PVF family is intermediate for $\alpha > 0$, allowing for a better fit, but also being more complicated to handle. The two parameters of the PVF model result in instability near independence. In the case of $\alpha < 0$, we have a model with some persons without risk. While this is possible in some cases and impossible in others, a negative estimate often reflects that we have very little information on the risk at late time points. In particular, with heavy censoring, we do not have the information on whether the dependence is higher or lower for late events than for early events. Assuming a given type, like gamma, apparently solves the problem, by substituting assumptions for lack of knowledge, but it does not add real information.

The lognormal frailty distribution is a one-parameter model, which only has one of the nice properties of Table 7.2, namely, infinite divisibility (of both the frailty and the logarithm to the frailty). Owing to its similarity with the inverse Gaussian distribution, it is expected to show the most important dependence at intermediate times. A further advantage is that a power transformation of the frailty still gives a lognormal distribution.

7.8.2   Comparison of fit

The fit and the flexibility of the models are also important factors in a comparison. The stable frailty distribution implies high early dependence, whereas the gamma frailty model describes high late dependence. The concept of early and late dependence was introduced informally in Sec-

Property	Gamma	PVF	Stable
No. of parameters	1	2	1
Selection family	Gamma	PVF	PVF
Selection	Scale change	→ homogen	→ homogen
Updating	Gamma	GIG ($\alpha = 1/2$)	
Weibull	Does not fit	Does not fit	Fits
Proportional hazards	No	No	Fits
Infinite divisibility	Yes	Yes	Yes
Infinite divisibility of log	Yes	No	Yes
Person of 0 risk	No	$\alpha < 0$	No
Likelihood	Simple	Acceptable	Acceptable
Time of importance	Late	Whole range	Early

Table 7.2. Key differences between frailty distributions. Blank means no simple result. The selection result for PVF is only valid for $\alpha > 0$.

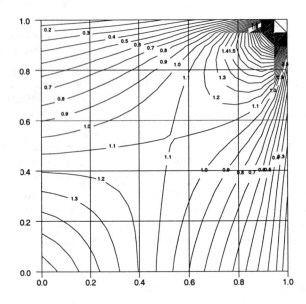

Figure 7.3. Contour curves for the density of a bivariate uniform distribution with gamma frailty dependence, with $\tau = 0.25$.

Subfamily	Parameters	Var(log Y)	τ	κ	ρ	Figures
Gamma	$\delta = 1.5$	0.935	0.25	0.247	0.3655	7.3, 7.7
Stable	$\alpha = 0.75$	1.279	0.25	0.247	0.3637	7.4, 7.8
Inverse Gauss	$\eta = 0.3899$	0.845	0.25	0.264	0.3669	7.5, 7.9
Lognormal	$\sigma = 0.882$	0.779	0.25			

Table 7.3. Parameters for examples used for illustrating dependence. For the lognormal, the values are based on approximations.

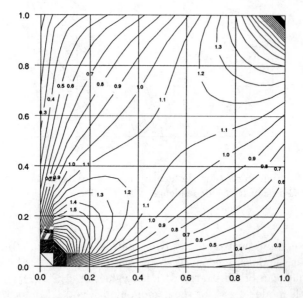

Figure 7.4. Contour curves for the density of a bivariate uniform distribution with positive stable frailty dependence, with $\tau = 0.25$.

tion 3.2.1. Here, the evaluation will be made explicit by means of contour curves. These are mathematically more correct than the motivating figures (Figures 3.2-3.4). To remove the effect of the marginal distributions, the marginal distributions will be assumed to be uniform over the unit interval. Thus under independence, the density will be 1 at any point. This corresponds to the descriptions of copulas (Section 13.5). To make figures that are comparable with respect to the degree of dependence, we have chosen frailty distributions with $\tau = 0.25$. Table 7.3 gives an overview of the parameter values for this comparison. For the gamma frailty model (Figure 7.3), the contour curves increase fastest near (1,1), showing a high late dependence. On the other hand, Figure 7.4 shows the contours for the stable frailty model. The density is above 1, near (0,0) and (1,1), but the contour curves increase fastest near (0,0), showing the high early dependence. Figure 7.5 shows the contour curves for the inverse Gaussian frailty

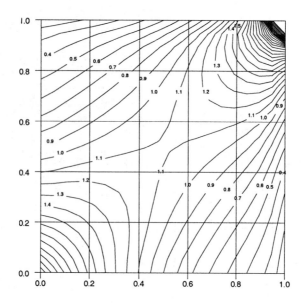

Figure 7.5. Contour curves for the density of a bivariate uniform distribution with inverse Gaussian frailty dependence, with $\tau = 0.25$.

model. The contour curves are not lying quite as close near (0,0) and (1,1), showing that the density is not as steep there. The density is higher in the interior, which can be illustrated with the values at (1/2,1/2), and is 1.107 for the stable model, 1.134 for the gamma model, and 1.116 for the inverse Gaussian model. In all cases, the value at this point is not far from 1. The inverse Gaussian frailty distribution is in both tails intermediate between the gamma and stable.

The lognormal is rather close to the inverse Gaussian model and therefore not shown. The only difference seems to be that the same value of τ is obtained with a slightly lower variance on the logarithm, as illustrated in Table 7.3.

This point becomes more clear by showing the density along the diagonal, which is done in Figure 7.6. This is the density at points (t, t), under a bivariate distribution with uniform marginals. Again, this shows that the density is high at the extreme points, but close to 1 in the central area. Also the close agreement of the lognormal and the inverse Gaussian is clearly shown.

As an alternative, the same figures can be made as three-dimensional plots. For the gamma model, this is done in Figure 7.7. For the positive stable model, this is done in Figure 7.8. For the inverse Gaussian model, this is done in Figure 7.9. These figures show, like the contour curves, the high early dependence for the stable model and the high late dependence

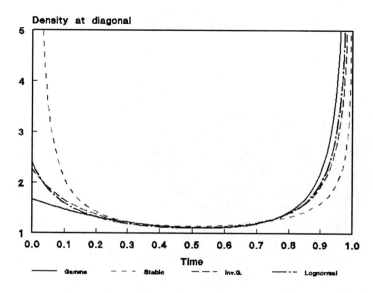

Figure 7.6. Density of bivariate uniform distributions at the diagonal (t, t) with stable, gamma, inverse Gaussian and lognormal frailty dependence, with $\tau = 0.25$. The lognormal is based on an approximation.

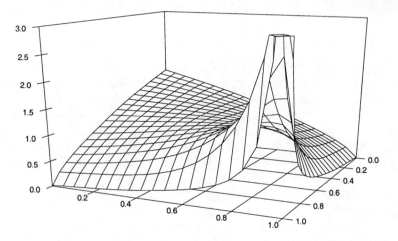

Figure 7.7. Density of a bivariate uniform distribution with gamma frailty dependence, with $\tau = 0.25$.

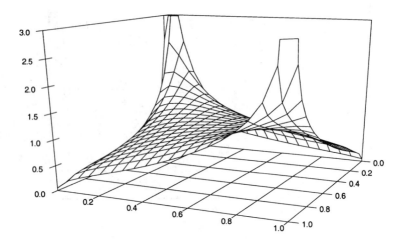

Figure 7.8. Density of a bivariate uniform distribution with positive stable frailty dependence, with $\tau = 0.25$.

for the gamma model. For points near $(0,1)$, corresponding to one early and one late event, the gamma model has almost 0 density, whereas the other distributions have a higher density.

A different illustration of the model fit based on a more dynamic evaluation is done in Figures 8.3 and 8.4 for one of the applications.

7.8.3   Quantification of dependence

To compare the various measures of dependence, Table 7.4 lists the expressions. All depend on the frailty distribution alone. This shows which measures are simple to evaluate, but not to which extent the measures are robust toward the choice of model. The agreement between the various measures can be calculated in one-parameter submodels. Kendall's τ and the median concordance are approximately equal. This is illustrated in Figure 7.10. Kendall's τ is simpler to evaluate, but has a more complicated interpretation, as it involves two pairs. The median concordance can be interpreted by means of a single pair. The measure called Corr. (marg.) is the integrated hazard correlation of Equation (4.15).

The relationship between the variance of the logarithm of Y and Kendall's τ is illustrated in Figure 7.11. For graphical purposes, this is done by considering the standard deviation of the logarithm of Y. There is a reasonable agreement on the relation between the two measures in the

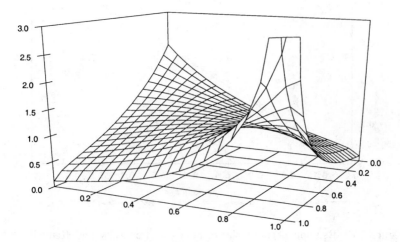

Figure 7.9. Density of a bivariate uniform distribution with inverse Gaussian frailty dependence, with $\tau = 0.25$.

Measure	Gamma	Stable	Inv.Gauss	PVF($\alpha > 0$)
$c.v.(Y)^2$	δ^{-1}	∞	$(2\eta)^{-1}$	$(1-\alpha)/\eta$
Var $(\log Y)$	$\psi'(\delta)$	$(\alpha^{-2} - 1)\psi'(1)$	Eq. (A.15)	Num. int.
Corr. (const. μ)	Known	$1 - h(1)/h(\alpha)$	Known	Known
Corr. (marg.)		$1 - h(\alpha)/h(\alpha^2)$		
Corr. $\log T$	Eq. (7.42)	$1 - \alpha^2$	Known	
τ	$1/(1+2\delta)$	$1 - \alpha$	Eq. (7.58)	Eq. (7.58)
κ	Eq. (7.36)	$2^{2-2^\alpha} - 1$	Eq. (7.59)	Eq. (7.59)
ρ	Eq. (7.37)	Num.int.	Num.int.	Num.int.
Max. τ	1	1	1/2	1

Table 7.4. Variability and dependence measures for various frailty models. Known means that a complicated, but known expression is available. Blank means that no reduced expression is available. $h(\cdot)$ is defined below Equation (7.53). Corr. $\log T$ refers to a Weibull model. Num.int. means numerical integration.

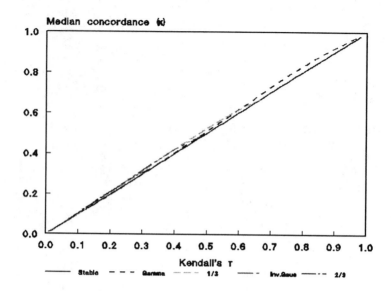

Figure 7.10. Relation between the median concordance κ and Kendall's τ in various submodels of the PVF family ($\theta = 0$ and $\alpha = 0$, 1/3, 1/2 and 2/3).

various submodels. The lognormal gives slightly larger values of τ than the inverse Gaussian model with the same variance on the logarithmic scale.

Figure 7.12 shows the relation between Spearman's ρ and Kendall's τ, for the bivariate models generated by the gamma, stable, and inverse Gaussian frailty distributions. For comparison also the relation for the bivariate normal distribution is included. All models give almost identical results, where for low values, τ is approximately 2/3 of ρ. Thus there is generally a good (but a non-linear) agreement between κ, ρ, and τ, whereas the frailty variation measure agree less well.

Figure 7.13 shows the relation between Spearman's ρ and the correlation of $\log T$ for bivariate Weibull models generated by the gamma, stable, and inverse Gaussian frailty distributions. Overall, one can conclude that there a fine agreement between these measures, which both make sense as correlation measures. Spearman's ρ is the correlation for uniform marginals and the other is the correlation for $\log T$ in a conditional Weibull model, in which case the model is linear, as follows from Equation 7.18. They show acceptable agreement, and none of them is uniformly higher than the other.

The overall conclusion is that except for the variance of Y, there is a good agreement between these dependence measures.

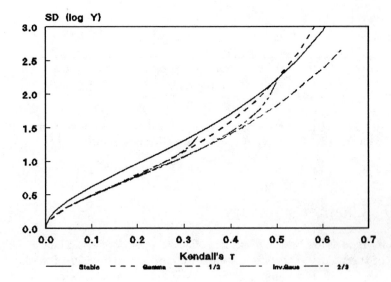

Figure 7.11. Relation between the standard deviation in the distribution of the logarithm of Y and Kendall's τ in various submodels of the PVF family ($\theta = 0$ and $\alpha = 0, 1/3, 1/2$ and $2/3$).

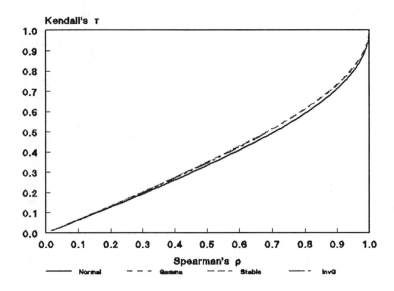

Figure 7.12. Relation between Spearman's ρ and Kendall's τ for various PVF frailty models ($\theta = 0$ and $\alpha = 0$ and $1/2$) and the normal distribution.

7.9 Chapter summary

Frailty models are basically random effects models for survival data, where one of the random effects is specified by means of the hazard function. In the case of matched pairs covariates, we do not need to specify a distribution for the group effect. In this case, we can simply evaluate the effect of the covariates, but not the degree of dependence. In order to evaluate the dependence, and to analyze models with more general covariates, we need to suggest a distribution for the frailty. From a theoretical point of view, the stable distributions are most satisfactory, as they are consistent regarding proportional hazards for the covariates, but unfortunately, the fit is in several of the applications not satisfactory. The stable model cannot be applicable when truncation is performed. The stable model might be the most sensible for regression models, whereas the gamma and the more general PVF models may give strange results for the effect of covariates, meaning that sometimes the non-proportional hazards have higher influence on the estimate than the degree of dependence and, therefore, one needs to interpret the results with care. The stable model implies high dependence early and the gamma model late, whereas the general PVF model and the lognormal model are intermediate. Dependence can be assessed by the rank-based correlation-type measures, Kendall's τ, Spearman's ρ and the median con-

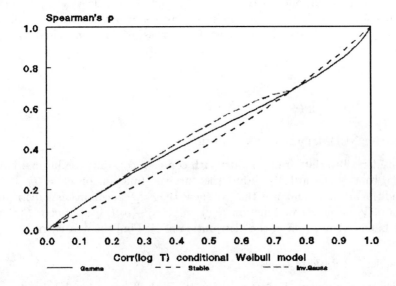

Figure 7.13. Relation between the correlation of $\log T$ for conditional Weibull models and Spearman's ρ for various PVF frailty models ($\theta = 0$, $\alpha = 0$, and $1/2$).

cordance (κ). All of these depend only on the frailty distribution (that is, are independent of the hazard function).

7.10   Bibliographic comments

The term *frailty* was suggested by Vaupel *et al.* (1979) for univariate data. The bivariate model based on gamma distributed frailty was derived by Clayton (1978). It was further studied by Oakes (1982a) and generalized to include covariates by Clayton and Cuzick (1985). The bivariate model based on stable distributed frailty was suggested by Hougaard (1986b), and further considered in Hougaard (1989) and Oakes (1989, 1994). In the case of exponential marginals (Equation (7.52)), the model was suggested by Gumbel (1960), but only very few properties were mentioned. Lee (1979) found the Equation (7.25) for the stable-Weibull model. This result was generalized to general frailty models by Genest and Rivest (1993), but formulated in a quite different way than presented here. Crowder (1989) studied the PVF models, from a different perspective. Review papers are Marshall and Olkin (1988), Hougaard (1995) and Liang *et al.* (1995). Whitmore and Lee (1991) suggest the multivariate model with inverse Gaussian frailty and exponential conditional distributions. Lu and Bhattacharyya (1990) presented several stable-Weibull model extensions, which here are described in the exercises. Some further dependence measures are considered by van den Berg (1997).

7.11 Exercises

Exercise 7.1 Distribution of sum of times

Consider a bivariate frailty model with common constant conditional hazards, that is, hazard $Y\mu$. Find the survivor function of $V = T_1 + T_2$ conditional on Y and use this to show that the unconditional distribution of V has survivor function $S(v) = L(\mu v) - \mu v L'(\mu v)$, where $L(s)$ is the Laplace transform of the distribution of Y. Find the density of V.

Exercise 7.2 Ratio of times

Consider a bivariate frailty model with Weibull conditional hazards, as described in Section 7.2.4. Derive the distribution of the ratio $V = T_1/T_2$ and show that this is stochastically independent of Y and that it is not influenced by the parameters of the distribution of Y. It may be convenient to work on a logarithmic scale for this evaluation.

Exercise 7.3 Number of survivors

Consider a shared frailty model for a group of k individuals, and assume the same distribution for all individuals. Find the probability that exactly m of them are alive at age t.

Exercise 7.4 General frailty updating

Consider a general shared frailty model for a group with k members, as in Equation (7.2). Find the mean and the variance expressed by the Laplace transform and its derivatives conditional on $T_j > t_j$, $j = 1, ..., k$. Find similarly the mean and the variance expressed by the Laplace transform and its derivatives conditional on $T_1 = t_1$, $T_j > t_j$, $j = 2, ..., k$.

Exercise 7.5 Derivation of Kendall's τ

Derive the formulas $\tau = 1/(1 + 2\delta)$ for the gamma model and $1 - \alpha$ for the stable model, using Equation (7.23).

Exercise 7.6 Alternative formula for Kendall's τ

Express Kendall's τ by means of $\int_0^\infty sL'(s)^2 ds$.

Exercise 7.7 Dependence assessment based on frailty variance

Make a figure like Figure 7.11, but using $SD(Y)$ instead of $SD(\log Y)$.

Exercise 7.8 Maximum correlation in Weibull models

Show that for each value of γ there is a maximum obtainable correlation
of times in Equation (7.20). Show that for the correlation of log times
(Equation (7.22)), the maximum is the trivial limit (1).

Exercise 7.9 Contours for $\tau = 0.5$

Make figures like Figures 7.7 and 7.8, but choosing $\tau = 0.5$. Why is it not
relevant to also make a figure for the inverse Gaussian model?

Exercise 7.10 Survivor function random variable

Consider a general shared frailty model without censoring. Let $W = S(T_1, T_2)$. Show that the distribution function for W is $w - q(w)/q'(w)$
using Equation (7.25), where q is the inverse to the Laplace transform.
What is the density for W?
    Specialize the results to the case of (T_1, T_2) being independent.

Exercise 7.11 Moments in gamma frailty Weibull models

Consider the model of Section 7.3.2. What is the mean and variance of T_1?
What is the correlation between T_1 and T_2? Compare this to the correlation
on the logarithmic scale (Equation (7.42)).
    For a more refined study of the dependence, we aim at evaluating
$\omega^2 = E\{T_2 - m(T_1)\}^2$. When $m(T_1)$ is restricted to be linear, the expression is minimized by the right hand side of Equation (4.2). In general,
the expression is minimized by $m(T_1) = E(T_2 \mid T_1)$. Find this function and
the value of ω^2. For comparing the general and the linear case, make a
figure of ω^2 as function of δ for two chosen values of γ.

Exercise 7.12 Gamma frailty probability results

What do Equations (7.25) and (7.26) tell when the frailty distribution is
gamma?

Exercise 7.13 Distribution of the bivariate maximum

Suppose the bivariate distribution is the Weibull model described in Equation (7.50). What is the distribution of the longest lifetime within a
pair?

Exercise 7.14 Conditional distributions in positive stable frailty models

Consider a bivariate model with positive stable frailty and conditional hazard functions $\mu_j(t)$. Derive the conditional distribution of T_1 given $T_2 = t_2$.

Evaluate the conditional mean $E(M_1(T_1) \mid T_2 = t_2)$. Derive the conditional distribution of T_1 given $T_2 > t_2$. Evaluate the conditional mean $E(M_1(T_1) \mid T_2 > t_2)$. This can be expressed by means of an incomplete gamma function integral.

Exercise 7.15 Trivariate stable-Weibull density

Find explicitly the density for a three-dimensional observation in the stable-Weibull model.

Exercise 7.16 Correlation for the stable-Weibull model

Make a figure like Figure 7.2, but draw curves for selected values of γ, the shape parameter in the conditional distribution.

Exercise 7.17 PVF frailty probability results

What do Equations (7.25) and (7.26) tell when the frailty distribution is in the PVF family?
    What does the result say in the stable frailty submodel?

Exercise 7.18 Truncated τ

Evaluate Kendall's τ for bivariate data after truncation at time t, under a PVF frailty model with conditional hazard $\mu(t)$. Show that it decreases over time, when $\alpha > 0$.

Exercise 7.19 PVF Gompertz model

Assume that the conditional hazard is $Y\varphi^t$ and that the distribution of Y is $\mathrm{PVF}(\alpha, \delta, 1/\log \varphi)$. Show that all parameters can be identified by means of bivariate data. Which parameter functions can be identified by means of univariate data? Conclude that this can serve a purpose as a Gompertz random effects model. Would you apply this model in practice?

Exercise 7.20 Correlation in the inverse Gaussian frailty model

Assume that the conditional distribution is exponential and that the frailty follows an inverse Gaussian distribution. Find the correlation of T_1 and T_2.

Exercise 7.21 Updating in the inverse Gaussian frailty model

Derive explicitly the density of the distribution of the frailty in a bivariate inverse Gaussian frailty model after observing a death at time t and knowing that the other pair member is alive at that time.

Exercise 7.22 Lognormal Weibull

Assume that the conditional distribution is Weibull and that the frailty follows a lognormal distribution. Find the correlation of T_1 and T_2 using Equations (7.19) and (7.20) and that if Y is lognormal, $Y^{-1/\gamma}$ is also lognormal. Show that it depends on γ, but is independent of λ_1 and λ_2. Compare to the value on the logarithmic scale (Equation (7.61)). This could be done by a figure similar to that shown in Figure 7.2.

Exercise 7.23 Lognormal contour plot

Make a figure like Figure 7.5, but for a lognormal frailty model using the approximate Laplace transform. Choose $\sigma = 0.882$, which was found to give $\tau = 0.25$ according to Table 7.3.

Exercise 7.24 Constant + gamma frailty

This is a continuation of an exercise in Section 2.9. Let the frailty be given as $Y = c + Z$, where c is a positive constant, and Z is gamma distributed. Derive the bivariate survivor function. What does the change in the coefficient of variation imply for the dependence? Consider only a single individual, and evaluate the distribution of Y giving the death time of the individual. Show that this is not of the form $c + \tilde{Z}$, where $\tilde{Z}$ is gamma distributed.

Exercise 7.25 Gamma-stable multiplicative frailty model

Suppose the frailty can be described as $Y = Z^{1/\alpha}U$, where Z and U are independent, Z is gamma distributed with parameters (δ, δ), and U follows a positive stable distribution of index α. This model is called an interior power family by Oakes (1994). Find the Laplace transform of Y. Let the conditional hazard be Weibull of shape γ, and suppose there is a vector of covariates z_j for the jth individual, so that the conditional hazard model reads $Y \exp(\beta' z_j)\lambda\gamma t^{\gamma-1}$. Find the marginal distribution of a lifetime. Find the bivariate survivor function. What is the correlation of $\log T_1$ and $\log T_2$? Show that Kendall's τ equals $1 - \alpha + \alpha/(1 + 2\delta)$.

   Show that it is not possible to identify all parameters from the marginal distributions. It is only possible to identify δ, $\alpha\beta$, λ^α, and $\alpha\gamma$. Show that the marginal distributions allow for determining a lower bound for the correlation of log times.

Exercise 7.26 Non-central gamma frailty

Let the frailty follow the non-central gamma distribution described in Section A.3.7. Find the relation between the marginal and conditional integrated hazard function. What is the distribution of the frailty among the survivors? For both univariate and bivariate data, evaluate the variance among the survivors in age t. Find the cross-ratio function extending Equation (7.39) of the central case. How does it change over time?

Exercise 7.27 Marshall-Olkin shared frailty combination

Let (U_0, U_1, U_2) follow a shared positive stable frailty model with Weibull conditional hazards of parameters $(\alpha, \epsilon_0, \epsilon_1, \epsilon_2, \gamma)$. Define $T_1 = \min(U_0, U_1)$, $T_2 = \min(U_0, U_2)$. Show that for $\alpha = 1, \gamma = 1$, this is the Marshall-Olkin model. Show that for $\alpha = 1$, this is the Marshall-Olkin extension described in Exercise 5.8. Show that for $\epsilon_0 = 0$, this is the bivariate shared stable frailty Weibull model of Section 7.4.3. Show that the marginal distributions of T_1 and T_2 are Weibull and describe the parameters. Show that the distribution of $T_{\min} = \min(T_1, T_2)$ is Weibull and describe the parameters. Find the probability that $T_1 = T_2$. Show that all parameters can be identified from bivariate data.

Exercise 7.28 A shared frailty-independence combination

Let U_1, U_2, and (V_1, V_2) be independent so that U_1 is Weibull (λ_1, γ), U_2 is Weibull (λ_2, γ), and (V_1, V_2) follow a shared positive stable frailty model with Weibull conditional hazards of parameters $(\alpha, \epsilon_1, \epsilon_2, \kappa)$. Define $T_1 = \min(V_1, U_1)$, $T_2 = \min(V_2, U_2)$. Assume that $\gamma = \alpha\kappa$. Find the bivariate survivor function. Show that if $\alpha = 1$, T_1 and T_2 are independent. Show that the marginal distributions of T_1 and T_2 are Weibull and describe the parameters. Show that the distribution of $T_{\min} = \min(T_1, T_2)$ is Weibull and describe the parameters. Show that the probability of $T_1 = T_2$ is 0. Show that all parameters can be identified from bivariate data.

Make an interpretation of this model as (U_1, U_2) representing one cause of death and (V_1, V_2) representing another cause of death.

Exercise 7.29 Exterior power families

Let T_{ij} follow a shared frailty model with frailty Y_i and thus with independence over i and dependence over j. Define the minimum across groups as $T_{\min,j} = \min(T_{1j}, ..., T_{nj})$. The aim of this exercise is to extend the results of Section 7.4.3 to more general frailty models. Show that the distribution of $(T_{\min,1}, ..., T_{\min,k})$ is a frailty model with the same conditional hazard and with frailty $Y = Y_1 + ... + Y_n$. This model has been denoted the exterior power family by Oakes (1994).

Exercise 7.30 Comparison of two reciprocal models

Let Y be stable distributed with $\alpha = 1/2$. Find the dependence measures τ, ρ, κ, $\text{Var}(Y)$ and $\text{Var}(\log Y)$ for a shared frailty model with Y as frailty. Show that $\tilde{Y} = 1/Y$ follows a gamma distribution and find the parameter value. Find the same dependence measures when $\tilde{Y}$ is the frailty. Compare to the values for Y.

8
Statistical inference for shared frailty models

This chapter considers the statistical inference for the shared frailty models described in the previous chapter. A main part of this is estimation procedures. Estimation difficulties have previously limited the applicability of the shared frailty models. There have, however, been a number of suggestions on how to estimate the parameters. Reasons for the many choices are, of course, that some formulas are complicated and that iteration can be time consuming. One basic direction to take is to integrate out the random frailties, but this is not the only possibility. Alternatively, one can use estimation routines where the frailties are included as unobserved random variables, similar to BLUP (best linear unbiased predictor) methods for normal distribution models. For non-parametric hazard functions, there is one parameter per time point with observed events. This can be specifically included in the model, or one can attempt to remove it from the likelihood, an approach that is inspired by the successful way of doing so in the Cox model. Also for the Nelson-Aalen estimate, it is easy to handle the hazard contributions, because there is a separate equation for each term allowing for an explicit solution. It is, unfortunately, not quite as easy in a frailty model; iteration is necessary as all expressions are non-linear and related to each other.

The general model used here is the frailty model with regression terms, as described in Equation (7.28). Parametric models make up the simplest approach and are described in Section 8.1. A simple alternative is to use a non-parametric dependence measure, like Kendall's τ, to estimate the dependence parameter (see Section 8.2). The EM-algorithm offers a reasonable simple approach (see Section 8.3), but the necessary number of iterations can be high. Another simple approach that partially accounts for a non-parametric hazard function is the three-stage approach described in Section 8.4. Without covariates or with covariates in a stable frailty model, the full non-parametric estimate can be found using the parametrization based on the marginal distribution (Section 8.5). The standard estimate can be found by a full maximization of the likelihood in the conditional parametrization (Section 8.6). An alternative procedure is the penalized likelihood approach (Section 8.7). This gives the same estimate as the conditional approach, but the calculated standard errors are different. Other approaches are mentioned in Section 8.8. Public software for these methods is briefly discussed in Section 8.9.

Methods to consider the goodness-of-fit are described in Section 8.10.

Asymptotic theory for these models is still under development. Recently, formulas for the Fisher information for several parametric models with gamma or stable frailties and Weibull hazards have been evaluated. These evaluations suffer from requiring uncensored data and are therefore not relevant for practical applications, but they allow for a better understanding of the models. Significant progress has also been made for semi-parametric models with gamma distributed frailty. Asymptotic evaluations are considered in Section 8.11.

Applications are considered in Section 8.12. Besides just illustrating that these methods can be applied, a number of key aspects of the theory are further discussed, covering the difference between the marginal and the conditional parametrization, including the interpretation of the corresponding regression coefficients, the difference between the various distributions of the frailty, the difference between the estimation procedures, quantification of dependence, and, finally, the difference between the relative risk and the accelerated failure time formulations for the effects of covariates in Weibull models.

Readers who are only interested in the applications may go directly Section 8.12.

8.1   Parametric models

A fully parametric model can be handled in the usual way, by differentiating the log likelihood, as described in Equation (7.6). Examples described in the previous chapter are the gamma-Weibull model and the stable-Weibull model. In principle, this presents no special problems in the bivariate case, but in the general multivariate case, one needs to code general formulas for the derivatives of the Laplace transform. We can use parameters from the conditional or marginal distribution as we like. The statistical models are not exponential families and thus there are no simple sufficient reductions.

An iterative solution is necessary. The matrix of second order derivatives can be found analytically or by numerical differentiation.

After the estimates and the variance matrix have been found, we can calculate the variance and correlation for a set of parameter functions. How this is done in practice is illustrated for one of the models in the application in Section 8.12.5.

An application using this approach is described in Section 8.12.2.

8.2 Simple estimates

In the simple case without covariates, one may evaluate some simple measure of dependence, like Kendall's τ by means of Equation (4.8). This is valid more generally than frailty models and allows for determining the degree of dependence. Within a frailty model, it can further be used for determining the frailty parameter. The equation for this is $\delta = (1/\tau - 1)/2$ in the gamma model and $\alpha = 1 - \tau$ in the stable case. The approach does not work for the PVF model, because this determination only allows for one parameter. This approach does not make sense when the frailty model is not known precisely and therefore this method seems applicable to obtain an initial estimate, but not relevant for the full estimate. Manatunga and Oakes (1996) consider the asymptotic efficiency of this approach and evaluate the moments for these estimates.

8.3 The EM-algorithm

The most commonly applied estimation method for parallel data with covariates is the EM-algorithm. This method does not use the observed likelihood of Equation (7.6), but the full likelihood, including both the observed quantities (T, D) and the frailty Y. Conceptually, it can be described as introducing the frailties into the likelihood (similar to the hazard function of Equation (7.1)) and then multiplying by the density of the frailties. We will describe this in the case of gamma distributed frailties, where we will take $\theta = \delta$ to obtain a mean of 1.

Formally, this gives a full likelihood of $L_{(T,D)|Y}L_Y$, where the first term is a standard survival likelihood given the frailties

$$\prod_i \prod_j Y_i^{D_{ij}} \mu_0(T_{ij})^{D_{ij}} \exp(D_{ij}\beta' z_{ij}) \exp\{-\int_0^{T_{ij}} Y_i \mu_0(u) \exp(\beta' z_{ij})du\}$$

$$(8.1)$$

extending Equation (2.33), and the second term is just a product of the gamma densities (Equation (A.8)):

$$\prod_i \delta^\delta Y_i^{\delta-1} \exp(-\delta Y_i)/\Gamma(\delta).$$

The approach alternates between an expectation step (E-step) and a maximization step (M-step). In the expectation step, the unobserved terms in the log likelihood are removed by substitution with the mean value given the observations. In the present case, this is the mean value in what we have previously called the updated distribution of Y, based on all information for the relevant group (Section 7.2.3). As described in Section 7.3.1, the conditional distribution is gamma with parameters $\tilde{\delta}_i = \delta + \sum_j D_j$ and $\tilde{\theta}_i = \delta + \sum_j M_j(T_j)$. Both Y_i and $\log Y_i$ enter the log likelihood. Therefore we insert

$$E(Y_i \mid F_\infty) = \frac{\tilde{\delta}_i}{\tilde{\theta}_i}, \quad E(\log Y_i \mid F_\infty) = \psi(\tilde{\delta}_i) - \log \tilde{\theta}, \qquad (8.2)$$

where the second term is found using Equation (A.10). In the maximization step, the frailty values are considered fixed and known. First, we observe the expected likelihood factors as $L_1(\beta)L_2(\delta)$. Correspondingly, we can maximize each term separately. The original formulation of this method moved the term originating from $Y_i^{D_{ij}}$ to the other factor, but as this is a likelihood constant in this step, it does not matter where it is placed. For δ the problem is a one-parameter maximization that can be done numerically. For β this is the same problem as a Cox model with known regression coefficients. The way this is seen is by formulating the Y_i term as $\exp(\zeta_i z_i)$, where $z_i = \log Y_i$, and ζ_i is a parameter, fixed at 1. The hazard function parameters are eliminated by

$$\hat{\lambda}_0(t) = \frac{1}{\sum_{(i,j)\in R(t)} \tilde{Y}_i \exp(\beta' z_{ij})}.$$

This gives an ordinary partial likelihood function of the same form as Equation (2.32), but including both ζ and β as parameters. Fixing ζ implies that β is estimated keeping the Y terms fixed. When β is found in this way, a new expectation step is performed. The procedure can be summarized in the following way:

1. Find estimates of β and $\Lambda(t)$ in the model without frailty. This corresponds to setting $\delta = \infty$.

2. (E-step) Insert the means evaluated by means of Equation (8.2) based on the current values of the parameters.

3. (M-step part 1) Maximize L_1 as function of β by means of the standard Cox evaluation. Evaluate the integrated hazard $\Lambda(t)$.

4. (M-step part 2) Maximize L_2 as function of δ.

5. Go to step 2 until the estimates have converged.

The EM-algorithm is simple, and easy to program, which are the main reasons for its popularity. It may, however, require a very large number of iterations. One advantage of this approach is that the death times contribute in a simple way, and only in the expectation step, as the maximization step (Step 3) is a Cox partial likelihood, where the parameters for the hazard at the death times are eliminated.

This approach does not allow for evaluation of the variance in the full model. It is, however, possible to use the EM-algorithm to obtain the parameter estimates and then use another approach for finding variance estimates.

8.4 The three-stage approach

As a parametric model might not give a satisfactory fit to the marginal distribution, we have also considered an alternative semi-parametric approach, which combines parametric models for the dependence with classical non-parametric estimates for the marginal distribution. This is based on Equation (7.9). The approach, which covers the model without covariates, and the positive stable frailty model with covariates, is a three-stage procedure, which approximates the full maximum likelihood estimate. In the first stage, estimates of the parameters of the marginal distributions are found, and this is done by a parametric model, a non-parametric Nelson-Aalen estimate in the case of no covariates, or a Cox partial likelihood in the case with covariates. This is called the independence working model (IWM), because we act as if the times are independent. The estimated integrated hazard then is $\hat{\Omega}_{ij}(t)$, which in the Nelson-Aalen case does not depend on i and j, and in the proportional hazards case is of the form $\hat{\Omega}(t)\exp(\hat{\beta}'z_{ij})$. In the second step, the marginal lifetime distributions are considered fixed and known and the dependence is estimated. In practice, this is done by transforming by the integrated hazard function, that is, observations T_{ij} are substituted for by

$$\tilde{T}_{ij} = \hat{\Omega}_{ij}(T_{ij}). \tag{8.3}$$

If the true value of $\Omega_{ij}(\cdot)$ was used instead of the estimate, this would give exponentially distributed variables of mean 1. As the hazard functions are estimated, $\tilde{T}_{ij}$ is only approximately exponentially distributed. However, one does not need to consider the scale of the transformed observations as fixed. It is simple to assume that the marginal hazards are proportional to the estimate found for the marginal distribution. In practice, this is done by applying a bivariate distribution with general exponential marginals instead of the unit exponential distributions expected after the time transformation in Equation (8.3). This is called step 3. Formally, this is an improvement the estimate by allowing the parameters to deviate from the

Step	Dependence parameter	Marginal distribution
1	Data assumed independent	Estimated
2	Estimated	Fixed
3	Estimated	Proportionality factor estimated

Table 8.1. Overview of the three-stage approach.

estimate under the hypothesis of independence. In practice, the difference is not big, but still it is beneficial to make this extension as the variance is less underestimated by choosing the largest possible model. For a positive stable frailty distribution, this makes only very little difference, both in the estimated dependence and the estimated variance for this quantity. For other distributions there difference is still only slight, although it is bigger than for the stable model. This approach does not account for the variance of the Nelson-Aalen estimate. The steps are summarized in Table 8.1.

One could also use a Weibull model instead of an exponential model for the marginal hazard, as this is a better approximation to the non-parametric estimate and gives a more correct variance estimate by relaxing the assumptions. In the case of the stable model, one could also include covariates in a regression model and fit the coefficients in the bivariate exponential model in order to improve the estimate, and to find a better estimate of the variability.

This approach is in some respects similar to the methods described in Chapter 13.

The three-stage approach is an approximation and therefore, it makes sense only when we are not able to calculate the full estimate. How to do that is described in the next section.

8.5 The full marginal estimate

It is also possible to use this as a step toward evaluating the full maximum likelihood estimate, which in light of the three-stage procedure will be called step 4. This requires the likelihood to be formulated with discrete contributions to the marginal hazard at the death times. This is done by using Equations (7.9) and (7.10), specifying the full distribution by means of the integrated hazard in the marginal distribution. The advantage of doing so is that it makes a good parametrization, that is, one where convergence is fast, as the various parameters are close to being independent. The disadvantage of this approach is that we do need to include a parameter for each death time. This means that there is no shortcut as in the partial likelihood approach, Equation (2.31), where the hazard terms cancel out.

Use of this method requires, of course, that the marginal distribution has a usable structure. This means that without covariates, this can be considered for any frailty distribution. Hazard functions can also differ in a stratified model. With covariates acting in a proportional hazards model, the approach, however, only makes sense from a random effects point of view, when the frailty distribution is the positive stable. Process-dependent censoring cannot be allowed, because in that case, the marginal estimate might be biased.

Specifically, in the case of a gamma model without covariates and common hazard function $\omega(t)$, we obtain by insertion in Equation (7.35) a likelihood contribution of a single group of

$$\{\prod_{j=1}^{k} \omega(T_j)^{D_j} \exp\{D_j\Omega(T_j)/\delta\}$$

$$[\sum_j \exp\{-\Omega(T_j)/\delta\} - (k-1)]^{-(\delta+D.)}\delta^{-D.}\Gamma(\delta+D.)/\Gamma(\delta). \qquad (8.4)$$

This function can be maximized by the same principles as will be described below for the conditional method of Section 8.6. That is, for each time of observed events, one parameter should be included giving a discrete contribution to $\Omega(t)$. The likelihood and its first two derivatives are evaluated and used in a Newton-Raphson procedure.

However, it is not necessary to evaluate the full matrix of second derivatives during iteration. Instead an approximation is used and therefore iteration can be done fast. In practice this is done by letting the mixed second derivatives with respect to the hazard contributions be approximated by 0, and then the second derivative matrix is inverted using the formula in the Appendix Equation (B.3). This is faster because there are fewer terms to evaluate, and the matrix inversion is simplified. When there are a large number of parameters, the matrix inversion is the slowest step. On the other hand, more iterations might be necessary, but in practice this makes only little difference, when the evaluations are done using the marginal parameters. Owing to the approximate independence, the approximation to the second derivative matrix is so good that it can often be used also for evaluation of the variance. This will be illustrated for the application to twins (Table 8.20).

8.6 The full conditional estimate

A more direct approach is to use Equation (7.6) and insert non-parametric expressions for the hazard, again assuming a discrete contribution, $\mu(t_j)$, at each time of event. The estimate equals that of the EM-algorithm. The formulas are reasonably simple, but the parameter estimates are clearly correlated. The consequence of this is that the approximation obtained by setting the mixed derivatives to 0, is not as satisfying as under the marginal parametrization. Therefore more iterations must be expected, and the approximate inverse is not as good a measure of the variability.

The same approach when used for the univariate proportional hazards models gives exactly the same results as the Cox partial likelihood, using the tie handling method of Breslow. In that case the mixed second derivatives with respect to the hazards at the death times are exactly 0, and therefore there is no approximation involved in the simple inversion method. We have gone through this anyway, because it gives a likelihood value that is comparable to the likelihood under the frailty models. The Cox partial likelihood values are not relevant here, because they do not account for the contribution of the hazard function.

The rest of this section describes in detail how to do this, and can be omitted by practically oriented readers. We will specify the actual formulas, to cover both the case of piecewise constant hazards and non-parametric hazard functions. Let index q correspond to interval number with interval endpoints $x_1, ..., x_m$ in the piecewise constant hazards case of Equation (2.12), respectively, death time number in the non-parametric case. In the latter case $x_1, ..., x_m$ denote the ordered death times. To simplify formulas, only a single group is considered, with times $T_1, ..., T_k$ and censoring indicators $D_1, ..., D_k$. We then define event indicators in each interval of the form $D_{jq} = D_j 1\{x_{q-1} < T_j \leq x_q\}$ and corresponding risk set variables, R_{jq}, which in the piecewise constant hazards case is given by Equation (2.13), and in the non-parametric case by $R_{jq} = 1\{T_j \geq x_q\}$. The integrated hazard function M_j is then given as $\exp(\beta' z_j) R'_j \mu$, where R_j is the vector with elements $(R_{j1}, ..., R_{jm})$ and μ the vector with elements $(\mu_1, ..., \mu_m)$. This is then inserted into Equation (7.6), with the modification that $\mu_j(t) = \exp(\beta' z_j)\mu(t)$.

8.6.1 The gamma model

In the gamma frailty case, the basis is Equation (7.34). After insertion of the model specified above, and letting $\delta = \theta$ to obtain identifiability, the expression for the log likelihood is

$$\left(\sum_q D_{.q} \log \mu_q\right) + \left(\sum_j D_j \beta' z_j\right) + \delta \log \delta - (\delta + D_{..}) \log(\delta + M.) +$$

$$\log \Gamma(\delta + D_{..}) - \log \Gamma(\delta). \tag{8.5}$$

The only parameter function that is not transparent in this formula is that $M.$ depends on β and μ. Thus M is a linear function of μ, but a non-linear function of β. From this expression, the derivatives with respect to all parameters are easily found.

$$\frac{d \log L}{d\delta} = \log \delta + 1 - \frac{\delta + D_{..}}{\delta + M.} - \log(\delta + M.) + \psi(\delta + D_{..}) - \psi(\delta), \tag{8.6}$$

$$\frac{d \log L}{d\beta_m} = (\sum_j D_j z_{jm}) - \frac{\delta + D..}{\delta + M.} \sum_j M_j z_{jm}, \tag{8.7}$$

$$\frac{d \log L}{d\mu_q} = \frac{D_{.q}}{\mu_q} - \frac{\delta + D..}{\delta + M.} \sum_j \exp(\beta' z_j) R_{jq}. \tag{8.8}$$

The second derivatives can be found by the same principle. They are

$$\frac{d^2 \log L}{d\delta^2} = \frac{1}{\delta} - \frac{2}{\delta + M.} + \frac{\delta + D..}{(\delta + M.)^2} + \psi'(\delta + D..) - \psi'(\delta), \tag{8.9}$$

$$\frac{d^2 \log L}{d\delta d\beta_\ell} = \{\frac{\delta + D..}{(\delta + M.)^2} - \frac{1}{\delta + M.}\} \sum_j M_j z_{j\ell}, \tag{8.10}$$

$$\frac{d^2 \log L}{d\delta d\mu_q} = \{\frac{\delta + D..}{(\delta + M.)^2} - \frac{1}{\delta + M.}\} \sum_j \exp(\beta' z_j) R_{jq}, \tag{8.11}$$

$$\frac{d^2 \log L}{d\beta_\ell d\beta_m} = -\frac{\delta + D..}{\delta + M.} \sum_j M_j z_{j\ell} z_{jm} + \frac{\delta + D..}{(\delta + M.)^2} (\sum_j M_j z_{j\ell})(\sum_j M_j z_{jm}), \tag{8.12}$$

$$\frac{d^2 \log L}{d\mu_\ell d\mu_q} =$$

$$-1\{\ell = q\}(\frac{D_{.q}}{\mu_q^2}) + \frac{\delta + D..}{(\delta + M.)^2} \{\sum_j \exp(\beta' z_j) R_{j\ell}\}\{\sum_j \exp(\beta' z_j) R_{jq}\}, \tag{8.13}$$

$$\frac{d^2 \log L}{d\beta_m d\mu_q} =$$

$$-\frac{\delta + D..}{\delta + M.} \sum_j \exp(\beta' z_j) R_{jq} z_{jm} + \frac{\delta + D..}{(\delta + M.)^2} (\sum_j M_j z_{jm})\{\sum_j \exp(\beta' z_j) R_{jq}\}. \tag{8.14}$$

As pointed out by Korsgaard and Andersen (1998), this likelihood function has a defect. Even though the probability model makes it impossible to identify the parameters from marginal data, the likelihood function depends on the frailty parameters also for univariate data without covariates. As a simple example take two independent individuals with observed times of t_1 and t_2, with $t_1 < t_2$. Then the maximum likelihood estimate is a hazard contribution of $1/2$ at t_1 and $1 + 1/(2\delta)$ at t_2. The profile likelihood is found by inserting this in the log likelihood (Equation (8.5)) and this turns out to be decreasing in δ, so that the estimate of δ is at the boundary corresponding to maximum dependence. This defect is introduced owing to the discrete extension of the hazard function used in the estimation. The marginal approach does not present the same problem.

During iteration, the second derivative may be approximated by using 0 for the value of Equation (8.13) when $\ell \neq q$.

8.6.2 The PVF model

In the PVF case, the expressions are more complicated and it is more difficult to handle the parameter restrictions. In order to cover both the stable and the non-stable case, we will wait to specify the parameter restriction to make the distribution identifiable. This is in order to be flexible later, regarding choice of restriction. So we use all parameters α, δ, and θ for the frailty distribution. That gives, together with Equation (A.18), the following specification of the logarithm of the likelihood:

$$\log L = (\sum_q D_{.q} \log \mu_q) + (\sum_j D_j \beta' z_j) - \frac{\delta}{\alpha}\{(\theta + M.)^\alpha - \theta^\alpha\} + \log Q, \quad (8.15)$$

where Q is given by

$$Q = \sum_{m=1}^{p} \{c_{pm}(\alpha)\delta^m(\theta + M.)^{m\alpha - p}\}, \quad (8.16)$$

where we use $p = D..$ to simplify formulas. The coefficients $c_{pm}(\alpha)$ are defined in Equation (A.19). Finding the derivatives with respect to all parameters is, in principle, elementary, from Equation (8.15), but because Q is a sum, depending on all parameters, it requires some care. The derivatives are

$$\frac{d \log L}{d\alpha} = \frac{\delta}{\alpha^2}\{(\theta + M.)^\alpha - \theta^\alpha\} - \frac{\delta}{\alpha}\{(\theta + M.)^\alpha \log(\theta + M.) - \theta^\alpha \log \theta\}$$

$$+ \sum_{m=1}^{p}\{c'_{pm}(\alpha)\delta^m(\theta + M.)^{m\alpha - p} + c_{pm}(\alpha)\delta^m(\theta + M.)^{m\alpha - p}m\log(\theta + M.)\}/Q$$

$$(8.17)$$

$$\frac{d \log L}{d\delta} = -\frac{1}{\alpha}\{(\theta + M.)^\alpha - \theta^\alpha\} + \sum_{m=1}^{p}\{c_{pm}(\alpha)m\delta^{m-1}(\theta + M.)^{m\alpha - p}\}/Q$$

$$(8.18)$$

$$\frac{d \log L}{d\theta} = -\delta\{(\theta + M.)^{\alpha - 1} - \theta^{\alpha - 1}\}$$

$$+ \sum_{m=1}^{p}\{c_{pm}(\alpha)\delta^m(m\alpha - p)(\theta + M.)^{m\alpha - (p+1)}\}/Q. \quad (8.19)$$

Finding the derivatives with respect to β and μ can be done jointly, by observing that most terms depend on these quantities via $M..$ Therefore, the expressions can be expressed by means of

$$D_M =$$

$$-\delta(\theta + M.)^{\alpha-1} + \sum_{m=1}^{p} \{c_{pm}(\alpha)\delta^m(m\alpha - p)(\theta + M.)^{m\alpha-(p+1)}\}/Q,$$

which is the derivative with respect to $M.$, ignoring the hazard terms that do not depend on the integrated hazard. Then

$$\frac{d \log L}{d\beta_m} = (\sum_j D_j z_{jm}) + D_M \sum_j M_j z_{jm} \qquad (8.20)$$

$$\frac{d \log L}{d\mu_q} = \frac{D_{.q}}{\mu_q} + D_M \sum_j \exp(\beta' z_j) R_{jq}. \qquad (8.21)$$

The second derivatives are derived in a similar way. This is left to the reader.

To apply this in practice, we need a restriction to make the parameters identifiable. In the case of the positive stable frailty distribution we would take $\delta = \alpha$ and let $\theta = 0$, but we can apply the restriction $\delta = \alpha$ also for positive θ. This means that the full parameter $\psi = (\alpha, \delta, \theta, \beta, \mu)$, where β and μ are vectors, should be specified as a linear function of the working parameter $\zeta = (\alpha, \theta, \beta, \mu)$, but this just implies that the vector of derivatives with respect to ζ are $(d \log L/d\alpha + d \log L/d\delta, d \log L/d\theta, d \log L/d\beta, d \log L/d\mu)$. This is the same approach as that of Equation (B.2) as this is just a fit, under an equality restriction for two parameters. As μ is a large dimensional parameter that is treated separately, when the second derivative is approximated, we do not include this in the formula below. Regarding β, we write the formula as it applies for a univariate covariate. To be specific,

$$G = \begin{pmatrix} 1 & 1 & 0 & 0 \\ 0 & 0 & 1 & 0 \\ 0 & 0 & 0 & 1 \end{pmatrix},$$

which is, in fact, just the transpose of $\frac{d\psi}{d\zeta}$. So, we evaluate the likelihood and its first derivatives with respect to the full parameter ψ, making sure that the value satisfies the restriction $\delta = \alpha$. To obtain the derivative with respect to the working parameter ζ, we combine the first two terms by addition, which alternatively can be formulated as multiplying the vector of derivatives with respect to $\alpha, \delta, \theta, \beta$ with the matrix G, and keeping the μ part of the derivative. For the second derivative, G, respectively, G' should be multiplied on either side of the second derivative matrix. Finally, the calculated parameter update should be applied on both α and δ, which is obtained by the first G' in Equation (B.2).

An alternative parametrization is to set $EY = 1$, that is, parametrize by means of (α, η), as described in Section 7.5. The derivatives with respect to the full parameter are found by the same formulas, but the matrix to be multiplied on the derivative vector is different. For the second derivatives, the formula is more complicated, because the function $\psi(\zeta)$ is non-linear in ζ. The function is $\psi(\zeta) = (\alpha, \eta^{1-\alpha}, \eta, \beta)$, again ignoring the μ term. The first and second derivatives of the likelihood are then found using the formulas for chain differentiation:

$$\frac{d \log L}{d\zeta} = \frac{d \log L}{d\psi}\frac{d\psi}{d\zeta}, \quad \frac{d^2 \log L}{d\zeta} = \frac{d\psi'}{d\zeta}\frac{d^2 \log L}{d\psi^2}\frac{d\psi}{d\zeta} + \frac{d \log L}{d\psi}\frac{d\psi^2}{d\zeta^2}$$

The last term is new owing to the non-linearity of the restriction.

The advantage of evaluating the derivatives with respect to the full parameter is that we have a choice of scale restrictions, making it possible to use the same code for the stable model as for the PVF model with the mean restricted to 1. This will also be beneficial for the more complex models to be presented in Chapter 10. The disadvantage compared to substituting the restriction into the likelihood function before differentiation is that we operate with a double parametrization and that some terms would simplify by substitution. However, it is only a few terms that simplify in this way and therefore the double parametrization solution is recommended.

8.7   The penalized likelihood approach

The penalized approach has some similarities to the EM-algorithm. It is based on a modification of the Cox partial likelihood (Equation (2.32)), so that both the regression coefficients and the frailties are included and optimized over. Specifically, the likelihood is described as a product, where the first term is the partial likelihood, including the frailty terms as parameters. The second term is a penalty introduced to avoid large differences between the frailties for the different groups. In practice, it is fitted by first setting the frailty values to 1. Then an iterative procedure is used with a first step of optimizing the partial likelihood, treating the frailties as fixed and known parameters. In the second step, the frailties are evaluated as the conditional means given their observations, using the formulas of Section 7.2.3, like the EM-algorithm. This is repeated until convergence. The advantage of this approach is that the contribution of the integrated hazard is controlled. It is not perfectly eliminated, but the calculations are so simple that the approach allows for a faster optimization. The major disadvantage is that it is difficult to obtain a valid estimate of the standard error, in particular of the frailty parameter. The approach works for the gamma model and approximately for the lognormal model.

8.8   Other approaches

A Markov chain Monte Carlo approach has also been suggested for the gamma frailty model. Instead of handling the complicated likelihood, frailties values are simulated from the distribution of the current step of the iteration. Similar to the EM-algorithm, the procedure interchanges between a step with simulation of the frailties based on the current parameters and the conditional distribution of the frailty given the data and a step, where the parameters are updated based on the frailty values.

Also for the lognormal frailty model, this approach can be performed.

It seems difficult to extend this to the stable model and the PVF model (except for $\alpha = 1/2$), because efficient simulation methods are not available.

8.9   Software

The unspecified frailty model of Section 7.1 is handled by means of the univariate stratified approach, as described in Section 2.4.7.

Splus is able to estimate in random frailty models by means of the penalized likelihood approach. For example, a program to fit the effect of a single covariate, using gamma frailty, can look like the following:

fit <-coxph(Surv(time,event) ~ (x1 + frailty(group)),
  data=dataset, method='breslow')

where time is the response time; event, the event indicator; x1, the covariate; group, the group number; and dataset, the data set stored as a data frame. The output is the variance in the frailty distribution and estimates of the regression coefficients. The standard error is only reported for the regression coefficients. To obtain the lognormal frailty distribution, the program should say

fit <-coxph(Surv(time,event) ~ (x1 + frailty(group,dist="gauss")),
  data=dataset, method='breslow')

The output is, in principle, the same as for the gamma model, but the frailty variance is substituted by the variance of the log frailty.

Klein has offered as SAS macro to estimate in the gamma and stable frailty models based on the EM-algorithm.

Most of the evaluations done in this book are made by the author's personally developed APL programs, which for the moment are not publicly available.

8.10   Goodness-of-fit

It is often relevant to check the assumptions of the model. Generally, this can be done in at least three different ways. One can fit a larger model and then formally or informally make a hypothesis test of the model to be checked. If the test is accepted, the original model is OK. Secondly, one can do additional calculations in the model, expecting specific results if the model is satisfactory. In the standard normal distribution linear model, this could consist of evaluating the residuals and comparing them in some way. Finally, one can fit a completely different model, in order to consider whether there is a satisfactory agreement. All these approaches will be discussed below.

There are quite a few possibilities for fitting larger models. If the frailty distribution of the model is a gamma model, one can fit a PVF frailty model instead. Alternatively, one can fit a bivariate frailty model (see Section 10.5.1). In order to check a parametric model for the hazard, one might instead find an estimate in a non-parametric model. In order to check the proportionality assumption in a regression model, one can stratify according to the covariate and compare the hazard functions. In order to check whether the dependence is of long-term time frame, one can fit a model with time-varying frailty (see Chapter 11). If one suspects that some variable is important, it can be included in the model as covariate. Whether the effect of a covariate is linear on the log hazard can be examined by including non-linear functions of the covariate.

The approach of doing additional calculations was suggested by Shih and Louis (1995a) in the parametric case and Glidden (1999) in the semi-parametric case. They suggested evaluating the conditional mean of Y as function of time in gamma frailty models, that is, the factors in Equation (7.38). These should fluctuate around 1 in the whole population. If the true frailty distribution is different, it deviates from this value.

Fitting a completely different model is possible by fitting a multi-state model for bivariate data. This approach is demonstrated for the twin data, where the ratio of hazards of Equation (7.60) is studied. The same ratio can be evaluated in a multi-state model, and this was done in Figure 6.4. According to the gamma frailty model, measures of dependence, like Kendall's τ, are unchanged by truncation, and in the PVF model, τ decreases over time to 0. This can be checked by evaluating a non-parametric estimate of τ as function of truncation time. Without covariates, this can be done by means of Equation (4.8). This was done for the twin data set by Hougaard, Harvald, and Holm (1992a). Another possibility without covariates is to evaluate a completely non-parametric estimate (see Chapter 14).

A natural question to consider at this point is what are the consequences of picking a wrong frailty distribution. For example, if the true model is generated by stable frailties and it is analyzed by a gamma frailty model, is the estimated τ then different from the true value of τ? With complete data and no covariates, using a wrong frailty model will generally lead to underestimating dependence. With censoring, the answer is not that simple. For example, if the correct model is the stable, and heavy censoring applies, using a gamma model, the estimation will consider the observed high early dependence and as the gamma model implies high late dependence suggest that the late dependence is enormous and overall lead to an overestimated dependence. On the other hand, if the correct model is the gamma, and we apply a stable model, we have the opposite problem: i.e., data appear to be independent even though they are not.

8.11   Asymptotic evaluations

For a valid statistical evaluation, it is important to know the asymptotical properties. This relates to questions like Are the estimates consistent? Do they asymptotically follow a normal distribution? What is the asymptotic variance? and can we estimate the asymptotic variance in a consistent way? A further, more specific, question is, Can we make a valid test of the hypothesis of independence? In a second round, we would like to ask more detailed questions: Are specific estimators preferable (this could both relate to asymptotic efficiency and to differences between asymptotically efficient estimators)? Are the asymptotic evaluations relevant to finite samples and are specific parametrizations better than others?

We have only a few answers to these questions. Clearly more work in this area would be desirable. In this section we report what is known for the moment.

The difficulties with the asymptotic calculations go along four themes – identifiability, boundary problems, censoring, and non-parametric hazards. More specifically, we can list some problems. The scale identifiability problem (for example, solved by restricting the mean frailty to 1) is so well understood that this is not a real problem. The univariate identifiability with finite mean frailty distributions and covariates is not a technical asymptotic problem (because an asymptotic evaluation does not consider whether a piece of information is relevant or irrelevant), but the asymptotic evaluations can show the importance of the problem in practice. By construction, frailty models have independence at the boundary, making it impossible to perform standard likelihood tests for this hypothesis. Some models can be extended to allow negative dependence; but others, like the stable model, have an infinite mean of the second derivative under the hypothesis, implying that the Fisher information does not exist and that it is impossible to extend the model. The PVF model has two parameters for the dependence, which both disappear under independence, creating an identifiability problem at the boundary. This problem also goes under the general name of a nuisance parameter, which is present only under the alternative. As estimation in this model becomes unstable near independence, it is not recommended to use this model for testing independence. The inverse Gaussian model has a boundary problem corresponding to maximal dependence, which is obtained at $\tau = 1/2$. If one experiences this problem, a different frailty model should be considered.

Censoring can lead to specific aspects' not being estimable. From the univariate case, we know, for example, that if the censoring distribution is not unbounded, any aspect of the distribution showing up after the upper limit cannot be estimated. Independent censoring is the most simple, but some sorts of process-dependent censoring are also possible; that is, censoring can depend on the history of the process, but should be independent of the unobserved part of the process, and independent of the frailty. There should furthermore be a positive probability of observing two or more events in each group in order to determine the degree of dependence. Also, censoring implies that variance calculations are based on the second derivative (the observed information) rather than the mean second derivative (the expected or Fisher information), just as in the univariate case, as discussed in Section 2.2.1. The non-parametric hazards require a more general asymptotic apparatus than the parametric models. For the univariate case, the martingale theory has been very successful as such, but more general methods are necessary for the multivariate case. A specific problem for non-parametric models is that the risk set will eventually be 0, meaning that each realization will have an upper bound for where the hazard can be determined. This problem is handled by only considering the estimated hazard function on a finite interval. For the marginal approaches, process-dependent censoring is not acceptable.

Two parametric and one non-parametric model are considered. The gamma-Weibull model with complete data is briefly described (Section 8.11.1). The stable-Weibull model with complete data is treated in detail (Section 8.11.2). Finally, some results for the gamma frailty non-parametric hazard model with as well as without covariates and with censoring are described (Section 8.11.3). Asymptotic results are also available for the estimate based on the first two steps of the three-stage approach (Section 8.11.4).

8.11.1 The gamma-Weibull model

For the gamma frailty bivariate Weibull model of Section 7.3.2 with complete data, the Fisher information can be evaluated by means of elementary functions, including the digamma function and its derivative. The specific formulas are given by Bjarnason and Hougaard (2000). As demonstrated in Section 2.2.7, it is possible to identify all parameters based on the marginals alone. This is similar to the univariate identifiability problem for regression models, but for this Weibull model, the problem is also present without covariates. In fact, the problem does not become worse when covariates are introduced. The paper quantifies how much information comes from the univariate model and how much from the bivariate part of the data. It is found that a marked proportion of the information comes from the univari-

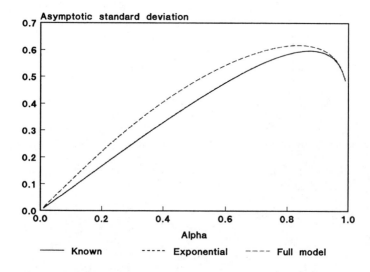

Figure 8.1. Asymptotic standard deviation for $\sqrt{n}(\hat{\alpha} - \alpha)$ in the bivariate stable frailty Weibull distribution, in the full model, under exponential marginals and under known marginals.

ate model, in particular, when the parameters are close to the independence hypothesis. Thus, it is concluded that the univariate identifiability problem is important also in practice.

Like the stable-Weibull model, the assumption of symmetry does not change the asymptotic variance of the dependence parameter.

8.11.2 The stable-Weibull model

The Fisher information can be evaluated in the stable frailty Weibull model, assuming complete data. This can give some theoretical understanding, but as data are typically censored, it is difficult to apply quantitatively to actual data. This section is more technical than the rest of the book. It can be omitted without loss for practical applications. This has been evaluated in the bivariate Weibull, allowing for different shape parameters. Thus it is a five parameter model, with parameters $(\omega_1, \omega_2, \rho_1, \rho_2, \alpha)$. The Weibull parameters used are those of the marginal distribution. At the hypothesis of independence ($\alpha = 1$), the mean of the second derivative with respect to α is infinite, implying that the usual Fisher information results, of the asymptotic variance being the inverse information, can only be applied in the interior of the parameter set. We describe here the relation in a slightly different parametrization than the above, using η_j, defined so that $\eta_j^{\rho_j} = \rho_j \omega_j$, $j = 1, 2$. This makes η_j a scale parameter on the time axis. To shorten formulas, we let $\varphi = 1/\alpha$. We use γ for Eulers constant $(\gamma = -\psi(1))$ and $\delta = \psi'(1) = \pi^2/6$. To simplify formulas, we introduce $H(\varphi) = e^{\varphi-1}E_1(\varphi-1)$, where E_1 is the exponential integral, see Appendix A.4.1. Then the information matrix of a single pair is given by

$$E(D_{\alpha\alpha}\ell) = \varphi^2(\frac{2}{3} - \frac{\pi^2}{9}) + \varphi - 2\alpha K_0 - \{\varphi^3 + \varphi^2 + (K_0-1)\varphi - 2K_0 + \alpha K_0\}H(\varphi),$$

where $K_0 = (15 - \pi^2)/18$. In the case of known marginals, this is the only term necessary. In general, the following terms must also be evaluated:

$$E(D_{\rho_1\rho_1}\ell) = \frac{1}{\rho_1^2}\{-\frac{4}{27}\alpha^3 + \frac{4}{9}\alpha^2(1-\gamma) - \frac{2}{27}\alpha(1-\alpha^2)H(\varphi) - \frac{2\alpha}{9}(3\delta + 3\gamma^2 - 6\gamma + 2)$$

$$+(\frac{2\gamma}{3} - \frac{23}{17}) + \frac{4}{9}\varphi\gamma - \frac{\varphi^2}{3}(\gamma^2 + \delta) + \frac{2}{9}\alpha(1-\alpha)^2 J_1(\alpha) - \frac{(1-\alpha)^2}{3}J_2(\alpha),$$

$$E(D_{\eta_1\eta_1}\ell) = -\frac{\rho_1^2}{3\eta_1^2}\{\varphi^2 + 2\alpha + (\varphi-1)^2\alpha H(\varphi)\},$$

$$E(D_{\rho_1\alpha}\ell) = \frac{1}{\rho_1}[\varphi(\frac{\pi^2}{18} + \frac{1}{6} - \frac{\gamma}{2}) - \frac{1}{2} + \alpha(\frac{\gamma}{2} - \frac{1}{2}) + \alpha^2(\frac{5}{6} - \frac{\pi^2}{18})$$

$$+(1-\alpha)H(\varphi)\{\frac{\varphi}{4} + (1-\alpha)(\frac{5}{12} - \frac{\pi^2}{36})\} - \frac{(\varphi-1)}{4}(2 + \alpha - \alpha^2)J_1(\alpha)],$$

$$E(D_{\eta_1\alpha}\ell) = -\frac{\rho_1\varphi}{4\eta_1}\{2\alpha^2 - 2 + (\varphi-1)(\alpha - \alpha^2 + 2)H(\varphi)\},$$

$$E(D_{\eta_1\rho_1}\ell) = \frac{1}{\eta_1}\{\frac{\gamma\varphi^2}{3} - \frac{2\varphi}{9} - \frac{1}{3} - \frac{2\alpha}{3}(1-\gamma) + \frac{2\alpha^2}{9}$$

$$+\frac{(\alpha-1)^2}{9}H(\varphi) - \frac{(1-\alpha)^2}{3}J_1(\alpha)\},$$

$$E(D_{\rho_1\eta_2}\ell) = \frac{\rho_2}{\rho_1\eta_2}\{-\frac{\gamma}{3}\varphi^2 + \frac{2}{9}\varphi - \frac{1}{6} - \frac{\alpha}{3}(1-\gamma) + \frac{5\alpha^2}{18}$$

$$+\frac{5}{36}(1-\alpha)^2 H(\varphi) - \frac{1}{6}(1-\alpha)^2 J_1(\alpha)\},$$

$$E(D_{\rho_1\rho_2}\ell) = \frac{1}{\rho_1\rho_2}[(\frac{\varphi^2}{3}(\delta + \gamma^2) - \frac{4}{9}\varphi\gamma + (\frac{\gamma}{3} - \frac{\pi^2}{18} + \frac{5}{27}) + \alpha\{-\frac{1}{3}(\delta + \gamma^2) + \frac{2}{3}\gamma - \frac{1}{18}\}$$

$$+\frac{5}{9}\alpha^2(1-\gamma) + \alpha^3(\frac{\pi^2}{18} - \frac{37}{54}) - \alpha(1-\alpha)^2(\frac{37}{108} - \frac{\pi^2}{36})H(\varphi)$$

$$+\frac{5}{18}\alpha(1-\alpha)^2 J_1(\alpha) - \frac{1}{6}(1-\alpha)^2 J_2(\alpha)],$$

$$E(D_{\eta_1\eta_2}\ell) = \frac{\rho_1\rho_2}{\eta_1\eta_2}\{\frac{\varphi^2}{3} - \frac{\alpha}{3} - \frac{1}{6}\alpha(\varphi-1)^2 H(\varphi)\},$$

where

$$J_m(\alpha) = \int_0^\infty e^{-x}(\log x)^m/(1-\alpha+\alpha x)dx$$

is needed for $m = 1, 2$. These functions have to be evaluated numerically.

To return to the original parametrization, we consider the parameter used for evaluating the Fisher information $(\alpha, \rho_1, \rho_2, \eta_1, \eta_2)$, say, ϑ, as a function of the original parameter $(\alpha, \rho_1, \rho_2, \omega_1, \omega_2)$, say, ζ. The only non-trivial components of this are $\eta_j = (\rho_j\omega_j)^{1/\rho_j}$, $j = 1, 2$. We then calculate the matrix of derivatives, $F = d\vartheta/d\zeta$, which is

$$\begin{pmatrix} 1 & 0 & 0 & 0 & 0 \\ 0 & 1 & 0 & 0 & 0 \\ 0 & 0 & 1 & 0 & 0 \\ 0 & \rho_1^{-2}\eta_1(1-\log\nu_1) & 0 & \nu_1^{1/\rho_1-1} & 0 \\ 0 & 0 & \rho_2^{-2}\eta_2(1-\log\nu_2) & 0 & \nu_2^{1/\rho_2-1} \end{pmatrix},$$

where ν_j is short-hand for $\rho_j\omega_j$. Then the information in the original parametrization is calculated as

$$I_\zeta(\zeta) = F'I_\vartheta(\vartheta(\zeta))F. \qquad (8.22)$$

One result of these calculations is that the asymptotic variance for $\hat\alpha$ depends on whether the other parameters are fixed or freely varying, but it does not depend on the actual values of these parameters. The reason for this is that on the logarithmic scale, the model is a location-scale model. The standard deviation for $\hat\alpha$ evaluated from the information matrix is shown in Figure 8.1. This standard deviation is evaluated in the five-parameter model, and in the three-parameter model, when ρ_1, ρ_2 are known, and in the one-parameter model, where all the other parameters are known. The three-parameter model corresponds to the bivariate exponential model. The one-parameter model corresponds to a bivariate unit exponential distribution, or to assuming that all marginal distributions are known. It is difficult to evaluate the numerical integrals near the independence assumption ($\alpha = 1$), where the information is infinite. The asymptotic variance is almost independent of whether ω_1 and ω_2 are known or unknown; the maximum relative difference is less than 0.2 %.

The assumption of shape symmetry $\rho_1 = \rho_2$, does not influence the asymptotic variance for α. Similarly, the assumption of scale symmetry $\eta_1 = \eta_2$ does not influence the asymptotic variance for α in the model with $\rho_1 = \rho_2$.

Equation (8.22) can also be used to evaluate the Fisher information in the conditional parametrization, by defining F correspondingly.

As described above, the mean of the second derivative does not exist on the boundary corresponding to independence. This clearly implies that one should be careful using the information near this hypothesis. It was, however, shown by Tawn (1988) that one could use the observed information, that is, the second derivative without taking means evaluated at the estimate, and still obtain valid tests. He also found that the convergence rate under the hypothesis was not the standard $\sqrt{n}$, but $\sqrt{n \log n}$.

The asymptotic variance of the maximum likelihood estimate of Kendall's τ is, of course, the same as that of α. Alternatively, one could estimate τ by Equation (4.7). Also in this case, it is possible to evaluate the mean and variance, from which the efficiency compared to the maximum likelihood estimate can be evaluated (see Manatunga and Oakes, 1996).

8.11.3   The non-parametric gamma model

The non-parametric shared gamma frailty model, allowing for censoring, but without covariates, was studied by Murphy (1994, 1995). The frame covers both parallel data and longitudinal data for recurrent events. She showed that the full maximum likelihood estimate in the conditional formulation is consistent and asymptotically normal. For the hazard this means that the estimated integrated hazard converges to a normal distribution stochastic process on a finite interval, $[0, t_m]$, where t_m is less than the upper limit of the censoring distribution.

Furthermore, the variance can be evaluated by inverting the matrix of second derivatives, when the model is parametrized by the frailty parameter and the contributions to the hazard at each single death time point. The censoring pattern was allowed to be process-dependent, but there should be a possibility of 2 or more events in a group, formulated so that there should be a positive probability that the group is under risk after the first event. So basically, these are positive answers to the first round of questions regarding the asymptotic results.

Later, Parner (1998) considered a multivariate gamma frailty model, including the shared gamma frailty model as a special case. This model included covariates, but considered only parallel data, allowing the group sizes to vary. There was no general requirement that there should be a possibility of 2 or more events in a group. Instead the frame considered included the information from the univariate identifiability due to the proportional conditional hazards. The censoring pattern was allowed to be process-dependent. The conclusions were the same, that is, that the full conditional maximum likelihood estimate is consistent and asymptotically normal and the variance can be estimated consistently by minus the inverse of the second derivative matrix.

8.11.4   The two-stage approach

Also the first two steps of the three-stage procedure can be handled asymptotically. Shih and Louis (1995b) consider the bivariate case with separate hazard functions for each coordinate, both with parametric and non-parametric hazards. For the frailty, they made general evaluations for one-parameter frailty models. Covariates were not considered. Specifically, they considered gamma and stable frailty distributions, as well as Frank's family of distributions for the bivariate times. For the censoring distribution, they allowed a bivariate time (C_1, C_2), independent of the bivariate survival time. In the first step, parametric models were handled by maximum likelihood for each margin separately, and for non-parametric models, the Kaplan-Meier estimates for each margin were evaluated. In the second step, the marginals were treated as known, and the dependence parameter estimated by maximum likelihood in this one-parameter model.

Under regularity conditions, the estimates are consistent and asymptotically normally distributed and they found an expression for the asymptotic variance as well as a method to estimate this. Under independence, this method was found to be efficient, but this is not the case when dependence is present. For the gamma and stable models, however, the method was close to being efficient.

8.12   Applications

The approaches described above will be studied by a number of examples. The matched pairs study of tumorigenesis is considered in Section 8.12.1, using both stratification and mixture models. The repeated measurements exercise data are considered in Section 8.12.2, both using stratification and mixture models. The kidney dialysis data are considered in Section 8.12.3 by mixture models. The amalgam fillings are considered in Section 8.12.4 by mixture models. The dependence for Danish twin data is a major example, and considered in Section 8.12.5. Some applications taken from the literature are described in Section 8.12.6.

The applications of this chapter are based on the assumption that the asymptotic theory works, that is, any parameter that is identifiable can be estimated consistently and have an asymptotic normal distribution, for which the variance can be evaluated by the inverse of minus the second derivative.

8.12.1   Tumorigenesis data

The unspecified frailty and the gamma and stable frailty approaches are illustrated with the litter data of Mantel, Section 1.5.3. The estimates of the regression coefficients in various models are shown in Table 8.2. In the

Model	Dependence	Tie-handling	Method	β(SE)	u
Weibull	Indep.		MLE	0.904 (0.317)	2.85
Weibull	Stable		MLE	0.944 (0.327)	2.89
Weibull	Gamma		MLE		
Cox	Indep.	Exact	MPLE	0.905 (0.318)	2.85
Cox	Indep.	Breslow	MPLE	0.898 (0.317)	2.83
Cox	Stratification	Exact	MPLE	0.985 (0.387)	2.55
Cox	Stable	Breslow	Two-stage	0.991	
Cox	Stable	Breslow	Conditional	0.931 (0.326)	2.85
Cox	Gamma	Breslow	Conditional	0.906 (0.323)	2.81
Cox	PVF	Breslow	Conditional		

Table 8.2. Estimates of the treatment effect for Mantel data, in various models. MLE, maximum likelihood estimation; MPLE, maximum partial likelihood estimation.

stable Weibull model, the estimated dependence parameter is $\hat{\alpha} = 0.906$ (SE 0.095), giving $\hat{\tau} = 0.094$, so the dependence is not statistically significant. In the two-stage non-parametric approach the parameter estimate is $\hat{\alpha} = 0.902$. The standard error not accounting for the variability in the marginal distribution is 0.092. The difference between the regression coefficients in the two Weibull models is not as large as we should expect, the factor ought to be the value of α, 0.902. In other words, in the stable-Weibull model, we can evaluate the regression coefficient in the marginal distributions as $\alpha\beta = 0.944 \cdot 0.902 = 0.853$, lower than the value found based on the marginal distributions (0.904). In the Cox model, the stratification approach (unspecified frailty) leads to a higher coefficient value, as expected, and also higher variability. The best measure of variability (that is, the measure most robust toward model choice) is the u-statistic, which decreases owing to the loss of information by the stratification approach. Under the gamma frailty model, the coefficient is only slightly increased. The estimated value of τ is 0.098 under the stable frailty model; it is 0.072 (0.097) in the two-stage model and 0.192 (0.151) under the gamma frailty model. The gain in likelihood compared to independence is 0.63 for the stable model, and 0.77 for the gamma model.

The PVF frailty model has the maximum corresponding to $\alpha = -\infty$. We have been able to fit the model for $\alpha = -45$, where the log likelihood is -207.98, which is not significantly better than the value found for the gamma model (-208.08). It is calculated that there is a proportion of 0.096 of the litters, where the risk of tumor is 0. Thus, there is, in no cases, a clear increase, and the approach assuming independence (no litter effect) is almost the same as the frailty model.

These data have also been studied by Klein and Moeschberger (1997) and Andersen et al. (1997). They do not obtain the same results owing to having modified the data.

Model	$\hat{\alpha}$ (SE)	$\hat{\tau}$ (SE)	$\log L$
Independence, no cov.	-	0	−999.95
Gamma, no cov.	0	0.459 (0.076)	−941.34
Stable, no cov.	0.622 (0.068)	0.378 (0.068)	−935.08
PVF, no cov.	0.589 (0.089)	0.366 (0.047)	−934.75
Independence, cov.	-	0	−978.19
Gamma, cov.	0	0.552 (0.070)	−886.53
Stable, cov.	0.498 (0.064)	0.502 (0.064)	−882.00
PVF, cov.	0.440 (0.090)	0.487 (0.057)	−881.23

Table 8.3. Key estimates and log likelihood values for various semi-parametric shared frailty models for the exercise data.

8.12.2 Exercise data

The exercise data of Section 1.8.2 contain data for a number of individuals who have tried several treatments and have performed exercise tests on ten occasions after these treatments. The purpose is to study the effect of the treatments and this is done by including a covariate for each occasion coordinate (except the first), describing the effect of the treatment compared to the sublingual placebo. These are then matched pairs covariates and they can therefore be analyzed by stratification. The likelihood from the stratified model is not comparable to those of the other models. Furthermore, they have been studied by the gamma, the stable, and the PVF frailty model. Estimates of key parameters and log likelihoods are shown in Table 8.3. This gives a Wald test for independence of $\chi^2 = (0.552/0.076)^2 = 62.18$ in the gamma frailty model. Thus, there is a clear person effect, as can also be illustrated by the likelihood ratio test for the same hypothesis, comparing the likelihood to that of proportional hazards and independence. The $-2 \log Q$ is 183.31. The PVF is a further improvement, corresponding to a $-2 \log Q$ test statistic of 10.60, and thus significantly better than the gamma frailty model. The dependence as expressed by τ is higher with covariates than without. This is because the covariates are of the matched pairs type. The effects of the various treatments, assuming independence and under the gamma and PVF frailty model, are illustrated in Table 8.4. Under the gamma frailty model, the estimates are larger, as expected. The estimates in the PVF frailty model are comparable. Also the standard errors are larger, but they are not increased as much as the estimates. This demonstrates that the experiment was successful in finding more precise effects of the various treatments, as can be seen by the u-statistics, shown in Table 8.6. The stratified analysis gives estimates close to those of the two frailty models, but the variances are larger due to the loss of information by stratification. The corresponding values in the stable frailty model are shown in Table 8.5, both as regression coefficients in the conditional distribution (β) and in the marginal distribution ($\alpha\beta$). The estimates in the conditional distribution are comparable to those of the PVF model,

Treatment	Prop. haz. $\hat{\beta}$ (SE)	Stratified $\hat{\beta}$ (SE)	Gamma $\hat{\beta}$ (SE)	PVF $\hat{\beta}$ (SE)
SNG	−0.79 (0.32)	−1.47 (0.39)	−1.51 (0.35)	−1.56 (0.36)
OP (0h)	0.25 (0.31)	0.54 (0.35)	0.65 (0.33)	0.65 (0.32)
OP (1h)	−0.02 (0.31)	0.03 (0.34)	0.00 (0.32)	−0.02 (0.31)
OP (3h)	−0.01 (0.31)	0.03 (0.35)	0.18 (0.33)	0.18 (0.32)
OP (5h)	0.13 (0.31)	0.52 (0.35)	0.58 (0.33)	0.58 (0.32)
Oral iso (0h)	−0.03 (0.31)	0.03 (0.35)	0.04 (0.33)	0.01 (0.33)
Oral iso (1h)	−1.39 (0.36)	−2.42 (0.49)	−2.38 (0.41)	−2.33 (0.41)
Oral iso (3h)	−0.94 (0.33)	−1.51 (0.41)	−1.40 (0.36)	−1.39 (0.36)
Oral iso (5h)	−0.42 (0.32)	−0.28(0.36)	−0.36 (0.34)	−0.34 (0.34)

Table 8.4. Estimates for log relative hazards (β) compared to sublingual placebo, for semi-parametric frailty models for exercise data. OP: Oral placebo; iso, isosorbide dinitrate; SNG, sublingual nitroglycerine.

Treatment	Conditional $\hat{\beta}$ (SE)	Marginal $\hat{\alpha}\hat{\beta}$ (SE)
SNG	−1.56 (0.36)	−0.78(0.20)
Oral placebo (0h)	0.65 (0.33)	0.33 (0.17)
Oral placebo (1h)	−0.03 (0.32))	−0.01 (0.16)
Oral placebo (3h)	0.17 (0.33)	0.09 (0.17)
Oral placebo (5h)	0.58 (0.33)	0.29 (0.16)
Oral iso (0h)	0.01(0.33)	0.00 (0.16)
Oral iso (1h)	−2.31 (0.40)	−1.15 (0.24)
Oral iso (3h)	−1.38 (0.36)	−0.69 (0.20)
Oral iso (5h)	−0.34 (0.34)	−0.17 (0.17)

Table 8.5. Estimates for log relative hazards (β, respectively, $\alpha\beta$) compared to sublingual placebo, for exercise data, using the semi-parametric stable frailty model. iso = isosorbide dinitrate; SNG = sublingual nitroglycerine.

Treatment	Prop. haz.	Stratified	Gamma	PVF
SNG	−2.45	−3.80	−4.30	−4.37
Oral placebo (0h)	0.80	1.53	1.94	1.94
Oral placebo (1h)	−0.08	−0.10	−0.01	−0.07
Oral placebo (3h)	−0.02	0.08	0.54	0.53
Oral placebo (5h)	0.42	1.50	1.75	1.76
Oral iso (0h)	0.09	0.09	0.12	0.04
Oral iso (1h)	−3.86	−4.96	−5.87	−5.76
Oral iso (3h)	−2.81	−3.73	−3.91	−3.86
Oral iso (5h)	−1.31	−0.80	−1.03	−0.99

Table 8.6. U-statistics for log relative hazards (β) compared to sublingual placebo, for various frailty models for the exercise data. iso = isosorbide dinitrate; SNG = sublingual nitroglycerine.

Model	$\hat{\alpha}$ (SE)	$\hat{\tau}$ (SE)	$\hat{\gamma}$ (SE)	log L
Indep., no cov.	-	0	2.00 (0.11)	−1260.47
Gamma, no cov.	0	0.452 (0.073)	3.39 (0.20)	−1189.54
Stable, no cov.	0.561 (0.066)	0.439 (0.066)	3.45 (0.20)	−1187.07
PVF, no cov.	0.475 (0.111)	0.409 (0.058)	3.44 (0.20)	−1186.04
Indep., cov.	-	0	2.30 (0.13)	−1232.46
Gamma, cov.	0	0.554 (0.068)	4.86	−1125.25
Stable, cov.	0.456 (0.060)	0.544 (0.060)	4.93 (0.29)	−1122.88
PVF, cov.	0.368 (0.097)	0.517 (0.053)	4.93 (0.29)	−1121.51

Table 8.7. Key estimates and log likelihood values for various shared frailty Weibull models for the exercise data.

and the same applies to the standard errors. The estimates in the marginal distribution are comparable to those of the proportional hazards independence model, but the standard errors are much smaller, owing to the error's now being evaluated toward the variability within individuals.

Similar analyses can be performed assuming that the conditional distribution is Weibull. Estimates of key parameters and log likelihoods are shown in Table 8.7. The results are reasonably close to those obtained in the semi-parametric case (Table 8.3). The Weibull assumption makes it possible to evaluate the hazard shape parameter (γ) as a measure of the unexplained variation, based on Equation (2.6). Without covariates and not accounting for the person variation, we have $\gamma = 2.0$. With covariates, but without person variation, we have $\gamma = 2.3$. Accounting for the person variation, but not the covariates (that is, we now consider the variation within individuals), γ is about 3.4. Finally, when we account for both the covariates and the person variation, we obtain γ about 4.9. Using a Weibull model makes it possible to use, not only the proportional hazards parameters (β in the conditional formulation and $\alpha\beta$ in the marginal formulation of the stable model), but also the accelerated failure time parameters (ν).

Treatment	Indep. $\hat{\nu}$ (SE)	Gamma $\hat{\nu}$ (SE)	Stable $\hat{\nu}$ (SE)	PVF $\hat{\nu}$ (SE)
SNG	0.369 (0.136)	0.311 (0.069)	0.313 (0.068)	0.313 (0.068)
OP (0h)	−0.138 (0.134)	−0.144 (0.068)	−0.144 (0.066)	−0.144 (0.067)
OP (1h)	−0.011 (0.134)	−0.029 (0.066)	−0.026 (0.065)	−0.027 (0.065)
OP (3h)	−0.003 (0.134)	−0.058 (0.068)	−0.055 (0.067)	−0.056 (0.067)
OP (5h)	−0.073 (0.134)	−0.132 (0.067)	−0.131 (0.066)	−0.132 (0.066)
OI (0h)	0.005 (0.134)	−0.031 (0.068)	−0.027 (0.066)	−0.028 (0.067)
OI (1h)	0.653 (0.150)	0.545 (0.079)	0.536 (0.078)	0.539 (0.078)
OI (3h)	0.424 (0.142)	0.282 (0.073)	0.278 (0.072)	0.279 (0.072)
OI (5h)	0.199 (0.138)	0.073 (0.072)	0.071 (0.070)	0.072 (0.071)

Table 8.8. Estimates for accelerated failure time parameters (ν) compared to sublingual placebo, for various shared frailty Weibull models for exercise data. OP=oral placebo; OP, oral isosorbide dinitrate; SNG, sublingual nitroglycerine.

Model	$\hat{\tau}$ without covariates	$\hat{\tau}$ with covariates
Shared gamma frailty	0.081 (0.128)	0.166 (0.082)
Shared stable frailty	0.092 (0.118)	< 0
Shared Inv.G. frailty	0.124 (0.140)	0.124 (0.080)
Shared PVF frailty	0.197 (0.120)	*
Spell specific gamma frailty	-	0.248 (0.121)

Table 8.9. Estimated values of τ for various frailty models, with and without covariates, for the catheter infections data. * means that $\alpha < 0$ and the distribution is partly discrete. - means that the value cannot be identified.

This parameter has the advantage that it is unchanged between the conditional and marginal formulations. The estimated values are listed in Table 8.8. There is a very fine agreement between the various frailty models. A major reason for this is that we consider matched pairs covariates, so that to a high extent the frailty value cancels out from the calculations. The values found under the assumption of independence are reasonably close, but, of course, the standard errors are too high, as they do not account for the covariates being of the matched pairs type.

8.12.3 Catheter infections

For the catheter infections data of Section 1.7.3, we similarly assume proportional conditional hazards effect of two of the covariates, sex and age, with various assumptions on the frailty distribution. Sex is a common covariate and age is almost a common covariate, as the persons are older at the start of the second spell. Table 8.9 shows the estimated values of τ with and without covariates. They are quite different for the various models. In the gamma model with covariates, the estimated value is higher with than without an effect of the covariates. Thus, the value is increased despite the

	Age $\hat{\beta}$ (SE)	Sex $\hat{\beta}$ (SE)	$\log L$
Proportional haz.	0.0022 (0.0092)	−0.82 (0.30)	−230.18
Spell-specific gamma frailty	0.0067 (0.0124)	−1.77 (0.61)	−228.07
Shared gamma frailty	0.0055 (0.0117)	−1.56 (0.50)	−227.58
Shared stable frailty	0.0021 (0.0089)	−0.81 (0.29)	−230.17
Shared Inv.G. frailty	0.0038 (0.0112)	−1.23 (0.41)	−228.54
Shared PVF frailty	0.0056 (0.0111)	−1.63 (0.48)	−227.15

Table 8.10. Estimates for log relative hazards and log likelihoods for various shared frailty models, for catheter infections data.

inclusion of common covariates in the model and we would expect that such common covariates explained a part of the dependence. The reason is that there is a non-proportional effect of the covariates. In a univariate gamma frailty model, that is, assuming independent frailties for the two spells for each individual, we can still estimate all the parameters. The value of $\hat{\delta}$ is 1.51, which corresponds to a value of τ of 0.248. Thus, this value appears to be almost as precise as that based on the paired data. For the inverse Gaussian model, the estimated values of τ are similar with and without covariates, but the calculated standard error is markedly reduced by the inclusion of covariates. Again, this is probably an effect of the univariate identifiability. The estimates in the models considered are shown in Table 8.10. Clearly, there are marked differences between the proportional hazards model and the individual frailty model, which are due to non-proportional hazards. Owing to higher frailty variance, the estimated regression coefficients are higher for spell-specific frailty than for shared frailty. The gain in likelihood owing to assuming shared frailty rather than spell-specific frailty is only slight, suggesting that what appears as dependence is, rather, non-proportional effects. This example illustrates that the marginal distributions contribute with information on the frailty variance and suggest a higher frailty variance than the bivariate model with shared frailty.

The PVF frailty model leads to a negative value (−1.25) of α, suggesting that some persons have zero risk of getting an infection. The estimated proportion with zero risk is 0.2 %. Three patients (7.9 %) have double censorings, and thus the model suggests that 0.2 % cannot get an infection, and 7.7 % can get an infection, but were not observed to experience one, owing to censoring. The PVF frailty model does not fit significantly better than the gamma frailty model. The stable frailty is only slightly better than the independence model, suggesting a negative dependence, as $\hat{\alpha} = 1.024$, with a standard error of 0.155. This suggests that there is no dependence, when the effect of sex is accounted for.

One way to overcome the determination of the dependence, caused by the covariates in the univariate case, is to stratify. As sex is the only impor-

	Age $\hat{\beta}$ (SE)	Sex $\hat{\beta}$ (SE)	$\log L$
Proportional haz.	−0.005 (0.007)	−0.52 (0.17)	−625.34
Shared gamma frailty	0.006 (0.012)	−0.51 (0.32)	−615.76
Shared stable frailty	0.008 (0.015)	−1.05 (0.36)	−618.64
Shared PVF frailty	0.006 (0.011)	−0.39 (0.30)	−614.99

Table 8.11. Estimates for log relative hazards and log likelihoods for various frailty models for amalgam fillings data.

tant covariate, we stratify by this variable and thus have separate hazard functions for each sex. In the gamma frailty model this leads to negative dependence and thus we conclude that the apparent dependence is due to a non-proportional effect of sex.

The penalized likelihood approach for the gamma shared frailty model gives the same estimates as in Table 8.10, but the standard errors are given as 0.0118 and 0.46. The frailty variance is estimated to 0.398. With a lognormal frailty, the estimated regression coefficients are 0.0049 (0.01249) and −1.39 (0.44). The frailty variance is 0.55. This is somewhat strange, because the lower regression coefficients for the lognormal model suggest a smaller dependence, but the frailty variance appears clearly higher. A partial explanation is that the frailty variances are evaluated on different scales. The variance of the log frailty for the gamma model is 0.487, making the two estimates more comparable.

In conclusion, it appears that all the dependence between the two spells can be explained by the sex, so that after inclusion of sex, there is no dependence.

8.12.4   Amalgam fillings

For the amalgam fillings data of Section 1.6.2, we fit the same models. The gamma frailty model without covariates gives τ=0.24 (0.08) and a log likelihood of −617.10. For the models with covariates, we obtain the results in Table 8.11. The frailty models give a significantly better fit than the proportional hazards model. This is not due to converging hazards, because the tooth-specific gamma frailty model cannot be fitted. The gamma model with covariates gives $\tau = 0.21$ (0.11), and is not significantly better than the model without covariates. The PVF model again gives negative estimates of α, without covariates we get $\hat{\alpha} = -3.04$ (5.89) and with covariates, we get −4.78 (13.92), and these models are not significantly better than the corresponding gamma frailty models. It suggests that the proportion of persons, who have no susceptibility to failure of a filling, is 0.069 without covariates and 0.074 in the model with covariates. The stable frailty model gives $\hat{\tau} = 0.22$ (0.09) without covariates, and $\hat{\tau} = 0.16$ (0.07) with

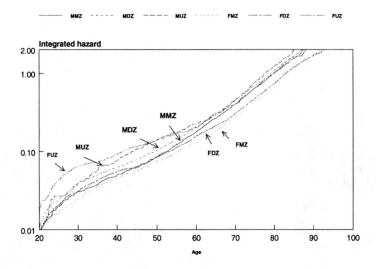

Figure 8.2. Nelson-Aalen estimate of the integrated hazard for Danish twin data, assuming independence.

covariates. It does not fit as well as the gamma model. The effect of sex is clearly larger than in the other models.

8.12.5   Danish twin data

The Danish twin data of Section 1.5.1 have been analyzed using a general hazard function, and gamma, stable and power variance frailty distributions, using the three-stage, the marginal, and the conditional estimation approaches. The effect of birth year is considered. Furthermore, the effect of grouping as well as of using piecewise constant hazard rates is considered, to reduce the size of the matrices involved. This is a long section, with illustration of many theoretical and practical points. Readers who are more interested in the conclusions regarding twin dependence should go directly to the summary at the end of the section.

Marginal and three-stage approach

First, the integrated marginal hazard functions are evaluated by the Nelson-Aalen approach assuming independence (see Figure 8.2). Step 2 evaluates the dependence assuming that the marginals are known, step 3 that the hazards are proportional to the Nelson-Aalen estimate. Finally, step 4 is a general estimate. Most of the results will be recorded as those of step 3. The estimated parameters of the frailty distribution are shown in Ta-

| | Stable | Gamma | | PVF |
	$\hat{\alpha}$ (SE)	$\hat{\delta}$ (SE)	$\hat{\alpha}$ (SE)	$\hat{\eta}$ (SE)
Males				
MZ	0.904 (0.021)	1.94 (0.32)	0.184 (0.292)	1.44 (1.34)
DZ	0.949 (0.014)	5.65 (1.62)	0.878 (0.056)	0.14 (0.14)
UZ	0.836 (0.038)	1.58 (0.41)	0.551 (0.41)	0.27 (0.23)
Females				
MZ	0.906 (0.020)	2.11 (0.42)	0 (-)	2.11 (-)
DZ	0.947 (0.014)	3.49 (0.73)	0.678 (0.232)	0.71 (0.82)
UZ	0.866 (0.032)	2.37 (0.69)	0.839 (0.052)	0.01 (0.03)

Table 8.12. Frailty distribution parameters estimated in step 3 for Danish twin data. The standard errors do not account for the variation in the marginal distribution.

	Gamma	Stable	Inv. Gauss	PVF
Males				
MZ	26.56	12.29	26.06	26.62
DZ	7.16	7.75	8.47	11.59
UZ	11.31	11.29	13.66	13.70
Females				
MZ	18.08	17.36	17.47	18.08
DZ	14.49	9.54	15.01	15.16
UZ	8.01	10.54	9.39	10.97
Sum	85.61	68.77	90.06	96.12

Table 8.13. Log likelihood values in step 3 of frailty models for Danish twin data, compared to the independence model.

ble 8.12. The scale factors for the marginal hazards are not described, but they range from 0.981 to 1.008, showing only little modification by allowing this parameter to vary. In the case of female monozygotic twins, the estimates in the PVF family is on the boundary, corresponding to the gamma mixture. A negative value of α has not been attempted in this estimation, as it is biologically impossible to have 0 risk of death. The extension is attempted in the marginal model below. Therefore the uncertainty has not been calculated. The value of the log likelihood functions, compared to the independence model, are shown in Table 8.13. These likelihood values can be compared to those found in Table 6.7, based on various multi-state models. The multi-state models give a better fit, which is due to the shared frailty model's suggesting a long-term dependence, where the multi-state models rather suggest short-term dependence. To illustrate this, see Figure 8.3, which is similar to Figure 6.4. This function is relevant for evaluating the prognosis for a person, as it studies the ratio of the hazard given the death time of the partner (if the partner is dead) to the hazard if the partner is currently alive. It is evaluated in the PVF frailty model (Equa-

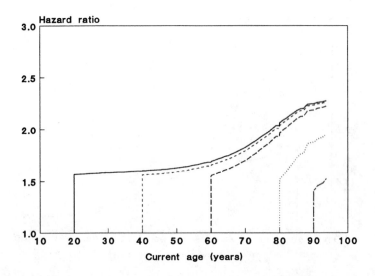

Figure 8.3. Relative hazards of death of a monozygotic male twin at age t, for various values (20, 40, 60, 80, and 90 years) of age at partners death t_1, compared to the partner's being alive, in the PVF frailty model.

tion (7.60)), but the course is close to the course seen in the gamma model. In the gamma model, the jump at the death time is the same whatever the death time is, after which an increase is seen. At old ages, there is a very high difference between the hazard of death for those whose partner is dead compared to those, whose partner is still alive. A somewhat different picture is seen for the dizygotic male twins (Figure 8.4). Here the course is more similar to the course seen for the stable frailty model. There is a very high relative mortality owing to death of partner during the young ages; but it decreases, and at old ages it seems almost irrelevant to include information on the status of the partner.

A second possibility of showing the dependence is Figure 8.5, which is similar to Figure 6.5, the figure that illustrates whether the dependence is short-term or long-term. In the multi-state Markov model these functions should be constant as functions of age at partners death. This is for monozygotic male twins. It is clearly seen that the dependence is long-term in this model.

The dependence can be quantified in various ways, as described in Section 7.8.3. Table 8.14 shows the values of the squared coefficient of variation in the distribution of Y. As expected, there are large differences between the various models. The value is always infinite for the stable model. Therefore, it could have been excluded from the table, but it is included to empha-

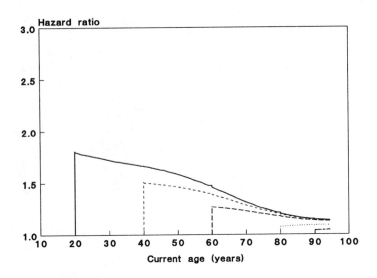

Figure 8.4. Relative hazards of death of a dizygotic male twin at age t, for various values (20, 40, 60, 80, and 90 years) of age at partners death t_1, compared to the partner's being alive, in the PVF frailty model.

size this point. It is not recommended to use this measure for evaluating dependence.

Table 8.15 shows the values of the variance in the distribution of $\log Y$. For the PVF model they are evaluated by means of numerical integration, except for the female monozygotic case, where the estimate is on the boundary. The differences between the various models are smaller than for the coefficient of variation. The stable model, which had infinite coefficients of variation, shows the smallest values for the variance of the logarithm. This model emphasizes the dependence in the young ages, but neglects dependence at old ages, and therefore gives smaller values for the dependence.

Sex	Data set	Gamma	Stable	Inv. Gauss	PVF
Males	MZ	0.52 (0.09)	∞	0.74 (0.17)	0.57 (0.20)
	DZ	0.18 (0.05)	∞	0.25 (0.08)	0.89 (0.63)
	UZ	0.63 (0.16)	∞	1.46 (0.54)	1.65 (0.92)
Females	MZ	0.47 (0.09)	∞	0.64 (0.17)	0.47 (-)
	DZ	0.29 (0.06)	∞	0.37 (0.09)	0.46 (0.23)
	UZ	0.42 (0.12)	∞	0.78 (0.30)	11.32 (20.25)

Table 8.14. Squared coefficient of variation in step 3 for the frailty distribution for Danish twin data.

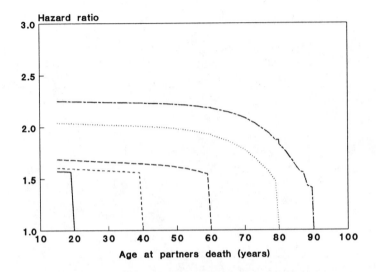

Figure 8.5. Relative hazards of death of a monozygotic male twin for various values (20, 40, 60, 80, and 90 years) of current age, compared to the partner's being alive, as function of age at partners death t_1, in the PVF frailty model.

Sex	Data set	Gamma	Stable	Inv. Gauss	PVF
Males	MZ	0.67 (0.14)	0.36 (0.09)	0.56 (0.10)	0.66
	DZ	0.19 (0.06)	0.18 (0.05)	0.22 (0.06)	0.22
	UZ	0.87 (0.29)	0.70 (0.22)	0.92 (0.23)	0.89
Females	MZ	0.60 (0.15)	0.36 (0.09)	0.50 (0.11)	0.60
	DZ	0.33 (0.08)	0.19 (0.05)	0.31 (0.07)	0.29
	UZ	0.52 (0.19)	0.55 (0.16)	0.58 (0.17)	0.53

Table 8.15. Variance of $\log Y$ in step 3 for the frailty distribution for Danish twin data.

	Gamma	Stable	Inv. Gauss	PVF
Males				
MZ	0.205 (0.027)	0.095 (0.021)	0.190 (0.024)	0.204 (0.028)
DZ	0.081 (0.021)	0.051 (0.014)	0.092 (0.021)	0.081 (0.019)
UZ	0.240 (0.163)	0.163 (0.038)	0.265 (0.040)	0.257 (0.049)
Females				
MZ	0.191 (0.031)	0.094 (0.020)	0.175 (0.027)	0.191 (-)
DZ	0.125 (0.023)	0.053 (0.014)	0.123 (0.021)	0.116 (0.024)
UZ	0.174 (0.042)	0.134 (0.032)	0.196 (0.041)	0.149 (0.038)

Table 8.16. Estimated value of τ in step 3 in the frailty models for Danish twin data.

Sex	Data set	Gamma	Stable	Inv. Gauss	PVF
Males	MZ	0.302	0.142	0.281	0.301
	DZ	0.122	0.076	0.138	0.121
	UZ	0.352	0.241	0.388	0.376
Females	MZ	0.283	0.140	0.260	0.281
	DZ	0.187	0.080	0.183	0.172
	UZ	0.258	0.198	0.289	0.220

Table 8.17. Estimated value of ρ in step 3 in the frailty models for Danish twin data.

Table 8.16 shows the values of the Kendall's τ among the lifetimes. Consistent with the variance of the logarithm, it shows that the stable model suggests the lowest dependence. In all other cases, there is a fine agreement between the various models. There is a much better agreement between the models than there was when the dependence was evaluated by means of the variation for Y.

Comparing the various types of twins, it is seen that the dependence is higher for monozygotic than for dizygotic twins, just as expected. This problem is not considered here, but is discussed and studied in Section 10.1.

The values of Spearman's ρ are shown in Table 8.17. As shown previously, they are about 1.5 τ, in the range of dependence present in these data. The interpretation of the Spearman's ρ is closer to an ordinary correlation coefficient than that of Kendall's τ, and therefore, we think, this measure is more satisfactory. However, ρ requires numerical integration.

Also the median concordance values are found and shown in Table 8.18. For understanding this measure, it is relevant also to include the median values seen. In the present study, survival was evaluated only for pairs, where both were alive at the age of 15 years, which should also be quoted for interpreting the median. The values are higher for monozygotic than for dizygotic twins. This is possibly due to the truncation at age 15 years, combined with the higher dependence for monozygotic twins.

Sex	Data set	Median	$\hat{p}$	$\hat{\kappa}$ (SE)
Males	MZ	76.0	0.602	0.204 (0.028)
	DZ	75.0	0.542	0.085 (0.021)
	UZ	74.1	0.636	0.272 (0.051)
Females	MZ	80.3	0.593	0.188 (0.035)
	DZ	79.3	0.561	0.122 (0.024)
	UZ	75.9	0.571	0.149 (0.041)

Table 8.18. Estimated value of probability of being on the same side of the median and κ in step 3 for Danish twin data, using the PVF frailty model ($\kappa = 2p - 1$).

	Gamma			Stable		
	Step 2	Step 3	Step 4	Step 2	Step 3	Step 4
Males						
MZ	26.48	26.56	26.73	12.29	12.29	12.73
DZ	7.12	7.16	7.32	7.75	7.75	7.91
UZ	11.31	11.31	12.00	11.28	11.29	11.57
Females						
MZ	17.95	18.08	18.31	17.35	17.36	17.51
DZ	14.35	14.49	14.72	9.53	9.54	9.67
UZ	8.00	8.01	8.29	10.54	10.54	10.66
Sum	85.21	85.61	87.37	68.74	68.77	70.05

Table 8.19. Log likelihood values in steps 2, 3, and 4 for Danish twin data, compared to the independence model. For gamma and stable distributed frailties.

A further point to be illustrated is whether the estimates of step 2 and 3, based on the marginal distribution, are acceptable. First, the likelihood values are described (Table 8.19). The estimates under step 2 (marginal assumed known, equal to the Nelson-Aalen estimate), step 3 (marginal integrated hazard assumed proportional to the Nelson-Aalen estimate), and step 4 (General) are given in Table 8.20 for the gamma frailty distribution. For comparison, the results are given by the value of τ. For step 2 and 3, we have an estimate of the standard error from the parametric model, but this is an underestimate, as it does not account for the variance of the non-parametric estimate found in step 1. For step 4, we can derive the full estimate, that is, the standard error found by inverting the full second derivative matrix, but as an approximation, we might use the inverse of the approximate matrix, where the mixed second derivatives with respect to the hazard parameters are set to 0. The same results, based on the stable frailty distributions, are given in Table 8.21. From these two tables, it can be seen that the estimated dependence increases with the steps, but only to a very limited degree for the stable model. In particular, steps 2 and 3 are very close for the stable model. This fits well to the results for the Fisher information that the scale parameter in the marginal distribution is almost independent of the dependence parameter. The gamma model gives higher

	Step 2		Step 3		Step 4		
	$\hat{\tau}$	SE[1]	$\hat{\tau}$	SE[1]	$\hat{\tau}$	SE[2]	SE
Males							
MZ	0.2026	0.0262	0.2052	0.0272	0.2095	0.0284	0.0285
DZ	0.0804	0.0210	0.0813	0.0214	0.0840	0.0221	0.0222
UZ	0.2395	0.0450	0.2402	0.0470	0.2641	0.0535	0.0529
Females							
MZ	0.1877	0.0298	0.1914	0.0309	0.1972	0.0324	0.0326
DZ	0.1231	0.0224	0.1254	0.0230	0.1292	0.0238	0.0239
UZ	0.1728	0.0407	0.1740	0.0420	0.1854	0.0460	0.0459

Table 8.20. Estimates of dependence (τ) for Danish twin data, based on the gamma frailty model, and various restrictions on the marginal distributions. SE[1], not accounting for the variance of Nelson-Aalen estimate; SE[2], approximation.

	Step 2		Step 3		Step 4		
	$\hat{\tau}$	SE[1]	$\hat{\tau}$	SE[1]	$\hat{\tau}$	SE[2]	SE
Males							
MZ	0.0952	0.0205	0.0952	0.0205	0.1022	0.0227	0.0225
DZ	0.0511	0.0139	0.0511	0.0139	0.0528	0.0145	0.0144
UZ	0.1627	0.0378	0.1632	0.0379	0.1744	0.0431	0.0427
Females							
MZ	0.0939	0.0198	0.0938	0.0198	0.0958	0.0212	0.0212
DZ	0.0535	0.0137	0.0535	0.0136	0.0553	0.0144	0.0144
UZ	0.1340	0.0323	0.1340	0.0323	0.1367	0.0346	0.0346

Table 8.21. Estimates of dependence (τ) for Danish twin data, based on the stable frailty model, and various restrictions on the marginal distributions. SE[1], not accounting for the variance of Nelson-Aalen estimate; SE[2], approximation.

values for τ than the stable model. This is because the stable model only recognizes the dependence in the young ages. This means that the estimate is determined on the basis of the initial course, whereas whether there appears to be dependence later has no or little influence on the estimate.

Conditional methods

The same models have also been studied by means of the conditional estimation approach. The likelihood gain compared to independence is shown in Table 8.22. The values are slightly lower than the step 4 values given in Table 8.19.

The conditional estimation method leads in the gamma frailty case to the estimates described in Table 8.23. The values are intermediate between those of steps 3 and 4 in Table 8.20. The approximation to the second derivative does not work as well in this case, because the parameters are not as close to be independent as they are in the marginal parametrization. The variances are very close to those reported for step 4 in the marginal

Sex	Data set	Gamma	Stable	Inv. Gauss	PVF
Males	MZ	26.10	12.16	25.56	26.10
	DZ	7.05	7.59	8.31	11.38
	UZ	10.63	10.59	12.73	12.84
Females	MZ	17.82	16.96	17.16	17.82
	DZ	14.39	9.34	14.84	14.98
	UZ	7.35	9.86	8.69	10.45
Sum		83.33	66.50	87.31	93.61

Table 8.22. Log likelihood values for the conditional parametrization of the frailty models for Danish twin data, compared to the independence model.

Sex	Data set	Gamma				Stable	
		$\hat{\tau}$	SE^2	SE	$\hat{\tau}$	SE^2	SE
Males	MZ	0.2068	0.0246	0.0285	0.0991	0.0206	0.0224
	DZ	0.0824	0.0200	0.0221	0.0515	0.0138	0.0144
	UZ	0.2493	0.0379	0.0536	0.1628	0.0365	0.0420
Females	MZ	0.1943	0.0291	0.0326	0.0930	0.0196	0.0210
	DZ	0.1276	0.0219	0.0239	0.0540	0.0136	0.0143
	UZ	0.1745	0.0355	0.0462	0.1292	0.0310	0.0341

Table 8.23. Estimates of dependence (τ) for Danish twin data, based on the gamma and stable frailty models and the conditional parametrization. SE^2, approximation.

approach. Corresponding results for the stable frailty model are also shown in Table 8.23.

Also the PVF frailty model can be examined using the conditional parametrization, The values of α and τ are shown in Table 8.24. The parameter α is a key parameter, and it appears that for the monozygotic twins, the value can be 0, corresponding to a gamma model, but for the other data sets, the value is significant positive. For the female monozygotic twins, the estimate is, in fact, $-\infty$, and it is suggested that a proportion of about 5 % has zero risk of death. As this is biologically impossible, it illustrates that the dependence is not well determined. Generally, it means that we have to take some action, and in this case, where it is known that all individuals will experience the event sooner or later, it is natural to use the estimate on the boundary corresponding to the gamma model.

As previously argued, the value of Spearman's ρ is easier to interpret like an ordinary correlation coefficient and therefore this value is calculated in this final model. The values are reported in Table 8.25. These are the best estimates of the degree of dependence, as evaluated at the start of the study, that is, at age 15 years. A more relevant quantity to evaluate would be the degree of dependence in total lifetimes, that is, as evaluated at birth. With the present data, it is impossible to evaluate this quantity. However, the problem can be discussed at the qualitative level. Under the gamma

Sex	Data set	$\hat{\alpha}$	SE^2	SE	$\hat{\tau}$	SE^2	SE
Males	MZ	0.149	0.456	0.494	0.2047	0.0271	0.0292
	DZ	0.880	0.050	0.051	0.0802	0.0181	0.0192
	UZ	0.583	0.140	0.162	0.2450	0.0351	0.0500
Females	MZ						
	DZ	0.674	0.231	0.243	0.1159	0.0243	0.0251
	UZ	0.844	0.049	0.053	0.1439	0.0353	0.0392

Table 8.24. Estimates of α and the dependence (τ) for Danish twin data, based on the PVF frailty model, and the conditional parametrization. SE^2, approximation.

Sex	Data set	$\hat{\rho}$	SE
Males	MZ	0.302	0.042
	DZ	0.120	0.029
	UZ	0.360	0.071
Females	MZ	0.287	0.047
	DZ	0.173	0.037
	UZ	0.213	0.057

Table 8.25. Estimates of Spearman's ρ for Danish twin data, based on the largest model (PVF frailty, except for female monozygotic, where the gamma model is used), and the conditional parametrization.

model, the degree of dependence is unchanged by truncation so in this model, there is no problem (at least not, when there are no covariates). However, under the PVF model (with $\alpha > 0$), and in particular under the stable model, the dependence decreases after truncation. This result can be used the opposite way to conclude that the degree of dependence for total lifetimes is higher than the value reported for truncated data in Table 8.25. Some further discussion of this problem follows in the subsection on combining the two sexes.

Combining the sexes

All the analyses above have studied the six data sets separately. The degree of dependence differs, of course, for monozygotic and dizygotic; and therefore these data sets should not be joined. More general models with different degrees of dependence will be separately considered in Chapter 10. But one could combine the two sexes and improve the precision. There were several reasons for not doing this previously. First, males and females do have a different mortality pattern and we would not assume proportional hazards in order not to suffer from the univariate identifiability problem. Second, truncation could have a differential influence for males and females. Finally, a more technical problem was that when the first analyses on this data set were made, computers were not able to handle data sets of the combined size in non-parametric hazard models. This latter problem is no longer a

	$\hat{\tau}$	SE^2	SE	$\log L$
MZ	0.2014	0.0188	0.0215	0.04
DZ	0.1033	0.0147	0.0163	0.96
UZ	0.2059	0.0259	0.0351	0.55

Table 8.26. Estimates of dependence (τ) for Danish twin data, based on the gamma frailty model, stratified by sex, using the conditional parametrization. SE^2, approximation. Change in $\log L$ compared to separate frailty parameters.

	$\hat{\alpha}$	SE^2	SE	$\hat{\eta}$	$\hat{\tau}$	SE^2	SE	$\log L$
MZ	−0.157	0.712	0.813	2.414				0.05
DZ	0.834	0.058	0.060	0.247	0.0926	0.0145	0.0152	0.81
UZ	0.740	0.089	0.131	0.102	0.1901	0.0324	0.0417	1.40

Table 8.27. Estimates of dependence (τ) for Danish twin data, based on the PVF frailty model, stratified by sex, using the conditional parametrization. SE^2, approximation. Change in $\log L$ compared to separate frailty parameters (2 d.f.).

problem for the estimation, but it can be for the evaluation of standard errors. The differential mortality pattern is handled by stratification.

First consider the gamma frailty model. If the frailty distribution for males and females were the same at birth, the truncation would imply that the δ parameters were the same after truncation and the θ-parameters were updated by the integrated hazard function. This change can, however, be absorbed in the hazard function and with stratification, it is not a problem if there is a differential change for the hazard function for the two sexes. The results are shown in Table 8.26, in the same setup as Table 8.23. This shows that the frailty parameters for the two sexes are not significantly different.

For the PVF model, the same evaluation is more complicated. First, consider the model, where the frailty parameters are the same at start of the study (that is, at age 15 years). The common estimates are listed in Table 8.27. Also in this model, we find that the frailty parameters for the two sexes are not significantly different.

However, in light of the truncation and the freely varying hazard functions, the PVF common parameter model above does not make sense. If the frailty distributions for males and females were the same at birth, the truncation at age 15 years will, in general, imply that the θ parameters differ, due to different hazard functions the first 15 years of life. On the other hand, the α parameter is unchanged by truncation. Therefore, we have fitted the model with common α, but separate θ parameters at age 15 for the two sexes, and separate hazard functions. The estimates are listed in Table 8.28. As the frailty distributions are normalized, this model is technically fitted using the η parameter instead of θ. Standard errors for $\hat{\eta}$ are not reported as we find it more relevant to consider the degree of dependence, as reported in Table 8.29. This gives in no cases a significant

	$\hat{\alpha}$	SE^2	SE	$\hat{\eta}_M$	$\hat{\eta}_F$	log L
MZ	−0.114	0.662	0.761	2.231	2.385	0.02
DZ	0.831	0.061	0.064	0.275	0.240	0.78
UZ	0.680	0.107	0.155	0.141	0.238	1.26

Table 8.28. Estimates of parameters for Danish twin data, based on the PVF frailty model, with the same value of α and separate values of η, stratified by sex, using the conditional parametrization. SE^2, approximation. Change in log L compared to separate frailty parameters (1 d.f.).

	$\hat{\tau}_M$	SE^2	SE	$\hat{\tau}_F$	SE^2	SE
MZ						
DZ	0.0907	0.0155	0.0170	0.0953	0.0182	0.0196
UZ	0.2192	0.0371	0.0593	0.1869	0.0274	0.0366

Table 8.29. Estimates of dependence (τ) for Danish twin data, based on the PVF frailty model, with the same value of α and separate values of θ, stratified by sex, using the conditional parametrization. SE^2, approximation.

improvement compared to the results of Table 8.27. However, it is theoretically more satisfactory, as it specifically accounts for the fact that the data are truncated. For the monozygotic twins, the fit is not better than for the gamma frailty model, and in fact, the estimates suggest that a proportion of the pairs cannot die. This proportion is in order of 10^{-7} and therefore not important in the big picture. However, it is natural to use the estimates in the gamma model, corresponding to a τ value of 0.2014, which is then also the value suggested at birth. For the dizygotic twins, the fit of the PVF model is significantly better than for the gamma model. This suggests a more early dependence, and that τ at birth is larger than the values quoted in Table 8.29, applicable at 15 years. The slightly lower value for males compared to females is consistent with the infant mortality's being higher for boys (and thus truncation more marked). However, it is impossible from these data to give a sensible estimate of the degree of dependence applicable at birth.

Grouping versus piecewise constant hazards

The dimension of these data sets, with up to 1916 death times, does create difficulties. Estimation is still possible by using the approximation to the matrix of second derivatives. Also the uncertainty of the dependence parameters can be found by a profile likelihood approach. But very often one would instead prefer a problem of lower dimension. In this section, we compare two such approaches. The conceptually simplest is the grouped data approach, where, for example, only the year of death is considered. This has the disadvantage that those who are censored during a year are given a survival advantage by letting them be censored at the end of the year. Instead one could let them be censored at the beginning of the year,

Sex	Data set	1 year piecewise		1 year grouping	
		$\hat{\tau}$	SE	$\hat{\tau}$	SE
Males	MZ	0.2081	0.0285	0.1778	0.0290
	DZ	0.0832	0.0221	0.0537	0.0222
	UZ	0.2594	0.0530	0.2063	0.0551
Females	MZ	0.1954	0.0326	0.1664	0.0332
	DZ	0.1297	0.0238	0.1054	0.0241
	UZ	0.1767	0.0462	0.1380	0.0471

Table 8.30. Estimates of dependence (τ) for Danish twin data, based on the gamma frailty model, and assuming piecewise constant hazards, or grouping into one year groups, using the conditional parametrization.

	1 year piecewise		1 year grouping	
	$\hat{\alpha}$ (SE)	$\hat{\tau}$ (SE)	$\hat{\alpha}$ (SE)	$\hat{\tau}$ (SE)
Males				
MZ	0.127 (0.501)		−0.230 (1.508)	
DZ	0.879 (0.051)	0.0808 (0.0192)	0.923 (0.037)	0.0560 (0.0179)
UZ	0.553 (0.169)	0.2552 (0.0498)	0.693(0.147)	0.2011 (0.0514)
Females				
MZ	-	-	-	-
DZ	0.648 (0.269)	0.1188 (0.0252)	0.689 (0.420)	0.0955 (0.0282)
UZ	0.844 (0.049)	0.1454 (0.0385)	0.868 (0.048)	0.1216 (0.0370)

Table 8.31. Estimates of α and the dependence (τ) for Danish twin data, based on the PVF frailty model, and assuming piecewise constant hazards, or grouping into one year groups, using the conditional parametrization.

but that would just be an error in the opposite direction. Alternatively, the hazard can be assumed to be piecewise constant in one-year age intervals. That would make it possible to account both for the precise death times as well as the precise censoring times. The results are shown in Table 8.30 for the gamma frailty case. This table shows that the piecewise conditional approach is reasonable, as it gives estimates comparable to those of Table 8.23. The grouping, however, leads to reduced estimates of dependence. The standard errors are in both cases comparable to those of the model based on actual days, which were shown in Table 8.23.

The same picture is observed for the PVF frailty model (see Table 8.31). In both cases, for female monozygotic twins, the estimate is at $\alpha = -\infty$, and therefore, no values are reported. For male monozygotic twins, the estimate of α is negative under grouping. So also in this case, the piecewise constant approach is satisfactory, whereas the grouping is not acceptable.

Effect of birth year

The effect of cohort (year of birth) can be similarly examined. We can evaluate the rate of mortality decline over time by including the year of

	Step1 $\hat{\beta}$ (SE^1)	Step 2 $\hat{\alpha}$ (SE^2)	Step 3 $\alpha\hat{\beta}$ (SE^2)	Step 3 $\hat{\beta}$ (SE^2)	Step 3 $\hat{\alpha}$ (SE^2)
Males					
MZ	−1.68 (0.31)	0.909 (0.021)	−1.67 (0.28)	−1.83 (0.30)	0.909 (0.021)
DZ	−1.62 (0.22)	0.952 (0.014)	−1.63 (0.19)	−1.71 (0.20)	0.952 (0.014)
UZ	0.74 (0.50)	0.839 (0.037)	0.79 (0.38)	0.94(0.46)	0.839 (0.037)
Females					
MZ	−2.60 (0.33)	0.914 (0.021)	−2.53 (0.30)	−2.77 (0.33)	0.913 (0.021)
DZ	−2.57 (0.23)	0.955 (0.014)	−2.57 (0.20)	−2.69 (0.21)	0.955 (0.014)
UZ	−0.34 (0.42)	0.866 (0.033)	−0.31 (0.36)	−0.36 (0.41)	0.866 (0.033)

Table 8.32. Estimated cohort effects (% per year) and the dependence parameter in the stable frailty model for Danish twins. SE^1 standard errors, calculated under the assumption of independence. SE^2, standard errors, which do not include all error components.

	$\hat{\tau}$	SE^2	SE	$\hat{\beta}$	SE^2	SE	$\hat{\alpha}\hat{\beta}$	SE^2	SE
Males									
MZ	0.0944	0.0214	0.0230	−1.83	0.35	0.36	−1.66	0.31	0.32
DZ	0.0484	0.0143	0.0148	−1.71	0.23	0.23	−1.63	0.22	0.22
UZ	0.1602	0.0365	0.0408	1.05	0.58	0.65	0.88	0.49	0.54
Females									
MZ	0.0842	0.0207	0.0220	−2.75	0.38	0.38	−2.51	0.34	0.35
DZ	0.0446	0.0144	0.0149	−2.68	0.25	0.25	−2.56	0.23	0.24
UZ	0.1293	0.0315	0.0343	−0.33	0.49	0.51	−0.29	0.43	0.44

Table 8.33. Estimates of dependence (τ) and cohort effect (β, % per year) for Danish twin data, based on the stable frailty model and the conditional parametrization. The regression coefficient is also evaluated in the marginal distribution ($\alpha\beta$). SE^2, approximation.

birth as a covariate. This is a common covariate. This is first evaluated assuming independence (step 1). The point is illustrated with the stable frailty model as this model is consistent with there being covariates showing proportional hazards. Assuming the cohort effect is known, we can evaluate the dependence parameter α. It is further possible to maximize over both α and the regression parameter in Step 3 of the marginal method. The regression parameter is evaluated both in the conditional distribution and in the marginal distribution, where it equals $\alpha\beta$. The results are described in Table 8.32.

Alternatively, the effect of cohort can be examined in the conditional model, still using the stable frailty distribution. This is shown in Table 8.33. Again, the approximate variance seems good for the regression coefficients, but not as good for the value of τ.

Also the gamma frailty model, with an effect of cohort is examined in the conditional model, see Table 8.34, with an arbitrary hazard function.

	$\hat{\tau}$	SE^2	SE	$\hat{\beta}$	SE^2	SE
Males						
MZ	0.1903	0.0239	0.0289	−1.66	0.35	0.36
DZ	0.0700	0.0193	0.0220	−1.66	0.23	0.23
UZ	0.2447	0.0391	0.0539	0.69	0.57	0.60
Females						
MZ	0.1642	0.0281	0.0332	−2.64	0.37	0.37
DZ	0.1062	0.0206	0.0234	−2.70	0.25	0.25
UZ	0.1732	0.0353	0.0462	−0.32	0.47	0.48

Table 8.34. Estimates of dependence (τ) and cohort effect (β) for Danish twin data, based on the gamma frailty model, and the conditional parametrization. SE^2, approximation.

	$\hat{\alpha}$	SE^2	SE	$\hat{\tau}$	SE^2	SE	$\hat{\beta}$	SE^2	SE
Males									
MZ	0.288	0.375	0.408	0.1887	0.0249	0.0284	−1.69	0.36	0.37
DZ	0.882	0.047	0.048	0.0784	0.0176	0.0192	−1.75	0.24	0.24
UZ	0.619	0.146	0.165	0.2342	0.0392	0.0515	0.78	0.61	0.66
Females									
MZ									
DZ	0.728	0.169	0.174	0.1031	0.0208	0.0227	−2.76	0.26	0.26
UZ	0.842	0.051	0.054	0.1450	0.0363	0.0399	−0.35	0.50	0.52

Table 8.35. Estimates of α, dependence (τ), and cohort effect (β) for Danish twin data, based on the PVF frailty model, and the conditional parametrization. SE^2, approximation.

The cohort effects are very close to those of the marginal distribution. The variance is increased, which was expected owing to it's being a common covariate. The approximate standard error is close to the estimate based on the full second derivative matrix. The value of τ is slightly lower than in Table 8.23, consistent with the cohort's explaining a part but only a small part of the dependence between twin pairs. The variance is increased in some cases compared to the value without cohort. The approximate standard error is not satisfactory in this case. It should be considered whether the estimate of the gamma parameters is influenced by the nonproportionality owing to the heterogeneity in the marginal distribution, and therefore, also a gamma frailty model with cohort has been applied assuming that the frailty is individual, thus assuming independence within pairs. In that case, the estimated value of δ diverges, suggesting that the hazards are proportional or diverging, as the gamma frailty model describes converging hazard functions.

Also, the PVF model is studied with a cohort effect. The results are reported in Table 8.35.

To illustrate how the variance and covariance of parameter functions can be evaluated, we consider monozygotic males. The estimation procedure finds the variance matrix for α, η, β, which is

$$V = \begin{pmatrix} 0.1663 & -0.4589 & 0.0241 \\ -0.4589 & 1.3398 & 0.0682 \\ 0.0241 & 0.0682 & 0.1334 \end{pmatrix}.$$

We further want the estimates of τ and ρ, which are functions of (α, η). The derivatives for τ at the maximum likelihood estimate are $(-0.299, -0.102)$, and those of ρ are $(-0.430, -0.147)$. Thus we consider the five-parameter functions $\varphi_1 = (\alpha, \eta, \beta, \tau, \rho)$ as a function of the three-dimensional parameter $\varphi = (\alpha, \eta, \beta)$, with variance matrix V. The variance matrix V_1 for $\hat{\varphi}$ is then $V_1 = GVG'$, where G is the matrix of derivatives of φ_1 with respect to φ. In this case, we find that the matrix is

$$G = \begin{pmatrix} 1 & 0 & 0 \\ 0 & 1 & 0 \\ 0 & 0 & 1 \\ -0.299 & -0.102 & 0 \\ -0.430 & -0.147 & 0 \end{pmatrix}.$$

From this, we derive standard errors of $(0.408, 1.157, 0.365, 0.0284, 0.0409)$ for $\hat{\varphi}_1$ and a correlation matrix of

$$\begin{pmatrix} 1 & -0.972 & -0.162 & -0.242 & 0.230 \\ -0.972 & 1 & 0.161 & 0.009 & -0.003 \\ -0.162 & 0.161 & 1 & 0.024 & -0.022 \\ -0.242 & 0.009 & 0.024 & 1 & 1.000 \\ -0.230 & -0.003 & -0.022 & 1.000 & 1 \end{pmatrix}.$$

The values of τ and ρ are clearly correlated, as expected. In a one-parameter frailty model, the two measures would be a function of each other, and thus have asymptotic correlation 1. The PVF model allows for a difference between the two measures For the example, the correlation is 0.9999, and it is even higher for the other data sets, implying that the measures of dependence are not in conflict to each other. The correlation between β and τ, respectively, ρ is almost 0, and this might appear surprising, given that the birth year explains a part of the dependence.

Finally, for comparison with the results for the lognormal distribution below, we also consider the inverse Gaussian frailty model with a cohort effect. The results are reported in Table 8.36.

The penalized likelihood approach

The penalized likelihood approach as found in Splus is based on gamma or lognormal distributions for the frailty. The procedure reports the frailty variance, which in the gamma case equals $1/\delta$. From this value, Kendall's τ can be evaluated. The estimates are reported in Table 8.37. The estimates

	$\hat{\mathrm{Var}}(Y)$ (SE)	$\hat{\mathrm{Var}}(\log(Y))$ (SE)	$\hat{\tau}$ (SE)	$\hat{\beta}$ (SE)
Males				
MZ	0.677 (0.166)	0.523 (0.102)	0.181 (0.025)	−1.73 (0.37)
DZ	0.220 (0.076)	0.199 (0.062)	0.084 (0.023)	−1.69 (0.024)
UZ	1.330 (0.505)	0.866 (0.229)	0.254 (0.042)	0.70 (0.64)
Females				
MZ	0.552 (0.169)	0.444 (0.112)	0.160 (0.030)	−2.72 (0.39)
DZ	0.311 (0.087)	0.272 (0.067)	0.109 (0.022)	−2.73 (0.26)
UZ	0.750 (0.301)	0.568 (0.177)	0.192 (0.042)	−0.36 (0.50)

Table 8.36. Estimates of frailty variances, dependence (τ), and cohort effect (β) for Danish twin data, based on the inverse Gaussian frailty model and the conditional parametrization.

Sex	Data set	$\hat{\mathrm{Var}}(Y)$	$\hat{\tau}$	$\hat{\beta}$(SE)
Males	MZ	0.463	0.188	−1.66 (0.35)
	DZ	0.119	0.056	−1.66 (0.23)
	UZ	0.647	0.244	0.69 (0.58)
Females	MZ	0.389	0.163	−2.64 (0.37)
	DZ	0.226	0.102	−2.69 (0.25)
	UZ	0.419	0.173	−0.32 (0.47)

Table 8.37. Estimates of dependence (τ) and cohort effect (β) for Danish twin data, based on the gamma frailty model and the penalized likelihood approach.

are the same as those of Table 8.34, but the standard errors are not. For the dependence parameter, the standard error is not evaluated and for the regression coefficient it is evaluated in a different way. The difference is not of major importance in this case.

For the lognormal frailty distribution, the program reports the variance of the log frailty. For comparison, we have further evaluated the coefficient of variation of the frailty and Kendall's τ using the approximation to the Laplace transform. The estimates are reported in Table 8.38. The lognormal model gives lower values of the variance compared to the inverse Gaussian

Sex	Data set	$\hat{\mathrm{Var}}(\log(Y))$	$\hat{\mathrm{Var}}(Y)$	τ	$\hat{\beta}$ (SE)
Males	MZ	0.476	0.610	0.179	−1.48 (0.35)
	DZ	0.187	0.206	0.084	−1.63 (0.23)
	UZ	0.747	1.111	0.244	1.05 (0.59)
Females	MZ	0.409	0.505	0.160	−2.49 (0.37)
	DZ	0.253	0.288	0.104	−2.62 (0.25)
	UZ	0.520	0.682	0.191	−0.13 (0.48)

Table 8.38. Estimates of dependence (τ) and cohort effect (β) for Danish twin data, based on the lognormal frailty model and the penalized likelihood approach.

model, both on the ordinary and logarithmic scale. However, the values of τ agree very well with the inverse Gaussian model.

Summary of the twin results

Survival data for twins are well suited for frailty models, as a major reason for dependence seems to be common risks. The degree of dependence is the interesting aspect of the bivariate distribution. The dependence is most conveniently quantified by the value of Spearman's ρ. The largest model examined is the PVF model using a non-parametric model for the hazard, for which the estimated dependence is quoted in Table 8.25. There is a higher dependence for monozygotic than for dizygotic twins. A part of the dependence is shown to be explained by the decreasing mortality trend over time, but this is only a small part of it. The data only include twin pairs, where both were alive at age 15 years. This truncation implies that the observed dependence is lower than it would be if lifetimes were considered at birth, according to the PVF shared frailty model. However, the importance of this aspect cannot be examined with the present data.

8.12.6   Other applications

The approach has also been considered for the leukemia data (Section 1.5.4), but the dependence is found to be negative in this case (Andersen et al., 1993). This is also what we found for the non-parametric estimate in Section 4.2.1. The stratified analysis can still be performed and gives a value of $\hat{\beta}=-1.79$ (SE 0.62) using exact tie handling, which is a slightly larger value than that obtained by neglecting pairing, $\hat{\beta}=-1.60$ (SE 0.42). There is a clear loss of precision by doing the stratified analysis.

For the adoption data of Section 1.5.2, Nielsen et al. (1992) did not find a significant dependence between the adoptee's lifetime and that of the biological or adoptive mother or father using the complete data. When they considered only early mortality, by introducing censoring at age 70 years, there was a significant dependence between the adoptee and the biological mother, corresponding to a value of $\tau = 0.16$.

Klein (1992) studied the survival patterns of whole families in the Framingham study by a gamma frailty model. The analysis included 3161 single individuals and 452 families with 1050 members. Kendall's τ was estimated to 0.09 for siblings.

Wassell, Kulczycki, and Moyer (1995) study the service lifetime of respirator safety devices, with gamma and stable frailty models with Weibull hazards. There were up to 34 devices from the same manufacturer. They found a clear dependence between devices from the same manufacturer.

Guo (1993) and Guo and Rodriguez (1992) study child mortality using gamma and binary frailty distributions to model dependence between siblings. They estimate τ to be 0.09.

Method	Hazard assumption	Estimate	Variance estimate
Parametric	Parametric	MLE	Full
EM	Non-parametric	MLE_c	No
Three-stage	Non-parametric	app. MLE_m	App.
Marginal	Non-parametric	MLE_m	Full
Conditional	Non-parametric	MLE_c	Full
Penalized	Non-parametric	MLE_c	Only covariates

Table 8.39. Summary of estimation procedures for the shared frailty model. c=conditional; m=marginal.

8.13 Chapter summary

Table 8.39 summarizes the various estimation procedures and also shows which of the estimates that agree. The EM-algorithm leads to the same estimate as the conditional model. The conditional and marginal non-parametric models, however, lead to different estimates, because the extensions to discrete time are not identical. The two estimates are compared for the application to twins, where they are slightly different. The marginal method is only applicable without covariates, or with covariates in a stable frailty model. The applications also consider the differences between the various frailty distributions. For some data sets, there has been a fine agreement between the various frailty distributions; for others there have been some difficulties. The stable frailty model is not satisfactory for the twin data, owing to the truncation at age 15 years. The gamma frailty model is not satisfactory for the kidney catheter data, because the effect of the sex interferes with the dependence.

Asymptotic theory still needs to be further developed, but some results are available for parametric models with complete data and for semi-parametric gamma models.

8.14 Bibliographic comments

Clayton and Cuzick (1985) suggested a procedure for estimating the parameters in the gamma model with covariates. The EM-algorithm was suggested by Klein (1992) and Nielsen et al. (1992) in a slightly simpler way regarding estimation of δ. It was further considered in Andersen et al. (1993). The three-stage procedure was suggested by Hougaard et al. (1992a) and further examined by Hougaard et al. (1992c).

Oakes and Manatunga (1992) derived the Fisher information in the bivariate stable-Weibull model. The results were generalized to the multivariate case by Shi (1995).

The kidney catheter data were analysed by McGilchrist and Aisbett (1991) using a lognormal frailty distribution.

The application to twins was done by Hougaard, Harvald, and Holm (1992a–c).

Tables 8.12, 8.13, 8.14, 8.15, 8.16, and 8.32 are based on material presented in Hougaard, Harvald, and Holm (1992a). Figures 8.2 and 8.3 are redrawn versions of figures first presented in Hougaard et al. (1992a). These are reprinted with permission. Tables 8.19, 8.20, and 8.21 are based on material presented in Hougaard, Harvald, and Holm (1992c). In a few cases, information has been added in these tables.

8.15   Exercises

Exercise 8.1 Different truncation times

Suppose the bivariate failure times for twins are generated by a shared frailty model, with gamma distributed frailty. Data are split in two groups. Group 1 is born in year x_1 and group 2 in year x_2. Actual data are truncated, so that only pairs, where both twins are alive in year x_3 are included ($x_1 < x_2 < x_3$). Discuss what parameters you can identify, with and without an assumption of proportional hazards between the groups.

Exercise 8.2 Gamma non-parametric likelihood

To discuss the defect of the conditional method for the gamma model, make a figure showing the profile log likelihood of δ (Equation (8.5)), for two univariate observations, $T_1 = 1$, $T_2 = 2$, without covariates and censoring. What is the difference between the minimal to the maximal value of the log likelihood? Show in the same figure the maximum value of the likelihood based on the marginal distribution, which turns out to be Equation (2.28. It might be easier to overview if you show it as function of τ rather than of δ. Make the same figure in the case where you add a third univariate observation $T_3 = 3$.

Exercise 8.3 EM-algorithm for inverse Gaussian frailty

How would you modify the EM-algorithm to work for an inverse Gaussian frailty model?

Exercise 8.4 Fisher information in the stable exponential model

From the results of Section 8.11.2 describe how you would derive the Fisher information of the positive stable frailty model, when the conditional distribution is exponential. Use this to derive the asymptotic variance of $\hat{\beta} = \log(\hat{\mu}_1/\hat{\mu}_2)$, corresponding to finding the effect of a matched pairs covariate.

This should now be compared to a simpler approach. It follows from Exercise 7.2 that the distribution of $V = \log(T_2/T_1)$ only depends on β.

What is the information about β in this variable? What is the efficiency of the simple approach?

Exercise 8.5 Model checking by censoring

One way to check a frailty model is to introduce artificial censoring at some specified time point. Which result would you expect if the frailty model were correct? Which result would you expect if you apply a gamma frailty model to data generated by a stable frailty model?

Exercise 8.6 Tumorigenesis data

Study the models and data of Section 8.12.1 using Splus or other available software.

Exercise 8.7 Comparison of Wald tests for independence

Table 8.3 reports $\hat{\tau} = 0.459$ (0.070) for the gamma frailty model without covariates. Find the estimated values and standard errors for δ, Var(Y) and the standard deviation of Y (using the restriction $EY = 1$). Use the latter two and τ to make Wald tests for independence. Why does this testing approach not make sense for δ? Evaluate the likelihood ratio test statistic from the values reported in Table 8.3. Which of the Wald tests gives the best agreement to the likelihood test statistic?

Exercise 8.8 Practical evaluation

Consider some other parallel data. To the extent possible, use the stratified model. Analyze the data by all the frailty models that the software allows. Compare the estimated regression coefficient. Compare the degree of dependence by means of Kendall's τ.

Some data you may consider are in Nelson (1982, p. 188) or in Le and Lindgren (1996).

9

Shared frailty models for recurrent events

Recurrent events are in several ways more complicated and in other ways more simple to analyze than parallel data of several individuals, and this is why the shared frailty models for such data are described in a separate chapter. This chapter treats the probability model as well as the statistical inference.

We have already seen how multi-state models can be used for the case of recurrent events, for example, by means of the state structure depicted in Figure 1.4. This is particularly relevant when the dependence is considered to be of the event-related type described in Section 3.1.3. Such models should be used when we think there are principal differences between the first and later events. How this can be done was described in Section 5.4.4 and 6.1.3.

The approach of this chapter covers such data where all events are of the same type and we do not think of the individual as moving between separate states. There might very well be many events (which is inconvenient when using the multi-state approach) or a highly varying number of events. For example, for fertility data a multi-state model seems most sensible because most women having less than four children and due to the event-related dependence as discussed in Section 3.3.1. Epileptic seizure rates, on the other hand, vary enormously between patients, with some patients having hundreds of seizures, and therefore it seems most sensible to use a frailty model. In the case of independent data, the event count corresponds to an ordinary Poisson process (Section 9.2). This means that future events are independent of previous ones, which inter alia requires that there be no random person variation. The process can be homogeneous as well as non-homogeneous. In the more general case of models with dependence over time, we think of models where conditionally on some individual values (frailty), the process evolves as a Poisson process or a Markov process. Thus the frailty model is a model for person variation.

The frailty models of this chapter are very similar to those for parallel data (Chapter 7) and many formulas are closely related. There are, however, major differences that make it relevant to consider them as two different cases. Even though there still are two random effects, they have a different interpretation. The frailty variation is not a group variation, but a variation between individuals, and the variation described by the hazard function is not an individual variation, but a variation within individuals, which for recurrent events alternatively could be called the Poisson variation. For parallel data, the risk set decreases at each event time, whereas for recurrent events data, the risk set is constant over the observation period. A consequence of this is that for parallel data, it is crucial to observe the times of events, whereas for recurrent events data, the frailty approach leads to variation in the number of events, even though the observation time is the same for all individuals. In the extreme case of a very long observation period, everybody will have died in the parallel case, so there is no variation in the number of deaths, in contrast to the recurrent events case, where the variation will be very large. For many purposes it is satisfactory to know the number of events within the observation period and the actual times are less important. This will, when the observation period is the same, be called period count data and treated as a special case. Another consequence of this is that in the recurrent events case, the stochastic process (the multi-state model of Figure 1.4) is Markov for frailty models, whereas the process for bivariate data (the multi-state model of Figure 5.12) is not Markov. The reason for this is that the risk set stays constant. For parallel data, it is relevant to evaluate Kendall's coefficient of concordance τ, and other bivariate measures of dependence, whereas for recurrent events data some essentially different measures seem more relevant. The assumption of constant hazards is often relevant for recurrent events, but rarely so for parallel data. For frailty models, the scale parameter of the frailty distribution might be treated differently, for parallel data, it is almost always treated by restricting the scale parameter to obtain identifiability, whereas for recurrent events, it is often convenient to restrict some other parameter instead.

This chapter starts by describing the notation, which is slightly different from the parallel data case (Section 9.1). Also the various observation plans are discussed in that section. The Poisson model is briefly described (Section 9.2). We will extend the Poisson approach to allow for overdispersion (Section 9.3). This is done by assuming a frailty common risks model, in which case a depiction like that of Figure 5.2 might appear equally informative. Even more intuitive is Figure 9.1, emphasizing individual differences, which are assumed to be random. The shared frailty model is a

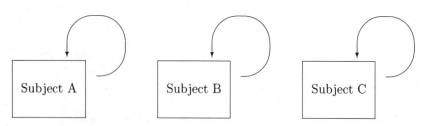

Figure 9.1. General model for recurrent events, suggesting individual differences.

model with common risk dependence. In this case it might be better denoted as constant risk dependence, as there is only a single individual for
each value of the random effect. This means that the term shared should
be interpreted as shared over time, that is, constant. Thus conditional on
a scalar valued frailty random variable, the model describes a Poisson process, where the frailty enters multiplicatively. As for the parallel data, we
specifically discuss gamma, stable, and PVF frailty distributions. Dependence measures like Kendall's τ and Spearman's ρ seem less relevant for
recurrent events. Other measures are discussed in Section 9.4. Regression
models are considered in Section 9.5. These are proportional hazards models for the conditional distribution given the frailties. Estimation methods
are described in Section 9.6. Asymptotic results are discussed in Section
9.7. Applications are described in Section 9.8.

9.1   Notation and observation plan

We will describe the data as there being one process for each individual studied and it will be assumed that the individuals are independent.
When only a single type of event is possible, the times of events for an
individual are ordered $0 < T_1 < T_2 < \dots$. The models used in this
chapter are continuous and thus there is probability 0 that two succeed-
ing observations coincide. If the eventual number of events is finite, we
define $T_{q+1} = T_{q+2} = \dots = \infty$, in which case, the times only satisfy
$0 \le T_1 \le T_2 \le \dots$. An alternative description of data is as the stochastic process describing the cumulative number of events, say, $K(t)$ at time t.
The whole process is denoted by means of brackets, $\{K(t)\}$, and defined in
the time interval $[0, \infty]$, with initial value $K(0) = 0$. The eventual number
$K(\infty)$ may be finite or infinite. This is a counting process and thus increasing over time, right-continuous and with values in $\{0, 1, \dots\}$. The event times
are the jump times of the process. These two approaches contain the same
information, as can be seen from the relations $T_j = \inf\{t; K(t) \ge j\}$ and
$K(t) = \sum_{j=1}^{\infty} 1\{T_j \le t\}$.

Design	Events	Obs. period	Risk set
Exact	Exact times	Individual	Constant
Exact, same period	Exact times	Common	Constant
Period counts	Number	Common	Constant
Interval counts	Number in intervals	Common	Constant
Alternating states	Exact times	Individual	$\{0, 1\}$

Table 9.1. Observation plans for recurrent events. Constant risk set means that it is constant (=1) until end of the observation period.

The observation period $(0, C]$ is finite and thus also the total observed number of events is finite, $K = K(C)$. That is, the number of events K is random, $K \in \{0, 1, ...\}$. The formulation above is slightly different from that used in the rest of the book. In the version used in this chapter, the use of event indicators (D) is avoided, meaning that $K \geq 0$ is the number of events, and not the number of times. The number of events was denoted E in Chapter 5. It is then necessary to separately define the time of end of observation (C). It is important to determine whether C is common to the individuals, because then some simplified approaches are available.

For some data sets, we do not have the exact times of events. This is natural, when the underlying process is assumed to have a reasonably constant hazard. In particular, when there can be several events per day, it is common with a summary describing the number of events that day. Also some insurance data do not consider data by the day, but only report the number of events during a year. In that case, the data are of the interval count form K_{ij}, $i = 1, ..., n$, $j = 1, ..., r_i$, where j describes the interval. The number of intervals (r_i) may be common to the individuals. Of course, an important special case is when there is only a single interval. Thus we only know the total number of events experienced for the various individuals. This will be called period count data and described as K_i.

More generally, there can be periods with missing data. In that case, it is necessary to define the subperiods of observations. This can be done by going back to a notation like that for the multi-state models, defining variables V_{ij}, X_{ij}, D_{ij}, so that there is one value of j for each event and for each observation interval without event. Then X_{ij} is the time of event/end of observation and D_{ij} an indicator of event at time X_{ij}. Finally, V_{ij} is the time of the previous event, or if observation is not complete, the time of the beginning of the actual observation interval. This is the case in an alternating state model (Figure 2.2). For example, if one studies recurrent infections in a catheter (like the problem described in Section 1.7.3, but assuming that we had complete information on all infections for all patients), the duration of the infection would be so long that it cannot be ignored. Then the person is only under risk of obtaining an infection in the healthy case. Then V_{ij} is the end of the $j - 1$th infection period (with $V_{i0} = 0$).

Table 9.1 summarizes the various observation plans. The alternating state observation plan is the most general. On the other hand, when the purpose is to assess the dependence (the variation between individuals) and the effect of common covariates, it greatly simplifies the methods when the observation period is common, because it is possible to reduce the data to the period counts.

9.2   Poisson processes

The basis for this model is Figure 1.4, with an assumption that the hazard of experiencing an event is $\lambda(t)$, independently of the current state. Clearly, this is a Markov model. In fact, the counting process has independent increments, which is a stronger condition than the Markov condition. Future events occur independently of the number of previous events. The distribution of the number of events $(K(t) - K(v))$ in the time interval $(v, t]$ is Poisson, with mean $\int_v^t \lambda(u)du$, say η. Thus, the probabilities are

$$Pr(K(t) - K(v) = j) = \eta^j \exp(-\eta)/j!. \tag{9.1}$$

In the constant hazards case, this was derived in Equation (5.25). Then the process is called a homogeneous Poisson process and the total number of events K is sufficient, with $K = K(C)$ following a Poisson distribution with mean $C\lambda$. This is an exponential family, where the canonical parameter is $\log \eta$. A consequence is that the variance in this distribution equals the mean, η. The distribution is unimodal and the mode is $[EK]$, the integer value of the mean.

The likelihood of the observed times follows directly from Equation (6.3), to be

$$\{\prod_{j=1}^{K} \lambda(T_j)\} \exp\{-\int_0^C \lambda(u)du\}. \tag{9.2}$$

This formula has a clear interpretation. There is a term with the hazard for each event observed and an exponential term describing the total integrated hazard experienced by the individual.

This model can be handled with a general hazard function and covariates acting via proportional hazards. This model specifies a hazard of

$$\exp(\beta' z_i)\lambda_0(t) \tag{9.3}$$

for the ith individual. This model is the same as that of Section 2.4, with the extension that each individual can experience several events.

Applications of this approach will be considered in Section 9.8.

9.2.1 Evaluation in SAS

The model above is easily handled by SAS, using the so-called counting process type of input, corresponding to the notation described above for periods of missing information. This is done by for each individual having $K + 1$ records. For each event, say $j = 1, ..., K$, there is a variable start equal to T_{j-1} (or more generally V_j), letting $T_0 = 0$, and a variable eventtim equal to T_j, and a variable event (event indicator) equal to 1. Furthermore, there is a record with start equal to T_K, eventtim C and event equal to 0. Then the model, in the case of two covariates x1 and x2, is fitted by the call

  proc phreg;
    model (start,eventtim)*event(0)=x1 x2;

This is then formulated in the same way as for truncated observations, but with a varying number of records per individual.

9.3 Constant frailty overdispersion models

In this section, the constant shared frailty model is applied to recurrent events data. The models are similar to those of Chapter 7, except that the risk set does not change by the events. Thus conditional on the frailty value Y, the process is assumed to follow a Poisson process, with hazard $Y\mu(t)$. Conditionally on Y, the probability is found by direct insertion in Equation (9.2), and after integration over Y, the likelihood contribution, based on observing K events before time t is

$$Pr(K = k, T_1 = t_1, ..., T_k = t_k) = (-1)^k \{\prod_{j=1}^{k} \mu(t_j)\} L^{(k)}(\int_0^t \mu(u)du),$$

(9.4)

which is very similar to Equation (7.6), but the total integrated hazard is here $M. = \int_0^t \mu(u)du$.

To get the distribution of the total number of events (K) during $(0, t]$, we integrate $t_1, ..., t_K$ over $(0, t)$, subject to the restriction $0 \leq t_1 \leq ... \leq t_K \leq t$. This integral can be evaluated by integrating over the product set $[0, t]^K$, and dividing by $K!$. The distribution of K is Poisson with mean $Y \int_0^t \mu(u)du$, conditionally on Y, and unconditionally, the distribution is given by

$$Pr(K = k) = (-1)^k \{\int_0^t \mu(u)du\}^k L^{(k)}(\int_0^t \mu(u)du)/k!.$$

(9.5)

The distribution of the event times conditional on the total number of events, K, is a distribution with density

$$f(t_1, ..., t_K \mid K) = 1\{0 \leq t_1 \leq ... \leq t_K \leq t\} \prod_{j=1}^{K} \{\mu(t_j)/\int_0^t \mu(u)du\}K!.$$
(9.6)

It follows from these results that the frailty distribution only enters in the distribution of the total number of events (Equation (9.5)), and this depends on the hazard only via the integrated hazard over the whole interval. The distribution of the times conditional on the number of events depends only on the relative hazard (that is, relative to the integrated hazard) (Equation (9.6)). This means that the number of events in any given interval, say, $(v, t]$ is a binomial distribution with probability parameter $\int_v^t \mu(u)du/\int_0^t \mu(u)du$, conditional on the total number of events.

In particular, when $\mu(t)$ is constant, we obtain the simple expression

$$Pr(K = k) = (-1)^k (t\mu)^k L^{(k)}(t\mu)/k!$$
(9.7)

and that the distribution of times conditional on the total number of events is the distribution of the ordered observations for K independent uniform random variables on the interval $(0, t]$.

From Equation (9.4), we can immediately derive the hazard rate of an event at time t, conditional on the history at that time. That is, we can update the frailty distribution. Suppose there have been k events at that time, then the hazard of a further event is

$$(-1)\mu(t)L^{(k+1)}\left(\int_0^t \mu(u)du\right)/L^{(k)}\left(\int_0^t \mu(u)du\right).$$
(9.8)

In particular, it is seen that the hazard is independent of the times of the previous events; only the number of events enters in the formula. This shows that the model is a Markov model, when considered as a multi-state model, illustrated in Figure 1.4. This means that the hazard in Equation (9.8) is of the form $\lambda_k(t)$. One consequence of this formula is that without covariates, the multi-state stratified approach of Section 6.1.3 is not in conflict with the frailty model. When covariates are included, however, the λ hazards will not be proportional for different values of the covariate, and therefore, a proportional conditional hazards model is different from the multi-state proportional hazards model.

9.3.1   Common observation period

The consequence of these results is that when the observation period is the same for all subjects, we can consider the model as two separate models, one for the total number of events and one for the distribution over the interval, conditional on the total number of events. The frailty distribution only enters in the first part. The hazard enters the first part only via the integrated hazard over the whole interval. In the second term, the hazard enters only relative to the integrated hazard. This implies that for evaluating person differences, the count over the whole interval is sufficient. Therefore, the models for the period count data where only the number of events within a common interval $(0, C]$ is observed will be separately considered. Where the previous section considered the event count at any time t, we now only observe $K = K(C)$. We may define the unit of time so that $C = 1$. Without loss of generality, we may assume that $\int_0^C \mu(u)du = 1$ in that case, because otherwise, this factor can be multiplied on Y to make some $\tilde{Y}$, and we can then consider the Laplace transform of $\tilde{Y}$ instead. This means that in this case, we do not want the mean of Y to be restricted to 1 as was done in the shared frailty model of Chapter 7, to make the parameters identifiable.

The mean of K equals that of Y. The variance is found by the formula $Var(K) = EY + Var(Y)$ derived from the classical formula $Var(K) = EVar(K \mid Y) + Var(E(K \mid Y))$. This formula has a clear interpretation, the first term is the Poisson variance and the second term is the extra variance due to the random individual level. Generally, the moments can be found using the factorial moment relation

$$E\{K(K-1)(K-2)...(K-r+1)\} = EY^r, \ r = 1, 2, ..., \qquad (9.9)$$

which is derived from the Poisson distribution by conditioning on Y.

The Laplace transform of K is easily described by means of the Laplace transform of Y by the expression

$$L_K(s) = L_Y(1 - e^{-s}).$$

9.3.2 Negative binomial models for period count data

In the case, where only the count of events during a fixed period $(0, C)$ is observed, we obtain a distribution, where the number of events is Poisson distributed, conditionally on Y. By using the observation period as the time unit (leading to $C = 1$), and absorbing the integrated hazard into Y, we formulate this problem as that conditionally on Y, the event count K is Poisson with mean Y. Alternatively, we can say that $\int_0^C \mu(u)du$ is restricted to 1 to obtain identifiability. When the distribution of Y is gamma with parameters δ and θ, the distribution of the number of events is

$$p(k) = \frac{\theta^\delta \Gamma(\delta + k)}{(1 + \theta)^{(\delta+k)} \Gamma(\delta) k!}, \qquad (9.10)$$

utilizing Equations (9.7) and (A.11). This is the negative binomial distribution, NB(δ, θ). For fixed δ, it is a natural exponential family in the parameter $\log(\theta + 1)$. The mean of K equals that of Y, which is δ/θ, and the variance is $Var(K) = \delta/\theta + \delta/\theta^2$. It is also possible to evaluate the

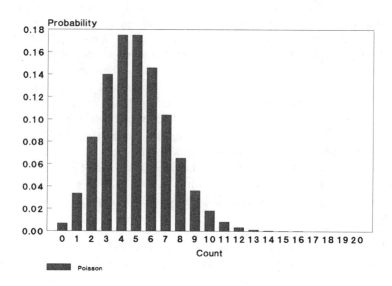

Figure 9.2. Probability distribution for the Poisson distribution with mean 5.

inverse factorial moment $E\{1/(K+1)\} = \{\theta - \theta^{\delta}(\theta+1)^{1-\delta}\}/(\delta-1)$, when $\delta \neq 1$. For $\delta = 1$, it can be found by continuity as $\theta \log(1 + 1/\theta)$. The distribution is unimodal. The mode is at $[EK - 1/\theta]$, where $[\cdot]$ denotes the integer part. Thus for a fixed value of the mean, overdispersion tends to reduce the mode. The masses are decreasing, that is, the mode is at 0, when $Var(K) > (EK)^2$. Thus large variation necessarily leads to decreasing masses. Furthermore, the masses are always decreasing, when $EK < 1$.

To illustrate how the distributions look, we first show a Poisson distribution with mean 5 (Figure 9.2). This distribution has a mode at 4-5 (meaning that the probability of 4 and 5 are equal, and are the highest values). A negative binomial with the same mean, but a variance of 15, is used for comparison, giving $\delta = 2.5$ and $\theta = 0.5$. This is shown in Figure 9.3. Thus the mixture distribution variance $(Var(Y))$ is 10. Clearly, the distribution is more spread out. In particular, the value at 0 is increased from a value of 0.0067 in the Poisson case to 0.0642 in the negative binomial case. The mode is at 2-3.

The Laplace transform of K is $L_K(s) = E(e^{-sK}) = \{\theta/(\theta+1-e^{-s})\}^{\delta}$.

Updating is particularly simple in this case, and given K events observed before time 1, the conditional distribution of Y is gamma with parameters $\delta + K$ and $\theta + 1$.

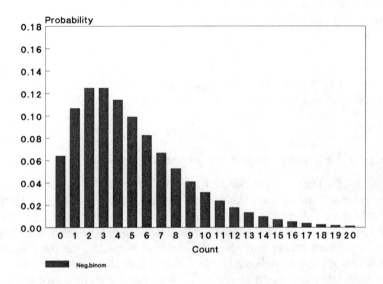

Figure 9.3. Probability distribution for the negative binomial distribution with mean 5 and variance 15.

9.3.3 Negative binomial models

This distribution is obtained by assuming that the frailty is gamma distributed, and that the process is observed continuously over an interval $(0, C]$. The end of observation C may differ for the individuals. Thus we have a conditional hazard of $Y\mu(t)$, where Y is gamma distributed with parameters δ and θ, and $\mu(t)$ describes the hazard as function of time. The distribution of $K(t)$ is negative binomial $\mathrm{NB}(\delta, \theta/\int_0^t \mu(u)du)$. In the constant hazards case, we can without loss of generality take $\mu(t) = 1$, in which case, the model is by definition the Polya process for the counting process, and the total number of events $K(C)$ is sufficient. This also implies that we cannot estimate all parameters based on a single process.

For period counts, we have found it convenient to restrict the integrated hazard to 1, in order to obtain identifiability. Alternatively, one could restrict the gamma mean to 1, in the usual way by setting $\delta = \theta$, and let the integrated hazard be a free parameter. The formulas could easily be generalized to cover both cases, for example, the conditional distribution of Y given the number of events $K(t)$ at time t is gamma with parameters $\delta + K(t)$ and $\theta + \int_0^t \mu(u)du$.

The ratio of hazards $\lambda_k(t)$ of Equation (9.8) is constant, making the formulas very simple. More precisely,

$$\frac{\lambda_k(t)}{\lambda_0(t)} = \frac{\delta + k}{\delta}. \tag{9.11}$$

This means that there are proportional hazards over the previous number of events, but not over covariates, as $\lambda_0(t) = \mu(t)\delta/\{\theta + M(t)\}$, as in the univariate case.

9.3.4   PVF frailty models for period count data

As we did for parallel data, we will consider what can be gained by using more general families than the gamma for the frailty distribution. In the case where we extend the gamma mixture to the power variance function family, it will be seen that many similar formulas can be derived for this case. In the case, where only the total count of events during the observation period is known, we consider the model where the number of events is Poisson distributed, conditionally on Y, with mean Y. The distribution of Y is assumed to be the PVF distribution with parameters (α, δ, θ). The distribution of K will be denoted P-PVF(α, δ, θ). The formulas in this section are correct for $\alpha \neq 0$, but only some of them are valid for $\alpha = 0$.

The probability of observing 0 events is $p(0) = \exp[-\delta\{(\theta+1)^\alpha - \theta^\alpha\}/\alpha]$. The general point probability is

$$p(k) = p(0)\{\sum_{m=1}^{k} c_{km}(\alpha)\delta^m(\theta + 1)^{m\alpha-k}\}/k! \tag{9.12}$$

The factors, c_{km}, are given in Equation (A.19). The mean $EK = EY$ is $\delta\theta^{\alpha-1}$, which is finite for $\theta > 0$. The variance is $Var(K) = \delta\theta^{\alpha-1} + \delta(1 - \alpha)\theta^{\alpha-2}$. Similar to the negative binomial model, the variation in count equals the Poisson variance plus the mixture variation.

Figures 9.4–9.6 show some possibilities for how the distribution can look. They have the same mean and variance as Figure 9.3. Figure 9.4 has $\alpha = 0.95$, and thus is extreme. The other parameters are $\delta = 4.1578$ and $\theta = 0.025$. It is rather similar to the Poisson case (Figure 9.2), but the difference in the interpretation is that most individuals have a risk slightly below the mean (5), leading to the mode at 4, but a few individuals have a markedly increased risk, leading to the mean's being 5, and the variance being clearly larger. Therefore, the tail is larger. The probability of zero events is 0.0129, close to the Poisson value. Figure 9.5 is based on the inverse Gaussian frailty distribution, that is, a PVF distribution with $\alpha = 1/2$. The other parameters are $\delta = 2.5$ and $\theta = 0.5$. This one is intermediate between that of the gamma mixture and the $\alpha = 0.95$ mixture, and has a mode at 3, and the probability at 0 is 0.0455. This is roughly similar to the gamma mixture, but with a lower left tail and a longer right tail.

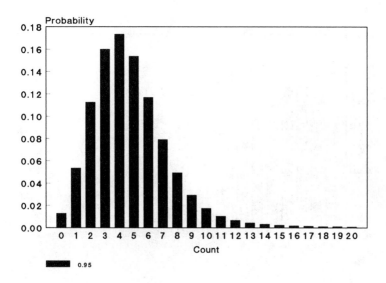

Figure 9.4. Probability distribution for the PVF Poisson mixture distribution with mean 5 and variance 15, with $\alpha = 0.95$.

Figure 9.6 assumes a negative value (-10) for α. The other parameters are $\delta = 6.97 \cdot 10^8$ and $\theta = 5.5$. In this case, the PVF model implies that there is a positive probability of Y being 0, or in other words some individuals are not vulnerable to experience the event under consideration. For $\alpha < 0$, the probability that $Y = 0$ is $\exp(\delta\theta^\alpha)$. In the example there is probability 0.064 for $Y = 0$ and 0.043 for $Y > 0$, but still observing no events, giving a total probability of 0.107 of observing no events. The mixture distributions are illustrated in Figure 9.7. This shows how the inverse Gaussian mixture appears more concentrated than the gamma owing to its smaller left tail and larger right tail. Except for the gamma distributions, the density starts out flat at 0. The $\alpha = 0.95$ mixture distribution is almost degenerate at a value slightly below 5. The negative α mixture distribution is multimodal.

This model is a natural exponential family in one parameter, but where θ is the canonical parameter in the PVF mixture distribution, it is slightly more complicated to derive the canonical parameter in the overdispersed count model. If we change the parametrization to (α, ρ, ω), where $\delta = \rho e^{-\alpha\omega}$ and $\theta = e^\omega - 1$, the model is a natural exponential family in $\omega = \log(\theta + 1)$ for fixed values of (α, ρ).

If K_1 and K_2 are independent, and K_j follows the distribution P-PVF $(\alpha, \delta_j, \theta)$, the distribution of $K_1 + K_2$ is P-PVF $(\alpha, \delta_1 + \delta_2, \theta)$. Thus for any n, the distribution P-PVF (α, δ, θ) can be derived as the sum of n

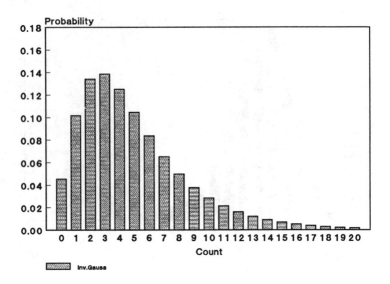

Figure 9.5. Probability distribution for inverse Gaussian mixture distribution with mean 5 and variance 15.

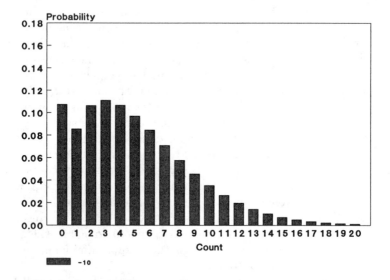

Figure 9.6. Probability distribution for PVF Poisson mixture distribution with mean 5 and variance 15, with $\alpha = -10$.

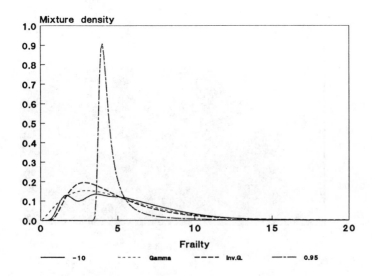

Figure 9.7. Mixture distributions with mean 5 and variance 10, for $\alpha = -10$, 0, 0.5 and 0.95. The $\alpha = -10$ distribution has a point mass of 0.064 at 0.

independent variables following the distribution P-PVF $(\alpha, \delta/n, \theta)$. Thus the distribution is infinite divisible in the parameter δ.

The Laplace transform of K is $L_K(s) = E(e^{-sK}) = \exp[-\delta\{(\theta+1 - e^{-s})^\alpha - \theta^\alpha\}/\alpha]$, when $\alpha \neq 0$.

When $\alpha \geq 0$, the distribution is unimodal, which follows from the mixture distribution's being unimodal. For fixed values of the mean and the variance, the mode seems to be an increasing function of α, from $[EK-1/\theta]$ at $\alpha = 0$ to $[EK]$ at $\alpha = 1$. For negative values of α, the distribution is typically not unimodal, owing to the point mass at 0, which may imply that there are several modes, one of them being at 0. The number of modes does not appear to be a simple function of the parameters. An example of a trimodal distribution is shown in Figure 9.8. The parameters in this case are $\alpha = -5$, $\delta = 3.82 \cdot 10^{-5}$, $\theta = 0.08$. There is a mode in 0 (probability 0.097), in 67 (probability 0.003928), and 102 (probability 0.003930). The local minimum of probabilities between 67 and 102 is at 82 (probability 0.003916). Thus the distribution is essentially flat between 67 and 102. In fact, this example was chosen to make the dip between the two larger values as large as possible, among the trimodal distributions found with $\alpha \geq -5$, so the other examples found are even more flat. Many period count data are zero-heavy, meaning that there many more observations of zero events than expected from simple theories, and therefore a distribution with $\alpha < 0$

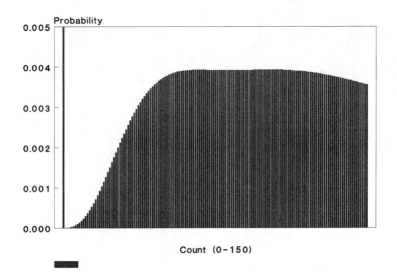

Figure 9.8. Trimodal probability distribution for PVF Poisson mixture distribution with modes 0, 67 and 102, with $\alpha = -5$. $p(0) = 0.097$.

might be relevant. For example, a proportion of epileptic patients who are well treated might have zero risk of experiencing a seizure.

In the special case of an inverse Gaussian mixture ($\alpha = 1/2$), there is a relation between the probabilities of any three consecutive counts, so that

$$p(k+1) = \frac{\delta^2 p(k-1)}{(\theta+1)k(k+1)} + \frac{(k-1/2)p(k)}{(\theta+1)(k+1)}. \qquad (9.13)$$

The advantage of using this expression is that the computational burden increases linearly with k, whereas the expression in Equation (9.12) implies that the number of computations increases with the square of k. It is also possible to evaluate the inverse factorial moment

$$E\{1/(K+1)\} =$$

$$1/2\delta^{-2} + \theta^{1/2}/\delta - \{1/2\delta^{-2} + (\theta+1)^{1/2}/\delta\}\exp[-2\delta\{(\theta+1)^{1/2} - \theta^{1/2}\}].$$

The case $\alpha = -1$ implies that Y follows a non-central gamma distribution of shape parameter 0. In this case, an explicit expression for the coefficients is also known, see the Appendix (Section A.3.4).

The limit for $\alpha \to -\infty$ is a scaled Poisson distribution for Y, meaning that it can be written as $Y = cQ$, where c is a constant and Q is Poisson distributed with mean, say η. The probability masses are

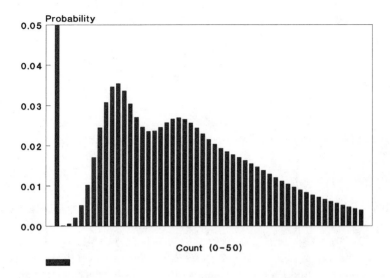

Figure 9.9. Probability distribution for scaled Poisson mixture distribution with mean 20 and variance 220.

$$p(0) = \exp\{-\eta(1 - e^{-c})\} \text{ and}$$

$$p(k) = p(0)c^k \{\sum_{m=1}^{k} w_{km}\eta^m e^{-mc}\}/k!, \qquad (9.14)$$

where the coefficients are given recursively by $w_{k1} = w_{kk} = 1$ and $w_{km} = w_{k-1,m-1} + m w_{k-1,m}$. The mean of K is $c\eta$ and the variance $c(c+1)\eta$. The count distribution can have many modes. Figure 9.9 shows such an example, where the Poisson distribution has mean 2, and the scale (c) is 10. The mean number of events is then 20. It is easy to see peaks in the distribution of K, corresponding to Y being 0, 10 and 20. The probability of 0 events is 0.135.

The hypothesis of no overdispersion (no person differences) is a hypothesis reducing the model by two parameters, and thus ordinary normal distribution methods are not applicable. The purpose of using this distribution is to obtain a good fit, particularly, when the there is a large overdispersion. For testing for the presence of overdispersion, it is recommended to fix α.

A few properties of these distributions are summarized in Table 9.2.

Case	Prob.mass	Mean	No. of modes	Mode position
General	Eq. (9.12)	$\delta\theta^{\alpha-1}$	≥ 1	
$\alpha \to -\infty$	Eq. (9.14)		≥ 1	
$\alpha = -1$	Eq. (9.12)	$\delta\theta^{-2}$	≥ 1	
$\alpha = 0$	Eq. (9.10)	δ/θ	1	$[EK - 1/\theta]$
$\alpha = 1/2$	Eq. (9.13)	$\delta/\sqrt{\theta}$	1	
$\alpha = 1$	Eq. (9.1)	δ	1	$[EK]$
$\theta = 0$	Eq. (9.16)	∞	1	

Table 9.2. Some properties of special cases of the PVF frailty model for period count data.

9.3.5 PVF frailty models

Also in this case, the conditional hazards model is $Y\mu(t)$, where Y follows the distribution $\mathrm{PVF}(\alpha, \delta, \theta)$. It follows directly that the distribution of $K(t)$ is $\mathrm{P\text{-}PVF}(\alpha, \delta\{\int_0^t \mu(u)du\}^\alpha, \theta/\int_0^t \mu(u)du)$. In the case of constant $\mu(t)$, this way of generating the process is similar to the Polya process for the gamma case, and therefore it is natural to denote this case the generalized Polya process. Also in this case, the total number of events is sufficient, and thus estimation cannot be performed on the basis of a single process.

For data on exact times, Equation (9.4) is used.

For interval count data, the probability of the observed response is most conveniently described by the distribution of the total number of events times the conditional distribution of the events in the intervals. Specifically, suppose that the frailty follows the distribution $\mathrm{PVF}(\alpha, \delta, \theta)$, and that there are two intervals, say, $(0, x_1]$ and $(x_1, x_2]$. The hazard contributions are $\mu_1 = \int_0^{x_1} \mu(u)du$ and $\mu_2 = \int_{x_1}^{x_2} \mu(u)du$. The distribution of the interval counts (K_1, K_2) is then given by $K = K_1 + K_2$ being $\mathrm{P\text{-}PVF}(\alpha, \delta\{\mu_1 + \mu_2\}^\alpha, \theta/(\mu_1 + \mu_2))$, and K_1 given K is binomial with probability parameter $\mu_1/(\mu_1 + \mu_2)$. The probability of observing 0 events is $p(0, 0) = \exp[-\tilde{\delta}\{(\tilde{\theta} + 1)^\alpha - \tilde{\theta}^\alpha\}/\alpha]$, where $\tilde{\delta} = \delta\{\mu_1 + \mu_2\}^\alpha$ and $\tilde{\theta} = \theta/(\mu_1 + \mu_2)$. The general point probability, $p(k_1, k_2)$, is

$$p(0,0)\{\sum_{m=1}^{k} c_{km}(\alpha)\tilde{\delta}^m(\tilde{\theta} + 1)^{m\alpha - k}\}\mu_1^{k_1}\mu_2^{k_2}/[(\mu_1 + \mu_2)^k k_1! k_2!], \qquad (9.15)$$

where $k = k_1 + k_2$.

9.3.6 Positive stable frailty models

The positive stable frailty model seems less relevant in this case than in the parallel data case, because the infinite mean of Y implies that the mean number of events in any interval is infinite. This model can be treated as a special case of the model of Section 9.3.4, but this section adds a few details. The probability masses are clearly simplified compared to Equation (9.12).

They are $p(0) = \exp(-\delta/\alpha)$ and

$$p(k) = p(0)\{\sum_{m=1}^{k} c_{km}(\alpha)\delta^m\}/k! \tag{9.16}$$

for $k > 0$.

The result (Equation (2.54)) regarding proportional hazards is still correct and implies that the model for the time to the first event follows a proportional hazards model, if the conditional model does. However, the model for later events is a complicated functions of the covariates, and therefore the proportionality result seems less important in this case.

Computationally, this case is covered by the results of Section 9.3.4.

9.4 Dependence measures

The dependence measures defined in Chapter 4 are parallel oriented and therefore not really useful for recurrent events data. The dependence between T_1 and T_2 is different, and positive owing to the order restriction $T_1 < T_2$ even in the Poisson model. It therefore seems that we have to return to the simple choice of the coefficient of variation $SD(Y)/EY$. It makes more sense in this case than for parallel data. This measure is evaluated in the frailty distribution, because the same measure in the count distribution changes nonlinearly over time. It can be evaluated non-parametrically with period count data, as $\{\text{Var}(K) - EK\}^{1/2}/EK$. For the PVF model, the quantity is $\sqrt{(1-\alpha)\theta^{-\alpha}/\delta}$, simplifying to $\delta^{-1/2}$ for the gamma model.

As an alternative, one could consider the variance on the logarithmic scale but this is more difficult to evaluate and cannot handle the case of $\alpha < 0$ owing to the point mass at 0.

9.5 Regression models

It is, of course, relevant to include covariates, in order to evaluate the effect of these variables, and second to examine whether they explain part of the variation between processes. If the covariates are known, it is preferable to include them in order to obtain a more precise description. The effect of the covariates will be modeled in a proportional hazards model. Thus the model describes that the hazard of experiencing an event at time t for the ith subject is

$$Y_i \exp(\beta' z_i)\mu_0(t) \tag{9.17}$$

conditional on Y_i. In this formulation z_i is a constant covariate (a common covariate in our general terminology), and the effect of this shows up in the variation between individuals. Alternatively, the covariate could describe treatment in a cross-over experiment and thus be a function of time, $z_i(t)$. This is also covered, but formally it cannot become a matched pairs covariate with exact times, because we do not know the number of events in the first period, and then the covariates are not functions of j.

Furthermore, one could have time-dependent covariates of the state-dependent type, that is, of the form z_{ij}. This could be useful for goodness-of-fit evaluations and for making more advanced models for the dependence. One should, however, be careful with such models as there basically are two different probability mechanisms creating dependence between the times.

The mathematical results regarding univariate identifiability in a proportional hazards model are still correct and imply that the variation between individuals can be identified from data on only the first event for each individual, and with arbitrary hazard functions as long as covariates are included. However, this seems less of a problem for recurrent events data, when we observe the process for a fixed time period. This intuitive comment is based on the number of events being more important than the timing of events in this case.

9.5.1 Period count data

Only constant covariates make sense for this observation plan. It follows from the general results above for the PVF model that the event count for an individual has the distribution P-PVF($\alpha, \delta \exp(\alpha\beta'z), \theta \exp(-\beta'z)$). This is, in principle, what is needed in order to continue with the model.

In the gamma frailty case, some further understanding of the model is possible. Regression covariates influence only the third parameter. One consequence of this is that for a binary covariate (say, with z having two levels u_1 and u_2) and fixed δ, the model is a two-dimensional exponential family, with canonical parameters $\log\{1 + \theta \exp(-\beta u_r)\}$, $r = 1, 2$. Thus, we can make use of exponential family theory in this case.

9.5.2 Interval count data

The covariates can be constant, or they can be time-dependent, but we will only consider the case where a time-dependent covariate changes at an interval endpoint.

For interval count data, the model specifies that conditional on Y_i, the number of events, K_{ij}, for individual i in interval j, follows a Poisson distribution with mean $Y_i \exp(\beta'z_{ij})\mu_j$. If the covariate depends only on j, the interval number, we still accept to call it a matched pairs covariate. Except for the unobserved nature of Y_i, this is a multiplicative Poisson model.

For the PVF frailty model (including the gamma model as a special case), the probabilities are most efficiently evaluated by the probability of the total number of events in the period, which follows the distribution P-PVF$(\alpha, \delta\{\sum_q \exp(\beta' z_q)\mu_q\}^\alpha, \theta / \sum_q \{\exp(\beta' z_q)\mu_q\})$ times the conditional distribution over the intervals, given the total number of events, which is a multinomial distribution with parameters $\exp(\beta' z_j)\mu_j / \sum_q \{\exp(\beta' z_q)\mu_q\}$. In this expression, it is necessary to implement a scale restriction as (δ, θ) and μ_j can both include a scale parameter, but this can be done in any of the ways previously described. The advantage of this expression is that it becomes clear that when the covariates are constant, they only influence the total number of events (which means they are compared to the variation between individuals) and when the covariates are of the matched pairs types, they only influence the relative distribution over the intervals (and are compared to the Poisson variation).

9.5.3 Gap times

An alternative model to that of Equation (9.17) is to use a time scale of time since the latest event. That is, when the subject has experienced precisely j events, the hazard of an event is $Y_i \exp(\beta' z_i)\varphi_0(t - T_j)$. This is a renewal process, where the distribution of gap times differs between individuals as a consequence of the individual frailties. The standard is to set $T_0 = 0$, but whether this makes sense must be judged specifically in each case. Estimates of dependence in this model are often smaller than in the model of Equation (9.17), because a decreasing hazard function $\varphi_0(t)$ is an alternative way of describing dependence. A further disadvantage of this model is that it is difficult to evaluate the distribution of the number of events at a given time point.

This formulation will make the data look more like parallel data than our standard recurrent events formulation. However, the number of times will vary between individuals.

9.6   Estimation

This will be considered separately for data on exact times, period count data, and for interval count data. The reason for this split is that the likelihood functions are very different. For exact times, we have observations in continuous time, a non-parametric hazard function, and censoring is an important possibility. For the other cases these problems are avoided. For period count data, the distribution is a parametric model for count data (observations on the non-negative integers). Interval count data are like period count data, but the count is multi-dimensional. The probability density is the period count expression supplemented with an extra factor describing the distribution over the intervals.

9.6.1 Data of exact times

This is, in principle, done in the same way as in Section 8.6. The model can be completely non-parametric or have piecewise constant hazards in some intervals. The number of events in the qth interval is D_q and similarly the index j can be omitted on M. As usual, the subject index i is neglected. The risk set is constant during the observation period, implying that for non-parametric hazards $M_q = 1\{x_q \leq C\}$ and for piecewise constant hazards $M_q = \min\{C, x_q\} - \min\{C, x_{q-1}\}$. With these slight formula modifications, the conditional method of Section 8.6 is applicable.

9.6.2 Period count data

In this section, the observations are assumed just to consist of counts of events, K_i, $i = 1, ..., n$, for some individuals, over the whole observation period, which without loss of generality can be assumed to have length 1. The individuals are assumed to be independent. First, the case of identically distributed variables is considered.

The Poisson case has just a single parameter, the mean, say, η. As this model is a one-dimensional natural exponential family, the estimate can be found by equating the observed and the theoretical mean, that is, $\hat{\eta} = \overline{K}$.

For the frailty models considered (without covariates), the model for the count contains a one-dimensional natural exponential family for fixed values of the other parameters. The canonical parameter does not involve α, which implies that both for α fixed and for α freely varying, the model contains a one-dimensional natural exponential family as submodel, and therefore the first moment equation is one of the maximum likelihood equations. This has as a consequence that the estimates will never be at the boundary corresponding to the positive stable mixture distributions ($\theta = 0$). It is, however, possible that the estimate is on the boundary corresponding to a Poisson distribution.

These results suggest using moment estimation, but that is, in general, not acceptable. It only makes sense for suggesting an initial estimate. This is because the second moment equation is not among the maximum likelihood equations. More specifically, for a gamma mixture, the left tail is very important for determining the frailty parameter, but the right tail is more important for evaluating the empirical variance. To use it as an initial estimate, we first evaluate the average $\overline{K}$, and the variance s^2, in the same way as done for normally distributed variables. The variance of the mixture distribution ($\mathrm{Var}(Y)$) is then found as $s_Y^2 = s^2 - \overline{K}$. If this quantity is negative, there is no overdispersion and the moment estimate is on the boundary corresponding to the Poisson distribution. When it is positive, we can with a chosen value of α derive $\theta = (1 - \alpha)\overline{K}/s_Y^2$ and $\delta = \overline{K}\theta^{1-\alpha}$ as the moment estimate. When α is freely varying, we can either include the third moment, or take $\alpha = 0.5$ for the initial estimate.

Maximum likelihood is preferable. This can also be done using the formulas of Section 8.6, but with a few more modifications. There is only one hazard value, so q is always 1. Similarly M_q equals 1. Finally, the factorial term $(k!)$ in Equation (9.5) is neglected because it does not involve the parameters.

Another standard approach for such data is a pseudo-likelihood evaluation, where the model is fitted in an exponential family framework (in this case using a Poisson model), including a dispersion parameter. This will not be considered here, because it is essentially a moment method, and cannot discriminate between a gamma and an inverse Gaussian model, for example.

Maximum likelihood is also recommended for regression models. For the gamma frailty model and a single covariate with two possible values, the three parameter model includes a two-parameter exponential family, as described in Section 9.5.1. The statistical consequence of this is that the maximum likelihood equations include a moment equation for each value of the covariate. Consequently, the estimate of the relative risk equals the empirical ratio of rates. For the general PVF model, the regression model modifies both δ and θ and therefore a similar result is not obtained.

9.6.3   Interval counts for several intervals

The above results (most spelled out in Section 9.5.2) imply that when the aim is to evaluate the frailty distribution and there are no covariates and the same intervals, the data can be reduced to the period counts over all intervals. Similarly for constant covariates, inference on both the frailty parameters and the regression coefficient is performed after reducing to the period counts.

In the case of matched pairs covariates, however, inference on the frailty parameters is done based on the period counts and inference on the regression coefficients is a multinomial regression on the relative distribution among the intervals. In the simplest cases, this is a logistic regression model. In fact, this has important consequences, because it says that modeling the overdispersion between individuals in a frailty model has no influence on the estimation of regression coefficients, which are determined within individuals.

9.7   Asymptotics

The asymptotic theory for the frailty model for recurrent events is less well developed than that for parallel data, described in Section 8.11. For data on exact times, we have the same problems for recurrent events. The results of

Murphy (1995) for the gamma frailty non-parametric hazard model apply also to recurrent events.

For period count data, the case is much simpler. Censoring is not a technical problem, because the observation period is fixed. The non-parametric hazard is not a problem, because what we observe is a consequence of the total hazard over the period. One more simplification is that there are only a countable number of possible outcomes, implying that the Fisher information can always be evaluated by considering all possible events up to some limit and adding the contributions, and this makes a much simpler approach than numerical integration, where we also need to consider the distance of points.

For gamma frailty regression models for period counts, it is possible to evaluate the Fisher information. This is most conveniently done using a mean value parametrization; that is, assuming that conditionally on Y, the distribution of the count is Poisson with mean $Y \exp(\beta' z)$, where Y is gamma(δ, δ) and z a vector of covariates, where we by definition have $z_1 = 1$. The information in a single observation with covariate z and $\mu = \exp(\beta' z)$ is

$$-Ed^2\ell/d\beta_m d\beta_r = \frac{\mu z_m z_r}{1 + \mu/\delta}, \quad -Ed^2\ell/d\beta_m d\delta = 0,$$

$$-Ed^2\ell/d\delta^2 = \left\{ \sum_{q=0}^{\infty} (\delta + q)^{-2} Pr(K \geq q) \right\} - \frac{\mu}{\delta(\delta + \mu)}. \tag{9.18}$$

The total information in a sample of independent observations is then obtained by summing over the individuals. A particular advantage of this expression is that it shows that the mean value parameters are asymptotically independent of the dispersion parameter δ. This result is consistent with the above-mentioned fact that in the one-sample and two-sample cases, the estimated mean equals the observed mean both in the case, where δ is known or unknown. Equation (9.18) can be used also to evaluate the information in interval count data and constant hazards models, but these evaluations are left as exercises.

The boundary problems described in Section 8.11 are also relevant in this case. The hypothesis of independence (no subject variation) is at the boundary. The PVF model has two parameters and thus becomes unstable near independence.

9.8 Applications

The applications include period counts, interval counts, and exact times for common periods. There are no examples for exact times and uncommon periods.

Claims	Policies	Poisson	Neg.bin.	P-IG	P-PVF
0	103704	102629.6	103723.6	103710.0	103704.6
1	14075	15922.0	13990.0	14054.7	14072.5
2	1766	1235.1	1857.1	1784.9	1769.3
3	255	63.9	245.2	254.5	255.2
4	45	2.48	32.29	40.42	41.98
5	6	0.08	4.24	6.94	7.58
6	2	0.002	0.557	1.258	1.459
≥ 7	0	0.00004	0.084	0.295	0.372
Total	119 853				

Table 9.3. Automobile claims data with fits in various Poisson overdispersion models.

9.8.1 Period count data

Automobile insurance data

The Swiss automobile insurance data of Section 1.7.4 is a one-sample example of period count data. The empirical mean is 0.1551 and the total empirical variance is 0.1793. Using the formula of Section 9.4, we calculate an empirical coefficient of variation for Y of 1.003, showing that this is a clear overdispersion.

The parameters of the Poisson distribution are easily found by the empirical mean to correspond to a mean of 0.1551 (SE 0.0011), and a log likelihood of -55108.46. The negative binomial distribution parameters are estimated to $\hat{\delta} = 1.033$ (SE 0.044), and $\hat{\theta} = 6.565$ (0.286), and the log likelihood is -54615.32, corresponding to an improvement of about 500, and thus gives a much better fit. The coefficient of variation of Y is estimated to 0.984. The inverse Gaussian parameters are estimated to $\hat{\delta} = 0.2784$ (SE 0.0063), and $\hat{\theta} = 3.220$ (0.148) and the log likelihood is -54609.76, clearly better than the negative binomial, even though it has the same number of parameters. These values are identical to those of Willmot (1987).

Here we supplement with the full PVF model, where the estimates are $\hat{\alpha} = 0.552$ (SE 0.083), $\hat{\delta} = 0.2490$ (0.0435), and $\hat{\theta} = 2.873$ (0.569), and the log likelihood is -54609.59. This is not significantly better than the inverse Gaussian mixture. The mean number of claims is identical to the estimate in the Poisson model, 0.1551, owing to the model's being an exponential family. The standard error of the mean is slightly increased compared to the Poisson model (from 0.0011 to 0.0012). The coefficient of variation for Y is 1.003, in practice the same as the empirical value. The observed and fitted distributions are shown in Table 9.3. Clearly, the fit of the Poisson PVF mixture is very fine.

Mammary tumors

The mammary tumors of Section 1.7.1 concern individuals who were all followed for a period of the same length. Thus the observation plan is exact times during a common period. In this section, the number of tumors experienced by the animals over the whole period is considered. In other words, the data are reduced to the total number of events, that is, period count data. The only covariate known is the treatment, which has two levels. This is first studied in a Poisson model, that is, without frailty. It is not necessary to assume a homogeneous Poisson process for this analysis, but it is only possible to determine the total integrated hazard over the period 60–182 days. According to the Poisson model, the sufficient statistics are the number of events in each treatment group, giving estimates of $149/25 = 5.96$ (SE 0.49) for the expected number of tumors during the observation period in the control group and $61/23 = 2.65$ (0.34) in the treatment group. The relative risk is directly evaluated as $\hat{\rho} = 2.65/5.96 = 0.44$. For the proportional hazards analysis, we evaluate this on log scale, $\hat{\beta} = \log \hat{\rho} = -0.810$, with standard error 0.152. The Wald test for no effect of the treatment then gives $u = -0.810/0.152 = -5.33$, showing a clear reduction of the tumor incidence by treatment. Alternatively, the hypothesis can be evaluated by the likelihood ratio test. In the full model, the log likelihood is -121.54, and under the hypothesis of no treatment effect, the log likelihood is -137.07, giving a test statistic of 31.07 and the same conclusion. The value is comparable to the squared Wald statistic, 28.40.

The gamma mixture model gives parameter estimates $\hat{\delta}=3.878$ (SE 1.600), $\hat{\theta}=0.651$ (0.282) and $\hat{\beta}=-0.810$ (0.211), which makes the means in both treatment groups agree with the empirical values. Thus the estimated relative risk is exactly the same as in the Poisson model, but the standard error is increased, reflecting the variation between individuals and that the treatment corresponds to a common covariate. The log likelihood is -113.47, corresponding to a likelihood test statistic for overdispersion of 16.13 clearly showing a better fit with the gamma frailty model.

The full PVF model no longer makes the means agree with the empirical values. The estimates are $\hat{\alpha} = -1.23$ (4.54), $\hat{\delta} = 16.48$ (117.31), $\hat{\theta} = 1.576$ (3.585) and $\hat{\beta} = -0.816$ (0.207). The estimated means are 5.978 and 2.644, respectively. As α is suggested to be negative, we can evaluate the probability of the animal having zero risk as 0.0005. As the response is tumor incidence, it is possible that a proportion of the animals were not susceptible. However, in this case, the proportion is so small that it is essentially 0. The log likelihood is -113.33, showing that the fit is not improved compared to the gamma frailty model.

Parameter	Poisson	Gamma	Inv. Gauss	PVF
Placebo				
α (SE)		0	0.5	0.719 (0.095)
δ (SE)		1.485 (0.379)	4.285 (0.639)	7.401 (1.988)
θ (SE)		0.0432 (0.0139)	0.0155 (0.0073)	0.0042 (0.0059)
Mean	34.39 (1.11)	34.39 (5.45)	34.39 (6.39)	34.39 (9.12)
Var (Y)	0	796 (324)	1,108 (695)	2,296 (3,233)
c.v.(Y)	0	0.67 (0.17)	0.97 (0.17)	1.39 (0.69)
$\log L$	-446.53	-126.36	-122.99	-121.72
Progabide				
α (SE)		0	0.5	0.548 (0.130)
δ (SE)		0.896 (0.213)	2.937 (0.445)	3.329 (1.239)
θ (SE)		0.0281 (0.0086)	0.0085 (0.0049)	0.0068 (0.0064)
Mean	31.84 (1.01)	31.84 (6.13)	31.84 (7.83)	31.84 (8.34)
Var (Y)	0	1,131 (511)	1,870 (1,485)	2,122 (2,071)
c.v.(Y)	0	1.06 (0.13)	1.36 (0.26)	1.45 (0.43)
$\log L$	-755.02	-138.65	-135.58	-135.52

Table 9.4. Estimates (standard errors) and likelihood for various frailty models for eight week epileptic seizure data.

Epileptic seizure count

The models can be applied to the epileptic seizure count of Section 1.7.2. These data are interval counts, with four intervals of two weeks. First the total number of events over the eight weeks is considered, corresponding to period counts. This is a typical set of data for overdispersion count models. The estimates are described in Table 9.4. These results were described by Hougaard, Lee, and Whitmore (1997), who present further evaluations than this book. The estimates of δ and θ vary markedly with the assumptions on α. A more robust choice of parameters is the mean and the variance. The estimated mean is in all cases identical to the observed mean, which is a consequence of the family's being a natural exponential family for fixed value of α and δ. The variance is not constant as function of α, but varies less than δ and θ. The estimated probability masses for the progabide group are shown in Figure 9.10 for the negative binomial distribution and in Figure 9.11 for the full estimate. A clear difference between these is that the mode is estimated as 0 for the negative binomial distribution and as 6 for the full model. In the gamma model, a zero mode is a consequence of the large variation, whereas the PVF model is more flexible. The PVF model fits clearly better than the negative binomial model. This example can also illustrate that the moment estimate is inferior. For the progabide group, the average is 31.84 and the empirical variance of K is 2809.55, from which the moment estimate in the negative binomial model is evaluated as $\delta = 0.365$, $\theta = 0.0114$, which has a likelihood value of -144.66, a decrement of 6 compared to the likelihood estimate. This is due to using a wrong model.

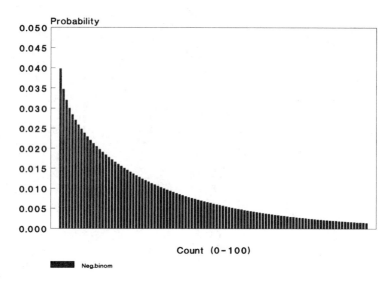

Figure 9.10. Estimated probability masses for the epileptic seizure data, Progabide group, assuming $\alpha = 0$.

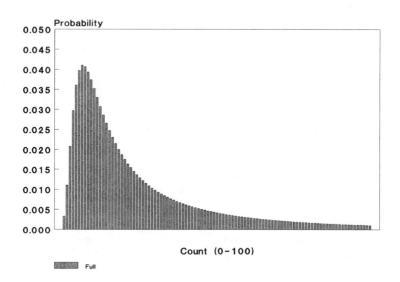

Figure 9.11. Estimated probability masses for the epileptic seizure data, Progabide group, in the full P-PVF model.

The large right tail has a major influence on the moment estimate, but less so on the maximum likelihood estimate in the negative binomial model.

A further point that can be illustrated is that testing for the Poisson model should be done by the likelihood ratio test. For the inverse Gaussian model for the placebo group, the likelihood ratio χ^2-value is 647, with 1 degree of freedom, but the Wald test based on the variance of Y gives a non-significant value of $W = 1.60$. The coefficient of variation for Y is a better parameter in this regard and gives a significant value of 5.74, but still this is far from the extreme significance of the likelihood test.

9.8.2   Time data for a fixed period

Mammary tumors

In this section, these data will be analyzed as exact times. Regarding the frailty distribution, it gives the same results, except that it now seems relevant to restrict the mean frailty to 1 and we obtain $\hat{\delta} = 3.878$ (SE 1.600) in the gamma model. For the treatment effect, the estimate is precisely the same $\hat{\beta} = -0.810$ (0.211). However, this approach gives separate hazard contributions at the 35 different event times. Thus, the analysis of the parameters of the frailty part can be found from studying the total number of events in the whole period.

The same applies under the PVF model. Thus the gain compared to the period count approach is only that the distribution over time is obtained. Regarding the treatment effect and the individual variation, there is nothing gained by studying the exact times.

9.8.3   Interval count data

Epileptic seizure count

When the aim is to consider the frailty distribution, there is nothing gained by using the interval count data compared to the period count data. The only difference is that the likelihood now includes an extra term, corresponding to the multinomial distribution of the counts over the intervals and that it is possible to determine separate hazard parameters for the four intervals.

To illustrate the implications of time-dependent covariates, we consider a comparison of first four and last four weeks of the epileptic seizure counts, for the placebo group. The aim of this comparison would be to study whether there is an increasing or decreasing trend in the seizure rate. An alternative phrasing is that the ratio of the separate hazard parameters is estimated, when the period is split into two intervals. The methods would be precisely the same if the two intervals concerned two different treatments and the aim was to compare the treatments.

In the Poisson model, the total number of events in each interval is sufficient. This gives 494 events for the first interval and 469 for the second. Thus the estimated rates in the two periods are found by dividing by the number of patients (28), and are 17.64 and 16.75, respectively. They can be compared by a likelihood ratio test, which gives a χ^2 test statistic of 2.90, implying that they are not significantly different. The relative hazard, say, ρ, in the second period compared to the first is simply estimated as $469/494=0.95$. The standard error on this ratio becomes 0.06.

For the frailty models, we have previously seen that the distribution can be formulated by the distribution of the total number of events and the conditional distribution of the two intervals given the total number of events. Introducing interval as a covariate is a reparametrization to the parameters of the total numbers, and an extension of the relative distribution between the two intervals. The probability of an event's being in the first interval then is $1/(1 + \rho)$. It follows from this result that the estimated ratio is again $\hat{\rho} = 0.95$ and the standard error is 0.06. Thus the results agree perfectly with those of the Poisson model, and this is true both for the gamma model, the inverse Gaussian model, and the full PVF model. This might appear surprising, but is due to the frailty describing the variation between individuals and the covariate describing variation within individuals. So the overdispersion has no consequences for the dispersion of the interval effect. In order to make a model with overdispersion also over time, a more general model is necessary, and this will be examined in Section 11.2.

9.8.4   Other applications

Kessing *et al.* (1999) study recurrence of psychiatric diseases trying to discriminate between a frailty and a multi-state model by suggesting a model that includes both, with a gamma distributed frailty term and proportional hazards over k. They use a gap time model and therefore the approach does not suffer from the identifiability problems following from Equation (9.11).

9.9   Chapter summary

This chapter describes frailty models for recurrent events data. There are many similarities, but also some important differences between the shared frailty model for parallel data and the (constant) frailty model for recurrent events. In particular, when the observation period is the same for all individuals, some evaluations can be based on only the number of events during the study period (called period count data). This leads to specific Poisson overdispersion distributions, for which a completely separate theory can be developed. Also, in the case of counts of events in various intervals, some simplification is possible along the same line as the period count data.

Property	Parallel data	Recurrent events data
Individuals sharing frailty	Several	1
Multi-state structure	Figure 5.12	Figure 1.4
Multi-state model	non-Markov	Markov
Risk set	$\{0, 1, ..., k\}$	$\{0, 1\}$
Number of events in interval	Not relevant	Poisson overdispersion
Dependence measures ρ, τ	Relevant	Not relevant
Dependence measure c.v.(Y)	Not relevant	Relevant

Table 9.5. Differences between the shared frailty applied to parallel data and recurrent events data.

Table 9.5 lists some differences between recurrent events and parallel data. One more difference in the way the models are presented here is that different restrictions are used to obtain identifiability. For the parallel data, a scale restriction is put on Y, whereas for period counts for recurrent events, it is more convenient to restrict the hazard. This difference is, however, not intrinsic to the problem and therefore not listed in the table.

Apart from these differences the analysis of shared frailty models for recurrent events data runs like it does for parallel data.

9.10 Bibliographic comments

The negative binomial distribution was derived as a gamma mixture of Poisson variables already by Greenwood and Yule (1920). The inverse Gaussian mixture models have been considered by a number of authors - Holla (1966), Sankaran (1968), Sichel (1971, 1973, 1974, 1982), Ord and Whitmore (1986), and Willmot (1987). Unimodality of period counts was considered by Holgate (1970).

The PVF overdispersion model for period count data was suggested in a review paper by Hougaard (1987). It was examined in detail by Hougaard, Lee, and Whitmore (1997).

Oakes (1992) also discusses frailty models for recurrent events.

Lawless (1987) derived Equation (9.18) as well as formulas for the variance of alternative estimates.

Table 9.4 is based on material first presented in Hougaard, Lee and Whitmore (1997).

9.11 Exercises

Exercise 9.1 Time to the kth event

Let $\mu(t)$ be constant and the frailty follow a general distribution. The density of T_k (the time to the kth event) can be derived in two ways. One

uses Equation (9.7) and the relation $T_k > t \Leftrightarrow K(t) < k$. The other is
by evaluating the survivor function of T_k conditional on Y using Equation
(A.29), then integrating Y out and differentiating with respect to t. Make
both evaluations.

Use the result to show that the distribution of T_2 in this case has the
same distribution as $T_1 + T_2$ in the bivariate case (Exercise 7.1).

Now, allow $\mu(t)$ to vary with t. Which of the two approaches can be used
to find the density of T_k? Make the derivation.

Exercise 9.2 Time to the kth event for gamma frailty

Specialize the results of the Exercise 9.1 to a gamma distribution,
gamma(δ, θ), assuming constant hazards. Check the calculations by observing that the density depends on μ and θ only via the scale parameter
μ/θ.

Exercise 9.3 Gamma frailty with probability of 0 risk

The gamma frailty model can be extended to allow for some individuals
having 0 risk. Let the frailty, Y, be 0 for a proportion p of the population
and chosen from a gamma distribution with parameters δ and θ for the rest
of the population. Find the Laplace transform of this distribution. Find the
mean and the variance of Y as well as of the period count K.

Exercise 9.4 Conditional distribution for interval count data

Consider a gamma frailty model (gamma (δ, δ)) with interval counts
(K_1, K_2) for two intervals, for which the hazards are μ_1 and μ_2. Evaluate
by two different methods the conditional distribution of K_2 given K_1.

Exercise 9.5 P-PVF as an exponential family

Find the probability masses of the P-PVF distribution using the parametriza-
tion (α, ρ, ω), where $\delta = \rho e^{-\alpha\omega}$ and $\theta = e^\omega - 1$ and prove that the model
is a natural exponential family in $\omega = \log(\theta + 1)$ for fixed values of (α, ρ).

Exercise 9.6 Skewness of P-PVF

Fix the mean EK to μ and the variance $\text{Var}(K)$ to σ^2 in the P-PVF
distribution for the period count. How does the skewness change with α?

Exercise 9.7 Moment estimate for P-PVF

Based on a period count sample, find the expression for the moment estimate for (α, δ, θ) in the P-PVF model based on the first three moments.
For which sample patterns does this estimate exist?

Exercise 9.8 Extended regression model

Consider a period count model with PVF frailty, where the frailty distribution is $\text{PVF}(\alpha, \delta \exp(\beta' z), \theta \exp(\gamma \beta' z))$. Which parameter restriction gives the standard model (Equation (9.17))? What is the advantage of this model compared to the standard model? Would you recommend this model for checking the standard model?

Exercise 9.9 Zero truncated period count data

Sometimes data are only available for persons with at least one event. For example, a hospital may only collect data for patients with at least one admission during a specified period. A data set on the number of prescriptions turned in by persons may only include those that have presented at least one prescription. Consider a period count frailty model for such data. Derive the probability masses, the mean and the variance for the number of recorded events by means of the Laplace transform.

Specialize the results to the PVF frailty model. Show that the distribution of the number of recorded events contains a one-dimensional natural exponential family.

Exercise 9.10 Generalized inverse Gaussian frailty model

Consider a period count observation, where the frailty follows the distribution described in Section A.3.6. Derive the probability masses $p(k)$ by means of Bessel functions.

Show that for the inverse Gaussian special case ($\gamma = -1/2$), the formula for the probability mass found by means of Equation (A.32) is the same as obtained from Equation (9.12).

Exercise 9.11 Information in the one-sample case

Use Equation (9.18) to derive the Fisher information about (δ, θ) in the distribution described in Section 9.3.2.

Exercise 9.12 Information in interval count data

Consider interval count data (K_1, K_2) for two intervals, with integrated hazards of $Y\mu_1$ and $Y\mu_2$ conditionally on Y, which is assumed to be gamma(δ, δ) distributed. Evaluate the Fisher information for δ, μ_1, μ_2 for a single individual. Suppose now that there are n_1 individuals with observations only for the first interval and n_2 individuals with observations for both intervals. What is the total information in the sample? Show that $\hat{\mu}_1$ is not asymptotically independent of $\hat{\delta}$. Hint: First reparametrize by $\mu = \mu_1 + \mu_2$ and $\rho = \mu_1/\mu$ and describe the distribution by the sum $K = K_1 + K_2$ and the conditional distribution of K_1 given K. Then use Equation (9.18).

Exercise 9.13 Information in a constant hazards model

Suppose we have observations for n individuals with exact times of all events during an observation period, which may vary from person to person, but is fixed by the design. Evaluate the Fisher information for the model, where the hazard is $Y\mu$ conditionally on Y, which is assumed to be gamma(δ, δ) distributed.

Exercise 9.14 Zero observed events

Consider a period count data set for n individuals in r groups $(r < n)$, where the covariate z_q is an indicator function for the qth group, $q = 1, ..., r - 1$. Besides this, the age of the individual is included as z_r. Suppose that no events are observed for group 1. Show that for the Poisson model this implies that the boundary estimate $\hat{\beta}_1 = -\infty$ is obtained and that the other regression coefficients and the maximal value of the log likelihood can be found by analyzing the data set, where the first group is deleted.

How can you handle the problem if there are no events for group r?

An alternative solution is to suggest a model with a frailty term for each group. Is it then a problem that one or more groups have no observed events? Does this approach make sense irrespectively of how the groups are defined?

Exercise 9.15 Automobile insurance

Fit the various models for the data set of automobile insurance from UK, described in Section 1.7.4.

10
Multivariate frailty models

The shared frailty model described in Chapter 7 is very useful for bivariate data with common risk dependence, but in many cases, we do need extensions. In particular, for truly multivariate data, that is, when there are three or more observations, we need more models with varying degrees of dependence. This general frailty approach can be used to create a random treatment by group interaction, or other models with several sources of variation. Secondly, combining subgroups with different degrees of dependence in a single model, for example, monozygotic and dizygotic twins, is difficult in a shared frailty model. Furthermore, this extension can be an improvement for the consideration of effects of covariates in frailty models.

The theory is less well developed than for shared frailty models, but there appears to be a great potential in these models. The main mathematical problem is that some nice probability results on mixtures are needed in order to obtain simple models. Compared to normal distribution models, the mixture probability results are more complicated and the models only have few of the many nice properties known for the multivariate normal models. Therefore it makes sense to consider several models in order to find out which properties are obtainable and in a second round when experience is gained, find out which properties are the most important. Owing to the many open ends in this theory, this chapter is more difficult to read than the previous chapters. It is, of course, possible to omit this chapter, but this is not recommended. It displays many difficulties and challenges, working with models for multivariate data, allowing not only to understand the shared frailty model better and to put that model in a broader perspective,

Problem	Reference
Different degrees of dependence	Sections 10.1, 10.4.2, and 10.5.3
Trivariate nested model	Sections 10.4.1 and 10.8
Treatment-center interaction	Sections 10.4.3 and 10.5.4
Alternating states	Sections 10.5.6 and 10.7
Full pedigrees	Sections 10.3, 10.5.5, and 10.6
General multivariate	Sections 10.3, 10.5.3, and 10.6
Bivariate fit improvement	Sections 10.2, 10.4.4, and 10.5.1
Negative dependence	Sections 10.2, 10.6, and 10.7

Table 10.1. Cases where multivariate frailty models can be useful.

but, I believe, there is also a more general inspiration for a closer study of complex models, also outside of the survival data field.

It is appropriate to consider a definition of a frailty model here, to make it clear exactly what is covered by such models. The definition used here consists of two requirements. First there is conditional independence. That is, conditional on the frailty, which may be a random variable, univariate or multivariate, or a stochastic process, the objects behave independently. It follows that in a frailty model there is some sort of dependence between the times, when the frailty is integrated out. Basically, this is a common risks model, but the multivariate formulation is more general, so that some individuals have risks that are more common than others and it also includes cases with negative dependence, which can strictly seen never be due to common risks. Secondly, we will require that the frailties act multiplicatively on the hazard, like Equation (2.16) in the univariate case. This condition is used to exclude more time-based models, like a lognormal accelerated failure time random effects model. Such models would be relevant to study and strongly needed, but should be assigned a different name.

Table 10.1 lists some cases where a multivariate frailty model can be appropriate, with references to sections where the problem is considered. On the general level, the models of this chapter can be described as random effects models for survival data, where there are more than two sources of variation. The first four problems of the table have three sources of variation. Full pedigrees and general models can have many sources of variation. For the fit improvement there are still only two sources of variation (group and individual variation), but they enter in a more complicated way. Finally, for negative dependence, we do not interpret the model as coming from several sources of variation.

The kind of data considered is parallel data of the form $T_1, ..., T_k$ in a single group (neglecting a group index). The overall model approach in this chapter is to substitute the shared frailty Y, with a multivariate random variable $(Y_1, ..., Y_k)$, so that Y_j applies to time number j. The shared frailty model is obtained when all frailties are equal ($Y_1 = ... = Y_k$) and the distribution of Y_1 is the same for all groups. This chapter still assumes that the frailties are constant. Time-varying frailties are considered in Chapter 11. This chapter is not structured according to the practical problem, but according to the mathematical model for the multivariate frailty.

This chapter contains a number of different approaches to handle this problem. Here follows an overview of these approaches. A simple problem that is placed in this chapter is the comparison of the degree of dependence among several bivariate samples. Where Chapter 7 considered a single univariate frailty distribution, this approach assumes that some subpopulations have different parameters for the frailty distributions. A major aim is then to make a hypothesis test whether these parameters are the same, that is, whether the subpopulations have the same degree of dependence. A prototype example is the twins data, where the key comparison is whether the monozygotic and the dizygotic twins show the same dependence. In this case, the three sources of variation are the shared effect for dizygotic twins, the effect shared by monozygotic, but not by dizygotic twins and the individual effect. This testing problem is considered in Section 10.1.

A slight extension of the shared frailty model, suggesting a univariate frailty variable having a differential effect for the various components is described in Section 10.2. This model may be relevant in cases, where the marginal distributions differ markedly.

A simple and pragmatic approach to handle different degrees of dependence for complicated multivariate data is to study each bivariate marginal separately by means of shared frailty models (Section 10.3). This is not a real multivariate model, but allows for discussing the degree of dependence and thus also for considering the goodness-of-fit of the shared frailty model.

From a purely theoretical point of view, the most interesting extension from the bivariate to the multivariate case is the multiplicative stable frailty model described in Section 10.4, because it allows for a multiple unobserved risk factor interpretation and bivariate models correspond to shared frailty models. Unfortunately, this model can only be used for nested dependence structures and the fit might not be satisfying. Furthermore, the likelihood becomes quite complicated. In case of truncation, a more complicated model is obtained.

By making an additive frailty model, that is, by creating a multivariate frailty variable, with one component for each individual, derived as sums of independent random variables, we can obtain more general dependence structures (Section 10.5). This appears to give more tractable models from a computational point of view, but is less satisfying theoretically. This corresponds to a hidden cause of death interpretation. In practice, the gamma distributions have been used for these models.

The multivariate lognormal distribution is conceptually attractive as a frailty distribution owing to its flexibility, but what can be calculated exactly in this model is more limited (Section 10.6). Instead estimation procedures based on various approximations are used.

Furthermore, it is interesting to examine the possibilities for models with negative dependence (Section 10.7). This topic is relevant to study not only for modeling actual data sets with negative dependence, but also to examine hypothesis tests for independence, because models allowing both positive and negative dependence avoid the problem that the hypothesis is on the boundary of the parameter space. The models considered are not really satisfactory and do need further development.

Nested data can be handled by two-level frailty models (Section 10.8). In the case of stable frailties this can be given a multivariate frailty interpretation, but the approach can be applied more generally.

For recurrent events, these models are not relevant; it is more relevant to consider the time development, as done in Chapter 11. However, for the more general alternating state model, a bivariate frailty model for the two hazards can be useful (Sections 10.5.6 and 10.6).

10.1   Comparison of dependence

For twins, a key question is whether the dependence is the same for monozygotic and dizygotic twins. This is not formally covered by the theory of Chapter 7, although a simple Wald test can be performed based on estimated values for the subgroups analyzed separately, as shown in the application. However, Wald tests are not satisfactory and depend on which parameter is used for describing the dependence. Therefore, a likelihood-based evaluation is more interesting. The frame considered here is a shared frailty approach, but where the parameters of the frailty distribution are not common to all groups.

A key problem is which assumptions to make regarding the hazard function. Theoretically, there are at least four possibilities for these assumptions. First, we can assume that the conditional hazards are the same. Technically, this is simple, when the frailty model is parametrized by means of Equation (7.6). This approach might from a superficial point of view appear as the most natural given the conditional construction of frailty models, but it implies that the marginal distributions are different, when the frailty distributions are different. Therefore, this is not satisfactory. An alternative approach is to let the marginal distributions be the same. This can be done when the model is parametrized by means of the marginal distribution (Equation (7.10)). This is easily done by means of the three-stage approach of Section 8.4. This approach implies that the conditional distributions are different, and thus is apparently in conflict with the conditional way of deriving frailty models. Although this method can make sense theoretically by using a multivariate frailty model (Section 10.4.2), in this section we just consider this as a pragmatic way of combining the data and as such it seems quite sensible. A more mathematical formulation of this approach is that we describe a model with three sources of variation as two data sets each modeled by two sources of variation, keeping the total variation common to the data sets. The third approach is to make some parametric relation between the hazards for the various types, e.g., proportional hazards. However, this does not really solve the problem and therefore has not been considered in further detail. Finally, we may stratify, so that the hazards for the various types vary completely independently of each other. In fact, the simple Wald test made initially is performed in this latter frame. This works fine, but is more difficult to interpret, because it might be difficult to understand how the frailty dependence should be the same, when the separate distributions are unrelated. It does make sense, however, for combining data on male and female twins.

Truncation is a special problem in this case. For example, the data on Danish twins only include pairs where both were alive by the age of 15 years, in order to know the zygosity. Under the hypothesis of the same hazard functions and equal dependence, truncation leads to the same selection, but in the general case, truncation might lead to differential selection in the groups and thus both the conditional and the marginal hazard functions differ between the two groups. In the case of the gamma frailty model, this works together with stratification regarding the hazard function. Truncation in the gamma frailty model leads to a change of scale for the frailty distribution, and this change is incorporated in the stratified hazard function. Therefore the normalized distribution of the frailty is independent of truncation. An application of this kind was presented in Section 8.12.5, combining data for male and female twins.

The approach considered in the rest of this chapter, the multivariate frailty, allows for the conditional and marginal distributions to be the same for the various types, see Sections 10.4.2 and 10.5.3.

10.1.1 Estimation

The two most promising approaches are the three-stage approach assuming common marginals, and the stratified approach, and they will be considered separately.

The first two steps of the three-stage approach are obtained by an approach similar to the step 2 estimate of Section 8.4. First, the Nelson-Aalen estimate based on both monozygotic and dizygotic twins of the same sex is evaluated. Then times are transformed according to Equation (8.3), and considered in a gamma frailty bivariate model with exponentially distributed marginals. The estimate under the hypothesis is found by considering all data simultaneously. The general estimate is obtained by considering the monozygotic and the dizygotic twins separately and then adding the log likelihoods. Continuing to find the step 3 estimate requires simultaneous fitting of monozygotic and dizygotic twins, and therefore more general software. The advantage of this approach is that the bivariate parts are parametric and thus there are only a few parameters to maximize over.

The stratified approach consists of non-parametric estimates. Under the hypothesis, the hazard function is stratified according to zygosity, so that monozygotic and dizygotic twins have separate hazard functions, and a common dependence parameter. The general estimate again consists of studying each type of twins separately, this time in a standard non-parametric frailty program. This approach has a large number of parameters, including one parameter for each death time in each stratum.

10.1.2 Application to twin data

The hypothesis of the same dependence for monozygotic and dizygotic twins can be simply tested by a Wald test using the difference in τ, evaluated in Table 8.16. For example, using the gamma frailty distribution, the difference is $0.205 - 0.081 = 0.124$ for males. The corresponding standard error is $(0.027^2 + 0.021^2)^{1/2}$, which is 0.034, from which the Wald test statistic is derived as $0.124/0.034 = 3.63$, which is clearly significant, using the normal distribution. Thus, there is a higher dependence for monozygotic than for dizygotic twins. Generally, this approach depends on which parametrization of the dependence (here τ) is used. This can be illustrated by using δ instead, as reported in Table 8.12. Then, the difference is $1.94 - 5.65 = -3.71$ (standard error 1.65), giving a test statistic of -2.25. In this parametrization the variance changes faster with the value of the parameter and therefore it is more difficult to detect the difference.

It is, however, more satisfactory to do this by means of a likelihood ratio approach, which then also requires fitting the model under the hypothesis. First, this problem is considered by assuming common marginals. The estimates in the three-stage approach with and without an assumption of the same gamma frailty distribution are given in Table 10.2. It is simple to do a likelihood-based comparison, by taking twice the difference in log likelihood, that is, 9.89 for males and 3.24 for females. The value for males is significant. This procedure does not account for the truncation, which in the general case can lead to differential selection for the two types of twins. In order to compare to the Wald test, we should apply the square root ($\sqrt{9.89} = 3.14$), and thus there is a reasonable agreement.

The alternative approach is to avoid the assumption of common hazard functions and use a stratified non-parametric approach, allowing for different hazard function for the two types of twins. This is reported in Table 10.3, where the parameters for separate values of δ are directly taken from Table 8.23. Comparing the likelihoods gives test statistics of 11.76 for males and 2.72 for females and the same conclusion as before.

	Common δ	Separate δ
Males		
τ(SE) for MZ	0.1287 (0.0168)	0.1938 (0.0259)
τ(SE) for DZ	0.1287 (0.0168)	0.0872 (0.0218)
Hazard scale	0.990 (0.019)	0.993 (0.019))
Log likelihood	-3039.16	-3034.22
Females		
τ(SE) for MZ	0.1490 (0.0184)	0.1939 (0.0303)
τ(SE) for DZ	0.1490 (0.0184)	0.1257 (0.0228)
Hazard scale	0.985 (0.021)	0.986 (0.021)
Log likelihood	-2633.54	-2631.92

Table 10.2. Estimates of dependence (τ) for Danish twin data, based on common or separate frailty distribution parameter in the gamma frailty model, assuming common marginals proportional to the Nelson-Aalen estimate based on both MZ and DZ twins. The standard errors do not account for the variability of the Nelson-Aalen estimate.

	Common δ	Separate δ
Males		
τ(SE) for MZ	0.1289 (0.0176)	0.2068 (0.0285)
τ(SE) for DZ	0.1289 (0.0176)	0.0824 (0.0221)
Log likelihood	-25167.24	-25161.36
Females		
τ(SE) for MZ	0.1507 (0.0193)	0.1943 (0.0326)
τ(SE) for DZ	0.1507 (0.0193)	0.1276 (0.0239)
Log likelihood	-22008.29	-22006.93

Table 10.3. Estimates of dependence (τ) for Danish twin data, based on common or separate frailty distribution parameter in the gamma frailty model, assuming non-parametric hazard functions using the conditional approach, and stratified according to zygosity.

10.2   Differential effect of a shared frailty

An extension of the shared frailty model, which is still a univariate frailty model, is created by the various responses being influenced by different functions of the frailty. That is, the hazard for individual j might be of the form $f_j(Y)\mu_j(t)$ in age t. To put this into the framework of the rest of this chapter, we define $Y_j = f_j(Y)$, so the hazard is $Y_j\mu_j(t)$. When $f_j(\cdot)$, $j = 1, ..., k$ do not depend on j, the model is a shared frailty model. Typically, the functions f_j are monotone, and we can, without loss of generality, define the first function as the identity for identifiability purposes. That is, the model is formulated by means of the first frailty term, $Y_1 = Y$. In the proportional hazards framework, the most natural class of functions are the power functions, because they fit into $Y_j = \exp(\psi_j' w)$, so that the original neglected covariates w have the same distribution, but the corresponding regression coefficients are allowed to vary. This is then an extension of Equation (2.50). The different functions f_j are obtained by having different values of ψ_j. This implies that the frailty is important for some responses and less so for other responses. It is unknown whether this is useful in practice, but it might be relevant when the hazard functions for the various values of j have markedly different shapes. If a frailty model is relevant for studying different events, this model might be an interesting choice.

The normal distribution counterpart to this model is a random coefficient regression model for repeated measurements. In that model, the various random effects can have different influence on the coordinates, implying inter alia that the total variation varies between the coordinates.

A specific approach to obtain negative dependence in such a model, is to assume that $Y_2 = 1/Y_1$, or formulated slightly differently, a bivariate frailty of $(Y, 1/Y)$. In the above formulation, this corresponds to $\psi_2 = -\psi_1$. This would, however, only allow negative dependence. To put this into precise distributional assumptions, one could assume the bivariate lognormal distribution (Section 10.6), with correlation of minus 1. This is considered in more generality in Section 10.6. Another possibility is the inverse Gaussian distribution, described in the Appendix, where the simultaneous Laplace transform of Y and $1/Y$ can be evaluated. The distribution of Y and $1/Y$ cannot be the same in this model, which appears as an inconvenient restriction. Therefore, it is an advantage to extend the model to Y following a generalized inverse Gaussian distribution, because in that case $1/Y$ will follow a distribution in the same family. This family has three parameters, (γ, δ, θ). In particular, when the parameter γ is 0, the distribution is log symmetric, implying that the distributions of Y and $1/Y$ only differ by a scale parameter. This model has never been examined in detail. In general, the Laplace transforms of the generalized inverse Gaussian distributions are given by means of Bessel functions. Whether this approach gives a useful model is unknown.

	Treatment	Control 1	Control 2
Treatment	-	1.22	0.81
Control 1		-	1.02
Control 2			-

Table 10.4. Estimates of α for the tumorigenesis data based on bivariate marginals and a proportional hazards model with frailty following a positive stable distribution. Values above 1 suggest negative dependence.

10.3 Shared frailty models for bivariate marginals

For multivariate data, where the degree of dependence is assumed to differ between the components, a simple approach is to consider each bivariate marginal separately, and analyze them by means of shared frailty models. This approach is inspired by the multivariate normal distribution with common covariates, where the bivariate marginal approach gives the same result as the estimate in the full multivariate distribution. For survival data, however, the bivariate approach typically leads to an estimate that does not correspond to a multivariate distribution. In fact, even the univariate marginals are expected to differ according to which bivariate marginal is considered. Therefore, this approach makes sense for its simplicity, not for its consistency properties. Furthermore, it makes sense in order to discuss the goodness-of-fit of the assumption of the same degree of dependence in all cases. So, it can be used for checking the shared frailty model in the multivariate case. The advantage of this approach is that it gives a simple way to overcome the theoretical and practical difficulties with first suggesting a multivariate model and second fit that particular model.

The disadvantage is the possible conflict between estimates obtained in the different marginals and the possible inefficiency of the approach.

In fact, this approach is similar to the separate handling of monozygotic and dizygotic twins.

10.3.1 Applications

The tumorigenesis data of Section 1.5.3 can be used to illustrate this approach. The approach can illustrate, whether there is a random treatment by litter effect, because such an effect would show up as smaller dependence between the treated animal and each control animal, than between the two control animals. First, the positive stable model is applied, assuming proportional hazards regarding the treatment effect. When the treated animal is among the two selected animals, there is a single covariate, but when the control animals are considered separately, no covariates are involved. In two of three cases, the estimated value of the dependence parameter α is above 1, suggesting negative dependence. Therefore, it makes no sense to report τ here. The estimates are given in Table 10.4. The gamma frailty

	Treatment	Control 1	Control 2
Treatment	-	neg.dep.	0.22 (0.19)
Control 1		-	0.26 (0.28)
Control 2			-

Table 10.5. Estimates of τ for the litter data based on bivariate marginals and a proportional hazards model with frailty following a gamma distribution.

Treatment	2	3	4	5	6	7	8	9	10
1 SP	0.49	0.43	0.54	9.45	0.57	0.48	0.27	0.29	0.36
2 SNG		0.46	0.48	0.45	0.50	0.43	0.48	0.59	0.51
3 OP (0h)			0.55	0.60	0.68	0.56	0.44	0.43	0.54
4 OP (1h)				0.54	0.60	0.45	0.33	0.38	0.47
5 OP (3h)					0.63	0.47	0.41	0.44	0.50
6 OP (5h)						0.52	0.42	0.51	0.57
7 OI (0h)							0.30	0.34	0.43
8 OI (1h)								0.58	0.60
9 OI (3h)									0.63
10 OI (5h)									

Table 10.6. Estimates of τ for the exercise data based on bivariate marginals and a proportional hazards model with frailty following a positive stable distribution. SP = sublingual placebo, OP = oral placebo, OI = oral isosorbide.

model can be similarly studied. The results are given in Table 10.5. In this case, one of three estimates corresponds to negative dependence. Overall, the dependence is only slight.

The exercise data of Section 1.8.2 is a typical example, where this approach makes sense. It gives a simple overview on whether the degree of dependence is the same for all responses. As some responses refer to two occasions under the same treatment, at the same days, it is expected that there are different degrees of dependence. Table 10.6 gives the values of $\hat{\tau}$, for the stable frailty model. The overall picture is that the last three responses, which are those 1, 3, and 5 hours after treatment with oral isosorbide, show a high dependence to each other and a lower dependence to the remaining seven responses. This seems understandable as these responses are measured after the same treatment, and at the same day.

10.4 The multiplicative stable model

The difficulty in making more complicated dependence structures is finding a mathematical model that is sensible, and at the same time can be handled computationally. Some sort of nice distributional mixture results are needed for both aspects. The model of this section is based on the probability result (see Section A.3.3) of the stable distributions that if X_1, X_2 are independent, X_1 follows Posstab(α), and X_2 follows Posstab(ρ), the distribution of $X_1^{1/\rho} X_2$ is Posstab($\alpha\rho$). Thus this gives a multiplicative mixture result, where the distribution stays within the family of positive stable distributions. The result makes it possible to evaluate some multivariate Laplace transforms for models with nested data.

Some models are described below, covering a trivariate model, a combined model for monozygotic and dizygotic twins and a model for center by treatment interaction. The advantage of this model is that it actually is a random effects model with three sources of variation, with simple results regarding marginal distributions and consistent with proportional hazards modeling. The disadvantages of this approach are first that the nested structure is a major restriction on the possible dependence structures. For example, a genetic model, including father, mother, and child, where the father and the child are dependent, and the mother and the child are dependent, but the father and the mother are independent, is not possible. The second disadvantage is that, as shown in Section 7.8, the stable frailty distribution leads to a high initial dependence, but almost no dependence at high ages, and this might imply a bad fit. Furthermore, handling truncation is difficult. Finally, the computational task is major.

10.4.1   The trivariate model

One of the tractable models is the nested trivariate parallel data model of (T_1, T_2, T_3), which is a model that would be applicable for a sibling group, where individuals 2 and 3 are twins and individual 1 is an ordinary sibling (single birth), so that T_2 and T_3 are strongly dependent, and T_1 shows a more modest dependence with (T_2, T_3). This is accomplished with three frailties Y_1, Y_2, Y_3 generated from powers of three independent stable variables, so that Z_0 is common to all individuals, Z_1 is for individual 1, and Z_2 is applicable for individuals 2 and 3, by the expressions

$$Y_1 = Z_0 Z_1, \ Y_2 = Y_3 = Z_0 Z_2. \tag{10.1}$$

It is assumed that Z_0^ρ is Posstab(α), and that Z_1, Z_2 are Posstab(ρ). To fit to the mixture result described in the beginning, Z_0 should correspond to $X_1^{1/\rho}$. By this construction, all the marginal distributions are identical. The marginal distribution of each Y is Posstab($\alpha\rho$). This construction makes it possible that both the conditional and the marginal distributions of lifetimes are common to the three individuals, but the degree of dependence is higher among (T_2, T_3) than among (T_1, T_2).

This is a random effects model with three sources of variation. Two of these sources, the group effect (Z_0) and the individual variation (modeled by the hazard $\mu(t)$) are like the corresponding quantities in the shared frailty model, and the third (described by Z_1, Z_2) model a source common to only a subgroup of the group under study.

It can be given a multiple unobserved risk factor interpretation, generalizing the model of Equation (2.49). The model is based on the covariates' being split in three parts, the observed covariates z, the common unobserved (neglected) covariates w, and the unobserved covariates that are common to individuals 2 and 3 only, u. Then the conditional model for individual j reads

$$\lambda_0(t)\exp(\beta'z + \psi'w + \phi'u_j). \qquad (10.2)$$

Then $Z_0 = \exp(\psi'w)$ and $Z_j = \exp(\phi'u_j)$, $j = 1, 2$. Now the rest follows from the assumptions on the distributions of Z_0, Z_1, Z_2. Two points become more clear by this evaluation. The assumed distribution for $\phi'u_j$ has a single parameter (ρ), but this parameter is not a scale parameter and therefore ϕ and u_j cannot be separately considered as a freely varying parameter and a specific distribution family for u_j. Second the assumed distribution for Z_0 implies that there are distributional assumptions for $\rho\psi'w$, so that the parameter for the distribution of u appears also in the distribution for the effect of the common covariates. These aspects are undesirable from a modeling point of view, but come as a consequence of the mixture results used for setting up the model.

The survivor function for the trivariate distribution is simply

$$S(t_1, t_2, t_3) = \exp(-[M_1(t_1)^\rho + \{M_2(t_2) + M_3(t_3)\}^\rho]^\alpha). \qquad (10.3)$$

The density is found by differentiation with respect to t_1, t_2 and t_3. This is tedious, but elementary.

This model can, if the conditional distributions are of Weibull form, alternatively be described by means of accelerated failure times. For doing so in the trivariate model, W_1, W_2 and W_3 should be independent, both mutually, and independent of (Z_0, Z_1, Z_2) and they should follow a Weibull distribution, Weibull(λ, γ). Then we obtain the multiplicative model

$$T_1 = Z_0^{-1/\gamma}Z_1^{-1/\gamma}W_1,\ T_2 = Z_0^{-1/\gamma}Z_2^{-1/\gamma}W_2,\ T_3 = Z_0^{-1/\gamma}Z_2^{-1/\gamma}W_3.$$
$$(10.4)$$

The marginal distributions of T_1, T_2, and T_3 are Weibull, of shape $\alpha\rho\gamma$. This model leads to the most simple formulas for the correlations of the logarithm to the times, which are

$$\mathrm{corr}(\log T_1, \log T_2) = 1 - \alpha^2,\ \mathrm{corr}(\log T_2, \log T_3) = 1 - \alpha^2\rho^2.$$

For considering the effect of truncation, we study the groups, where all individuals are alive by age t_0. Thus the residual lifetimes are $\tilde{T}_1 = T_1 - t_0$, $\tilde{T}_2 = T_2 - t_0$, $\tilde{T}_3 = T_3 - t_0$. Correspondingly, we define $\tilde{M}_1(t_1) = M_1(t_1 + t_0) - M_1(t_0)$, $\tilde{M}_2(t_2) = M_2(t_2 + t_0) - M_2(t_0)$, $\tilde{M}_3(t_3) = M_3(t_3 + t_0) - M_3(t_0)$, in order to describe the integration from time t_0 to t. The survivor function for the residual truncated lifetime generally is

$$\tilde{S}(t_1, t_2, t_3) = S(t_1 + t_0, t_2 + t_0, t_3 + t_0)/S(t_0, t_0, t_0). \qquad (10.5)$$

To simplify the formulas and to show the expression as a model for the observed truncated data, we define $\theta_1 = M_1(t_0)$, $\theta_2 = M_2(t_0)$, $\theta_3 = M_3(t_0)$. Using Equation (10.3), the expression for $\tilde{S}(t_1, t_2, t_3)$ becomes

$$\exp(-[\{\theta_1 + \tilde{M}_1(t_1)\}^\rho + \{\theta_{23} + \tilde{M}_2(t_2) + \tilde{M}_3(t_3)\}^\rho]^\alpha + \{\theta_1^\rho + \theta_{23}^\rho\}^\alpha), \quad (10.6)$$

where $\theta_{23} = \theta_2 + \theta_3$. Thus, truncation changes the distribution in a nontrivial way. It introduces two extra parameters, θ_1 and θ_{23}. In the symmetric case, there is only one more parameter owing to the relation $\theta_{23} = 2\theta_1$. It follows from this that updating becomes clearly more difficult than in the shared frailty model. However, there could be some potential in this model as a generalization of the trivariate stable model, allowing for truncation.

This approach leads to a theoretically very interesting model for trivariate data, but the computations seem cumbersome.

10.4.2 Combined model for monozygotic and dizygotic twins

Another purpose that this approach can satisfy is a unified model for monozygotic and dizygotic twins. This could be considered as bivariate marginals in the above trivariate example. Monozygotic twins have high dependence, and could correspond to the bivariate marginal distribution of (T_2, T_3), whereas the dizygotic twins have smaller dependence, and could correspond to the bivariate marginal distribution of (T_1, T_2). An alternative description of this model is that the frailty is of the form $Z_0 Z_j$, where there is a term that is always common, Z_0, and terms (Z_1, Z_2), which are common ($Z_1 = Z_2$) for monozygotic twins, and separate, independent for dizygotic twins. The conditional and the marginal distributions are common to all twins. Thus, in the case of monozygotic twins, it is a shared frailty model, with the frailty Y_2, which follows a positive stable distribution of index $\alpha\rho$. In the case of dizygotic twins, it is a shared frailty model, with frailty Z_0^ρ, which follows a positive stable distribution of index α. This statement is not trivial, but is derived by means of the bivariate survivor function, where we first condition on Z_0, Z_1, Z_2. It is

$$Pr(T_1 > t_1, T_2 > t_2 \mid Z_0, Z_1, Z_2) = \exp\{-Z_0 Z_1 M_1(t_1) - Z_0 Z_2 M_2(t_2)\}.$$

We then integrate Z_1 and Z_2 out, to obtain

$$Pr(T_1 > t_1, T_2 > t_2 \mid Z_0) = \exp\{-Z_0^\rho M_1(t_1)^\rho - Z_0^\rho M_2(t_2)^\rho\},$$

showing that this is a shared frailty model with Z_0^ρ as frailty and $M_1(t_1)^\rho$ and $M_2(t_2)^\rho$ as integrated hazard functions. This result is important, because it demonstrates that the individual terms (Z_1, Z_2) contribute to the variability by combining with the simple random error described by the hazard function, into a different hazard function. The individual terms then have no influence on the dependence as such. It is just a different parametrization of the same model. In summary, all the bivariate marginals are shared stable frailty models. This gives a very strong interpretation, and it also gives various possibilities for estimation of the dependence. It also means that the correlations and other measures of dependence are easily derived, using this fact. In particular, Kendall's coefficient of concordance (expressed in the trivariate model) is $\tau(T_1, T_2) = 1 - \alpha$, $\tau(T_2, T_3) = 1 - \alpha\rho$.

Instead of using the nested parametrization, we can use the parameters corresponding to the bivariate models. This is a reparametrization to (α, ϵ), where $\epsilon = \alpha\rho$. This means that the monozygotic twins have dependence parameter ϵ, and the dizygotic twins have dependence parameter α. This makes a more symmetric model, but the parameter set is $\epsilon \leq \alpha \leq 1$. In this formulation, it appears natural to extend the parameter set, to have ϵ and α varying independently, $\epsilon \leq 1$, $\alpha \leq 1$, which is symmetric. The formulation of the frailty as a product of Z values is then impossible, but the model is completely symmetric, it just makes the degrees of dependence different for the two subpopulations, and the marginals common to all observations. Another way to say this is that the multivariate frailty approach makes no improvement compared to the shared frailty model for each subpopulation separately, regarding fit to the data. The only difference is that it assumes that all marginal distributions are the same.

In the case of truncation, the two subgroups still show shared frailty models, but the frailty distributions are of the PVF type. Making formulas like that of Equation (10.6), we obtain for monozygotic twins,

$$\tilde{S}_{MZ}(t_1, t_2) = \exp[-\{2\theta + \tilde{M}(t_1) + \tilde{M}(t_2)\}^{\rho\alpha} + (2\theta)^{\rho\alpha}]$$

corresponding to a frailty of $PVF(\rho\alpha, \rho\alpha, 2\theta)$, and for dizygotic twins

$$\tilde{S}_{DZ}(t_1, t_2) = \exp(-[\{\theta + \tilde{M}(t_1)\}^{\rho} + \{\theta + \tilde{M}(t_2)\}^{\rho}]^{\alpha} + 2\theta^{\rho\alpha}),$$

which corresponds to a frailty of $PVF(\alpha, \alpha, 2\theta^{\rho})$, and a conditional integrated hazard of $\{\theta + \tilde{M}(t)\}^{\rho} - \theta^{\rho}$. In summary, this is a three-parameter frailty model, with two hazard functions that are different, but related parametrically. Interestingly, the first parameter of the PVF distribution α, respectively $\alpha\rho$ are unchanged by truncation. It should be possible to fit this model, but it is not recommended as a standard model. In fact, the model should be applied with extreme care, if it should ever be applied, because the assumptions regarding the period before start of the study are impossible to justify and crucial for the evaluation. It is much simpler to fit the larger model with 4 frailty parameters obtained by letting the third PVF parameter vary independently for the two types of twins, and using stratified hazard functions. That is, completely separate estimations for the two types of twins. This was, in fact, the approach used in Section 8.12.5. Further discussion of these models follows under the application.

Of course, this approach can be used more generally than for twins, to compare whether the dependence is the same in two subgroups of the data.

An application is considered in Section 10.4.6.

10.4.3   Treatment by center interaction

A more general model could have multiple observations having Y_1 as frailty and multiple observations having Y_2 as frailty, using notation from the trivariate model above. This could model a random treatment by group interaction, as Y_1 might be the value for the control treatment and Y_2 for the new treatment. Then Z_0 would be the real group effect, and Z_1 and Z_2 the random treatment influence for that group. This is handled by a generalization of Equation (10.3). There should also be a variable describing the systematic treatment effect, as the frailty part only describes the random effects. A particular case for such a model is treatment by center interaction, with center corresponding to the groups above. This then makes the model a random effects model with three sources of variation, the center effect, the center by treatment interaction, and the individual variation.

An application where the effect is treatment by litter interaction is considered in Section 10.4.6.

10.4.4   Goodness-of-fit

As described above, for the bivariate model, for example, obtained as the first two coordinates of the trivariate nested model, the model is not more general than the shared stable frailty model of Section 7.4. This is an advantage in the sense of random effects models, because it demonstrates how individual frailty components combine with the simple random error described by the hazard function, but seen from a goodness of fit point of view, it is a disadvantage, because it means that this approach does not give a more general model in the bivariate case. The random effects properties are the most important, and therefore we should not be disappointed by not obtaining a better fit.

10.4.5   Estimation

The combined monozygotic/dizygotic twin model can be analyzed by a three-stage procedure similar to that described in Section 8.4, that is, by first evaluating the marginal distribution, in the case of no covariates, by a Nelson-Aalen estimate. Then the dependence is evaluated, assuming the marginals are either fixed and known, equal to the Nelson-Aalen estimate (Step 2) or proportional to the Nelson-Aalen estimate (Step 3). In this case, the data can be completely analyzed by computer programs that can handle the shared stable frailty model with fixed respectively exponential marginals, because the first step is a standard univariate analysis, the Nelson-Aalen estimate for the two twin types combined, and in the second step, each data set is studied separately in the shared frailty analysis. However, this is not completely satisfying. Therefore, the full semi-parametric estimate is also found. This requires extension of programs for the shared

| Sex | Data set | MZ twins | DZ twins |
		$\hat{\tau}$ (SE)	$\hat{\tau}$ (SE)
Males	MZ	0.0952 (0.0205)	
	DZ		0.0511 (0.0139)
	MZ+DZ	0.1004 (0.0212)	0.0506 (0.0135)
Females	MZ	0.0938 (0.0198)	
	DZ		0.0535 (0.0136)
	MZ+DZ	0.0965 (0.0203)	0.0535 (0.0134)

Table 10.7. Estimates of dependence (τ) for Danish twin data, based on the multiplicative stable frailty model, assuming the marginals proportional to the Nelson-Aalen estimate based on the data set, described in the first column.

frailty models, but it can be done by combining results from several calls of the same program if the original program is based on parametrizing by means of the marginal distribution, like that of Section 8.5. That is, first death times of the total material are found. An initial estimate is found, for example, as the shared frailty model based on all data combined. In each step of the iteration, one evaluates the log likelihood and its derivatives for the monozygotic twins. Similar evaluations are performed for the dizygotic twins. The derivatives with respect to the two frailty parameters are kept separate, whereas the derivatives with respect to the hazard parameters are added over the two subpopulations (which, in fact, corresponds to the use of a large-dimensional G as in Equation (B.2)). These derivatives are then used for updating the estimate in the usual Newton-Raphson way.

The trivariate case is handled by using Equation (10.3) and its derivatives with respect to t_1, t_2 and t_3. The treatment by center interaction model is studied analogously, but differentiating a higher number of times, corresponding to the number of events in the two groups, and therefore, this becomes complicated.

10.4.6   Applications

The Danish data on monozygotic and dizygotic twins have been analyzed by this combined approach. Owing to the model's being a shared frailty model for each type of twin separately, the only real difference compared to the results of Chapter 7 is that the marginal distributions are assumed common to monozygotic and dizygotic twins.

First, we consider the results with a simple handling of the marginal distribution, that is, the three-stage procedure. The results are reported in Table 10.7 for the combined data set of monozygotic and dizygotic twins. For easy reference the results from step 3 of Table 8.21 are included. These are in the table described as based only on a single data set. As described in Chapter 7, the standard errors are underestimated by this approach, and the restriction on the marginals is purely a computational restriction

Sex	Data set	MZ twins $\hat{\tau}$ (SE)	DZ twins $\hat{\tau}$ (SE)
Males	MZ	0.1022 (0.0227)	
	DZ		0.0528 (0.0145)
	MZ+DZ	0.1049 (0.0220)	0.0532 (0.0141)
Females	MZ	0.0958 (0.0212)	
	DZ		0.0553 (0.0144)
	MZ+DZ	0.0988 (0.0210)	0.0551 (0.0139)

Table 10.8. Estimates of dependence (τ) for Danish twin data, based on the multiplicative stable frailty model with arbitrary common marginals.

to simplify the estimation. Therefore, Table 10.8 gives the corresponding estimates in the full model, that is, when the marginals are allowed to vary freely in a semi-parametric model, but, of course, being the same for monozygotic and dizygotic twins. It is clear that the estimated standard errors are higher, although owing to the approximate independence of the dependence parameter to the marginal distributions not that much higher compared to the step 3 estimation method. Also the estimates of τ are higher. The standard errors are slightly lower for the combined data set, than for the single data sets, illustrating the variance reduction by assuming common marginals.

The above evaluation does not account for the truncation at 15 years and it is known that a large proportion of the twins pairs were lost before this. We have not applied the truncated combined model with three parameters for the frailty, but the application in Section 8.12.5 fitted the larger four-parameter model. Just looking at the estimates of α (Table 8.24) for males for monozygotic (0.149) and dizygotic (0.880) translates into $\hat{\alpha} = 0.149$ and $\hat{\rho} = 0.169$, suggesting an extremely strong dependence for total lifetime (that is, from birth) of monozygotic twins. For females the same evaluation falls outside of the possible parameters, but suggests an even stronger dependence. These numbers are, of course, an overinterpretation of the data and are included here only for more theoretical reasons. It emphasizes that truncation is an aspect that should be taken seriously as it can have dramatic influence on the interpretation of the dependence. Truncation may imply a reduction in dependence. In particular, in stable frailty models, the dependence decreases very fast initially and implies that we may overlook an important dependence if data are truncated.

The litter data of Section 1.5.3 can be used to illustrate treatment by litter interaction that is, the model of Section 10.4.3, which in this case corresponds to the trivariate model of Section 10.4.1.

Pickles and Crouchley (1994) analyzed a subset of the exercise test data of Section 1.8.2, covering the measurements before and 1 and 3 hours after treatment with oral isosorbide. The idea was that the treatment variation should not affect the time before treatment, leading to a larger dependence between the 1 and 3 hours measurement, and lower between the before measurement and the other ones. This almost corresponds to the trivariate model of Section 10.4.1. The only difference is that they believed that the variation was larger after treatment, and therefore ignored the Z_1 term. For the hazard a Weibull distribution was used. The estimate was found as $\hat{\alpha}=0.425$ and $\hat{\rho} = 0.662$. From these we derive that the estimates for τ are 0.58 and 0.72, which are somewhat higher than the values of Table 10.6 found by the bivariate marginal approach. The likelihood ratio test for the same dependence between all measurements ($\rho = 1$) gave $-2 \log Q = 12.35$, confirming the expected differential dependence.

10.5   Additive models

The above-mentioned multiplicative result is unique to the stable distributions. In general, it is much more tractable to handle additive frailty models. This was noted already by Vaupel and Yashin (1985), for gamma models for univariate data. Here it will first be considered more generally than the gamma distribution. This will be introduced by the bivariate model. Similar to the other sections, we assume that the conditional hazard for individual j is of the form $Y_j \mu_j(t)$, given the bivariate frailty (Y_1, Y_2). The approach is based on letting the frailty (Y_1, Y_2) be given by the expressions

$$Y_1 = Z_0 + Z_1, \; Y_2 = Z_0 + Z_2, \qquad (10.7)$$

where Z_0, Z_1, Z_2 are independently distributed variables. Conceptually, this is similar to the first two components of the trivariate multiplicative stable model, where the product is substituted by an addition, and the stable distributions with general or gamma distributions. The term Z_0 generates dependence, and Z_1 and Z_2 are independent individual terms, generating only extra variance. However, in this model, the effect of Z_1 and Z_2 cannot easily be combined with the hazard function. Contrary to the multiplicative stable model, the model is a true extension corresponding shared frailty model in the bivariate case. The positive phrasing of this is that the model can be used to improve the fit for the data. This is why the model is introduced by the bivariate case, rather than the trivariate used in the multiplicative stable model.

   This model can be given an interpretation as a hidden cause of death model. Suppose there are two causes of death, with proportional hazards $c_1 \mu(t)$ and $c_2 \mu(t)$, and corresponding frailties, U_1 and U_2. If cause number 1 was genetically influenced, but cause number 2 was unrelated to genetics, it could be so that U_1 was shared between family members, whereas the U_2-term was individual, that is of the form U_{2j} for individual j. If the actual cause of death is unknown, this gives exactly an additive model, with $Z_0 = c_1 U_1$, $Z_1 = c_2 U_{21}$ and $Z_2 = c_2 U_{22}$. It is crucial for this evaluation that the hazards are proportional and thus the model is somewhat simpler than we expect the reality is. An extension to non-proportional hazards is considered in Section 11.5.

The calculations are most transparent if we write the expressions by means of the Laplace transform, and they are then correct for general distributions. The conditional survivor function in the bivariate case is

$$S(t_1, t_2 \mid Z_0, Z_1, Z_2) = \exp\{-(Z_0 + Z_1)M_1(t) - (Z_0 + Z_2)M_2(t_2)\}. \quad (10.8)$$

By collecting terms corresponding to Z_0, Z_1, Z_2, respectively, the expression becomes a product of independent terms and then the bivariate distribution integral is easily derived by means of the Laplace transform $L_m(s)$ for $Z_m, m = 0, 1, 2$ as

$$S(t_1, t_2) = L_0(M_1(t_1) + M_2(t_2))L_1(M_1(t_1))L_2(M_2(t_2)). \quad (10.9)$$

The density is derived by differentiation with respect to t_1 and t_2. It is

$$\mu_1(t_1)\mu_2(t_2)\{L_0''L_1L_2 + L_0'L_1'L_2 + L_0'L_1L_2' + L_0L_1'L_2'\} \quad (10.10)$$

where all L_0 terms are evaluated at $M. = M_1(t_1) + M_2(t_2)$, all L_1 terms at $M_1 = M_1(t_1)$, and all L_2 terms at $M_2 = M_2(t_2)$. There is a clear structure in this formula. There are two derivatives in each term, one derivative in either L_0 or L_1, and one, which is either in L_0 or L_2. It can be described as a matrix product in the following way:

$$\mu_1(t_1)\mu_2(t_2) \, (L_1' \ L_1) \begin{pmatrix} L_0 & L_0' \\ L_0' & L_0'' \end{pmatrix} (L_2' \ L_2)^T, \quad (10.11)$$

where the symbol T is used for transpose in order not to confuse it with differentiation ($'$). This equation has a strong interpretation. Each event is assigned either to the shared part or the individual part (implying that a derivative is taken for the relevant part), and the probabilities for the various possibilities are then added. In the case of an event for individual 1 and a censoring for individual 2, the expression is

$$\mu_1(t_1)\{L_0'L_1 + L_0L_1'\}L_2, \quad (10.12)$$

with the interpretation that the first term corresponds to assigning the event to the common part and the second to the individual part.

It is common to restrict the parameters so that the marginal distributions of Y_1 and Y_2 are simple. The reason is that to obtain a relation similar to the univariate formula (Equation (7.7)), we find

$$S_j(t) = \tilde{L}_j(M_j(t)), \quad (10.13)$$

where $\tilde{L}_j(s)$ is the Laplace transform of Y_j. When the distribution of Y_j is simple, it is much more easy to handle this expression. This relation is particularly relevant, when using the marginal parametrization, as it is simpler to combine Equation (10.10) with the inverse relation found from Equation (10.13).

When the conditional distribution is Weibull, this model can also be given an accelerated failure time interpretation, by means of the expression

$$T_1 = (Z_0 + Z_1)^{-1/\gamma}W_1, \ T_2 = (Z_0 + Z_2)^{-1/\gamma}W_2,$$

where W_1 and W_2 are Weibull (λ, γ). This is not as elegant as the multiplicative stable model, Equation (10.4), as it is rather a hyperbolic type expression and the contributions of the various terms do not separate.

This model might appear as a more detailed model for dependence, but there is only one term, Z_0, common for the individuals, and the more detailed model is rather for the variance, as both (Z_1, Z_2) and the hazard function describe the individual variation. Thus the model can be interpreted as a model with three random effects describing the effect of two sources of variation. Having two random effects for the same source of variation, of course, implies that it will be difficult or impossible to separate the random effects.

Truncation is easily handled, using Equation (10.9), which shows that the conditional distribution again corresponds to an additive model, but the relation between the parameters might become more complicated. More specifically, in the conditional distribution giving survival of both individuals to time t, there will still be an additive relation like Equation (10.7), but each component will be updated like in Equation (7.12). The θ parameters will be different for the common component Z_0 than for Z_1. More general updating expressions can be found, but in that case the additive structure, Equation (10.7), does not hold (a simple example follows from Exercise 7.24).

10.5.1   Bivariate additive gamma models

The applications of additive frailty models have exclusively used the gamma distribution for Z and to make the marginal distributions simple, the distributions have been restricted to have the same value of the parameter θ. This model leads to the marginal distributions of Y_j being gamma. The model goes under the name of correlated frailty. The term used here (additive gamma) is more specific. Symmetry has been obtained by letting the distributions of Z_1 and Z_2 be the same, so that the distributions of Y_1 and Y_2 are the same. Thus, the parameters are δ_0 and θ for Y_0 and δ_1 and θ for Y_1 and Y_2, with the restriction that $\delta_0 + \delta_1 = \theta$ to secure a mean of 1 for Y_1 and Y_2. Therefore, an alternative parametrization is (θ, ξ), where θ describes the marginal distribution of Y_1 and Y_2, and ξ is the correlation between them, which is the reason for the name correlated frailty. Thus $\delta_0 = \xi\theta$, $\delta_1 = (1 - \xi)\theta$ and $\xi = \delta_0/(\delta_0 + \delta_1)$. In this framework, we can generalize Equation (7.31) to

$$S(t_1, t_2) = \frac{S_1(t_1)^{1-\xi}S_2(t_2)^{1-\xi}}{\{S_1(t_1)^{-1/\theta} + S_2(t_2)^{-1/\theta} - 1\}^{\xi\theta}}. \tag{10.14}$$

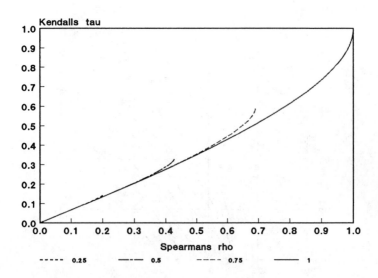

Figure 10.1. Relation between Spearman's ρ and Kendall's τ for the additive gamma frailty model, with various values of ξ (0.25, 0.5, 0.75 and 1).

When $\theta \to 0$, the survivor function converges to the model

$$S(t_1, t_2) = S_1(t_1)S_2(t_2) \max(S_1(t_1), S_2(t_2))^{-\xi}. \qquad (10.15)$$

Thus there is maximum dependence obtainable for a fixed value of ξ.

Kendall's τ has not been evaluated theoretically, but it can be derived numerically, as well as Spearman's measure. Regarding the median concordance, a very simple formula is obtained, based on Equation (4.14) and (10.14):

$$\kappa = 2\{2(2^{1+1/\theta} - 1)^{-\theta}\}^{\xi}2^{-(1-\xi)} - 1,$$

which has a much stronger interpretation, when written in the form of the bivariate survivor function $p = S(S_1^{-1}(1/2), S_2^{-1}(1/2))$, where $\kappa = 4p - 1$. We obtain

$$p(\theta, \xi) = p(\theta, 1)^{\xi}p(\theta, 0)^{1-\xi},$$

which is a linear interpolation in ξ, on logarithmic scale, of the value in the shared frailty model with θ as parameter (corresponding to $\xi = 1$), and the value 1/4 under independence. Figure 10.1 shows corresponding values of Spearman's ρ and Kendall's τ. Generally, the agreement between these two measures of dependence is the same, but near the maximal dependence for each value of ξ, that is, for low values of δ_0, τ is larger than expected from the shared frailty model ($\xi = 1$).

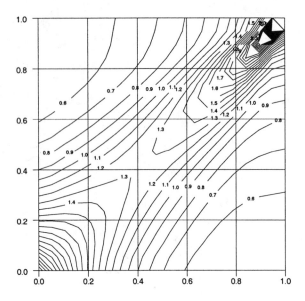

Figure 10.2. Contour curves for the density of a bivariate uniform distribution with additive gamma frailty dependence, with $\xi = 1/2$ and $\tau = 0.25$.

How the distribution looks, can be illustrated by means of contour curves like those of Section 7.8. The parameter values were selected to have $\tau = 0.25$ like the gamma model of Figure 7.3, but with frailty correlation ξ 0.5. This is obtained for $\theta = 0.2758$. Using uniform marginal distributions, this is done in Figure 10.2, and it is seen that where the shared gamma frailty model leads to high dependence at high ages, this model makes the time of importance more intermediate. Alternatively, the density is illustrated in Figure 10.3. In the shared frailty model it is almost impossible to have one low and one high time within a pair, but in the additive model, the density never gets really low. In the figure, the density comes down to 0.5. Generally, this value is $1 - \xi$. This is a relevant point in light of the cause of death interpretation. The person might die early owing to "independent" causes, even though the person has inherited a low risk of death of other important shared causes of death. For example, a person might have inherited a strong heart, but he can still die prematurely owing to accidental causes. In particular, the additive gamma frailty model leads to an increase in the density along the diagonal, that is, for $t_1 = t_2$. This is illustrated in Figure 10.4, where the density is illustrated for five different choices of ξ, with a fixed value of Kendall's τ (0.25). The reason for not including $\xi = 0.25$ is that such a distribution does not exist. This figure shows that the additive gamma frailty model leads to the time of importance being more intermediate than the shared gamma frailty model. The figure can be

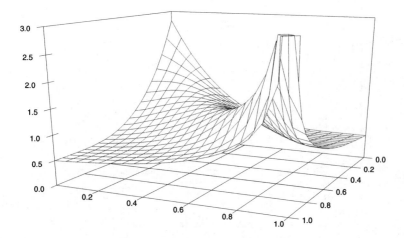

Figure 10.3. Bivariate density of a uniform distribution with additive gamma frailty dependence, with $\xi = 1/2$ and $\tau = 0.25$.

ξ	δ	ρ	κ
0.41	0.0353	0.340	0.315
0.45	0.1494	0.352	0.304
0.5	0.2758	0.358	0.293
0.75	0.8823	0.365	0.262
1	1.5	0.366	0.247

Table 10.9. Parameter values and dependence measures for additive gamma frailty models of Figure 10.4. The parameters are chosen to have $\tau = 0.25$.

compared to Figure 7.6 showing that the additive gamma model is better to create a high density along the diagonal than the shared PVF model. In fact, the limiting distribution (Equation (10.15)) places a probability of $1 - \xi$ precisely at the diagonal and thus is not continuous. A few properties for the parameter values are listed in Table 10.9. In this case, there is a differential development between τ and κ.

Truncation is easily handled, using Equation (10.9), which shows that the conditional distribution again corresponds to an additive gamma model. However, the differential change for the θ-components, by $M_1 + M_2$ for Z_0 and M_1 alone for Z_1, and similarly M_2 for Z_2, implies that the restriction that the θ parameters are common for all contributions is violated. The consequence of this is that the dependence decreases over time. That is, there is early dependence. More general updating formulas can also be

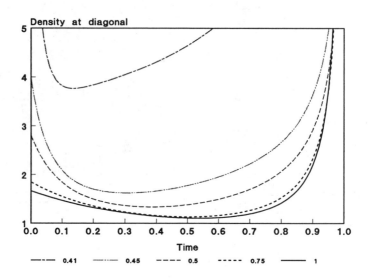

Figure 10.4. Density at the diagonal of bivariate uniform distributions with additive gamma frailty, with $\tau = 0.25$ and ξ 0.41, 0.45, 0.5, 0.75 and 1.

derived, but they are clearly more complicated than for the shared frailty model. If one wants to fit this model, it appears to be convenient to make a different identifiability restriction on the parameters, namely, that the $EZ_0 = 1$. By normalizing the hazard function, this may be obtained also after truncation. This means that after truncation the parameters of Z_0 are (δ_0, δ_0) and those for Z_1 and Z_2 are (δ_1, θ_1).

Independence can be obtained both for $\xi = 0$ and as a limit for $\theta \to \infty$. In the latter case, ξ cannot be identified and therefore standard test statistics cannot be used for testing the hypothesis of independence.

In general, this model is identifiable by means of bivariate data. That is, except for the boundary cases corresponding to independence, no two sets of parameter values give rise to the same bivariate distribution. However, the values are not well determined. This is because there are two terms that basically describe individual variation, the individual frailties (Z_1, Z_2), and the hazard function.

This model may be used for checking the assumptions of the shared gamma frailty model. It is, however, somewhat unclear exactly which assumption of the model is checked, but by comparing Figure 10.3 with Figure 7.7, it is related to the density near the diagonal and to the density when one observation is low and one is high. A more relevant place for these models might be for regression models, because only θ can be identified by means of univariate data, and thus the dependence in form of the combined effect of θ and ξ, measured, for example, by τ, cannot be identified. However, we cannot be certain that the problems for regression models are completely solved. Identifying θ from the marginals implies that a non-trivial upper limit to the dependence is found and thus there is some sort of information in the marginals. The model does not allow for a multiple risk factor interpretation, like that of Equation (10.2). Until this problem is better understood, some reservations are appropriate.

10.5.2   Compound symmetry model

The model above is easily generalized to a multivariate model, similar in idea to the compound symmetry models for normally distributed data. That is, $Y_j = Z_0 + Z_j$, $j = 1, ..., k$. This model has never been considered in the literature, so we can just mention a few immediate aspects. The bivariate marginals are all bivariate additive frailty models, like those of Section 10.5.1. The density can be expressed by a formula similar to Equation (10.10), but involving a sum over k dimensions. This extension does not solve the problem that there are two random effects describing the individual source of variation.

10.5.3   Combined model for monozygotic and dizygotic twins

This model can easily be extended to more general dependence structures. One such case is the combination of monozygotic and dizygotic twins in one model, similar to what was done in the multiplicative stable model. The simplest way to do so is to assume that Z_0 in Equation (10.7) is a common term for both monozygotic and dizygotic twins, but Z_1 and Z_2 are terms that are common for monozygotic and individual (independent) for dizygotic twins. This leads to a model where the conditional as well as the marginal hazards can be the same, but the degree of dependence is higher for monozygotic than for dizygotic twins. Specifically in the gamma model, θ is common and ξ is 1 for monozygotic and a free parameter for dizygotic twins. This idea, which was fine for the multiplicative stable model, is not satisfactory for the additive gamma frailty case, because it allows all parameters to be determined from the data on dizygotic twins alone, as will be demonstrated in the application. To avoid this problem, we must extend the model by specifying that both types of twins follow the model (10.7) with independent terms, but with the same value of θ for both types of twins, and separate values of ξ, say, (θ, ξ_M) for monozygotic and (θ, ξ_D) for dizygotic twins. An alternative formulation of this model is as

$$Y_1 = Z_0 + Z_1 + Z_3, \quad Y_2 = Z_0 + Z_2 + Z_4, \tag{10.16}$$

where Z_0 describes terms that are common in any case; Z_1 and Z_2 are terms common to monozygotic and independent for dizygotic twins and Z_3 and Z_4 are environmental terms that are individual for both types of twins. To obtain gamma distributions for Y_1 and Y_2, the value of θ is the same for all terms, and owing to symmetry, we assume that the distributions of Z_1 and Z_2 are the same and that the distributions of Z_3 and Z_4 are the same, giving a total of three parameters to describe the two levels of dependence. The parameters are related so that $\xi_M = (\delta_0 + \delta_1)/\theta$ and $\xi_D = \delta_0/\theta$. Thus this model requires one parameter more than the corresponding multiplicative stable frailty model. Alternatively, this can be interpreted that we have four random effects describing three sources of variation, as both (Z_3, Z_4) and the hazard function describe individual variation.

Truncation leads to a differential change in the θ parameters and to a reduction in dependence (see Section 10.5.1). To express this change, θ is subscripted by the component to which it refers. The parameter θ_0 is updated by the sum of the integrated hazards, whereas θ_3 is updated by the individual value. However, θ_1 is updated by the sum for monozygotic, but by the single values for dizygotic twins, implying that the parameter restrictions are not satisfied after truncation.

10.5.4   Treatment by center interaction

Another case is random treatment by center effect, where multiple persons (the control group at a center) have Y_1 as frailty, and multiple persons (the treatment group at the center) have Y_2 as frailty. Then Z_0 describes the center effect and Z_1 and Z_2 describe random center-specific treatment effects. The model should also include a systematic effect of the treatment in general. Thus there is a high dependence between patients on the same treatment on the same center, and a positive, but smaller dependence between patients on different treatments on the same centers. Patients on different centers are independent.

Also for data covering recurrent events for similar organs, like implantation of artificial hips for right and left hips for a set of patients, this model could be applied with Y_1 the frailty for organ 1 (right hip) and Y_2 the frailty for organ 2 (left hip).

10.5.5   Father-mother-child model

A further model that can be considered in this way is a father-mother-child model, where some genetic terms are common to the father and the child, and some for the mother and the child, and there possibly also are environmental terms common to all of them. The approach will be illustrated with such a model. One point to note first is that we should be aware of the marginal distribution, and that means that the standard case should be constructed so as to lead to common marginals. To obtain this, there must be corresponding terms for all individuals. This means, for example, that if there is a term common for the mother and the child, we should assign an independent contribution for the father, with the same distribution. To construct the model, we first take Z_1 as a term common to all individuals, to cover common environmental effects. Then Z_2 is common for the father and the child. This requires a corresponding term Z_3 for the mother, following the same distribution as Z_2. Furthermore, there should be a term Z_4 common for the mother and the child, with a corresponding term Z_5 for the father. There may further by individual terms Z_6, Z_7, Z_8, but we will not do this here. These terms might be beneficial, to avoid determination of all parameters from a subset of the data, similar to the combined model for monozygotic and dizygotic twins. Letting T_1 be the lifetime of the father, T_2 of the mother and T_3 of the child, the model for the vector of frailties is

$$\begin{pmatrix} Y_1 \\ Y_2 \\ Y_3 \end{pmatrix} = \begin{pmatrix} Z_1 + Z_2 + Z_5 \\ Z_1 + Z_3 + Z_4 \\ Z_1 + Z_2 + Z_4 \end{pmatrix} = \begin{pmatrix} 1 & 1 & 0 & 0 & 1 \\ 1 & 0 & 1 & 1 & 0 \\ 1 & 1 & 0 & 1 & 0 \end{pmatrix} (Z_1\ Z_2\ Z_3\ Z_4\ Z_5)'.$$

(10.17)

The model then typically specifies that there is a common scale parameter θ, and values $\delta_1, ..., \delta_5$ for the components, with the restrictions of symmetry ($\delta_2 = \delta_3$ and $\delta_4 = \delta_5$) and the scale restriction ($\theta = \delta_1 + \delta_2 + \delta_4$), leaving three parameters ($\delta_1, \delta_2, \delta_4$).

This can be expressed by the Laplace transforms of $Z_1, ..., Z_5$ in a way similar to Equation (10.9). The large sums involved in differentiating the expression are a main limitation of this approach.

For the model of Equation (10.17), the bivariate marginal model of the lifetimes of the father and the mother is a bivariate additive model with Z_1 as common component, whereas the bivariate distribution of the father and the child is a bivariate additive model with $Z_1 + Z_2$ as the common component. The bivariate distribution of the mother and the child is a bivariate additive model with $Z_1 + Z_4$ as the common component.

This model can be identified, when the censoring patterns allows for multiple events in a group. This is seen by considering the bivariate marginals, which show that it is possible to identify θ, δ_1 and $\delta_1 + \delta_2$, from which all the other parameters can be derived.

Alternatively, the same model could describe a purely genetic model for father, mother, and child; that is, the environmental term (Z_1) in (10.17) is deleted.

10.5.6 General models

One can make a similar model for the lifetime of an adoptive child and its biological and adoptive parents. For simplicity, we only consider the child and the mothers. Then the lifetime of the biological mother, the adoptive mother and the child can follow a model as that of Equation (10.17), except that the Z_1-term is deleted. A term common to all individuals is no longer relevant. The genetic dependence between the biological mother and

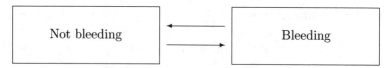

Figure 10.5. Bleeding episode model.

the child is described by Z_2 (and Z_3) and the environmental dependence between the adoptive mother and the child is described by Z_4 (and Z_5).

In order to cover the fathers also, the model becomes more complicated because the shared environment between the child and the adoptive parents need not follow a compound symmetry model. Regarding the biological fathers, they may or may not live together with the biological mother and this does influence the degrees of shared environment for these. Giving the complexity of these problems, it is understandable if one prefers to analyze such data by the bivariate marginal approach (Section 10.3).

In general an expression like Equation (10.17) can be described as QZ, where Q is a known matrix of constants, which are positive or 0. The bivariate marginals are of the same type, taking the relevant rows of Q, and where columns corresponding to components of Z that are not present can be deleted. Like the father-mother-child model of Section 10.5.5, the standard model should include matching terms so that the total variation is the same for all components. Estimation appears to be quite complex.

Some data on recurrent events are based on a switch between two alternating states. Previous examples include epileptic seizures (Figure 2.2), where we typically do not model the period with active seizure, and the pregnancy-birth model (Figure 5.4). Xue and Brookmeyer (1996) present an example of repeated psychiatric admissions, where the two states are in hospital and outside hospital. We will discuss bleeding episodes for hormone-treated post-menopausal women, corresponding to the model in Figure 10.5, as introduced in Section 3.3.7. We will assume a conditional Markov model. That is, there is a bivariate frailty variable, say, (Y_1, Y_2), for each woman, so that the hazard of starting a bleeding episode is $Y_1 \lambda(t)$, and the hazard of ending a bleeding episode is $Y_2 \mu(t)$. As distribution for (Y_1, Y_2), one could pick one of the bivariate frailty models described above. It appears as if the additive model is the most applicable in this case, because it allows for explicit evaluation, and the stable model might lead to some persons' having extremely many events. However, both these models suggest positive dependence and whether this is the case is unknown.

The evaluations above have been based on the gamma model but could be extended to the PVF distribution family. Formulas like Equations (10.9) and (10.11) are general and can be applied to the PVF family as well. This family has not been considered in the literature. The identifiability problems present for the bivariate fit improvement will be amplified as there are still two random effects describing the individual variation, and there are more parameters to describe these effects. More specifically, both the shared PVF and the additive gamma models lead to the dependence happening earlier, and thus it will be difficult to identify all parameters in an additive PVF model.

There might, however, be a place for such models for more complicated types of data, like combining monozygotic and dizygotic twins.

10.5.7 Estimation

For the bivariate fit improvement model, it is possible to utilize Equation (10.14), when there are no covariates. This is then differentiated according to t_1 and t_2.

In the general case, however, we can come further by using Equation (10.11) and appropriate generalizations. The advantage of that expression is that by means of computer programs for shared frailty models, it is possible to evaluate all terms from L_0, L_1, and L_2 separately. The only extension needed is that such a program should not implement the identifiability restriction $\delta = \theta$, but include both parameters. A shared frailty model can still use such a program, implementing the restriction by means of a matrix G as shown in Equation (B.2). For the additive frailty model, such a program typically evaluates the log likelihood and its derivatives. This log likelihood should include all relevant terms so that probabilities can be evaluated. From this, the probability (that is, the likelihood, not the log likelihood) is evaluated together with the derivatives for each Z component separately, using the relevant values for θ and δ. Equation (10.11) is then applied to find the likelihood for the model, in the case of a double event. In the case of no or a single event, simpler formulas along the same line, like Equation (10.12), can be used. Iteration then is based on a more complicated G, parametrizing by δ_0 and δ_1, and using that $\theta = \delta_0 + \delta_1$ is a linear function of these parameters.

10.5.8 Asymptotic evaluation

Parner (1998) considered the bivariate additive gamma model with possibly time-dependent covariates and showed that the distribution is identifiable. The conditions are few. One thing is that there should be a frailty component; in our parametrization this means that θ should be finite. If this is not the case, it is impossible to identify ξ. There should be a positive probability that at least two persons are at risk initially. The hazard can, of course, only be estimated at times when there is positive probability that some individuals are at risk. Similarly, the covariates must vary in the full dimension in order to determine β. When $\xi = 0$, the observations are independent and therefore covariates having a non-zero effect are a must in order to determine θ, by what we have previously called the univariate identifiability. He showed that the full conditional estimate is consistent

	$\hat{\delta}$ (SE)	$\hat{\xi}$ (SE)	$\hat{\omega}$ (SE)	$\hat{\tau}$ (SE)	$\log L$
Males					
MZ	0.912 (0.733)	0.630 (0.283)	0.988 (0.034)	0.1991 (0.0287)	0.33
DZ	0.337 (0.152)	0.194 (0.055)	0.995 (0.023)	0.0826 (0.0188)	5.04
UZ	0.374 (0.177)	0.534 (0.132)	1.004 (0.061)	0.2463 (0.0502)	2.96
Females					
MZ	0.286 (0.159)	0.334 (0.094)	0.990 (0.036)	0.1552 (0.0328)	1.02
DZ	0.121 (0.072)	0.159 (0.044)	0.996 (0.025)	0.0798 (0.0202)	2.48
UZ	0.063 (0.036)	0.200 (0.059)	1.004 (0.050)	0.1073 (0.0329)	2.53

Table 10.10. Estimates in additive gamma frailty models for Danish twin data, and the improvement of the log likelihood compared to the shared gamma frailty model, using the three-stage approach.

and asymptotically normal and that the variance can be estimated consistently by minus the inverse of the second derivative matrix based on one parameter per observed event time.

10.5.9 Applications

Twins – bivariate data

First the additive gamma model is used as a way of improving the fit for the data on Danish twins. That is, each of the six data sets is analyzed separately by the additive model. This is first done by an approach similar to the three-stage approach for the shared frailty model, where first the data are transformed by the Nelson-Aalen estimate and second an additive gamma frailty model is used, with exponential marginal distributions. The parameter ω is the marginal hazard scale, which naturally is close to 1. The estimates from the third stage are shown in Table 10.10, together with the improvement in likelihood compared to the shared gamma frailty model based on the same handling of the marginal distribution (Table 8.13). The estimates of δ and τ in the corresponding shared frailty model are shown in Tables 8.12 and 8.20. There is a significant improvement compared to the shared gamma model for dizygotic twins and twins of unknown zygosity, but there is no significant improvement for monozygotic twins. Compared to the shared gamma model, the additive gamma model leads to the time frame of the dependence being earlier. Therefore, the improvement is roughly comparable to the improvement in Table 8.13, where the PVF model gives an earlier dependence compared to the gamma model. The additive gamma frailty model gives a better fit than the shared PVF frailty model, which probably is due to the density's being more concentrated along the diagonal, as seen by comparing Figures 7.6 and 10.4. The value for ξ is lower for dizygotic twins than for monozygotic twins. The values for τ are comparable to the shared gamma model estimates of Table 8.23

	$\hat{\delta}_0$ (SE)	$\hat{\delta}_1$ (SE)	$\hat{\xi}$ (SE)	$\hat{\tau}$ (SE)	$\log L$
Males					
MZ	1.918 (-)	0 (-)	1 (-)	0.2068 (-)	0
DZ	0.183 (0.152)	0.507 (0.241)	0.265 (0.084)	0.0882 (0.0192)	2.00
UZ	0.752 (0.678)	0.207 (0.136)	0.784 (0.240)	0.251 (0.0504)	0.20
Females					
MZ	2.073 (-)	0 (-)	1 (-)	0.1943 (-)	0
DZ	0.544 (0.953)	0.631 (0.330)	0.463 (0.319)	0.1208 (0.0241)	0.26
UZ	2.159 (3.684)	0.083 (1.410)	0.963 (0.665)	0.1745 (0.0459)	0.001

Table 10.11. Estimates in the non-parametric additive gamma frailty models for Danish twin data using the conditional parametrization, and the improvement of the log likelihood compared to the shared gamma frailty model.

for the first four data sets, but for dizygotic females and for females of unknown zygosity, the values are lower than for the shared frailty model.

The full non-parametric estimate can also be found (Table 10.11). For the monozygotic twins, the estimates are on the boundary corresponding to only common frailty. The values of τ are quite close to those of the shared frailty model (Table 8.23). Regarding the values of ξ, the values are clearly different from those of Table 10.10. The reason is that the individual frailty terms Z_1 and Z_2 describe simple random variation in competition with the hazard function, and therefore the separate contributions of the terms are not well determined. This is clearly illustrated by the very large standard errors on the parameters δ_0, δ_1 and ξ. The standard error on τ is not equally large. The non-parametric estimates of τ are larger than those of the three-stage approach. This is probably due to the more general phenomenon that the most flexible model gives the highest degree of dependence, like that observed in Tables 8.20 and 8.21.

Having truncated data, it is difficult to argue that the θ parameters for the common and the individual frailties should be the same. As described in Section 10.5.1, the θ parameters change differentially over time. To identify the parameters, we use the restriction that $EZ_0 = 1$, implying that the distribution of Z_0 is gamma (δ_0, δ_0) and that of Z_1 and Z_2 is gamma (δ_1, θ_1). For all six data sets, the iterative procedure converged to the boundary of the parameter set. In two cases, δ_1 converged toward 0; and in four cases, δ_1 and θ_1 converged toward ∞. In two of the latter cases, the fit was significantly improved. It is not surprising that there are technical problems in fitting such a model, because it actually includes three different quantities to describe individual variation, δ_1, θ_1 and the hazard function. Whether the problems are due to a theoretical identifiability problem or a practical problem badly determined parameters is unknown.

Sex	Data set	$\hat{\theta}$ (SE)	$\hat{\xi}$ (SE)	$\hat{\omega}$ (SE)
Males	MZ	1.937 (0.323)	1 (-)	0.986 (0.034)
	DZ	0.337 (0.152)	0.194 (0.055)	0.995 (0.023)
	MZ+DZ	1.979 (0.313)	0.472 (0.112)	0.993 (0.019)
Females	MZ	2.113 (0.422)	1 (-)	0.981 (0.036)
	DZ	0.121 (0.072)	0.159 (0.044)	0.996 (0.025)
	MZ+DZ	2.000 (0.375)	0.646 (0.136)	0.986 (0.021)

Table 10.12. Estimates of parameters for Danish twin data, based on the additive gamma frailty model with common marginals (Step 3), with $\xi = 1$ for MZ twins, and arbitrary for DZ twins.

Sex	Data set	MZ twins $\hat{\tau}$ (SE)	DZ twins $\hat{\tau}$ (SE)
Males	MZ	0.205 (0.027)	-
	DZ	0.597 (0.108)	0.083 (0.019)
	MZ+DZ	0.203 (0.013)	0.086 (0.019)
Females	MZ	0.191 (0.031)	-
	DZ	0.805 (0.094)	0.080 (0.020)
	MZ+DZ	0.200 (0.030)	0.121 (0.023)

Table 10.13. Estimates of dependence (τ), for Danish twin data, based on the additive gamma frailty model with common marginals with $\xi = 1$ for MZ twins, and arbitrary for DZ twins (Step 3).

Twins – combined model for monozygotic and dizygotic

In order to unite the monozygotic and the dizygotic twins into one analysis, we have to make similar two-stage estimates for the combined model, where the same marginals are assumed for monozygotic and dizygotic twins, and a shared gamma frailty model for the monozygotic twins (which corresponds to an additive gamma frailty model with frailty correlation 1), and an additive gamma frailty model for dizygotic twins, using the same parameter θ. The parameters are determined as far as possible based on both MZ and DZ twins, and based on each data set separately. The results are reported in Table 10.12. The results based on monozygotic twins are taken from Table 8.12, whereas those for dizygotic twins are from Table 10.10. There is a clear difference between the value of ξ for dizygotic twins, whether monozygotic twins are included in the data or not. The ω parameters are not comparable, as they refer to different Nelson-Aalen estimates. In the combined data set, the value of ξ is roughly 1/2; but otherwise, it is somewhat difficult to make sense out of such a set of parameters, and therefore Table 10.13 gives estimates of the dependence, Kendall's τ. This requires numerical integration in the additive model. There is a fine agreement for the various models for both monozygotic and dizygotic twins, as long the corresponding data are included in the estimation. However, the value

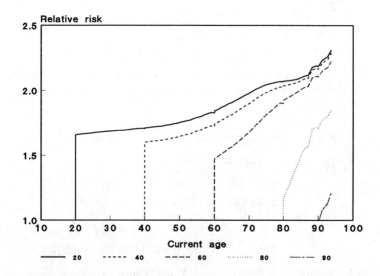

Figure 10.6. Relative hazards of death of a monozygotic male twin at time t, for various values (20, 40, 60, 80 and 90 years) of age at partners death t_1, compared to partner being alive, in the additive gamma model.

for monozygotic twins, calculated on the basis of only dizygotic twins, is clearly wrong. For comparison, the value of $\hat{\tau}$ for dizygotic twins based on the shared frailty model are 0.081 (0.021) for males and 0.125 (0.023) for females. This means that even though the estimates of the parameters in the additive gamma model are difficult to compare with the shared frailty model, the estimated degree of dependence is comparable. This illustrates the difficulties owing to the two ways of modeling the individual variation. The dependence can also be evaluated in the same way as Figure 8.3. This is shown in Figure 10.6. At old ages, the additive models suggest lower dependence than the shared gamma frailty model.

Obviously, it is unsatisfactory that the degree of dependence for monozygotic twins should be identifiable for dizygotic twins. One way to avoid this problem is to also let the monozygotic twins have arbitrary ξ, still assuming that the θ parameter is common for the two types of twins. In that case, the estimates for single data sets are those reported in Table 10.10. For the combined data set, the estimates are described in Table 10.14. The estimated degree of dependence, measured by Kendall's τ is shown in Table 10.15. These results appear more satisfying. In particular, it is noted that the standard error for the MZ value is the same, when based on MZ twins alone, as when based on both MZ and DZ twins. This is in contrast to Ta-

Data set	$\hat{\theta}$ (SE)	$\hat{\xi}_{MZ}$ (SE)	$\hat{\xi}_{DZ}$ (SE)
Males	0.463 (0.191)	0.441 (0.099)	0.227 (0.060)
Females	0.283 (0.147)	0.338 (0.091)	0.221 (0.063)

Table 10.14. Estimates of parameters for Danish twin data, based on the additive gamma frailty model with common marginals (Step 3), and separate ξ for MZ and DZ twins.

Sex	Data set	MZ twins $\hat{\tau}$ (SE)	DZ twins $\hat{\tau}$ (SE)
Males	MZ	0.199 (0.029)	-
	DZ	-	0.083 (0.019)
	MZ+DZ	0.182 (0.028)	0.088 (0.019)
Females	MZ	0.155 (0.033)	-
	DZ	-	0.080 (0.020)
	MZ+DZ	0.158 (0.033)	0.099 (0.022)

Table 10.15. Estimates of dependence (τ), for Danish twin data, based on the additive gamma frailty model with common marginals (Step 3), and arbitrary ξ for both MZ and DZ twins.

ble 10.13, where there appears to be a slight change in precision, probably due to the undesired information on MZ twins in the DZ twin data.

Catheter infections

For the kidney infections data of Section 1.7.3, the additive gamma frailty model has been used with covariates. Regarding the effect of the covariates, the results are shown in Table 10.16, which is comparable to Table 8.10. These results are roughly comparable to the individual frailty model and with a slightly better fit. The shared frailty value appears to be biased upward owing to the strong non-proportionality. With bivariate data, the value is estimated to $\tau = 0.136$ (0.101) and thus lower than the shared gamma frailty model, although it is still higher than the shared gamma frailty model without covariates. Also the standard error is higher, apparently due to this method obtaining less information on the dependence from the marginal distributions.

In a bivariate additive gamma model without covariates, the dependence cannot be estimated from the marginal distributions, except that the model requires the dependence to be between independence $\tau = 0$ and the value found from the spell-specific model, that is, $\tau < 0.248$.

Without covariates, the additive gamma model for the bivariate data has the estimate at the boundary corresponding to $\xi = 1$, which then suggests a value of τ of 0.081, as described in Table 8.9.

	Age $\hat{\beta}$ (SE)	Sex $\hat{\beta}$ (SE)	$\log L$
Additive frailty	0.0068 (0.0126)	-1.69 (0.57)	-227.41

Table 10.16. Estimates for log relative hazards and log likelihoods for kidney catheter data in the additive gamma frailty model.

Tumorigenesis data

The treatment litter interaction can be studied for the tumorigenesis data of Section 1.5.3. The estimate in the interaction model of Section 10.5.4 turns out to be on the boundary corresponding to the shared frailty model, that is, no variation in Z_1 and Z_2.

10.6 Multivariate lognormal frailty

The simplest way to construct a valid multivariate frailty model is to use a multivariate lognormal distribution. Thus in the bivariate case, the frailty (Y_1, Y_2) is given by $(\log Y_1, \log Y_2)$, say, (X_1, X_2), following a bivariate normal distribution, where we may choose the mean to be 0, and then the variance to be a general 2 by 2 variance matrix. However, it is difficult to do explicit calculations, as simple expressions for the Laplace transform are not available. As described in Section 7.6, there are several ways to handle this problem. One can perform numerical integration, one can apply an approximation to the integral as described in Section A.3.5 or one can perform simulations according to the distributions and base inference on those. Finally, one can use a penalized likelihood approach for estimation. For more complicated dependence structures, this approach is more promising that the additive approach. The bivariate marginals of the times in a multivariate lognormal frailty model are bivariate lognormal frailty models. Negative dependence is easily modeled as described in Section 10.2.

A special case of this model is $X_1 = U_0 + U_1$, $X_2 = U_0 + U_2$, which gives a multiplicative model of the same form as Equation (10.1), but with other distributional assumptions. This model is also covered by Equation (10.2) and thus also carries an interpretation by means of multiple unobserved risk factors, that is as neglected covariates.

The finite mean of the frailty in this case implies that the parameters of the marginal frailty (that is the variances, not the means and the covariances) can be identified from univariate data. The practical consequences of this have never been studied in this model.

There have been very few applications of this model. Korsgaard, Madsen, and Jensen (1998) applied a Bayesian lognormal frailty model to data on 1635 bulls using the genetic relations between the bulls to determine the relations between the individual frailties. The estimation was done by means of Gibbs sampling. Ripatti (1999) used it for the analysis of hip replacement data, where patients could have multiple hip operations on both sides. The likelihood was evaluated by means of an approximation to the multivariate Laplace transform generalizing that of Section A.3.5.

10.7   Negative dependence models

Almost all cases considered show positive dependence, which is the most sensible owing to the random effects interpretation. It is, however, useful to have models also showing negative dependence. First of all, we must be able to evaluate whether the dependence is positive, absent or negative. This could be obtained by a extending a model with positive dependence to also allow for negative dependence. Second, we need models, for the few cases of negative dependence. A particular case where negative dependence is quite possible is the model describing recurrent data from an alternating state process (Section 10.5.6). Otherwise, negative dependence could be due to competition for limited resources. The shared gamma frailty model of Section 7.3 can be extended to allow for negative dependence, but it has the peculiar feature that the probability mass is concentrated on a subset of $(0, \infty)^2$, and the restrictions become more tight with increasing dimension.

The multivariate normal frailty model is a simple model that adapts to negative dependence equally well as to positive dependence.

Another approach is due to Aalen (1987). He suggested a distribution, where (Y_1, Y_2) is the diagonal in a Wishart distributed matrix. The marginal distributions are then of gamma form, but it is a different distribution than the additive gamma model. In most cases, this model gives a positive dependence, but for some parameter values, the dependence is negative. This model, however, seems difficult to analyze, and it is complicated to specify when the dependence is negative. The example considered in that paper was a conditional Markov multi-state model, which includes the alternating state model as special case.

10.8   Other approaches

Two-level frailty models cover nested data, and thus cases like the trivariate model described above. It is generated as an extension of Equation (7.8). Let $L_0(s)$ be the Laplace transform of the common frailty term, and let there be a further frailty term, with Laplace transform $L_1(s)$, in order to describe further dependence between individual 2 and 3, as above. Then the survivor function is modeled as

$$S(t_1, t_2, t_3) = L_0(L_0^{-1}(S_1(t)) + L_0^{-1}(L_1(L_1^{-1}(S_2(t_2)) + L_1^{-1}(S_3(t_3))))).$$
$$(10.18)$$

The idea is that conditional on the shared frailty Y_0 individual 1 is independent of individuals 2 and 3. Furthermore, conditional on more specific frailties, individuals 2 and 3 are independent. It is, however, difficult to specify how the frailties enter in the model, except in the case of positive stable distributions. In this case, this approach gives the trivariate model of Section 10.4.1. In the case of gamma distributions, it leads to a model not previously described.

Sastry (1997) and Sargent (1998) considered a multiplicative model, similar to the treatment by center interaction model of Section 10.4.3, where the distributions of Z_0 and Z_1 are of gamma form. Maximum likelihood evaluation has not been performed, but it is possible to estimate the parameters by means of Markov chain Monte Carlo methods or an EM algorithm approach. These approaches are convenient in this framework. The probabilistic properties of this multiplicative gamma frailty model have not been considered.

10.9 Chapter summary

This chapter has considered how to construct models with more complicated dependence structures over individuals, but not more complicated structures over time. From a theoretical point of view, the multiplicative stable models are the most interesting, because they have more satisfactory properties regarding which parameters can be estimated from which data subset and the number of parameters in the frailty distribution equals the necessary number of dependence parameters. However, the fit is not necessarily satisfactory and not all dependence structures can be handled. Therefore, the additive models are more operational, it is easy to derive multivariate Laplace transforms, and the possible dependence structures are more flexible.

Truncation in the multiplicative stable leads to structures with PVF-like terms. In particular for combining monozygotic and dizygotic twins, the truncated data follow PVF models. For the additive gamma, truncation leads to a differential development in the θ parameters.

The multivariate lognormal frailty models have fewer nice theoretical properties, but it is easier to develop more complicated dependence structures, and depending on the estimation method used, we may avoid the rather complicated combinations of the terms in the additive models.

A disadvantage of the additive model is that we need more parameters to make models where the parameters cannot be identified from subsets of the data. For example, to describe two degrees of dependence, it is necessary to have three parameters. Table 10.17 shows models and properties that can be obtained by the multiplicative stable, the additive gamma and the lognormal model. The multiplicative models can be given a multiple

	Multiplicative stable	Additive gamma	Lognormal
Model			
MZ+DZ combination	x	x	x
(No. of parameters)	2	3	3
Random interaction	x	x	x
Pedigrees	-	x	x
Nested models	x	x	x
Non-nested models	-	x	x
Bivariate fit improvement	-	x	x
Negative dependence	-	-	x
Property			
Interpretation	MURF	HCD	MURF
Fits Weibull	x	-	-
Fits proportional hazards	x	-	-
Explicit evaluation	x	x	-
Truncation	PVF model	Non-common θ	Unknown

Table 10.17. Models covered and properties obtained by three multivariate frailty models. x, yes; -, no; MURF, multiple unobserved risk factors; HCD, hidden cause of death.

unobserved risk factor interpretation, whereas the additive models have an interpretation as hidden causes of deaths. The lognormal is the most flexible regarding the unobserved covariates.

Generally, these models appear to be in their infancy, with a large potential for further development and applications and a great need for experience.

10.10   Bibliographic comments

Most of these models are quite recent and are only described in a few papers. The trivariate multiplicative stable model was suggested by Hougaard (1986b). The additive gamma frailty model was considered by Vaupel and Yashin (1985) for the univariate case, and later Yashin and Iachine (1995) for the bivariate case. Parner (1998) has studied the consistency and asymptotic normality in the additive gamma model. Petersen (1998) studied the additive gamma frailty model and analyzed a data set on the lifetimes of biological and adoptive mothers and the adoptive child.

Aalen (1987) suggested bivariate frailty distributions for a Markov chain alternating state model, and considered particularly, when the dependence is positive or negative.

Lindeboom and van den Berg (1994) suggested the bivariate lognormal model. Xue and Brookmeyer (1996) consider a bivariate lognormal model for the alternating states model.

The two-level frailty models were described by Bandeen-Roche and Liang (1996).

10.11   Exercises

Exercise 10.1 Lognormal Weibull model moments

Consider a general bivariate lognormal frailty model with a Weibull conditional distribution. Find variances and covariances of the times and their correlation. Find variances and covariances of the log times and their correlation. What is the range of the correlations?

Exercise 10.2 Differential effect of a shared lognormal frailty

Consider a frailty model for bivariate data, with a differential effect of a shared lognormal frailty. That is, $Y_2 = Y_1^c$, where c is a real number. Describe two submodels that imply independence of times. For which values of c is the dependence positive, respectively negative? Show that the bivariate Laplace transform can be expressed by means of the univariate Laplace transform of Y_1. Use this to evaluate the density of bivariate times.

Specialize the results above to $c = -1$.

Exercise 10.3 Lognormal father-mother-child model

Make a multivariate lognormal frailty model for data on lifetimes of father, mother, and child. You need only consider the genetic dependence here. This can be done along two lines: you can let the dependence between father and child, respectively, mother and child vary freely, or one can use genetic laws for the correlation of frailties supplemented with a common variance parameter. The latter is easier to extend to general pedigrees. Make both models.

To which extent can the parameters be identified by means of bivariate data on mother and child?

Extend the model to allow for two children in each family.

Discuss the necessary truncation for such a dataset.

Exercise 10.4 Multiplicative stable gamma model

This is related to an exercise in Section 7.11. Suppose the frailty for individual j, $j = 1, 2$ can be described as $Y_j = Z^{1/\alpha} U_j$, where Z, U_1, and U_2 are independent, Z is gamma distributed with parameters (δ, δ) and U_1, and U_2 follow positive stable distributions of index α. Let the conditional hazard be Weibull of shape γ, and suppose there are covariates z_j for the jth individual, so that the conditional hazard model reads $Y_j \exp(\beta' z_j) \lambda \gamma t^{\gamma-1}$. Find the marginal distribution of a lifetime. Find the bivariate survivor function. What is the correlation of $\log T_1$ and $\log T_2$? Show that it is not possible to identify all parameters even with complete bivariate data. It is only possible to identify δ, $\alpha\beta$, λ^α, and $\alpha\gamma$.

Exercise 10.5 Trivariate multiplicative stable gamma model

The model above can be extended to the trivariate case. Suppose the frailty for individual j, $j = 1, 2, 3$ can be described as $Y_j = Z^{1/\alpha} U_j$, where Z, U_1, and U_2 are independent, $U_2 = U_3$, Z is gamma distributed with parameters (δ, δ) and U_1 and U_2 follow positive stable distributions of index α. Show that this is a special case of Equation (10.18). Find Kendall's τ for (T_1, T_2) and for (T_2, T_3). Hint: You may need results of Exercise 7.25.

Exercise 10.6 Additive stable model

Find the bivariate density of the lifetimes, when the frailty model is that of Equation (10.7), with positive stable distributions for Z_0, Z_1, Z_2, assuming the same value of α and $\delta_1 = \delta_2$.

Exercise 10.7 Marshall-Olkin frailty model

As the bivariate Laplace transform of the Marshall-Olkin model is known (see Equation (5.26)), this can also be used as a bivariate frailty distribution. For the most generality, also introduce a convolution parameter, say, δ, so that (Y_1, Y_2) are obtained as the sum of δ independent copies of the Marshall-Olkin distribution. Start with δ integer and show it can be extended to all positive values. How would you restrict the parameters in order to avoid the scale parameter? Which model is obtained in the special case $\varphi_1 = \varphi_2 = 0$? Which model is obtained in the special case $\varphi_0 = 0$?

Exercise 10.8 Median concordance for twins

Evaluate the dependence measure κ for the estimates of Table 10.11. Compare to the estimated values of τ.

11

Instantaneous and short-term frailty models

Dependence has previously been classified into three time frames: instantaneous, short-term, and long-term (Section 3.2). Almost all the standard models studied until now lead to long-term dependence. Important examples are the Markov multi-state models and the shared frailty models. Only a single standard model, the Marshall-Olkin model of Section 5.5.4, displays instantaneous dependence. No standard models show short-term dependence, even though we have argued that many common subject matter problems possibly or probably display short-term dependence. Therefore, it makes sense to develop models that can be used to discuss whether the dependence is of short-term or long-term time frame. Multi-state models can easily be constructed to model short-term dependence by releasing the Markov assumption, substituting with a Markov extension model as shown in Chapter 5, but they have no interpretation, whereas a frailty model has an interpretation as a random effects model. In particular for frailty models, it is an advantage to have short-term dependence models for checking the fit of the ordinary shared frailty model. The aim of this chapter is to extend the frailty models to describe both instantaneous and short-term dependence.

On the general level, these models are random effects models with three sources of variation. For parallel data, these are group effects and individual random effects, as in the shared frailty model, and besides this, there is a random group by time interaction effect. For recurrent events, the corresponding random effects are individual variation and simple variation, which in this chapter is supplemented with a random variation over time.

This chapter describes the models both for parallel data and recurrent events.

The models of this chapter do require further development and further application before they can be applied routinely. The aim of this chapter is to present the concepts and the ideas and open up a new area of research. This chapter is more difficult to follow and includes fewer ready-to-use expressions than the rest of this book. Consequently, readers who are only interested in the better-established models may prefer to omit this chapter.

A major problem with these models is their mathematical complexity. It is not possible to handle the most interesting models; that is, it is necessary to consider models that are simpler than desired, which is disappointing from a practical point of view. For example, we would prefer a model with the frailty varying in continuous time, but it is easier to study models, where the frailty is piecewise constant. A consequence of this is that the model is not truly a short-term dependence model, within each interval the dependence is rather of long-term time frame. Another point along this line is that we would prefer a multiplicative model rather than an additive, but multiplicative models appear to be more complicated computationally. Also the models considered here will often assume constant hazards in order to simplify the evaluations.

Instantaneous dependence can be obtained by the frailty being modeled as an independent increments process (Section 11.1). This is a continuous time model for a randomly varying environment. In that case, the common risks are independent for disjoint time intervals, implying the possibility of several events' happening at the same time. In the case of recurrent events, this model can also be derived by means of a subordinated stochastic process. This derivation corresponds to a randomly varying speed of time. Furthermore, this process can be added to a constant frailty process, giving a model containing both the constant frailty model and the independent increments frailty model so that the relevance of both models can be tested in a proper way (Section 11.2).

Short-term dependence is mathematically more complicated to handle than instantaneous dependence, but more relevant in practice. It can be introduced by models similar to the additive models described in Chapter 10, but having the additive structure over time rather than over individuals (Section 11.3). This gives a model with piecewise constant frailty. Section 11.4 describes a moving average model, which is a model intended for reducing the jumps in the dependence in the piecewise constant frailty model of Section 11.3.

Another idea that can be used to generate short-term dependence is a hidden cause of death model (Section 11.5), which is still a shared frailty model. This is based on the idea that each person has a constant, but multivariate frailty, with one coordinate for each cause of death. This makes it possible to have a more smooth change over time. However, this model requires major development before it can be applied in practice.

Also, the frailty can be described as a diffusion process (Section 11.6). This offers the advantage that the frailty varies smoothly over time. There is a lot of potential in this idea, but the computational difficulties are huge. This model has only been considered theoretically for the univariate case, so it is still unknown whether it can be used in the bivariate case.

11.1 Independent increments frailty model

This model is a model leading to instantaneous dependence, that is, simultaneous events. Compared to the shared frailty models of Chapter 7, it substitutes the constant frailty, Y, with a stochastic process common to all individuals in the group. This describes a common risks model in a randomly changing environment. It will be formulated so that it is the increments of the process $\tilde{Y}(t)$ that describe the risk at time t. The tilde refers to the process's being an integrated value. To be precise, the integrated conditional hazard is $\tilde{Y}(t)$ conditional on the frailty process. This generalizes the expression $YM(t)$ from the shared frailty model. Thus, the time-dependent frailty formulation allows for a combination of the frailty and the hazard term. It is assumed that $\{\tilde{Y}(t)\}_{t \geq 0}$ constitutes an increasing stochastic process, with $\tilde{Y}(0) = 0$. The process is assumed to have independent increments; that is, that $\{\tilde{Y}(t) - \tilde{Y}(s)\}_{t \geq s}$ is independent of $\{\tilde{Y}(t)\}_{0 \leq t \leq s}$. It can have stationary increments, in which case $E\tilde{Y}(t) = t\mu$, or non-stationary increments. In general, this makes a process with jumps. For parallel data, this model is considered in Section 11.1.1, and for recurrent events in Section 11.1.2.

11.1.1 Bivariate parallel data

The individuals in a group are assumed to share the same realization of $\tilde{Y}(t)$, and the groups are assumed independent, but have the same distribution of the stochastic process. As usual, the individuals are assumed independent, given the frailty stochastic process. Then it is assumed that the conditional survivor function for two individuals in a group is

$$S(t_1, t_2 \mid \tilde{Y}(u), 0 \leq u \leq \infty)) = \exp[-\{\tilde{Y}(t_1) + \tilde{Y}(t_2)\}] \tag{11.1}$$

As the right-hand side only depends on $\tilde{Y}(t)$ up to the largest time point, this is equivalent to

$$S(t_1, t_2 \mid \tilde{Y}(u), 0 \leq u \leq \max\{t_1, t_2\}).$$

The marginal distribution for a single individual is found in the usual way, and turns out to be the Laplace transform of $\tilde{Y}(t)$ evaluated at 1, that is,

$$S_1(t) = E \exp(-\tilde{Y}(t)). \tag{11.2}$$

Similarly, the bivariate survival function is found by integrating $\tilde{Y}(t)$ out. At the diagonal, we simply find $S(t,t) = E\exp\{-2\tilde{Y}(t)\}$, that is, the Laplace transform of $\tilde{Y}(t)$, evaluated at 2. More generally, we find

$$S(t_1, t_2) = E\exp\{-2\tilde{Y}(t_1)\}E\exp[-\{\tilde{Y}(t_2) - \tilde{Y}(t_1)\}] \qquad (11.3)$$

when $t_1 \leq t_2$, with a corresponding expression for $t_2 < t_1$, utilizing the independent increments assumption. The consequence of the independent increments assumption is that the risks of events in any two intervals are independent given the risk set. In other words, the probability of a given individual's failing in an interval given that he was alive at the beginning of the interval is independent of the history regarding the other individuals in the group. As we will see below, the dependence is obtained by there being a chance of simultaneous events, and thus this is conceptually the same idea as the Marshall and Olkin model (Section 5.5.4). This makes the model relevant for data on similar organs, but less so for several individuals.

The most commonly used process is the gamma process. For the gamma process with independent stationary increments, the increment $\tilde{Y}(t) - \tilde{Y}(s)$, say, ΔY, from time s to time t is gamma distributed, with parameters $(t-s)\delta$ and θ. This gives a mean increase of $(t-s)\delta/\theta$. The model for the hazard is a constant at 1, so that the integrated hazard for that interval is ΔY. From Equation (11.2), we find that the univariate survivor function is $S_1(t) = \{\theta/(1+\theta)\}^{\delta t}$, from which we derive the hazard as $\omega(t) = \delta\log(1 + 1/\theta)$, which turns out not to depend on t, and thus is shortened to ω. To find the probability of simultaneous events for two individuals, we first evaluate the bivariate survivor function on the diagonal, $S(t,t) = \{\theta/(2+\theta)\}^{\delta t}$. The probability of both dying before time t is found using Equation (5.6). The hazard does not depend on t, when the risk set is fixed. Letting $t \to 0$, we find that there is a hazard of $\omega_2 = \delta\{2\log(1+1/\theta) - \log(1+2/\theta)\}$ for simultaneous events, and $\omega_1 = \omega - \omega_2$ for death of a specific single individual when the risk set is 2. The conditional distribution of a single event given that one or two has failed is independent of δ. It is not precisely the Marshall-Olkin model (Section 5.5.4), but is a special case of the combined multi-state model (Section 5.5.5).

11.1.2 Recurrent events

In principle, the same evaluations can be performed for recurrent events. Whether instantaneous dependence is relevant for recurrent events data depends on the actual case considered. In some cases, it is physically impossible to experience two events simultaneously; in other cases it is possible. Even when it is physically impossible to experience several events simultaneously, this model may make sense as an approximation, when the dependence is extremely short-term. Overall, the theory is simpler for instantaneous dependence compared to short-term dependence, but less often relevant in practice. The formulas turn out to be different from those of parallel data, because the risk set is constant. In fact, they are simpler and mathematically nicer.

An alternative formulation is as a subordinated time model, using $\{\tilde{Y}(t)\}$ as time process. As before, it is a real-valued increasing stochastic process in continuous time, starting at 0. The idea is that this process describes the real time scale, in which the events happen independently, so that $\{N(y)\}$ is a homogeneous Poisson process. As there is a scale parameter in the time process, we can without loss of generality take the rate parameter of the Poisson process as 1. For example, the time process describes the accumulated use of the object. A standard example is the risk of car accidents, where risk depends on the distance driven, with $\tilde{Y}(t)$ as the cumulative mileage, but as this process is not monitored we have to observe the number of events over calendar time t, so we observe the process given by $K(t) = N(\tilde{Y}(t))$. The time process considered here is a process with stationary independent increments, an assumption that leads to the count process $K(t)$ having stationary independent increments. The distributions of the increments $(\tilde{Y}(t) - \tilde{Y}(s))$ will be either gamma or general PVF, $\text{PVF}(\alpha, \delta(t - s), \theta)$. For interval count data given by interval end points, $0 < x_1 < ... < x_m$, the number of events in each interval are independent and the distribution of the number in the jth interval, $K(x_j) - K(x_{j-1})$ is $\text{P-PVF}(\alpha, \delta(x_j - x_{j-1}), \theta)$.

The event process $K(t)$ is an overdispersed Poisson model with independent increments, two properties that appear conflicting. It is, however, possible because the count process has clusters, that is, multiple events happening simultaneously. To see this, we first find the hazard of any event at time t, as $\omega = \lim_{\Delta t \to 0} 1 - Pr\{K(t + \Delta t) - K(t) = 0\}/\Delta t$, independently of t. This probability evaluation is, for the gamma process case, found by Equation (9.10) with parameters $\delta \Delta t$ and θ. The hazard of precisely r events is found as $\omega_r = \lim_{\Delta t \to 0} p(r)/\Delta t$. The number of events, R, in a cluster, is a distribution on the numbers $\{1, 2, ...\}$, and the probability mass is found as ω_r/ω , which in the gamma process case is

$$q(r) = (\theta + 1)^{-r}/[r\{\log(\theta + 1) - \log \theta\}]. \tag{11.4}$$

In the general PVF case $(\alpha \neq 0)$, the probabilities are

$$q(r) = \alpha(\theta + 1)^{\alpha - r}\Gamma(r - \alpha)/[r!\Gamma(1 - \alpha)\{(\theta + 1)^\alpha - \theta^\alpha\}]. \tag{11.5}$$

In both cases, the parameter δ cancels out. The probabilities are decreasing in r when $\theta > -(1 + \alpha)/2$, which for $\alpha \geq -1$ is satisfied for all θ. In particular, the masses decrease for the gamma and positive stable special cases. Generally, the mass decreases only for $r \geq -(1 + \alpha)/\theta$. The distribution is always unimodal.

The distribution of the number of events at a time with events is an exponential family with canonical parameter $\log(\theta + 1)$. The mean in this distribution is $ER = 1/[\theta\{\log(\theta + 1) - \log \theta\}]$ for $\alpha = 0$ and $\alpha\theta^{\alpha-1}/\{(\theta + 1)^\alpha - \theta^\alpha\}$ for $\alpha \neq 0$, $\theta > 0$. In the case of $\theta = 0$, the distribution has infinite

Property	Generalized Polya	Indep. increments
Parameters of P-PVF	α	α
distribution of $K(t)$	$t^\alpha \delta$	$t\delta$
	θ/t	θ
$E\{K(t)\}$	μt	μt
$\mathrm{Var}\{K(t)\}$	$\mu t + \sigma^2 t^2$	$\mu t + \sigma^2 t$
Jump sizes	1	$1,2,...$
$K(t)$ indep. increments	No	Yes

Table 11.1. Similarities and differences between the generalized Polya and the independent increments PVF frailty process. Moments exist for $\theta > 0$, in which case $\mu = \delta\theta^{\alpha-1}$, $\sigma^2 = \delta(1-\alpha)\theta^{\alpha-2}$.

mean. The Laplace transform of this variable is

$$E(e^{-sR}) = \frac{s + \log(\theta+1) - \log\{e^s(\theta+1)-1\}}{\log(\theta+1) - \log\theta},$$

when $\alpha = 0$ and

$$E(e^{-sR}) = \frac{(\theta+1)^\alpha - (\theta+1-e^{-s})^\alpha}{(\theta+1)^\alpha - \theta^\alpha},$$

when $\alpha \neq 0$.

The clusters arrive according to a Poisson process, the rate of which, say λ, can be derived as $E\tilde{Y}(1)/ER$, which gives $\delta\{\log(\theta+1) - \log\theta\}$ for $\alpha = 0$ and $\delta\{(\theta+1)^\alpha - \theta^\alpha\}/\alpha$ for $\alpha \neq 0$, $\theta > 0$. Thus the arrival process depends only on the parameter function λ, and the cluster distribution depends only on the two parameters (α, θ).

When $\alpha = -1$, $R - 1$ follows a geometric distribution, which in the present terminology means that $R - 1$ follows P-PVF$(0, 1, \theta + 1)$.

As mentioned above, the distribution of $K(t)$ is in the P-PVF family both for the generalized Polya process of Chapter 9 and the independent increments process, but the parameters change in different ways over time. Table 11.1 gives a comparison of the two processes. The mean increases linearly in both cases, but the variances have different developments. One term (the Poisson error) increases linearly, but the term depending on the frailty increases linearly for the independent increments model, and quadratically for the generalized Polya process. Asymptotically, the two processes can be discriminated when exact times of events are recorded, because the independent increments process allows for simultaneous events, and the generalized Polya does not.

11.1.3 Estimation for recurrent events

If the processes are observed in continuous time, data consist of times of event clusters and for each cluster, the number of events in the cluster. In the case of a set of identically distributed homogeneous stochastic processes, the cluster process parameter λ can be estimated as the number of clusters divided by the total time studied. The parameters (α, θ) can be found just by considering the distribution of the number of events in the clusters. This is just a parametric model describing discrete outcomes, $1, 2, \dots$. As the cluster size distribution is an exponential family for α fixed, the first moment equation will be included in the maximum likelihood equations, both when α is known and unknown.

If the observations are not recorded in continuous time, but describe the number of events in some intervals of the same length, they can be analyzed in the same way as the period count data (Section 9.3.4), with the modification that there is a single observation for each interval and intervals are independent. Thus each combination of subject and interval corresponds to a subject in the count data approach.

11.1.4   Estimation for parallel data

This case has never been considered in the literature. In the bivariate constant hazards case, however, this makes a parametric model, which is a submodel in the multi-state model combining the Marshall-Olkin model and the Freund model (Section 5.5.5), so at least a sufficient statistic is the number of single and double events when the risk set is 2 and the number of events, when the risk set is 1, and the total times for all periods when the risk set is 1 and 2. The symmetric version of the combined model has 3 parameters, as has the PVF frailty model, suggesting that the estimate can be found directly. Of course, it is possible that there are points, which do not correspond to a PVF solution.

11.1.5   Asymptotics

For the parametric models considered here, there are no unexpected asymptotic problems. Owing to the independence over time, observing a single process is sufficient to identify all parameters in the case of recurrent events, both when the observations are done in continuous time and when they consist of interval counts. It can be difficult to identify all parameters in the case of interval count data, if the intervals are so long that each interval contains many clusters.

When observations are recorded in continuous time, it is possible to evaluate the Fisher information in the case of $\alpha = 0$, which will be left as an exercise.

For interval count data, the asymptotic theory is completely covered by Section 9.7.

11.1.6 Application

The epileptic seizure data of Section 1.7.2 are interval count data with four intervals of two weeks. According to the independent increments frailty model, the distribution of the number of events in an interval is P-PVF(α, δ, θ), if the time unit is chosen as two weeks. All event counts are independent and it follows that we can estimate the parameters by means of the methods for period count data (described in Chapter 9). For the placebo group, the data are then structured as 112 intervals rather than as 28 patients. For the gamma model applied to the placebo group, assuming the same parameter values for all intervals, the estimates are $\hat{\delta} = 1.130$ (0.166) and $\hat{\theta} = 0.1314$ (0.0239), implying a mean of 8.60 (0.81) events per two weeks, in perfect agreement with the empirical mean. The likelihood is -358.91.

For the full independent increments PVF frailty model, the estimates are $\hat{\alpha} = 0.581$ (0.102), $\hat{\delta} = 2.06$ (0.36) and $\hat{\theta} = 0.0333$ (0.0193), implying a mean of 8.60 (1.02) events per two weeks. Again the estimated mean is in perfect agreement with the empirical mean. The likelihood is -353.81. Thus, this model fits significantly better than the gamma model. The estimate is rather close to the inverse Gaussian submodel.

For showing the use of covariates, we also consider the data as two periods of four weeks, in order to find out whether there is a trend over time, that is, whether the seizure rate is the same during the last four weeks as during the first four weeks. As above, the placebo data set can be fitted as 56 independent observations for count data, but in this case with two different scale parameters. For the gamma model, the estimates are $\hat{\delta} = 1.311$ (0.248) and $\hat{\theta} = 0.0743$ (0.0190), referring to the first interval and a ratio for the second interval of 0.949 (0.230). The estimated means in both intervals agree with the empirical means, 17.64, respectively, 16.75; and correspondingly the ratio agrees with the empirical ratio and the ratio in the constant frailty models (Section 9.8). However, the standard error on the ratio is clearly increased. The likelihood for these bivariate counts is -215.90, which is not comparable to the values above because the intervals used are different. In the PVF model the estimates are $\hat{\alpha} = 0.661$ (0.094), $\hat{\delta} = 3.847$ (0.878), and $\hat{\theta} = 0.0116$ (0.0103) and a ratio of 0.973 (0.222). In this case the estimated means in the two intervals (17.42 and 16.96) do not agree perfectly with the empirical means. The log likelihood is -210.40.

11.2 Polya and independent increments additive model

The generalized Polya model of Section 9.3 had a constant frailty value, (with a linearly increasing stochastic process, $\tilde{Y}(t) = Yt$, in the frailty process terminology of this chapter) leading to long-term dependence. The independent increments frailty model of Section 11.1.2 is another extreme, displaying instantaneous dependence. A compromise between these extremes appears to be more useful. The aim of this section is to construct a model for recurrent events that includes both models and makes it possible to quantify the fit of both. From a mathematical point of view, the easiest way to do so appears to be in an additive model.

Specifically, the constant frailty part leads to a count process $K_P(t)$, (P for Polya) following P-PVF($\alpha, \delta_P t^\alpha, \theta_P/t$) and the independent increments process leads to a count process $K_I(t)$ (I for independent increments) following P-PVF($\alpha, \delta_I t, \theta_I$). Then the total number of events accumulated to time t is $K(t) = K_P(t) + K_I(t)$. If $\theta_P = \theta_I = 0$, the frailty processes are stable processes and $K(t)$ follows P-PVF($\alpha, \delta_P t^\alpha + \delta_I t, 0$). In general, however, this additive process will not have simple marginal distributions, because the last parameter has different behavior with t. When θ_P and θ_I are positive, there will only be a single time point $t = \theta_P/\theta_I$, where $K(t)$ is in the P-PVF family.

When $\theta_P = \theta_I$ and the observations consist of period count data (length 1), the marginal distribution of the number of events is P-PVF($\alpha, \delta_P + \delta_I, \theta$). Thus δ_P and δ_I cannot be separately identified, only their sum. Without the restriction on θ, all parameters can be identified, except that there is a symmetry relation so that it is impossible to find out whether a given θ refers to the Polya part or the independent increments part. Thus, from an identifiability point of view the restriction $\theta_P = \theta_I$ seems natural, but as said above, for the whole process there is only a single time point, where this is satisfied and generally, there is no reason to believe that this happens exactly at the interval end point.

In particular, for interval count data, we can define Z_0 as the frailty for the Polya part and Z_q as the increase in the qth interval of the independent increments frailty process. With intervals of the same length (without loss of generality length 1), Z_0 is PVF($\alpha, \delta_P, \theta_P$) and Z_q is PVF($\alpha, \delta_I, \theta_I$), $q = 1, ..., m$. Furthermore, $Z_0, Z_1, ..., Z_m$ are assumed independent. This gives a similar additive structure to that of Equation (10.7). The data will be of the form $K_{iq}, q = 1, ..., m$, where individuals are denoted by i and intervals by q. The probability distribution can be derived by means of a convolution formula, which in the case of two intervals is

$$p(k_1, k_2) = \sum_{r=0}^{k_1} \sum_{s=0}^{k_2} p_0(r, s) p_1(k_1 - r) p_2(k_2 - s), \qquad (11.6)$$

where $p_0(r, s)$ is the probability distribution of the interval counts based on only the Polya process, Equation (9.15), and the p_1 and p_2 are the distributions of the events owing to $K_I(\cdot)$ in the two intervals.

In the more general case of exact times, the convolution formula is similar to Equation (10.11).

When there are several intervals, there is no computational advantage of the assumption $\theta_P = \theta_I$, because θ enters in different ways for the p_0 as for the p_1 and p_2 terms in Equation (11.6).

With all parameters varying freely (and with α fixed), the model contains a one-dimensional natural exponential family. As the submodel of the one-dimensional exponential family is not a particularly interesting model, the advantages of this result are limited. The advantages are that the first moment equation is contained in the maximum likelihood equation and consequently that the estimated mean equals the observed mean. Under the restriction $\theta_P = \theta_I$, the model does not include a one-dimensional natural exponential family.

11.2.1 Application

The data on epileptic seizures, of Section 1.7.2, cover count data for four periods of two weeks. Thus they can be analyzed by the additive model of Equation (11.7), and it is possible to evaluate whether there are time-varying random effects.

Suppose first that the frailty is constant, that is, corresponding to the generalized Polya process. Then the total number of events for each individual $(K_{i\cdot})$ is sufficient. In fact, the results are quoted in Table 9.4. However, that section uses a time unit of eight weeks and here we use a time unit of two weeks, corresponding to a parameter transformation, $\delta_8 = \delta_2 4^\alpha$ and $\theta_8 = \theta_2/4$. The likelihood employs a different observation dependent constant, describing the multinomial conditional distribution of the events in the intervals given the total number of events, Equation (9.15). This implies that the estimates using the unit of two weeks are $\hat\alpha = 0.719$ (0.095), $\hat\delta = 2.73$ (0.43) and $\hat\theta = 0.0168$ (0.0235). The likelihood becomes -355.23.

If the independent increments frailty model applies, the results are quoted in Section 11.1.6.

The additive model of this section gives a full estimate of $\hat\alpha = 0.611$ (0.126), $\hat\delta_0 = 1.615$ (0.446), $\hat\delta_1 = 0.617$ (0.355) and $\hat\theta_0 = 0.0332$ (0.0386) and $\hat\theta_1 = 0.0270$ (0.272). The log likelihood becomes -327.33. The mean of the number of events is 8.60 (1.72), equal to the empirical mean. In fact, one can derive means and variances for the two processes separately. Thus the mean for the Polya process and the independent increments part over a two-week interval are 6.08 and 2.52, respectively, whereas the standard deviations for are 8.45 and 6.02, respectively. From this we conclude that the Polya part is the most important.

One might employ the restriction $\theta_I = \theta_P$. The advantage of this is that then the marginal distributions of $Z_0 + Z_q$ is in the PVF family, with a distribution of the form $\text{PVF}(\alpha, \delta_0 + \delta_1, \theta)$. It follows that the degree of dependence, modeled by $\delta_0/(\delta_0 + \delta_1)$ cannot be estimated by data from only a single interval for each patient. In this model, the full estimate is

$\hat{\alpha} = 0.616$ (0.118), $\hat{\delta}_0 = 1.583$ (0.391), $\hat{\delta}_1 = 0.651$ (0.274) and $\hat{\theta} = 0.0291$ (0.0242). The estimated mean in this model is 8.69 (1.68). As this model no longer contains a one-parameter natural exponential family, the estimated mean can and does differ from the empirical mean. The log likelihood is -327.34. Thus this model does not fit significantly worse than the full model.

For studying whether there is a trend over time, the data are considered as two intervals of four weeks with a covariate being 0 for the first interval and 1 for the second interval. In the gamma model, we obtain estimates $\hat{\delta}_0 = 1.354$ (0.414), $\hat{\delta}_1 = 0.124$ (0.105), $\hat{\theta}_0 = 0.0896$ (0.0312) and $\hat{\theta}_1 = 0.0343$ (0.0263), describing the distribution in the first interval and the ratio is 0.847 (0.094). The ratio is somewhat lower than the empirical ratio. A more detailed study has shown that this is due to the estimate being less dependent on patients and intervals with an extreme number of events. The standard error lies between the value found for the Poisson and shared frailty model (0.06) and the value found for the independent increments model (0.23). This is just as expected as the model now includes all sources of variation. The log likelihood is -203.88. For the PVF model, the estimates are $\hat{\alpha}_0 = 0.668$ (0.111), $\hat{\delta}_0 = 3.155$ (0.973), $\hat{\delta}_1 = 0.124$ (0.105) and $\hat{\theta}_0 = 0.0111$ (0.0149), $\hat{\theta}_1 = 0.0095$ (0.0155) and the ratio is 0.843 (0.087). The log likelihood is -200.51. Thus the PVF model fits significantly better than the gamma model. The two models agree well regarding the ratio.

In this model, it does not make sense to assume that $\theta_0 = \theta_1$, because that would imply that the marginal distribution of the number of events in the first interval is in the P-PVF family, but the corresponding distribution for the second interval would not be in the family.

Overall, we conclude that it is possible to fit this model, when the number of intervals is small.

11.3   Piecewise gamma model

The model to be suggested is an attempt to make a short-term dependence model, but due to mathematical complexity, it is not developed in continuous time and therefore does strictly speaking not make a short-term dependence model. This piecewise gamma model uses a similar additive description as covered by what we will here call the subject based model of Section 10.5 shown in Equation (10.7), but instead of letting the subscript correspond to persons, it corresponds to time intervals. This can then be called a time-varying shared frailty model. To be specific, define interval cutpoints $0 = x_0 \leq x_1 \leq ... \leq x_m = \infty$, and assume that there is a general frailty Z_0 valid for all intervals, and interval specific frailties Z_q, $q = 1, ..., m$, where Z_q applies for the period x_{q-1} to x_q, and the hazard at time t for all the individuals in the group is

$$(Z_0 + Z_q)\mu(t), \text{ for } x_{q-1} < t \le x_q. \tag{11.7}$$

Thus the frailty is $Y(t) = Z_0 + Z_q$, when $x_{q-1} < t \le x_q$. The frailty process defined above then is $\tilde{Y}(t) = Z_0 t + \sum_q Z_q\{\min(t, x_q) - \min(t, x_{q-1})\}$. This will be called a stochastic process, even though it is piecewise linear and the number of slopes over time can be as low as two. There might very well be more than two intervals. Despite the appearance of the model formula being like the additive gamma model, it has a completely different interpretation. The piecewise gamma approach theoretically makes much more sense than the additive subjects model in the parallel case, because we do not mix the unobserved individual random variation (described by Z_1 and Z_2 in the subject based model) and the simple random variation described by the hazard function. This is due to the frailty value being common to several individuals. In the piecewise model, the individuals in the group share the whole frailty term and thus all individual variation is described by the hazard function. Similarly, for recurrent events, there can be many events in each interval, making it possible to identify all parameters.

This model is inspired by a model with the same name suggested by Paik, Tsai and Ottman (1994), but it is rather different in the sense that the present model has the time-dependent quantities, $(Z_1, ..., Z_m)$, common to the individuals, whereas the model of Paik *et al.* assumes that they are independent, similar to Section 10.5. The Paik model is not a time-varying shared frailty model.

In the simplest case we take $m = 2$, so the only quantity we need to decide upon is x_1, the limit so that before time x_1 the shared frailty is $Y_1 = Z_0 + Z_1$ and after this time point, it is $Y_2 = Z_0 + Z_2$. The simplest approach is to take all distributions of Z_0, Z_1, Z_2 as gamma variables with the same scale parameter θ. This implies that the distributions of Y_1 and Y_2 are also gamma with the same scale parameter. Again, it is necessary to restrict the distribution in some way to obtain identifiability and the simplest choice is $\delta_0 + \delta_1 = \theta$. This secures that the mean frailty before time x_1 is 1. It is more difficult to say what to do regarding the second interval. As the initial model, we might take $\delta_2 = \delta_1$, which means that the mean of Y_2 will also be 1, when evaluated at birth. The correlation of (Y_1, Y_2) is $\delta_0/(\delta_0 + \delta_1)$.

This should, however, not necessarily be the final model, because, one of the aspects we are interested in examining is whether the degree of dependence changes over time, which is then not possible. For example, the early failures can be random (or you could say individual), that is, Z_1 has no variation, and there is no dependence initially, whereas the inherited diseases show up in the old ages, implying a higher variation in Z_2.

11.3.1 Bivariate parallel data

To calculate the likelihood in this model, we need a derivation similar in scope to Equation (10.9), but necessarily more complicated as we need to separate the contributions for each interval for each individual. Let $M_{jq}(t)$ be the contribution to the integrated conditional hazard for individual j, in interval q. This can be written as the shorthand notation $M_{jq} = M_{jq}(t_j) = \int_{\min(x_{q-1},t_j)}^{\min(x_q,t_j)} \mu_j(u)du$. The bivariate survivor function is calculated similar to Equation (10.8) and after rearranging the terms, we obtain

$$S(t_1, t_2 \mid Z_0, Z_1, Z_2)$$

$$= \exp\{-Z_0(\sum_{jk} M_{jk}) - Z_1(M_{11} + M_{21}) - Z_2(M_{12} + M_{22})\}. \qquad (11.8)$$

This is integrated over the frailties to give

$$S(t_1, t_2) = L_0(M_{11} + M_{12} + M_{21} + M_{22})L_1(M_{11} + M_{21})L_2(M_{12} + M_{22}), \qquad (11.9)$$

similar to Equation (10.9), but with more terms in the arguments. This can be differentiated with respect to t_1 and t_2 to give the density, but there will be more terms than in Equation (10.10), as we need the double derivatives of $L_1(s)$ and $L_2(s)$. It is convenient to write the equation in the same way as Equation (10.11). If both events are in the first interval, M_{12} and M_{22} are 0 and the formula looks like

$$\mu_1(t_1)\mu_2(t_2)\{L_0''L_1 + 2L_0'L_1' + L_0L_1''\},$$

where we have abbreviated the formula by excluding the arguments to the Laplace transforms. The arguments are specified in Equation (11.9). If there is one event in the first and one in the second, the formula is

$$\mu_1(t_1)\mu_2(t_2)\{L_0''L_1L_2 + L_0'L_1'L_2 + L_0'L_1L_2' + L_0L_1'L_2'\},$$

which is close to that of Equation (10.11), except that the arguments are different. If both events are in the second interval, the formula is

$$\mu_1(t_1)\mu_2(t_2)\{L_0''L_1L_2 + 2L_0'L_1L_2' + L_0L_1L_2''\}.$$

An alternative way to perform these calculations is to observe that it corresponds to the nested model of Section 10.5.4. All the data of the first interval are considered as coming from subgroup 1. If no events are observed, the data are censored at x_1. The survivors of the first interval contribute with their experience in the second interval as coming from subgroup 2, with truncation at time x_1. If no events are observed, the data are censored at x_2. This approach is then continued for all intervals. This approach is then continued for all intervals. This implies that with bivariate data for two intervals, the approach gives a likelihood corresponding to those of Section 10.5 for four individuals in two subgroups, allowing for truncation, but at most experiencing two events in any group.

It is somewhat more difficult to evaluate properties for this model than for the shared frailty model, but one thing that can be noticed immediately is that up to time x_1, the data will behave exactly like those of a shared frailty model, with frailty Y_1. In the case mentioned above, this will be a shared gamma frailty model, with Y_1 being gamma distributed, with mean 1 and parameter θ. This, inter alia, implies that an initial estimate for θ can be obtained by censoring all individuals at time x_1 and using a shared frailty model. If x_1 is chosen to be after the median this implies that the median concordance follows the same formula (Equation (7.36)) as derived for the shared gamma frailty model.

A similar approach cannot be used to study Y_2, because the distribution of the common component Z_0 changes over time, and thus is different at time x_1 than it was initially.

11.3.2   Recurrent events

Of course, the natural intervals over which to perform interval count data are the intervals during which the frailties are constant. In that case, the observed data follow the model described in Section 11.3. As said above, when the data are observed in intervals, it is the same as the additive independent increments model. However, when observation is done on the basis of the exact times, they disagree. The piecewise gamma model does not allow for simultaneous events, but in the additive model, there could be such events owing to the independent increments process. With interval count data, it is impossible to discriminate between simultaneous events and event happening at different times in the same interval.

11.3.3   Applications

For the data on twins of Section 1.5.1, we start with a gamma frailty model, with $m = 2$ and the same value of the θ parameter, and with $\delta_1 = \delta_2$. For normalization, we take the mean at the start equal to 1, that is, $\delta_0 + \delta_1 = \theta$. That leaves us with only two parameters, θ, δ_0. Table 11.2 gives the estimates from the shared piecewise gamma frailty model, with two intervals. The first columns report the results of the constant shared frailty model of Table 8.23 for comparison purposes, but here listing δ rather than τ. The other columns give the results for the piecewise gamma model, using a threshold of x_1=20,000 days, corresponding to about 54.8 years. Monozygotic and dizygotic female twins show a significant improvement compared to the constant frailty model. The estimate for males of unknown zygosity is on the boundary corresponding to the constant frailty model. For the other three data sets, the model is insignificantly improved compared to the constant frailty model.

To illustrate the robustness towards the choice of x_1, we have done the same calculations using an interval end point of 30,000 days, corresponding

	$\hat{\theta}$ (SE)	$\hat{\delta}_0$ (SE)	$\hat{\theta}$ (SE)	$\Delta \log L$
Males				
MZ	1.918 (0.334)	1.327 (0.556)	1.728 (0.333)	0.46
DZ	5.570 (1.632)	3.768 (2.899)	4.981 (1.657)	0.14
UZ	1.506 (0.431)	1.506	1.506	0
Females				
MZ	2.073 (0.431)	0.436 (0.356)	1.488 (0.293)	4.09
DZ	3.419 (0.773)	0.861 (0.605)	2.448 (0.498)	3.14
UZ	2.365 (0.758)	0.787 (0.872)	1.852 (0.597)	0.80

Table 11.2. Estimates of parameters in constant and piecewise gamma frailty model for Danish twin data, with a threshold of $x_1 = 20,000$ days.

	$\hat{\delta}_0$ (SE)	$\hat{\theta}$ (SE)	$\Delta \log L$
Males			
MZ	1.783 (0.661)	1.903 (0.335)	0.03
DZ	0	4.225	4.13
UZ	0	1.300	3.09
Females			
MZ	2.073	2.073	0
DZ	1.333 (1.400)	3.068 (0.635)	1.06
UZ	1.304 (1.241)	2.236 (0.595)	0.31

Table 11.3. Estimates of parameters in the piecewise gamma frailty model, for Danish twin data, with a threshold of $x_1 = 30,000$ days.

to 82.1 years. This is shown in Table 11.3. It makes no sense directly to compare these models, because they are in conflict to each other. However, the robustness of the approach can be illustrated by evaluating Kendall's τ in the various models. This is done in Table 11.4. This shows that the piecewise gamma model gives values of Kendall's τ that are rather close to those of the shared frailty model. Even though the piecewise model increases the likelihood, it probably is not really well fitting owing to the abrupt change in dependence at the threshold between the two intervals. It suggests high dependence within each interval, and smaller dependence between intervals. A more continuous model would be more appropriate.

In order to consider whether the dependence increases over time, we relax the assumption $\delta_1 = \delta_2$. This is done just by letting δ_2 be a freely varying parameter. The estimates using a threshold of 20,000 days are given in Table 11.5. For two datasets, the iterative procedure converges to a point on the boundary. In one of these cases (dizygotic males), and no other, the fit is significantly improved compared to the model with $\delta_1 = \delta_2$. In that case, the estimated value of τ is slightly lower than evaluated in Table 11.4.

	Shared frailty	20,000 days	30,000 days
Males			
MZ	0.2068	0.2073	0.2052
DZ	0.0824	0.0830	0.0985
UZ	0.2493	0.2493	0.2572
Females			
MZ	0.1943	0.2031	0.1943
DZ	0.1276	0.1353	0.1182
UZ	0.1745	0.1648	0.1698

Table 11.4. Estimates of τ in constant and piecewise gamma frailty model, for Danish twin data, with a threshold of $x_1=20{,}000$ and $30{,}000$ days.

	$\hat{\delta}_0$ (SE)	$\hat{\delta}_1$ (SE)	$\hat{\delta}_2$ (SE)	$\hat{\tau}$ (SE)	$\Delta \log L$
Males					
MZ	1.228 (0.691)	0.344 (0.443)	0.526 (0.694)	0.2068	0.48
DZ	1.717	0	5.163	0.0775	2.65
UZ	0.918	0	0.825	0.2326	0.57
Females					
MZ	0.405 (0.382)	0.965 (0.640)	1.099 (0.476)	0.2025	4.10
DZ	0.672 (0.516)	1.146 (0.674)	1.922 (0.718)	0.1326	3.37
UZ	0.554 (0.597)	0.409 (0.612)	1.783 (0.949)	0.1636	1.69

Table 11.5. Estimates of parameters in the piecewise gamma frailty model, for Danish twin data, with a threshold of $x_1=20{,}000$ days. With δ_2 varying freely. $\Delta \log L$ is increase compared to shared gamma frailty model.

11.4 Moving average model

The model above implies long-term dependence within each interval, and at the same time, time points in different intervals show low dependence even though such time points can be close to each other. This section suggests a model that is closer to be a model in continuous time, and thus with smaller jumps between intervals. A model that can be considered in the additive framework is the moving average model, where the frailty Y_q in the q-th interval has the form $c_1 Z_{q-1} + c_0 Z_q$, where then the $Z_0, ..., Z_m$ are independent with some common distribution, and c_0, c_1 are parameters. This would correspond to shared frailties within each intervals, some degree of dependence among neighboring intervals, and independence between intervals that are not neighbors. In the case of $m = 2$, it is a special case of the model of Section 11.3 with Z_1 as the common term and Z_0 and Z_2 as period specific terms. The advantage compared to the piecewise gamma model of Section 11.3 is that there would be better control of for how long the dependence lasts, and there would be dependence between neighboring intervals.

The density would be a generalization of Equation (11.9).

The model can be extended by also including a constant term in the sum. This makes it possible to test the hypothesis of the shared frailty model. The properties of this model are unknown.

11.5   Hidden cause of death model

The piecewise gamma model above requires the definition of interval end points, where there is an abrupt change in frailty. Thus the conditional hazard will also change abruptly, which is inconvenient. In this section, a model for parallel data will be discussed, similar conceptually to the piecewise gamma model, but avoiding the selection of cutpoints and the sudden changes in hazard. This section should serve as inspiration for developing models of this type. The model is not fully developed. It is a completely different principle for creating short-term dependence and therefore it is theoretically interesting to consider.

To derive the model, we suggest that there are m causes of death, each with a separate hazard function, say, $\mu_p(t)$, for the pth cause, and a separate (cause-specific) frailty, shared by all individuals in the group, say Z_p. First, we will assume that the cause-specific frailties are independent. This is a hidden cause of death model, which implies that the actual causes of death are unknown, generalizing the ideas of Section 2.2.5. Therefore the relevant quantity to consider is the total hazard for the individual, which, conditional on $Z_1, ..., Z_m$ is $\sum_{p=1}^{m} Z_p \mu_p(t)$. If the cause-specific hazards are proportional, say $\mu_p(t) = c_p \mu(t)$, the total hazard is $(\sum_{p=1}^{m} c_p Z_p)\mu(t)$, which is just an ordinary shared frailty model with frailty $\sum_{p=1}^{m} c_p Z_p$ and conditional hazard function $\mu(t)$. Thus, the interesting case is when the hazard functions are non-proportional. Only this case is considered below. When the ratio of hazards changes gradually, there will be a shift from causes of death of the young to causes of death of the old, leading to a dependence more concentrated in time than the shared frailty model, that is, a short-term dependence. This is first performed in a Weibull model. Thus the shape parameters are γ_p, describing the non-proportionality and c_p giving an absolute level of the hazard. Generally, no two values of γ_p can be equal, because in that case, the hazards are proportional and the terms can be combined. It is convenient to order the values $\gamma_1 < ... < \gamma_m$, as the order cannot be identified.

Extension to the non-parametric case is relevant, but the completely general case, where all hazards are allowed to vary freely, gives a model that is too large. It is more sensible to suggest a common non-parametric component, letting the cause-specific hazards deviate by factors similar to the Weibull model. This implies that the hazards differ by a factor changing smoothly by time. The first hazard $\mu_1(t)$ is taken as a basis, and it is assumed that the others are given by $\mu_p(t) = c_p t^{\gamma_p - 1}\mu_1(t)$, $p = 2, ..., m$.

These expressions are greatly inspired by the Weibull distribution, but the marginals will be completely arbitrary. To write common formulas we may set $c_1 = \gamma_1 = 1$.

The assumption that the cause-specific frailties are independent might seem restrictive. But, this is not the case. Suppose that there is an additive frailty relation between the first two causes of death so that $Z_1 = c_1 U_0 + U_1$, $Z_2 = c_2 U_0 + U_2$, then the total hazard from these two causes of death equals $U_0(c_1\mu_1(t) + c_2\mu_2(t)) + U_1\mu_1(t) + U_2\mu_2(t)$, which is also a hidden cause of death model, the only change is that there are three hidden causes of death, rather than two.

This evaluation depends on the causes' being unknown. If they were known, we could look for such a structure, but that would require a more detailed study.

One problem with this suggestion is that there is some degree of identifiability from univariate data. Precisely what can be estimated from such data, and it implications for the complete approach, requires a more detailed study.

11.6   The Woodbury-Manton model

It would be desirable to have a model where the frailty varies smoothly with time. The only model suggested in the literature is the diffusion process given by the stochastic differential equation,

$$dZ_t = a(t)dt + b(t)Z_t dt + cdW_t,$$

where W_t is a Brownian motion. The parameter $a(t)$ describes a fixed change with time, $b(t)$ is a factor in a term describing a change dependent on the value of the process, and c a scale factor. If the frailty at time t is defined as $Y_t = Z_t^2$, so that the hazard is $Y_t\mu(t)$, it is possible to derive the population hazard (the univariate case) by the formula

$$\omega(t) = \mu(t)\{m(t)^2 + \sigma(t)^2\},$$

where $m(t)$ and $\sigma(t)^2$ are the mean and variance of Z_t conditional on survival until time t. These functions are the solutions to the differential equation

$$dm(t)/dt = a(t) + b(t)m(t) - 2m(t)\sigma^2(t)\mu(t),$$

$$d\sigma^2(t)/dt = 2b(t)\sigma^2(t) + c^2 - 2\sigma^4(t)\mu(t). \tag{11.10}$$

The problem with this approach is that the computational work can be difficult. Even in the univariate case, we need to use a numerical solution to Equation (11.10). The model has never been considered for bivariate data, and therefore, it is not known how much more difficult the equations are in that case. As long as both individuals are alive, the bivariate case can be handled by setting a factor of 2 on $\lambda(t)$, but it is unknown what happens when one person dies. So the conclusion on this model is that it needs to be developed further and studied in more detail before we can discuss the applicability of the approach.

11.7   Chapter summary

Instantaneous dependence has a mathematical appeal allowing for many theoretical evaluations. It is obtained by using a frailty varying randomly over time, where the hazard is described by the independent increments of the process.

Short-term dependence models seem to be a more relevant (for the practice) extension of the frailty model and from a mathematical point of view, there seems to be a lot of potential in these models. The key problem is the computational burden.

Models with time-varying frailties seem particularly important for recurrent events data, but unfortunately, most such models can treat only additive piecewise constant frailties and with a limited number of intervals.

The hidden cause of death model gives an alternative approach to obtain short-term dependence, by means of constant, but multidimensional frailties for each individual.

These models require much further study and application before they can become routine models.

11.8   Bibliographic comments

There are only a few papers on instantaneous dependence. Kalbfleisch (1978) suggested the independent increments gamma model as a Bayesian model for non-parametric hazards, implying that there was only a single realization of the process. This was extended by Burridge (1981).

Lee and Whitmore (1993) introduced the independent increments PVF frailty model. Hougaard, Lee, and Whitmore (1997) described the statistical analysis of it.

There are even fewer papers on short-term dependence. Paik, Tsai, and Ottman (1994) suggested a piecewise gamma model, but with independent piecewise contributions.

The only paper that has taken the short-term dependence approach seriously in frailty models for parallel data seems to be an unpublished work by Self (1993), who considered a smoothed gamma process.

The Woodbury-Manton model was suggested by Woodbury and Manton (1977). It is described in a frailty frame in Aalen (1994). The model has been further considered by Yashin, Manton, and Stallard (1986, 1989) and by Yashin, Manton, and Lowrimore (1997).

11.9   Exercises

Exercise 11.1 Regression model for the independent increments model

You may suggest two regression models for the stationary independent increments frailty model of Section 11.1.2. Either $\tilde{Y}_1(t, z) = \exp(\beta' z)\tilde{Y}(t, 0)$ or $\tilde{Y}_2(t, z) = \tilde{Y}(\exp(\beta' z)t, 0)$. Give an interpretation of these models. Show that the two models have the same mean, but are different. Find the cluster distribution in the models. Which of the cluster distributions does not depend on z?

Exercise 11.2 Updating in independent increments model

Consider the independent increments frailty model, where $\tilde{Y}(t)$ is gamma distributed with parameters $(M(t), \theta)$. Let the observed events be given by the counting process $K(t)$. Show that the process $\tilde{Y}(t)$ given the process $K(t)$ is an independent increments gamma model with parameters $M(t) + K(t)$ and $\theta + 1$.

Exercise 11.3 Information in independent increments process

Consider the homogeneous process of Section 11.1.2 for $\alpha = 0$. Make the reparametrization to λ as described in the section and $\psi = \log(\theta + 1)$. Show that the information obtained in complete observation on the event process during the interval $(0, t]$ is

$$-Ed^2\ell/d\lambda^2 = t\lambda^{-1}, \quad -Ed^2\ell/d\lambda d\psi = 0,$$

$$-Ed^2\ell/d\psi^2 = \lambda t e^\psi \{\psi - \log(e^\psi - 1)\} - 1.$$

Exercise 11.4 Additive frailty model for recurrent events

Consider an additive frailty model for interval count recurrent events with two intervals, as described in Section 11.2. Let the distribution of Z_1 and Z_2 be the same. Based on moments for Z_0 and Z_1, derive the correlation between Y_1 and Y_2. Derive also the correlation between K_1 and K_2. Which one is the larger?

Exercise 11.5 Interval counts in piecewise gamma model

Consider the model for recurrent events described in Section 11.3, observing interval counts for $2m$ intervals, giving counts K_{ij}. Consider the reduction of the data by combining the intervals two and two, $G_{ij} = K_{i,2j-1} + K_{i,2j}$. Show that this is also an interval count observation in a piecewise gamma model and find the relation of the parameters of the two cases. Is the reduction sufficient?

Exercise 11.6 Truncation in hidden cause of death model

Consider the non-parametric hazard model of Section 11.5. Show that if lifetimes are truncated, it is still a model of the same type (that is, additive frailty hidden cause of death model with frailty distributions in the same family), if each frailty term follows a distribution in a natural exponential family.

Exercise 11.7 Variance for epileptic data

Evaluate the empirical mean and variance for the four-interval version of the placebo data of Section 1.7.2 assuming independence and the same distribution for all patients and intervals. What is the variance of the frailty component? Evaluate the estimated variances for both the gamma and the PVF independent increments process based on the results of Section 11.1.6.

12
Competing risks models

The term *competing risks* refers to cause of death models. Competing risks have been introduced and illustrated as a multi-state model in Figure 1.7 and discussed previously, in Sections 1.10, 3.3.9, and Chapter 5; but such data present special challenges, and therefore are considered separately in this chapter. It differs from the rest of this book in that only one event is possible for each individual, and in that sense, the concept of dependence seems irrelevant. However, two problems stand out as particularly important for competing risks data, the possibility of classification error and, more important, the desire to study the effect of modifying the hazards for some causes of death. Therefore, dependence is the key problem for such data. We would like to discuss aspects where dependence is important, but it is impossible to estimate the degree of dependence. In fact, it is impossible even to give a specific interpretation of dependence. The problem is caused by competing risks not being a truly multivariate survival problem. This has been discussed for centuries, since Bernoulli considered what the eradication of smallpox would imply for the mean lifetime.

The data consist, for each individual, of the lifetime T, and the cause of death, D, among a list of k possible causes. In many medical applications, there is a single cause of death that is particularly interesting, typically death of the disease under study, and then all other causes are combined, whereas in public tables for population data, there are a large number of possible causes, which are treated on an equal basis. We then define the cause-specific hazard at time t by the expression,

$$\lambda_j(t) = \lim_{\Delta t \searrow 0} \frac{Pr(t \leq T < t + \Delta t, D = j \mid t \leq T)}{\Delta t}, \tag{12.1}$$

for the jth cause, $j = 1, ..., k$. These are precisely the transition hazards, when the model is considered as a multi-state model. The hazard corresponding to the lifetime, irrespective of cause of death, is the sum of the cause-specific hazards. For recording data, it is convenient to code censoring as $D = 0$.

For obtaining cause of death data, there are generally definition problems. It is difficult to state a single cause of death in all cases. To address this problem, death certificates give a primary, secondary, and tertiary cause of death, where the primary cause of death is the immediate cause of death, and the others describe diseases or conditions that contribute to the death process. For example, a diabetic has a risk of dying from hypoglycemia, and if that happens, hypoglycemia is the primary cause of death, and diabetes is a pre-existing condition that should be listed as a secondary cause of death. The classifications for describing the cause of death have been changed over time. International cooperation started in 1893, and in 1948 WHO took over and introduced standardized international classifications, which are basically those used today. Before WHO, that is, just 50 years ago, it was common to die of old age, a cause of death that is now eliminated by definition. Instead the persons are now said to die of other, more specific, causes, e.g. from heart disease. Similarly for infants, there has been a trend over time from unspecific to specific causes of death. Therefore, the interpretation of competing risks data must include also the circumstances, like the risk of death of other causes.

Secondly, it is not in all cases that the cause of death is known, and the doctor has to consider the most probable cause of death. This probably leads to an overassignment to common causes, with no clear signs, typically heart disease. This problem is not common for other multi-state models. Typically, when there is an event, it is clear which event it is.

The competing risks models have been used to discuss the effect of removing a cause of death. This is extremely difficult to evaluate, because it has to be decided how the other causes of death will develop. The standard choice is to assume that the cause-specific hazards of death of all other causes remain the same, a choice that might appear sensible at a first glance, but is, in fact, a quite critical assumption, and rarely satisfied. This problem is more general than for solely cause of death data. It will be illustrated with a number of examples in Section 12.1.

One standard method for competing risks data is to consider the lifetime as a multivariate random variable. That is, interpret the problem in a parallel frame. That is, each person should have a "lifetime" for each cause of death. Then the ordinary (or realized) lifetime would be the minimum of the cause-specific lifetimes. This is described in Section 12.2, which also describes the limitations of the approach. A multi-state model should be used in this case and how this is done is described in Section 12.3. The dependence can be modeled by a frailty approach, as described in Section 12.4. This model is helpful in illustrating the difficulties in discussing the topic of removing some causes of death, but again cannot solve the basic problem. Section 12.5 discusses what can be estimated by means of competing risks data. Section 12.6 discusses the relation between cause-specific hazards for dependent individuals, illustrated by twins. Finally, Section 12.7 presents a couple of applications.

The presentation in this chapter is directed toward the biological case, where the competing risks describe the various causes of death of the individual. In the technical reliability case, the latent multivariate approach makes much more sense, because the components of the system can be tested separately.

The advice to give from these evaluations is that it is fine to analyze competing risks data, but if one wants to consider the effect of removing or reducing some specific cause, one should be very careful, and include suitable reservations and discussions. Similarly, if one wants a more detailed interpretation one should keep in mind all the causes, and not only the cause under specific study.

12.1   Effects of changing cause-specific hazards

This section discusses the practical aspects for changing cause-specific hazards. How can this be done in practice, and what are the consequences for the quantities considered in the model? These problems will be illustrated with some examples. Suppose first that we want to reduce the hazard of death of heart disease. How should we do that? One possibility is improvement in heart disease surgery techniques, so that we could repair hearts or transplant new hearts, whenever needed. This would increase the surgery related deaths but not affect the extent of any other vascular disease. But as the persons having heart disease often also present with other vascular disease, this would mean that many more people would die of other vascular diseases. If instead, we were able chemically to clean the blood vessels for cholesterol (including both the heart and other vessels), this would decrease the incidence of both heart disease and other vascular disease. Another, more simple, possibility is to change the diet of the population to include more vegetables, rather than fat. This would also have an impact on other vascular disease and, furthermore, on some cancers. Also reduction of smoking would have an effect, not only on heart disease, but on many other causes of death.

As a further example, consider another cause of death, suicide. If we were able to remove shooting weapons, suicide by shooting would disappear. The total suicide hazard will decrease, but suicide by other means would probably increase. Another point regarding suicide is that some of the people that commit suicide have serious health problems. A particular example is alcoholism. If we could make suicide impossible, the death hazard for selected other causes would increase owing to this.

It is also possible that reducing one cause of death directly increases another. For example, treatment to reduce the risk of stroke owing to thromboses could consist of blood clot dissolving, and this would increase the risk of hemorrhage. As another example, a diabetic patient is treated intensively to avoid the late complications owing to high blood glucose, but such treatment increases the risk of hypoglycemia.

Several cancers have common causes. Thus some ways of reducing the risk would reduce the risk of all such cancers, whereas screening might lead to treatment of only the specific cancer, and instead the patients, still having the same risk factors, might experience some other cancer owing to the same causes.

One further example is shown in Section 12.2.

In fact, this problem is present in multi-state models in general, but we discuss the effect of changing hazard functions less often. Still, it is important. One such example is the disability model of Figure 5.10. If we change the requirements for obtaining status of being disabled, or start a new program to reactivate disabled, the hazard of death among the disabled and the healthy might change, even though the individual mortality as well as the total mortality in the population are unchanged. This is due to the disabled group's consisting of a mixture of people with varying degrees of disability, and thus varying degrees of mortality, and changing the status of some people, probably will have highest impact for the lowest degrees of disability, whereas the most severe cases stay in the disabled state.

12.2   The multivariate parallel approach

A standard approach is to consider competing risks data as originating from a multivariate parallel random variable, $(T_1, ..., T_k)$, giving separate lifetimes of cause $1,...,k$. The realized lifetime is then the minimum of these, $T = \min\{T_1, ..., T_k\}$. This is basically a wrong approach, because there is a conceptual conflict with such times' being speculative. The formulation implies that for any given person we have a potential observation that he dies of any cause. To make an explicit example, suppose the person dies of a traffic accident at age 20, develops alcoholism and dies from it at age 50, dies of heart disease at age 75, and dies of lung cancer at age 85. Thus, what really happens is that he dies from the traffic accident. Taken literally, an action toward reducing traffic accidents, may rescue him from the accident and then lead to the person dying of alcoholism. However, one action toward traffic deaths could be directed specifically toward drunk driving by fighting alcoholism. Would that change his risk of death of alcoholism? If he is not allowed to drink, would he then instead smoke more and die earlier of heart disease and/or lung cancer? Such discussions illustrate the speculative aspects of this formulation and the lesson to be learned from this is that the multivariate approach is misleading.

All that can be estimated are the cause-specific hazard rates, which do not determine the total multivariate distribution. Some people conclude from this that when many multivariate distributions lead to the same cause-specific death hazards, we can as well apply the simplest multivariate distribution having the cause-specific hazards, that is, the multivariate distribution with independence. Any set of cause-specific hazards has a corresponding multivariate distribution with independence, given by the survivor functions $S_j(t) = \exp\{-\int_0^t \lambda_j(u)du\}$, for T_j. The assumption has no consequences when the aim is to derive, say, the asymptotic distribution of a given estimator, but for the interpretation, it is still misleading. Therefore, the approach is not recommended. Solving a basic identifiability problem by making arbitrary assumptions just hides the problem, and in the present case, it apparently makes it possible to estimate quantities that it should not be possible to estimate.

When there are covariates in a proportional hazards model, it is possible to identify the full multivariate distribution based on competing risks data. This was shown by Heckman and Honore (1989). There are a few necessary regularity conditions, e.g., the regression coefficients should not be the same for all causes, and the covariates should vary between $-\infty$ and ∞. This evaluation is, of course, critically dependent on the assumption of proportional hazards.

12.3   The multi-state approach

The multi-state approach consists of assuming the model of Figure 1.7 and the cause-specific hazards of Equation (12.1). When there are separate parameters for each cause of death, the hazard of death of cause j can be estimated simply by considering the deaths of the actual cause as the events and deaths of all other causes as censorings, precisely as described in Section 6.3. This might appear as if we do the same thing as assuming independence in the multivariate approach, but it is not, because there are no assumptions made requiring existence of the speculative other cause-specific lifetimes.

The limitation of this approach is that it offers no hints toward solving the special problems for competing risks data. Each transition hazard function has to be interpreted in the full model and is not valid after changing some other hazard functions.

The identifiability problem can be illustrated by the Freund model (Section 5.5.3). With competing risks data, it is possible to identify λ_1 and λ_2, but it is impossible to determine μ_1 and μ_2. The assumption of independence implies $\mu_1 = \lambda_1$ and $\mu_2 = \lambda_2$ and thus makes the hazard functions identifiable.

12.4 The frailty approach

The frailty approach is normally formulated as a multivariate approach and therefore not advisable to use for estimation. It can, however, be used for more clearly illustrating the problems with competing risks data. For example, the bivariate Weibull model based on positive stable frailty of Section 7.4.3 displays the unidentifiability problems. In the bivariate model, there are four parameters – α, γ, ϵ_1 and ϵ_2 – but with competing risks data, only three parameter functions can be identified – $\alpha\gamma$, which was denoted ρ in the marginal parametrization; and $(\epsilon_1 + \epsilon_2)^\alpha$ and $\epsilon_1/(\epsilon_1 + \epsilon_2)$, as these are the only parameters that enter in the cause-specific hazards. For the jth cause, the hazard is

$$\lambda_j(t) = \epsilon_j(\epsilon_1 + \epsilon_2)^{\alpha-1}\alpha\gamma t^{\alpha\gamma-1}. \tag{12.2}$$

This can be contrasted by the hazard for the minimum, which is

$$\lambda_{\min}(t) = (\epsilon_1 + \epsilon_2)^\alpha\alpha\gamma t^{\alpha\gamma-1}.$$

One application using frailty models was the Swedish population data studied by Vaupel, Manton, and Stallard (1979), the paper that introduced the term *frailty*. Here, the example will be given a competing risks interpretation, but with hidden causes of death, that is, the actual cause of death is unknown. Suppose there are two causes of death and that conditional on the frailty, Y, they are independent with cause-specific hazard $Y\mu(t)$, that is, the same hazard for both causes. The total hazard is then $2Y\mu(t)$. If one of these causes could be removed without affecting the conditional hazard of the other one, the new total hazard would be $Y\mu(t)$. The example assumed that the frailty was gamma distributed and found out that the population hazard (the unconditional hazard) would be reduced to one-half the original hazard at lower ages, but there would only be a smaller decrease at older ages, and eventually there would be no change in the population hazard. The formula is similar to that in Equation (2.51). The reason for this development over time is that those saved by the reduced hazard are frailer than the original survivors and this fact counteracts the hazard reduction. If the parameter δ is small, the population hazard would be unchanged, whereas if δ is large, the population hazard would be reduced by a factor of $1/2$, over the whole range. The parameter δ cannot be identified by the original data and therefore the approach can only be used to illustrate the point.

In fact, it is not necessary to assume the existence of the full multivariate observation to evaluate the data in a frailty model. It can be formulated as a conditional multi-state model (Section 5.9) for the competing risks multi-state model of Figure 1.7. Thus, the hazard of death of cause j is $Y\mu_j(t)$ conditional on Y. This model gives exactly the same distributions of the observed quantities as competing risks data in the frailty model for the full multivariate time. However, the model does not assume the existence of a multivariate time observation behind the observed quantities. Furthermore, there will be parameters that cannot be identified. So, this is similar to the Freund model example in Section 12.3. Applying the Freund model to competing risks data requires no assumptions neither regarding μ_1 and μ_2 nor regarding independence of non-existing times. The question is, of course, what do we gain from considering such a model? In terms of modeling observed cause-specific hazard functions, we do not gain anything, but we might gain something on a more intellectual level in the sense that we better understand the limitations of competing risks data.

12.5   What can be estimated?

As described above, the cause-specific hazard functions can be estimated. One way to do this is to evaluate the integrated cause-specific hazards, by a Nelson-Aalen estimator, or include covariates in a Cox model.

One could suggest making a Kaplan-Meier curve for each cause of death, but it is difficult to give this a survival function interpretation and therefore this is not recommended. It is, however, possible to make a generalization of the Kaplan-Meier by including all causes on a single figure. This is just the Aalen-Johansen estimator of Equation (6.7). At each time of death, the probability of death is estimated by the Kaplan-Meier estimate and assigned to the cause of death for the person dying at that time (in the case of ties the probability is distributed according to the relative distribution among those dying at that time). Only dropouts are then considered as censorings. How to do this will be illustrated in the application.

It is possible to evaluate the overall probability of death of a specific cause. If the various cause-specific hazards are proportional, these probabilities are easily estimated by the observed distribution of causes. However, it is difficult to argue that hazards of death of two different causes should be proportional so it much more interesting in the general case.

12.6   Competing risks for twin data

In the case of competing risks data for twins (or more generally for a group or family of individuals), there is hope that we can identify more quantities

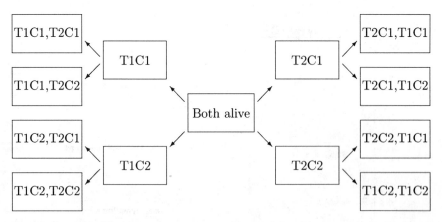

Figure 12.1. Multi-state model for competing risks data for twins. T1, twin 1; T2, twin 2; C1, dead of cause 1; C2, dead of cause 2.

than in the case of individuals, but we cannot solve the basic problem. In the multi-state frame work the observable process is as illustrated in Figure 12.1 in the simplest possible case, with just two causes of death. To make it easier to overview the figure, it is illustrated as a progressive model. Alternatively, one could combine states (T1C1,T2C1) and (T2C1,T1C1) and so on. Just for the purpose of discussing the model, we will state the hazards as Markov hazards. It would be no problem to use more general hazard functions. Also, for simplicity, we will assume the model is symmetric in the twins. This means that there are hazards $\lambda_j(t)$ for death of cause j, when both are alive. There is hazard $\mu_j(t)$ for death of cause j, when the partner has died of cause j; and finally, there is hazard $\omega_j(t)$ of death of cause j, when the partner has died of the other cause. One could then define independent causes of death as the hypothesis $\omega_j(t) = \lambda_j(t)$; that is, the risk of death of cause j is not influenced by knowing that the partner died of some other cause. If this is not the case, it suggests that there are some risk factors or other mechanisms that create dependence. Therefore, this hypothesis should always be considered. However, most people would probably find the other comparison, $\mu_j(t) = \lambda_j(t)$, the most interesting hypothesis; that is, is the risk of death of a specific cause changed by knowing that the partner has died of that cause?

The hazard functions $\lambda_j(t)$, $\mu_j(t)$ and $\omega_j(t)$ are the observable quantities. This means that we cannot even with twin data identify a full multivariate distribution. This will be illustrated in an exercise. Correspondingly, we cannot tell what happens if some cause of death is eradicated.

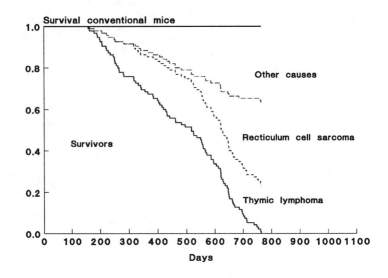

Figure 12.2. Generalized Kaplan-Meier estimate for conventional mice.

Data set	Model	RCS	TL	Other causes
Conventional	Proportional hazards	0.40	0.23	0.37
	Freely varying	0.40	0.23	0.37
Germ-free	Proportional hazards	0.35	0.20	0.47
	Freely varying	0.35	0.20	0.47

Table 12.1. Probabilities of death of the various causes. RCS=recticulum cell sarcoma; TL=thymic lymphoma.

12.7 Applications

For the data on radiation exposed mice of Section 1.10.1, Figure 12.2 shows the Kaplan-Meier generalization for conventional mice and Figure 12.3 for germ-free mice. The total mortality can be read off the curves, and the estimate equals the Kaplan-Meier estimate based on the lifetimes, not accounting for the cause of death. The estimated distribution of the causes of death are given in Table 12.1. Under the assumption of proportional hazards, the estimates are just the observed frequencies among the deaths, for example, 38 of 95 deaths among conventional mice are of recticulum cell sarcoma, giving a probability of 0.40. In the general case, the same applies because there are no censorings. The evaluation now is 38 of 95 mice (rather than 38 of 95 deaths). Generally, this will not be the case as some individuals are censored.

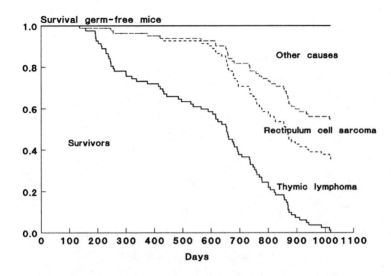

Figure 12.3. Generalized Kaplan-Meier estimate for germ-free mice.

For comparing the two types of mice, we use a proportional hazards model for each cause of death, completely as in Chapter 6. We obtain regression coefficients for the germ-free mice compared to the conventional mice. For death of thymic lymphoma, the regression coefficient is 0.31 (SE 0.29). For death of recticulum cell sarcoma, the regression coefficient is −2.03 (0.35). For death of other causes, the regression coefficient is −1.10 (0.33). Thus there are no significant differences for death of thymic lymphoma and the germ-free mice have a decreased hazard of death of recticulum cell sarcoma and of other causes.

For the data of malignant melanoma of Section 1.10.2, we first evaluate the probability of dying of the disease, not accounting for covariates. Assuming that the cause-specific hazards of death of the disease and death of other causes are proportional, the overall probability of death of the disease is $57/71 = 0.80$. However, this proportionality assumption seems unrealistic, it is quite possible that death of the disease happens early after diagnosis, whereas long-term survivors are more probable to die of other causes. Based on the cause-specific Kaplan-Meier approach, shown in Figure 12.4, we can find out that at the time of the last observation (that is, 9.5 years), there is probability of 0.34 of having died from the disease and 0.11 of having died of other causes, whereas for the survivors (proportion 0.56), the cause is undeterminable. At a first glance, it is quite annoying that we cannot estimate the overall probability of death of the disease, but it is clear that it has to be so. Without assumptions like proportional hazards

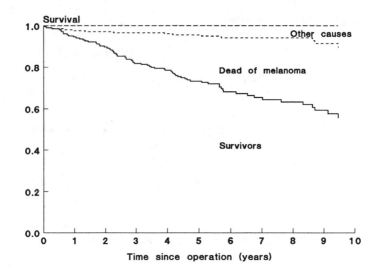

Figure 12.4. Generalized Kaplan-Meier estimate for melanoma patients.

Covariate	Disease $\hat{\beta}$ (SE)	Other causes $\hat{\beta}$ (SE)
Sex	0.55 (0.27)	0.37 (0.54)
Age (year)	0.012 (0.008)	0.073 (0.022)
Thickness (1/100 mm)	0.155 (0.033)	0.055 (0.083)

Table 12.2. Regression coefficients for a competing risks model for melanoma data.

of the cause-specific hazards or parametric models for the hazards, it has to be impossible to predict the cause of death for individuals alive after the time of the last observed event.

With covariates, it is possible to make more detailed models regarding the influence of clinical variables. The regression coefficients for the cause-specific hazard for death of the disease was described in Section 2.4.8, based on a proportional hazards model. Here, the same covariates are used to explain the risk of death of other causes. For both causes, the regression coefficients are described in Table 12.2. The regression coefficients are as expected, age has a large influence on death of other causes, but only a small effect for death of the disease, whereas severity of disease, as measured by the tumor thickness, has a large effect on the hazard of death of the disease and no significant effect on death of other causes.

12.8   Chapter summary

In one sense, cause of death data are simpler than the general multivariate survival data, as there is at most one event for each individual. However, it is misleading to consider the data as observing only the first time in a multivariate parallel data problem. What we can estimate is the cause-specific hazards, which can be interpreted in a descriptive way. The generalized Kaplan-Meier estimate is one way to make this clear. As a consequence, we cannot quantitatively consider the effect on the lifetime of reducing the hazard of death of some specific cause.

A second, more practical, problem is that in some cases it is difficult to classify the event, that is, to find out what cause of death was acting in the actual case.

12.9   Bibliographic comments

The limitations of competing risks data were made clear by Prentice *et al.* (1978). David and Moeschberger (1978) describe various models for competing risks data.

There have, of course, been applications studying the relation between cause-specific hazard functions for twins, but it has never been treated systematically,

12.10   Exercises

Exercise 12.1 Combining causes of death

Suppose we in a competing risks case want to combine several causes of death. For example, we may have separate hazards for cancer at various sites and now want the overall cancer death risk. For simplicity suppose we want to combine causes 1 and 2. Show that theoretically, the desired hazard is $\lambda_1(t) + \lambda_2(t)$ and that all other causes are not influenced. For estimating the hazard, there are two possibilities: one can add the estimates or one can reanalyze the data using a death indicator combining the two causes. Show that the two approaches give the same results for the cause-specific Nelson-Aalen estimate. Show that the same applies for a piecewise constant hazard model with separate parameters for the causes and the same interval end points. What happens, when the hazards are of Weibull form?

Exercise 12.2 Conditional Weibull gamma frailty model

Consider the model defined in Equation (7.41). Show that it is possible to identify all four parameters with competing risks data.

Exercise 12.3 Cause-specific Weibull gamma frailty model

Consider the gamma frailty model defined by the cause-specific hazards being of Weibull form $\lambda_j(t) = \xi_j \gamma t^{\gamma-1}$, $j = 1, 2$, and the frailty following a gamma(δ, δ) distribution. Derive the bivariate survivor function and the marginal survivor functions. Show that it is possible to identify all parameters from bivariate data, but only a three-dimensional parameter function with competing risks data.

Exercise 12.4 Marginal Weibull gamma frailty model

Consider the bivariate model giving by the marginal distributions being of Weibull form $\lambda_j(t) = \xi_j \gamma t^{\gamma-1}$, $j = 1, 2$ and the bivariate distribution being giving by Equation (7.31). Show that it is possible to identify all 4 parameters with competing risks data.

Exercise 12.5 Gamma frailty models

Consider the gamma frailty model with completely arbitrary cause-specific hazard functions $\lambda_j(t)$. Show that it is not possible to identify the parameter of the frailty distribution.

Consider this result together with the results of the three previous exercises. Which model would you prefer and why?

Exercise 12.6 Twin data

The purpose of this exercise is to illustrate identifiability problems for the twin data competing risks model of Section 12.6. For simplicity, you may assume that there are only two causes of death and that the conditional hazards are of the form $Y_{ijm}\lambda_j \gamma t^{\gamma-1}$, where j is the cause of death and m denotes the individual twin. We will assume that all pairs are independent and neglect the index i. Consider the following models: Model A (shared frailty): $Y_{jm} = Y$. Model B (individual effect): $Y_{jm} = Y_m$, with values independent for m, Model C (cause of death effect): $Y_{jm} = Y_j$, with values independent for j. Assume that the frailties follow positive stable distributions with parameter α. Derive the hazard functions $\lambda_j(t)$, $\mu_j(t)$, and $\omega_j(t)$, for each model. Show that the parameters can be identified for Model A and Model C, but not for Model B.

Then consider the same questions for Model D, $Y_{jm} = Z_0 Z_j$, using the multiplicative stable distribution of Section 10.4.

13
Marginal and copula modeling

Marginal modeling is a term used for an approach where the effect of explanatory factors is estimated based on considering the marginal distributions. The dependence is not the interesting aspect and is not considered in detail. Afterwards, the variability of the regression coefficient estimators is determined by a procedure that accounts for the dependence between the observations. For parallel data, there are in practice two versions of this general idea. The coordinate-wise (CW) approach considers each marginal separately and estimates the regression coefficients in each marginal. The covariance matrix of these estimates is estimated and used for combining the estimates from the coordinates by means of a weighted average. The estimated covariance matrix is further used to evaluate the variance of the combined estimate. The second version of the approach is the independence working model (IWM) approach, where the estimate is found under the (incorrect) assumption of independence between the coordinates. This yields directly the final estimate of the regression coefficients. The uncertainty of the regression coefficient estimate is evaluated by means of an estimator that accounts for the dependence between the coordinates. This is typically done by a "sandwich estimator" (see below). The independence working model approach is closely related to the so-called generalized estimating equations. For recurrent events, there is an approach similar in concept to the IWM approach.

The marginal modeling approaches are model-free regarding dependence assumptions. It can be seen as an advantage that we do not have to specify and rely on a specific model; but on the other hand, it is unknown whether the approaches are particularly good or bad for specific models.

In terms of purpose of the analysis these approaches may be useful for finding the effect of covariates, but do not make sense for assessment of dependence, goodness-of-fit, or for prediction. In fact, it is further limited, as the coordinate-wise approach cannot handle matched pairs covariates.

The CW and IWM approaches are derived in a frame of parallel data for several individuals. They are less good for recurrent events data, as such data show an order restriction $T_1 < T_2$, which means that the observations are concentrated on a subset of $(0, \infty)^2$. The marginal modeling approach does not use this fact, but is based on some asymptotic normal approximations. The approaches furthermore have difficulties handling the varying number of observations. I think, these approaches should be used only when the observations vary in a product set and when the marginal model includes the hypothesis of independence between the observations. The approaches do not appear relevant for event-related dependence and multi-state models, because they do not recognize this type of dependence. None of the methods should be used for longitudinal data on different events, where one of the events is death, first because the methods do not accept the process-dependent censoring owing to death; and second, because there is no reason to suggest that the covariate should have the same effect for all events. Furthermore, it seems relevant only to consider continuous data, ruling out data showing instantaneous dependence. The coordinate-wise approach is described in detail in Section 13.1. The independence working model approach is described in Section 13.2. The two approaches are discussed and compared in Section 13.3. A similar approach to studying recurrent events is described in Section 13.4.

A somewhat complementary approach to the marginal modeling is the concept of copulas (Section 13.5). The purpose of this approach is purely to study the dependence, removing all effects of the distribution as function of time and covariates. This is obtained by assuming that the marginal distributions are known. For standardization a uniform distribution on the unit interval is chosen. If the distribution is another continuous distribution, it can be transformed to the uniform case. Then the dependence is evaluated by specifying a family of distributions for the bivariate observations. It can, however, be discussed to which extent this approach is useful as the marginal distributions are rarely known. Typically, there will be some parameters also in the marginal distributions and then we do need a larger model for the analysis. In the terminology for purposes introduced in Section 1.14 this approach can be used for assessment of the dependence and for evaluating the goodness-of-fit of specific models. Furthermore, the copula approach is relevant for probability evaluations made for understanding the dependence pattern.

However, the marginal and copula approaches can be combined so that the effect of the covariates and the time scale is modeled by means of the marginal hazard functions and the dependence is modeled by the copula approach (Section 13.6). In this way, we get the advantages of both procedures. Compared to the marginal modeling, we have a specific way of studying the dependence and compared to the copula approach, we do not assume that the marginal distributions are known. On the other hand, it is also more complicated than either of the approaches. In particular, the interpretation is more difficult, because even though a frailty model is used for deriving the model, it does not necessarily allow for a random effects interpretation because the model is not described by means of conditional distributions.

13.1   The coordinate-wise approach

The idea of this approach is to make an analysis of all regression coefficients for each coordinate separately using a standard Cox proportional hazards model. In the standard notation of this book, this is an analysis for each value of j. This gives a number of estimates of each regression coefficient. The standard partial likelihood approach gives estimates of the variances of these coefficients, but the covariances are not obtainable by this approach. The second step in the marginal modeling approach therefore evaluates an alternative variance estimate, including covariances, but does not improve the estimator. The third step in the marginal modeling approach is a unification of the coordinate-specific estimates of the same effects by weighting the separate estimators.

By studying each coordinate separately, we do not necessarily assume independence. This is well known from the normal distribution models with multivariate response, the multivariate Gauss-Markov model, where all estimates (except the correlation parameters) are found by studying the coordinates separately. This type of analysis corresponds to the first two steps of the marginal modeling approach. The third step is included in order to obtain a common estimate of the regression coefficient. The multivariate Gauss-Markov model does not attempt to obtain a common estimate.

The real advantage of this approach is that it is simple and operational, and can be implemented in SAS with a few extra statements besides the procedure calls. It can be seen as a pragmatic approach, because it delivers an estimate of the important quantity (if the purpose is to find the effect of a covariate) in a quick way, and it also gives a valid estimate of the standard error. It does, however, not have the scientific support of being based on a specific model.

The approach is not always possible because it is necessary that the covariates vary for each coordinate, thus excluding matched pairs covariates. This is further discussed in Section 13.3.

The final estimates do not account for the extra variation owing to having estimated the weights. This effect disappears asymptotically, but it is unknown what the implications are for small samples. Based on general evaluations, it is expected that estimated weights lead to overestimation of precision.

The rest of this section is a more technical description of how the estimation is performed. The first step is a coordinate-wise estimation, which is easily done using the methods described in Section 2.4. It is an advantage to formulate this as a stratified Cox model, with separate regression coefficients, because that makes it possible to evaluate all parameters of the first stage in a single call to the procedure. This means that for observation T_{ij}, the hazard at time t is $\lambda_{0j}(t) \exp(\beta_j x_{ij})$ in the case of a univariate explanatory variable x. To make this into the standard framework, we define covariates $z_{ijq} = 1\{j = q\}x_{ij}$, so that for each j, the correct component (β_j) is selected. This fitting gives estimates of the regression coefficients and their standard errors, but not the correlations. The second step is to derive the variances, and, in particular, covariances between the regression coefficients. This is based on a different variance estimate of the regression coefficients, based on the generalized residuals in the Cox model. This is based on the univariate formulation of the likelihood in Equation (2.39). This is done separately for each coordinate, implying that for the j-th coordinate of the ith group, and for covariate q, the quantity is

$$W_{ijq} = D_i\{z_{ijq} - \bar{z}_{jq}(t_i)\} - \sum_m \frac{D_{mj} R_{ij}(t_{mj}) \exp(\beta' z_{ijq})}{\sum_r R_{rj}(t_{mj}) \exp(\beta' z_{rjq})}\{z_{ijq} - \bar{z}_{jq}(t_{mj})\}.$$

(13.1)

The variance matrix V of the score vector then is found by an extension of Equation (2.46)

$$v_{qm} = \sum_i \sum_j \sum_\ell W_{ijq} W_{i\ell m}.$$

(13.2)

The variance matrix B of the regression coefficients then is found by the sandwich expression in Equation (2.47).

Combining the estimates is technically the same as finding an estimate in a normal distribution model with common mean and known variance. Defining $J = (1, ..., 1)'$ as a vector of ones, the formula for the weights is $H = (J'B^{-1}J)^{-1}J'B^{-1}$, and then the combined estimate is $H\hat{\beta}$, and the estimated variance of this is HBH'.

13.1.1   Recurrent events

Wei, Lin, and Weissfeld (1989) specifically suggest this procedure also for recurrent events. The time of event number j should then be the jth coordinate. Surprisingly, they suggested that the observation time for all coordinates should start at 0, contrary to the multi-state model of Section 5.4.4, where the time is considered truncated at T_{j-1}. For using Equation (13.2), it is necessary to include only a fixed number of events for each individual. Therefore a person who at time C has experienced k events should have time $T_{k+1}, T_{k+2}, \ldots$ included as censored observations at C. This is inefficient, when the number of events vary greatly between the individuals. This approach invalidates independent censoring, because knowledge of the number of observed events influences the distribution of the hazard of future events. Instead, one should use the method of Section 13.4.

13.1.2 Computational aspects

This approach can easily be handled by SAS. How to do this is shown in the program below, which is a modified version of the program found in *SAS/STAT Software: Changes and Enhancements, Release 6.10*. Allison (1995) contains a macro for the same purpose. The program below is designed for the twin data, assuming that there are variables pair (pair number, to identify the pair), member (1,2, number within pair), lifetime (the response time), death (death indicator), and cohort (year of birth, the covariate to study). First, a standard analysis is performed, one for all the twin 1's, and one for all the twin 2's. This can be done by separate calls to proc phreg or by means of a by statement, but it is most convenient to make it in a single analysis, by stratification, and use separate covariates for each coordinate. The regression coefficients are stored for later use, and the influence diagnostics are evaluated and saved. This is done by the following lines of codes:

```
data a; set twindata;
cohort1=cohort*(member=1);
cohort2=cohort*(member=2);
proc sort;
by pair;
proc phreg outest=est1;
   model lifetime*death(0)=cohort1-cohort2;
output out=out1 dfbeta=dt1-dt2/order=data;
strata member;
id pair;
```

The variables dt1 and dt2 contain the $A^{-1}W_{ij}$ terms, where W_{ij} is the vector of terms W_{ijk}. These influence statistics are then summed over j, by the code:

```
proc means data=out1 noprint;
by pair;
var dt1-dt2;
output out=out2 sum=dt1-dt2;
```

Finally, proc iml is called, the variance matrix of the regression coefficients is derived, the common estimate is found, and a combined test of

$\beta_1 = \beta_2 = 0$ is performed.

```
proc iml;
use est1;
read all var{cohort1 cohort2} into coh;
b=t(coh);
use out2;
read all var{dt1 dt2} into x;
v=t(x)*x;
nparm=nrow(b);
se=sqrt(vecdiag(v));
reset noname;
stitle={"Estimate", " Std Error"};
vname={"coh1", "coh2"};
tmpprt= b || se;
print, tmpprt[colname=stitle rowname=vname format=10.5];
print, "Estimated covariance matrix",,
v[colname=vname rowname=vname format=10.5];
/* H0: beta1=beta2 =0*/
chisq=t(b)*inv(v)*b;
df=nrow(b);
p=1-probchi(chisq,df);
print ,,"Testing H0: no cohort effects", ,
"Wald Chi-square = " chisq, " DF = " df,
"p-value= " p[format=5.4],;
/* Estimate common value */
e=j(2,1,1);
isi=inv(v);
h=inv(t(e)* isi*e)*isi *e;
b1=t(h)*b;
se=sqrt(t(h)*v*h);
zscore=b1/se;
chisq=zscore*zscore;
p=1 - probchi(chisq,1);
print ,"Estimation of the common parameter for cohort",,
"Optimal weights = " h,
"Estimate = " b1,
"Standard error = " se,
"z-score =" zscore,
"chi-square =" chisq,
"2-sided p-value = " p[format=5.4];
quit;
```

13.1.3   Asymptotic results

The first point to consider is whether the estimates are consistent. This requires that the marginal model is correctly specified and that the censoring is independent. For the first two steps, this is described by Spiekerman and Lin (1998). The third step offers no difficulties.

That process-dependent censoring is not acceptable can be seen easily by considering multivariate data censored at the time of first event. This is similar to competing risks data, but in this case, there is an actual multivariate observation in the first place. If we use the bivariate stable frailty Weibull model with a matched pairs covariate (in the competing risks terminology with proportional cause-specific hazards), the cause-specific hazards will have the same ratio as the conditional hazards, as demonstrated in Equation (12.2), whereas the factor in the marginal distribution is the power α of the ratio in the conditional hazards (Equation (2.54)). Thus, the true marginal and the theoretical value of the fitted marginal hazards deviate by a factor of α.

The next point is to show that the estimates are asymptotically normal with a variance matrix that can be estimated consistently. This was done by Wei *et al.* (1989), who basically showed that the vector of derivatives of the log likelihood function can be reformulated as a sum of independent terms, with a variance matrix estimated by the expression of Equation (13.2). The estimated regression coefficient is approximately a linear function of this, with derivative matrix A^{-1}, giving the variance matrix B by the sandwich formula in Equation (2.47).

13.1.4   Applications

Twin data

The twin data, of Section 1.5.1, is a typical example of how the methods can be used to find the effect of the year of birth. The overall aim of this study was to assess the dependence, which is not possible by the marginal approach. In this section, we instead consider the problem of finding the effect of the covariate. All the twin 1's are analyzed separately and an effect found. Similarly, all the twin 2's are analyzed and an effect of cohort found. The robust variances and covariances are then found (Table 13.1). It appears that the standard errors found by the marginal modeling approach are slightly lower than those found by the partial likelihood for these data. In the Gauss-Markov normal distribution models, the correlation between the estimates is the same as the correlation between the observations and therefore we expected that the correlations should be similar to the Spearman correlations. However, the values are clearly smaller than the corresponding values found by the gamma frailty model (Table 8.34). There are clear differences between the coordinate specific estimates and thus a need for a combined estimate. The optimal weights and the combined estimate of

	$\hat{\beta}_1(\mathrm{SE}^c)$	SE^r	$\hat{\beta}_2(\mathrm{SE}^c)$	SE^r	corr.
Males					
MZ	−2.218 (0.443)	0.443	−1.171 (0.424)	0.413	0.141
DZ	−2.016 (0.307)	0.301	−1.225 (0.304)	0.302	0.077
UZ	1.012 (0.722)	0.695	0.387 (0.696)	0.673	0.262
Females					
MZ	−2.100 (0.474)	0.449	−3.081 (0.470)	0.459	0.085
DZ	−2.578 (0.332)	0.326	−2.571 (0.321)	0.313	0.099
UZ	0.047 (0.596)	0.561	−0.744 (0.590)	0.585	0.188

Table 13.1. Cohort effect (% per year) for Danish twin data. SE^c: Standard error in Cox model, SE^r: robust standard error.

	Weight$_1$	β_m
Males		
MZ	0.460	−1.653 (0.323)
DZ	0.502	−1.622 (0.221)
UZ	0.478	0.686 (0.543)
Females		
MZ	0.513	−2.578 (0.335)
DZ	0.478	−2.574 (0.237)
UZ	0.527	−0.327 (0.441)

Table 13.2. Cohort effect (% /year) for Danish twin data. β_m combined estimate in marginal model. Weight$_1$ is weight for $\hat{\beta}_1$.

the cohort effect are shown in Table 13.2. The weights are roughly equal to 1/2. The results look sensible and show for the monozygotic and dizygotic twins that the mortality decrease depends on sex and not on zygosity. The estimates correspond well to the pattern seen in the general population over the same period. The approach is unable to use the assumption of symmetry, but is based on allowing different hazard functions for twins numbered 1 and 2. As the numbering is arbitrary, this implies that the method may be inefficient.

Kidney catheter infections

The kidney catheter infection data of Section 1.7.3 can also be analyzed in this way. In this case, sex will be included as the only covariate. The coordinate-wise approach first considers the first and second spell separately. The sex effects found in the Cox model are −1.409 (0.420) and −0.535 (0.456), respectively. The standard errors found by the marginal modeling approach are slightly larger for the first spell (0.438), but clearly larger (0.634) for the second spell. The correlation is evaluated to 0.728. The optimal weights found are 1.003 for the first, and −0.003 for the second, which leads to a combined estimate of −1.412, with a standard error of 0.438, slightly below the value for the first spell alone. Thus, in this case, it is suggested that only the first spell is informative, in the sense that the second gives no additional information. In fact, the second spell gets a negative weight, which is because the covariance (0.1928) is larger than the smallest of the variances (0.1922). The dependence between the two regression coefficients is surprisingly high, as calculations by other approaches (Section 4.2.1 and Table 10.16) have shown small or negative dependence between the times, when sex is accounted for in the model.

Other data

Data sets like the tumorigenesis data of Section 1.5.3 and the exercise data of Section 1.8.2 cannot be analyzed in this way, because the covariates vary within groups rather than between groups, and thus cannot be determined in the coordinate specific analysis.

13.2   The independence working model

As the name suggests, this method will employ some calculations assuming independence, but do other evaluations in a more general frame in order to make the whole approach statistically valid.

The approach consists of two stages. In the first stage the dependence is neglected. That is, a full analysis is made of all data, assuming that all times are independent. The estimate of the regression coefficients obtained in this way is used as the final estimate. This might be sensible, but the variability of the estimate must not be based on the independence assumption. For common covariates that would underestimate variability and for matched pairs covariates, it would overestimate variability. Therefore, the second stage consists of evaluating a valid uncertainty estimate by means of the robust variance matrix, not relying on the assumption of independence. The terms for the robust estimator are basically the same as for the coordinate-wise approach, except that now all individuals are in the same stratum and thus contribute to the evaluation of all scores. One consequence is that the index j can be deleted on $\bar{z}$. In this section, we will allow for a multivariate covariate and thus have an index q on $\bar{z}$. Thus the expression for W_{ijq} is

$$D_i\{z_{ijq} - \bar{z}_q(t_i)\} - \sum_m \sum_\ell \frac{D_{m\ell} R_{i\ell}(t_{m\ell}) \exp(\beta' z_{ijq})}{\sum_r \sum_s R_{rs}(t_{m\ell}) \exp(\beta' z_{rs})} \{z_{ijq} - \bar{z}_q(t_{q\ell})\}.$$

(13.3)

It might not appear obvious from this formula, but the terms are just the influence diagnostics obtained from studying all individuals in a univariate analysis, neglecting relationships between the times. The variance is then evaluated by the sandwich formula of Equations (13.2) and (2.47). The first of these equations accounts for the relationship between individuals.

The approach is basically a GEE (generalized estimating equation) approach, where the estimates are found by using an estimating equation, which is simpler than the correct likelihood equation. In this case, the equation is the likelihood equation in a simpler model (that is, under independence).

At first glance this seems similar to the two-stage approach used for the frailty model applications (Section 8.4), but there are major differences. The first step is the same, but the second step is different. The approach of Section 8.4 aims at improving the estimate and the marginal modeling approach aims at improving the variance evaluation, without modifying the estimate.

The results above have been formulated as all covariates having a proportional hazards effect, and thus with the same hazard function. However, this is not necessary and one can allow stratification.

Another aspect is that the independence working model weighs all observations equally. However, individuals (groups) with matched pairs covariates are more informative than those with common covariates so that if the data set includes subpopulations with either type of covariates, it will be more efficient to weigh them unequally. Furthermore, if dependence is high, it will be inefficient to weigh the data as if they are independent. Instead, one can weigh according to the degree of dependence. The basis for this evaluation is the likelihood formulation of Equation (2.40). The independence working model approach consists of adding a subscript j and summing over both i and j in Equation (2.40). Weights are then introduced by inserting a weight matrix,

$$\sum_i \sum_j \sum_m z'_{ijk} w_{ijm}(\beta)\{D_{im} - \exp(\beta' z_{imk})\Lambda(T_{im})\}, \qquad (13.4)$$

Setting $w_{ijm} = 1\{j = m\}$ gives Equation (2.40), except for the use of a double subscript. This is formulated as a vector equation over j to be written as

$$\sum_i z'_{ik} w_i(\beta)\{D_i - \exp(\beta' z_{ik})\Lambda(T_i)\}. \qquad (13.5)$$

The weights are allowed to depend on time, but they must be predictable; that is, at time t, they must be based on the information collected strictly before time t. This approach can be beneficial if the dependence is high, whereas if the dependence is low, there is no gain in using it. In practice, estimates have to been inserted.

13.2.1 Asymptotic evaluation

The asymptotical evaluations have shown that as long as the marginal models are correctly specified and censoring is independent, the estimates are consistent and asymptotically normally distributed. Process-dependent censoring is not acceptable as described in Section 13.1.3.

A simulation study of Gao and Zhou (1997) finds that the independence working model approach (which they wrongly attribute to the paper suggesting the coordinate-wise approach) underestimates variance. This is evaluated in a bivariate gamma frailty model, both with independent covariates and with matched pairs covariates.

As there is not a full model underlying the approach, likelihood ratio test statistics cannot be correctly evaluated, so it is necessary to use Wald tests. However, it is possible to use the likelihood ratio test statistic under the independence working model, using a modified asymptotic distribution. The asymptotic distribution of the likelihood can be approximated by the distribution of a linear function of independent χ^2-distributions. The coefficients are found as the eigenvalues of a matrix. In the case of a simple hypothesis $\beta = \beta_0$, the matrix is $A^{-1}V$, where A is the second derivative as used in Equation (2.41) and V is defined in Equation (13.2). This equation can be generalized to the weighted case and to a composite hypothesis (see Cai, 1999)).

13.2.2 Software

This approach can be fit directly by Splus using the following code:
```
fit <-coxph(Surv(time,event) ~ (x + cluster(group)),
data=dataset)
```
where time is the response time, event the event indicator, x the covariate, group the group number, and dataset the data set stored as a data frame. The cluster term implies that the robust standard error is evaluated.

13.2.3 Applications

Twin data

For the Danish twin data, the estimates based on the independence working model approach are shown in Table 13.3. The estimate assuming symmetry joins both twins into a single analysis, neglecting pairing, that is, assuming independence. The robust standard errors are higher than those based on assuming independence. This was expected as the covariates are common covariates. The results are comparable to those of the coordinate-wise approach. A major reason for this is the low dependence.

Kidney catheter infections

If the pairing and order are ignored for the infection data of Section 1.7.3, that is, assuming symmetry and independence, the estimated regression coefficient for sex is -0.870 (0.297). The robust standard error is 0.483, markedly higher than the value assuming independence. In this case, the

	$\beta_i(SE^i)$	Robust SE
Males		
MZ	−1.677 (0.306)	0.322
DZ	−1.619 (0.216)	0.221
UZ	0.739 (0.501)	0.547
Females		
MZ	−2.601 (0.334)	0.335
DZ	−2.573 (0.231)	0.237
UZ	−0.335 (0.418)	0.438

Table 13.3. Cohort effect (% per year) for Danish twin data. β_i estimate assuming symmetry and independence, SE^i, standard error, assuming independence.

Treatment	Independence. $\hat{\beta}$ (SE)	Robust SE	u-statistic
SNG	−0.791 (0.322)	0.175	−4.52
Oral placebo (0h)	0.249 (0.310)	0.146	1.71
Oral placebo (1h)	−0.025 (0.309)	0.130	−1.89
Oral placebo (3h)	−0.007 (0.310)	0.174	−0.04
Oral placebo (5h)	0.131 (0.310)	0.126	1.03
Oral iso (0h)	−0.028 (0.309)	0.146	−0.19
Oral iso (1h)	−1.389 (0.360)	0.325	−4.27
Oral iso (3h)	−0.940 (0.334)	0.251	−3.74
Oral iso (5h)	−0.416 (0.318)	0.212	−1.96

Table 13.4. IWM estimates for log relative hazards (β) compared to sublingual placebo, for exercise data. Iso, isosorbide dinitrate; SNG, sublingual nitroglycerine.

IWM approach appears to perform badly compared to the coordinate-wise approach. This is because the coordinate-wise approach finds that only the first time is informative. The IWM approach uses a more equal weighting of the two times. If we force the CW approach to weight the two times equally, the estimate will be −0.972, and with a standard error of 0.485.

Tumorigenesis data

For the litter matched tumorigenesis study of Section 1.5.3, the estimated treatment effect under independence is 0.898 (0.317). The robust standard error of this is 0.300, slightly lower owing to the covariates' being matched pairs covariates and the fact that the dependence is low.

Exercise data

For the exercise data of Section 1.8.2, the covariates are also of the matched pairs type. Under independence, the estimates are as already reported in Table 8.4. These are repeated in Table 13.4. The robust variance values are clearly below those based on the independence assumption. Again, this is due to the covariates' being of the matched pairs type, so that treatment comparisons are made within individuals. The u-statistics are roughly comparable to those obtained using the frailty models (Table 8.6).

Leukemia remission

The covariates for the leukemia remission data of Section 1.5.4 are also of the matched pairs type. The estimate of the treatment effect is, as found earlier, -1.509 (SE 0.410). The robust standard error is 0.376. This is lower than the value found under independence, which implies that the marginal modeling approach suggests that the dependence is positive. This is surprising, because evaluations in Sections 4.2.1 and 8.12.6 suggest that the dependence is negative.

13.3   Discussion of marginal modeling

The approach is useful for finding the effect of covariates in parallel data. It is, however, somewhat restricted. The first requirement for the marginal modeling approach to make sense is that the parameters we are interested in are influencing the marginal distributions. In practice, this means regression parameters in a Cox-type fashion. The parameters describing the dependence, however, are difficult or impossible to estimate by this approach; and therefore the approach is most relevant when the dependence parameters are nuisance parameters. The CW approach does not work for all regression models. It is necessary that the covariates vary for each coordinate. This excludes the cases with matched pairs covariates and it is better suited for common covariates. However, repeated measurements studies with a crossover design can still be considered, if the coordinates correspond to the first and second time. This means that when there are two treatments, say, A and B, some patients receive them in the order AB and some in the order BA. The coordinate $j = 1$ should then correspond to the first period; and by studying this period alone, we can estimate the treatment effect. Similarly, $j = 2$ is the second period. Then the two estimates of the treatment effect are combined as described. Thus, to apply the procedure, the data should not be reduced to the responses for each treatment, that is, $j = 1$ for treatment A and $j = 2$ for treatment B. For matched pairs drug trials, this trick may not work. If this should work for the leukemia remission data, we should create a numbering of individuals and this appears artificial.

The approach seems sensible for several individuals and repeated measurements, where the dependence is generated by common risks. Mathematically, it is best suited to the positive stable frailty model, because in that model it is possible to have proportional hazards both in the con-

Property	CW	IWM	Stable frailty
Model for covariate effect	Yes	Yes	Yes
Model for dependence	No	No	Yes
Covariates allowed	Restricted	General	General
Negative dependence accepted	Yes	Yes	No
Recurrent events data	??	??	Yes[1]
Simple estimation	Yes	Yes	No
Estimate assumes indep.	No	Yes	No
Dependence estimable	No	No	Yes
Valid SE	Yes	Yes	MD
Test statistics	Wald	Wald	Wald and LRT

Table 13.5. Aspects of marginal modeling approaches compared to the stable frailty model. Yes[1], possible, but other frailty models are recommended (Section 9.3). MD, method dependent (see Chapter 8); LRT, likelihood ratio test.

ditional and the marginal distributions (see Section 7.4). Previously, this has been interpreted as a bias in the regression coefficients, so that the parameters of the marginal distributions are closer to no effect than the parameters in the conditional distribution. Alternatively, one can formulate this as the conditional and marginal hazard parameters' being two different parametrizations of the same model. Interestingly, the parameters of the marginal distributions are more robust toward the precise assumptions on the dependence. Thus the marginal modeling can be considered as a pragmatic way to avoid the identifiability properties of frailty regression models with a frailty distribution with finite mean (Section 7.2.7). By formulating the model with proportional hazards in the marginal distribution, we avoid the univariate identifiability problems, but at a price of obtaining a model that is more difficult to justify from a random effects point of view. One advantage of the marginal modeling approach is that it is more consistent with the univariate methods than the multi-state models and the frailty models, in the sense that univariate models are just a special case of the multivariate model. The univariate methods then correspond to the first step. The approach is relevant for parallel studies only. Application to recurrent events are discussed in Section 13.1.1 and 13.4.

Technically, the first step of the CW approach is contained in the IWM approach, as stratification is acceptable and it is acceptable to create covariates that only influence some events.

Table 13.5 summarizes some key aspects of the marginal modeling approaches, and to put them in perspective, the stable frailty model (Chapters 7 and 8) is also included in the comparison.

13.4 Recurrent events

It appears inconvenient to apply the independence working model of Section 13.2, when the independence assumption can not in any case be satisfied. This is the case for recurrent events, where the times are increasing, $T_1 \leq T_2 \leq ... \leq T_k$. Instead it makes more sense to use a procedure, which could be named Poisson process working model. This approach has many similarities to the above procedures, but instead of using the times to the events as the basic quantities, it uses $K(t)$, the number of events until time t, just as was done in Chapter 9. So the overall idea is to estimate the parameters for the mean process by means of the Poisson process likelihood method, and then evaluate the variability in a robust way by means of a sandwich estimator.

First, we consider the case without covariates, so we basically assume that $EK(t) = \Lambda(t)$ and want to estimate $\Lambda(t)$ based on a sample of n independent individuals. This is done by means of the Nelson-Aalen estimate (Equation (2.29)), extended to allow for multiple events for each person and that the risk indicator stays at 1 until end of study or censoring. Using the notation of Section 9.1, we write the estimated integrated hazard as

$$\hat{\Lambda}(t) = \sum_{ij} \frac{1\{T_{ij} \leq t\}}{\sum_m 1\{C_m \geq T_{ij}\}}.$$

This notation, however, becomes quite heavy, when we want to present the variance formula, and therefore we change to the alternative notation described in Section 9.1, which is more of a counting process notation. In this notation, the above formula is

$$\hat{\Lambda}(t) = \int_0^t \frac{K.(du)}{R.(u)},$$

where the denominator is just the number of persons at risk, which can be calculated from $R_i(t) = 1\{t \leq C_i\}$ and the dots mean summing over the index. The expression $K(dt)$ is the increase at time t, defined as $K(dt) = K(t) - K(t^-)$. The variance of this estimate is then evaluated to

$$\hat{\text{Var}}(\hat{\Lambda}(t)) = \sum_i [\int_0^t \frac{R_i(u)}{R.(u)} \{K(du) - \hat{\Lambda}(du)\}]^2. \tag{13.6}$$

This can be extended to regression models. Suppose that there is a constant covariate z included in a model with $E\Lambda(t) = \exp(\beta'z)\lambda_0(t)$. In the standard semi-parametric frame, this is formally considered as a discrete time multiplicative model at all time points and it is seen that at time points without events, the hazard function is estimated to 0, so that only time points with events contribute. The parameters are estimated using a working Poisson model. First, it is seen that the hazard function is estimated as $\hat{\lambda}_0(dt) = K(dt)/\sum_i R_i(t)\exp(\beta'z_i)$. If this is inserted in the working likelihood function, we obtain a profile log likelihood for β of the form

$$\sum_i \int_0^C R_i(t)K_i(dt)\{\beta' z_i - \log\{\sum_m R_m(t)\exp(\beta' z_m)\}.$$

This is precisely the Cox partial likelihood, generalized to recurrent events. The derivative of this equation is

$$\frac{d\ell}{d\beta_r} = \sum_i \int_0^C R_i(t)K_i(dt)\{z_{ir} - \frac{\sum_m R_m(t)z_{mr}\exp(\beta' z_m)}{\sum_m R_m(t)\exp(\beta' z_m)}\}.$$

The estimate of β is found by solving this equation. In order to derive an expression for the variance, which does not assume the Poisson distribution, we define W_{ir} as

$$\int_0^{C_i} \{z_{ir} - \frac{\sum_m R_m(t)z_{mr}\exp(\beta' z_m)}{\sum_m R_m(t)\exp(\beta' z_m)}\}\{K_i(dt) - \frac{\exp(\beta' z_i)K_{\cdot}(dt)}{\sum_m R_m(t)\exp(\beta' z_m)}\}.$$

and A_{irm} as

$$\int_0^{C_i} z_{ir}\exp(\beta' z_i)[\frac{z_{im}}{\sum_q R_q(t)\exp(\beta' z_q)} - \frac{\sum_q R_q(t)z_{qm}\exp(\beta' z_q)}{\{\sum_q R_q(t)\exp(\beta' z_q)\}^2}]K_{\cdot}(dt).$$

Here the term $R_i(t)$ is avoided by integrating only over the set where it is 1. From these expressions we can now calculate the estimated variability of $\hat{\beta}$ by the sandwich approach of Equations (2.46) and (2.47), after summing A over i. Similar to the parallel case above, it can be shown that the estimate solving the working model equation is asymptotically normally distributed and the variance can be estimated by the matrix B.

This approach seems closely related to that of the independent working model. In fact, many of the formulas are rather similar. However, the basic quantities that are entered in the formulas are quite different and therefore the results are not comparable. Just to compare them we consider a case with a single covariate. For the IWM approach one needs to choose a maximum number, say, k, of events to include. Then there are k W-variables for this case. For the recurrent events model, there are no limits to the number of events, and in this case only a single W is defined for each person. This makes the recurrent events approach much more sensible, when the number of events vary markedly.

When the true distribution is a frailty model, the efficiency of the approach will be high for the mean value parameters. As will be shown in an exercise, in some cases the estimated mean will be identical to the maximum likelihood estimate. This implies that the method is fully efficient in those cases. However, it is not possible to estimate the subject variation by the marginal modeling method.

13.5   Copulas

The idea behind copulas is to study the dependence, when the influence of the marginal distributions is removed, that is, by considering the marginals fixed. As long as the distribution is continuous, the actual marginals are unimportant, because changing the known marginals is only a matter of applying a specific transformation of the time. For standardizing this approach, uniform marginal distributions are assumed.

Strictly speaking, copulas are not important from a statistical point of view. It is extremely rare that the marginal distributions are known. Assuming the marginals are known is in almost all cases in conflict with reality. Copulas make sense, however, in a more broad perspective, first of all as part of the combined approach (Section 13.6), where the model is parametrized by means of the marginal distributions and the copula. Secondly, they make sense for illustrating dependence, as we have already done, for example, in Figures 3.2 and 7.7.

This approach has only been used in the bivariate parallel case. Let the survivor function be $S(t_1, t_2)$. The requirements on the uniform marginal distributions imply that $S(t_1, 0) = 1 - t_1$ and $S(0, t_2) = 1 - t_2$. A special case is the so-called Archimedian copula, where the survivor function has the following form:

$$S(t_1, t_2) = \phi(\phi^{-1}(1 - t_1) + \phi^{-1}(1 - t_2)). \tag{13.7}$$

Thus for frailty models where the marginals are assumed fixed, this is just a different formulation of Equation (7.8), using $\phi(s) = L(s)$. It is, however, slightly more general as ϕ does not need to be a Laplace transform. For example, it covers the extension of the gamma frailty model allowing for negative dependence (Section 7.3.3). In the gamma frailty case, the density is

$$(1 + 1/\delta)(1 - t_1)^{-1-1/\delta}(1 - t_2)^{-1-1/\delta}\{(1 - t_1)^{-1/\delta} + (1 - t_2)^{-1/\delta} - 1\}^{-2-\delta}.$$

In the stable frailty case, the survivor function is found by inserting in Equation (7.46), giving directly

$$S(t_1, t_2) = \exp(-[\{-\log(1 - t_1)\}^{1/\alpha} + \{-\log(1 - t_2)\}^{1/\alpha}]^\alpha),$$

from which the density is found by differentiation with respect to t_1 and t_2. The density is

$$S(t_1, t_2)\{Q^{2(\alpha-1)} + (1 - \alpha)Q^{\alpha-2}\}\{-\log u_1\}^{\varphi-1}\{-\log u_2\}^{\varphi-1}u_1^{-1}u_2^{-1},$$

where $\varphi = 1/\alpha$, $u_1 = 1 - t_1$, $u_2 = 1 - t_2$ and $Q = \{-\log u_1\}^\varphi + \{-\log u_2\}^\varphi$.

13.6   The combined approach

The idea of this approach is that the marginals are modeled by standard Cox models, and the dependence is modeled by some sort of copula. The copulas used are those corresponding to frailty models. It is a multivariate approach that is more consistent with the univariate model than the multi-state and frailty models. This is an approach that gives us the frailty models in simple cases. Without covariates, it corresponds to using the marginal parametrization, as described in Equation (7.9). In the case of a positive stable frailty model, proportional hazards in the conditional distribution lead to proportional hazards in the marginal model, as shown in Equation (2.54). There is, however, a change in the regression covariates, so that those of the marginal distribution are the regression coefficients in the conditional distribution multiplied with the positive stable index (α). The multivariate model is described by the survivor function in Equation (7.47). For other frailty distributions, the marginal modeling approach gives a way of avoiding the univariate identifiability problems in regression models.

In the case of Weibull marginal distributions and positive stable frailty dependence, we obtain the model of Section 7.4.3.

If one applies a gamma frailty model together with Weibull marginal hazards, a model is obtained that is different from the gamma Weibull frailty model described in Section 7.3.2. Again, the problem of being able to identify all parameters from univariate data is avoided. When there are covariates, we may assume proportional hazards in the marginal distributions. For a gamma frailty distribution, this leads to diverging conditional hazards. This is seen by inserting a proportional hazards model in Equation (7.30), which gives the hazard function

$$\exp(\beta' z)\omega(t)\exp\{\exp(\beta' z)\Omega_0(t)/\delta\}.$$

The divergence of these functions follows by dividing the expressions for two different values of z.

Quantifying the dependence can be done by means of Kendall's τ, Spearman's ρ, and κ. As these measures are independent of the hazard function, they can be directly transferred from Chapter 7.

There is a clear need for experience with this approach. Some applications are presented below.

13.6.1   Estimation

For parametric models, one just inserts the expressions into Equation (7.11). For non- or semi-parametric models, one can base estimation on the three-stage approach of Section 8.4 or use the full marginal approach of Section 8.5. For the latter approach, the only difference to the shared frailty model described in that section is that more general hazard functions are used, incorporating covariates. The dependence between the frailty parameter and the other parameters is smaller in this model and, therefore, convergence is faster.

The EM-algorithm can also be used, but it is more complicated than the approach of Section 8.3, because the maximization step cannot be used directly owing to the more complicated expressions for the conditional hazards. Glidden and Self (1999) suggested a way to overcome this problem by modifying this step. Estimation in that model is only approximate regarding $\Lambda(t)$.

13.6.2 Asymptotics

It is possible to evaluate the Fisher information both in the stable-Weibull and the gamma-Weibull models, when there is no censoring. For the stable-Weibull model, this follows directly from Section 8.11.2. In fact, the information was formulated in the marginal parametrization of the model.

This was done for the gamma frailty model with marginal Weibull distributions by Bjarnason and Hougaard (2000). They found expressions for the information for complete data, being explicit, except for two terms that require numerical integration. Assuming symmetry, either as common shape parameters or as common scale and shape parameters, does not change the asymptotic variance of the dependence parameter. Compared to the conditional Weibull model (Section 8.11.1), the variance of the dependence parameter is larger as a consequence of the conditional model gaining information from the marginal distributions.

Using Equation (2.48), we can study the amount of information lost by using the IWM approach for a given model.

13.6.3 Applications

Twin data

For the Danish twins of Section 1.5.1, the results are described in Table 13.6. This table can on the one hand be compared to Table 8.34, which presents the similar results in the shared frailty model. The combined copula approach suggests a higher dependence, whereas the effect of the covariates is similar. In particular, we cannot see the expected result that the regression coefficients should be higher in the shared frailty model.

Furthermore, it can be compared to the results obtained by the IWM approach, described in Table 13.3. The results are similar, but not identical.

Catheter infection data

For the time to infection data of Section 1.7.3, with sex as the only covariate, the regression coefficient is -0.876 (0.314). Thus the estimate is similar to the IWM approach, but the standard error is clearly smaller. The estimated value of Kendall's τ is 0.099 (0.092), suggesting a positive

	$\hat{\tau}$	SE^2	SE	$\hat{\beta}$	SE^2	SE
Males						
MZ	0.1985	0.0285	0.0285	-1.626	0.325	0.326
DZ	0.0740	0.0219	0.0219	-1.618	0.222	0.222
UZ	0.2622	0.0534	0.0530	0.715	0.532	0.540
Females						
MZ	0.1769	0.0327	0.0328	-2.568	0.350	0.352
DZ	0.1105	0.0233	0.0233	-2.595	0.239	0.240
UZ	0.1850	0.0460	0.0459	-0.343	0.443	0.444

Table 13.6. Estimates of dependence (τ) and cohort effect (β, in %/year) for Danish twin data, based on the combined copula-marginal gamma frailty model. SE^2, approximation.

Treatment	$\hat{\beta}$ (SE)	u-statistic
SNG	-0.43 (0.12)	-3.74
Oral placebo (0h)	0.30 (0.10)	3.16
Oral placebo (1h)	0.07 (0.09)	0.80
Oral placebo (3h)	0.04 (0.09)	0.46
Oral placebo (5h)	0.19 (0.09)	2.23
Oral iso (0h)	0.06 (0.09)	0.63
Oral iso (1h)	-0.77 (0.16)	-4.70
Oral iso (3h)	-0.42 (0.12)	-3.65
Oral iso (5h)	-0.15 (0.10)	-1.52

Table 13.7. Combined copula gamma frailty results for log relative hazards (β) compared to sublingual placebo, for exercise data. Iso, isosorbide dinitrate; SNG, sublingual nitroglycerine.

dependence, although the effect is not significantly positive. Compared to the gamma shared frailty model presented in Table 8.9, the dependence in the marginal model is smaller. Also the standard error of τ is smaller in the marginal model, in fine agreement with the conditional model, including too much information.

Tumorigenesis data

For the litter-matched study of Section 1.5.3, the estimated treatment effect under independence is 0.859 (0.287). Thus, the estimate is a little smaller than the IWM approach, and the standard error is clearly smaller.

Exercise data

The combined approach is also useful for the exercise data of Section 1.8.2. The estimated regression coefficients are described in Table 13.7. The estimated regression coefficients are also somewhat low, compared to the previous estimates describing the relation in the marginal model, the proportional hazards models, the $\hat{\alpha}\hat{\beta}$ of the stable frailty model in Table 8.5, and the independence estimates of Table 13.4. The standard errors are markedly lower. Overall this amounts to the u-statistics' being in the same range as in the two tables. Kendall's τ is estimated as 0.576 (0.068), slightly higher than in the conditional model (Table 8.3).

Leukemia remission

For the leukemia remission data of Section 1.5.4, the dependence is suggested to be negative.

13.7 Chapter summary

Marginal modeling is a simple descriptive approach to determine the effect (and its significance) of a regression coefficient in the presence of dependence in the data. The coordinate-wise approach for parallel data has the advantage that in the first stage it does not base evaluations on an incorrect model. However, disadvantages are that it cannot handle matched pairs covariates and that the estimation in the second stage uses weights that are estimated from the data. The independence working model accepts more designs, including matched pairs covariates, but implies that the estimates are derived in a model that is incorrect. The real advantage of these approaches is the simplicity of the calculations.

There are different approaches to handling parallel data and recurrent events.

Copulas models are not relevant by themselves owing to their having the marginals fixed, but the combined approach of marginal models and copulas for parallel data has the advantage that it is based on a detailed model, implying, for example, that it is possible to estimate the dependence and to discuss whether the model is satisfactory. A more technical point is that there is a proper likelihood to use. The disadvantage of this approach is that the computations are more complicated.

13.8 Bibliographic comments

The coordinate-wise marginal modeling approach is described in Wei, Lin, and Weissfeld (1989). The independence working model approach is described by Lee, Wei, and Amato (1992). Huster, Brookmeyer, and Self (1989) have suggested a similar approach in a parametric setting. Reviews of the approaches are Lin (1994) and Liang et al. (1995). The most complete description of asymptotic results is Spiekerman and Lin (1998). Clegg, Cai, and Sen (1999) discussed the IWM model with partial stratification.

Manatunga and Oakes (1999) criticized the independence working model on the basis of efficiency evaluation in the stable frailty model.

Using weights for the contributions was suggested by Cai and Prentice (1995) and further considered by Cai and Prentice (1997) and Cai (1999).

The method for recurrent events was suggested by Lawless and Nadeau (1995), extending a one-sample approach by Nelson (1995).

The copula approach has been studied by Genest and MacKay (1986a,b), Genest and Rivest (1993), and Oakes (1989).

A two-step estimation method for the combined approach was suggested by Hougaard (1986b) in the stable case and used more generally by Hougaard, Harvald, and Holm (1992a). The methods are considered in more detail by Mahe and Chevret (1999). Glidden and Self (1999) considered the model for gamma frailty and suggested a modified EM-algorithm for the estimation in the semi-parametric models.

13.9   Exercises

Exercise 13.1 Comparison of Poisson processes by the IWM approach

Consider a Poisson process with rate μ. What is the hazard in the distribution of the time to the first event T_1? What is the distribution of the time from start to the second event T_2 (that is, not including any information on T_1)? What is the hazard in this distribution?

Consider also a second Poisson process, with rate $\rho\mu$. Confirm that the ratio of hazards for the two processes is ρ for T_1, as expected. Find the ratio of hazards for T_2 and show that the limiting value is ρ^2 at time 0. Are the hazards proportional?

Exercise 13.2 Recurrent events with same observation period

Suppose that for n independent individuals, we have information for recurrent events consisting of all events times from time 0 to time C (common to all individuals). Show that $\hat{\Lambda}(C) = \sum_i K_i(C)/n$ and that the estimated variance is the empirical variance $\sum_i \{K_i(C) - \hat{\Lambda}(C)\}^2/n^3$.

Exercise 13.3 Analysis of mammary tumor data

Apply the procedure of Section 13.4 to the mammary tumor data described in Section 1.7.1. Compare to the results reported in Section 9.8.

Analyze the data also by the method described in Section 13.1.1. Try to vary the number of events included in the analysis. Discuss the results.

Exercise 13.4 Gamma frailty Weibull marginal model density

Consider a gamma frailty model with marginal Weibull distributions. Derive the density in the bivariate case.

Exercise 13.5 Gamma frailty Weibull marginal model derived quantities

Consider a gamma frailty model with marginal Weibull distributions. Make precise, what distributional results are obtained from Equations (7.25) and (7.26) and consider which moments can be evaluated by means of these results.

Exercise 13.6 Conditional quartiles

An alternative way to assess dependence is to evaluate conditional fractiles in a copula model. Do this in the gamma frailty as well as in the stable frailty model. Make a figure of the quartiles in the two models, choosing the parameters to have $\tau = 0.25$.

Exercise 13.7 Marshall-Olkin model copula

Derive the copula corresponding to the Marshall-Olkin model of Section 5.5.4. Find the set, where the density has a singularity.

14
Multivariate non-parametric estimates

It is desirable to have a completely non-parametric estimate of a multivariate survival distribution. This has the advantage of not requiring distributional assumptions, but it does, of course, require some structural assumptions, namely, independence of groups and identical multivariate distributions for the groups. It could serve as a baseline for evaluating the fit of more specific models. In principle, it allows for assessment of the dependence, but it may be inefficient compared to a fully parametric or semi-parametric estimate.

There is, at present, no final solution to this estimation problem. The available solutions are mathematically complicated, in particular, much more complicated than the univariate Kaplan-Meier estimate that they aim to generalize. It is, however, not because the estimates are difficult to compute. The available suggestions are in some cases explicit and, in fact, simple to evaluate. The problems rather are that we have no experience in graphically judging bivariate survivor functions, that the actual estimates have some undesirable features, and that the mass is spread out over many points, making it difficult to report the estimate. Therefore, this approach is, at present, not of major practical importance. One consequence is that this chapter can be read independently of the other chapters, or in other words, practitioners can omit this chapter.

For univariate data, the Kaplan-Meier estimate of Section 2.3.1 is a non-parametric estimate of the survivor function in the case of independent identically distributed data. It allows for censoring, and in the case where there are no censored data, it gives the empirical distribution as result. It is interesting and relevant to generalize this to multivariate survival data.

This is, however, not simple. Therefore, we restrict ourselves to the case of bivariate parallel data, corresponding to lifetimes of two individuals or the failure times of two components of a unit. Some of the methods can be extended to cover data for two different events, say, heart disease and death, modeled by the disability model (Figure 1.5), but then one needs to account for the time of heart disease being undefined if death occurs without heart disease. This can be done and we have such an example. For recurrent events data no completely non-parametric estimate exists. The approach here can be used for the first two events, but doing so requires that all persons will eventually experience the event at least twice. If there are persons who do not experience the event at all, it is difficult to formulate the problem in this framework.

So we try to estimate a bivariate survivor function $S(t_1, t_2)$. There are several problems. One problem is already present with the Kaplan-Meier estimate as it has the technical shortcoming that if the largest time value, say $T_{(n)}$, corresponds to a censoring, the value of the survivor function is undefined after this time point. An alternative interpretation is that it assigns the probability to the interval $(T_{(n)}, \infty)$ rather than to a single point. Thus the estimate assigns probability to the observed death times plus possibly the interval from the largest time value to infinity. In the univariate case, this is easily handled by not considering the survival function after the last time point. In the bivariate case, this problem is, however, grossly amplified and may lead to the estimate's being undefined in a large part of the bivariate plane. It also makes it difficult to evaluate some measures of dependence. Another problem is related to the so-called curse of dimensionality. For the univariate estimate, it is sufficient to evaluate the function at the observed death times, meaning that with n observations, the estimate can be reported in a table with at most n time values and n values for the survivor function. In the bivariate case, however, we need to evaluate the function on a grid. With observations on n pairs, this requires an estimate of the survivor function at n^2 points, making it impossible to handle large data sets. However, the number of support points is at most n for some of the estimates considered.

Some requirements we would like to discuss for a multivariate survival distribution estimate are listed in Table 14.1. Most of the properties are desirable, but whether it is desirable that the marginal distributions equal the Kaplan-Meier estimates is an open question. Some of the properties seem so natural that we might not even think they should be mentioned, but it turns out that several of the suggested estimates have difficulties satisfying even the first two requirements. Some are only defined in a small subset of the relevant set and other estimates put negative probability mass at some points. Equivariant under increasing transformations means that if $\hat{S}$ is the estimate based on a sample, $T_{ij}, i = 1, ..., n, j = 1, 2$ and $\tilde{S}$ the estimate of based on the transformed observations $f(T_{ij}), i = 1, ..., n, j = 1, 2$, where f is an increasing function, the estimates should satisfy the relation

Properties
Well-defined in a large set
Proper joint survivor distribution
Explicit estimation
Without censoring the empirical distribution is obtained
The marginal distributions equal the Kaplan-Meier estimates
Equivariant under common increasing transformations
Equivariant under reversal of coordinates

Table 14.1. Properties for consideration of bivariate non-parametric survival distribution estimates.

$\hat{S}(t_1, t_2) = \tilde{S}(f(t_1), f(t_2))$, meaning that the two estimates are essentially the same. We will not require the same property satisfied with different functions for the two coordinates, because in many cases, the time axis is the same for both coordinates and transforming with different functions would invalidate the common time scale interpretation. Equivariant under reversal of coordinates means that if we define $Y_{ij}, i = 1, ..., n, j = 1, 2$ by $Y_{i1} = T_{i2}, Y_{i2} = T_{i1}$, the estimate based on the Y-observations, say, $\tilde{S}$, should satisfy $\tilde{S}(t_1, t_2) = \hat{S}(t_2, t_1)$. For example, if the estimate is derived by means of the marginal distribution of T_1, and the conditional distribution of T_2 given T_1, it will not automatically be equivariant under reversal of coordinates. Dabrowska (1988) termed this property symmetry, but we will not use this term as we prefer symmetry to mean that the distribution is symmetric, that is, $S(t_1, t_2) = S(t_2, t_1)$, by assumption. All the estimates considered here are equivariant under reversal of coordinates.

A major disadvantage of a completely non-parametric estimate is that it is difficult or impossible to quantify any aspect of the distribution. One specific problem is that there are point masses corresponding to one or both coordinates belonging to intervals near ∞. This is similar to the univariate case, but the problem turns out to be much more influential in the bivariate case. In this case, we can easily obtain estimates of the marginal distributions, but it is difficult to quantify the dependence and discuss concepts like whether the dependence time frame is short-term or long-term. The only directly available estimate of the degree of dependence is the median concordance (see Section 4.4).

At present, only independent censoring has been considered, but process-dependent censoring patterns can be acceptable, see Pruitt (1993a).

A further disadvantage is that it is not directly possible to include co-variates in order to make a semi-parametric model. However, just as the Cox model is a semi-parametric extension of the Nelson-Aalen approach, it is possible that we, at a later stage, can suggest a sensible semi-parametric model extending the simple approach.

In the statistical literature, there is very little experience on how to illustrate and consider bivariate survivor functions. This is a major problem and this chapter also tries to build up this experience. We, of course, want a way where we can detect important features of the distribution. The absence of this experience makes it more difficult to satisfy the purposes of the study. In the univariate case, we can easily discuss features like position, made explicit by the median, that is, where the function crosses $1/2$ and we can find points where the density is high or low by differentiation by eye. In the bivariate case, we can, of course, do the same thing, which is covered by the purpose prediction in the terminology of Section 1.14. But we are particularly interested in more bivariate features, corresponding to the purpose of assessing the dependence, by means of questions like Is there dependence? Is it positive or negative? Finally, the purpose of checking a more specific model can be illustrated by questions like Is the model a Markov model? as discussed in Section 5.3.3 and Is the dependence of short-term or long-term time frame?

Some ways of illustrating a bivariate survivor function are three-dimensional plots; contour plots; bivariate plots where one coordinate takes selected values; evaluation of selected distributions conditional on survival; evaluation of distributions conditional on one coordinate's being in selected intervals; and the ratio of the bivariate function to the product of the marginals. One possibility to remove the dependence on the marginal distributions is to transform by the marginal estimates, basically corresponding to finding the actual copula distribution, see Section 13.5.

Section 14.1 does basic evaluations of the survival function and the hazard in bivariate distributions, and discusses the notation and the censoring patterns. In Section 14.2 we illustrate some basic estimation problems with bivariate censored data and discuss the estimate suggested by Hanley and Parnes. The estimate suggested by Dabrowska is described in Section 14.3. An estimate suggested by Pruitt designed to repair the problem of the Hanley and Parnes method is considered in Section 14.4. These estimates are compared in Section 14.5. Other estimates and multivariate extensions are considered in Section 14.6. Asymptotic results are discussed in Section 14.7. The problem of illustrating a bivariate survival function is discussed in Section 14.8. Section 14.9 discusses how to give a quantitative summary of the distribution, in order to discuss not only the degree of dependence, but also whether the dependence is early or late and whether it is of short-term or long-term time frame. Model checking is specifically considered in Section 14.10. Section 14.11 applies the various methods to several data sets. In particular, the Danish twin data are used in order to compare the various estimates and to discuss how to illustrate and quantify the bivariate survivor function in the best way. Other data sets are used to discuss the general applicability of the approaches.

Observation type	Observation	Restriction
Double death	(T_1, T_2)	None
Single death	(T_1+, T_2)	$T_1 \geq T_2$
	(T_1, T_2+)	$T_1 \leq T_2$
Double censoring	(T_1+, T_2+)	$T_1 = T_2$

Table 14.2. Observation types and their restrictions for homogeneous censoring.

14.1   Distribution concepts and observations

Handling probabilities is more complicated in the bivariate case than in the univariate. In the univariate case, the probability of an interval (a, b), that is, $Pr(T \in (a, b))$, is found as $S(b) - S(a)$, but in the bivariate case, the corresponding formula is

$$Pr(T_1 \in (a_1, b_1), T_2 \in (a_2, b_2)) = S(b_1, b_2) - S(a_1, b_2) - S(b_1, a_2) + S(a_1, a_2).$$
(14.1)

We may define a bivariate hazard function as

$$\lambda(t_1, t_2) = f(t_1, t_2)/S(t_1, t_2),$$
(14.2)

which describes the probability that both coordinates will experience an event given that they are both alive. This naturally extends the univariate expression $\lambda(t) = f(t)/S(t)$, which alternatively can be written as $-d \log S(t)/dt$. Thus $\lambda(t_1, t_2)$ equals $\{d^2/dt_1 dt_2 S(t_1, t_2)\}/S(t_1, t_2)$, but it cannot be simply formulated by means of the derivative of $\log S(t_1, t_2)$. In fact, the relation is

$$\frac{d^2}{dt_1 dt_2} \log S(t_1, t_2) = \lambda(t_1, t_2) - \{\frac{d}{dt_1} \log S(t_1, t_2)\}\{\frac{d}{dt_2} \log S(t_1, t_2)\}.$$
(14.3)

The last term in this formula is one cause of the difficulties in finding a non-parametric estimate of the bivariate survivor function.

Where the univariate expression can be inverted by the classical formula $S(t) = \exp\{-\int_0^t \lambda(u)du\}$, the bivariate case is more complicated. The expression is

$$S(t_1, t_2) = S(t_1, 0)S(0, t_2) \exp\{\int_0^{t_1} \int_0^{t_2} \lambda(u, v)dudv\}.$$
(14.4)

Observations are described in the standard parallel way, as (T_1, T_2) with corresponding death indicators (D_1, D_2). There are three types of observations - the double deaths, that is, known times; single deaths, where one individual is observed to die and the other is censored; and double censorings. These cases are listed in Table 14.2, where the restrictions placed owing to the homogeneous censorings are also described. As an illustrative example consider the observations of five pairs shown in Figure 14.1. The double deaths just give a single point of observation. The double censorings correspond to a quadrant in the homogeneous case, translated along the

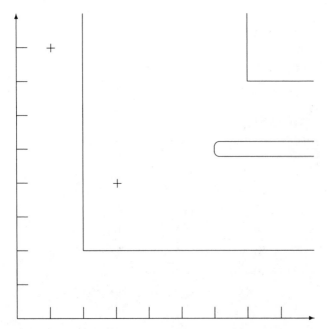

Figure 14.1. Artificial data on five pairs, illustrating bivariate data under homogeneous censoring. Observations: (1,8), (3,4), (6+,5), (2+,2+), (7+,7+).

diagonal. The single deaths correspond to a univariate interval in the bivariate plane, extending to ∞. These intervals do not cross the diagonal in the homogeneous case. These observations correspond to homogeneous censoring, which implies that the sets generated by the censoring pattern are jointly either nested or disjoint. For example (1,8) and (6+,5) are disjoint, whereas (2+,2+) and (6+,5) are nested.

An example, showing three observations that are not possible under homogeneous censoring are given in Figure 14.2. It is clear that the sets no longer satisfy the relation that they are either nested or disjoint.

14.2   The Hanley and Parnes estimate

Hanley and Parnes (1983) suggested this estimate and made an explicit evaluation under homogeneous censoring and described an iterative solution in the general case. Their estimation method for the homogeneous case has an interpretation like the multi-state model of Figure 5.13, because they split the problem into the distribution of the minimum, the distribution of which component(s) fails at the minimum given the minimum, and then an arbitrary distribution for the second event given the first. When the censoring pattern is not homogeneous, this simple derivation is not possible. Therefore, the two cases are treated separately.

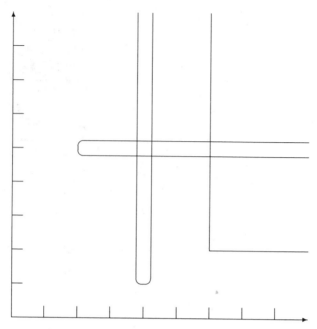

Figure 14.2. Artificial data on 3 pairs, illustrating bivariate data under heterogeneous censoring. Observations: (2+,5), (4,1+), (6+,2+).

14.2.1 Homogeneous censoring

The marginal distribution does not equal the Kaplan-Meier estimate based on the marginal data, but the probability of both being alive (corresponding to $S(t,t)$) equals the Kaplan-Meier distribution based on the marginal distribution of the first event in each pair.

Based on the knowledge we have from the univariate case, the Kaplan-Meier estimate, the redistribution to the right algorithm, and the interval censored case, we can, in the homogeneous censoring case, immediately describe the bivariate non-parametric estimate of the bivariate distribution. We first need to find out which sets will have positive mass. At each time point of a double death, there will be a positive estimated mass. For each double censoring there will typically be some observations completely contained in the set, in which case we can apply the redistribution to the right algorithm, implying that the mass is taken over by the observations within the set of possible lifetimes consistent with the censoring times, as done for the observation (2+,2+). In case there are no deaths observed, the set will keep the mass, as done for the observation (7+,7+). There can at most be one such observation. The single deaths create the real problems, because for continuous data, they will with probability 1 have no overlap to other observations, and thus the sets should keep the mass, like what we saw for interval censored data. This means that a univariate interval gets

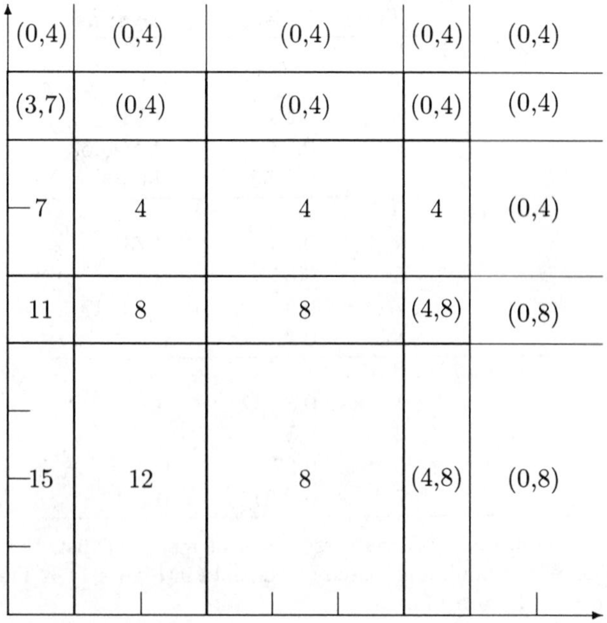

(0,4)	(0,4)	(0,4)	(0,4)	(0,4)
(3,7)	(0,4)	(0,4)	(0,4)	(0,4)
-7	4	4	4	(0,4)
11	8	8	(4,8)	(0,8)
-15	12	8	(4,8)	(0,8)

Figure 14.3. Bivariate survival estimate for the artificial data on five pairs, in multiples of $1/15$. Observations: (1,8), (3,4), (6+,5), (2+,2+), (7+,7+).

a positive mass. Typically, there are many such intervals. This makes it impossible to evaluate the survival function at some bivariate points and is a major problem. In the illustrative example, we obtain the estimate shown in Figure 14.3. It gives a mass of $1/5$ at the points (1,8), $4/15$ at (3,4), and $4/15$ to the univariate interval (6+,5) and $4/15$ to the bivariate interval (7+,7+). This implies that the survivor function estimate is unknown in large areas of the plane. For example, the mass at the (7+,7+) implies that the survivor function cannot be evaluated for the sets (0,7+) and (7+,0). More important is that with continuous data, each single censoring implies that there is an area (like a shadow), in which the survivor function cannot be estimated. For example, an observation (t_1+, t_2) implies that the survivor function cannot be determined on the set $(t_1, \infty) \times (0, t_2)$. In the example, the interval (6+,5) implies that the probability cannot be evaluated in the set $(6, \infty) \times (0, 5)$. When there are ties in one coordinate, say, t_2, it is more complicated; there will only be a shadow if t_1 is maximal among the observations with the actual value of t_2. However, we can see that the survivor function is known on the diagonal from time 0 until some maximum time. Along the diagonal, it equals the Kaplan-Meier estimate evaluated on the basis on the minimums within each pair, that is, based on $T_{(1)} = \min(T_1, T_2)$. Generally, we may find a bivariate interval within which the estimate is well defined. In the example this is the interval from (0,0) to (6,7). The marginal distributions can be read off the figure. Sim-

Coordinate	Time	Univariate	Bivariate
Marginal 1	0	1	1
	1	0.8	0.8
	3	0.53	0.53
	6	0.53	0.27-0.53
	7	0-0.53	0-0.53
Marginal 2	0	1	1
	4	0.75	0.73
	5	0.5	0.47
	7	0.5	0.2-0.47
	8	0-0.5	0-0.27
Minimum	0	1	1
	1	0.8	0.8
	3	0.53	0.53
	5	0.27	0.27
	7	0-0.27	0-0.27

Table 14.3. Univariate and bivariate estimates of marginal distribution and of the distribution of the minimum, based on the data in Figure 14.1. The bivariate estimate is read off Figure 14.3.

ilarly, the distribution of the time to the first event in the pair, that is, the minimum lifetime, can be seen on the figure. The values are described in Table 14.3, and compared to the univariate estimates. The univariate estimates are the Kaplan-Meier estimates based on only the observations corresponding to that marginal. There is a reasonable agreement between the univariate and the bivariate marginal estimates, but it can be seen that the bivariate estimates in more cases lead to the values being unknown.

To be precise, the estimation in the homogeneous censoring case goes along the following way, which has many similarities to the approaches in Section 6.3. First calculate the minimum within each pair, that is, $T_{(1)} = \min\{T_1, T_2\}$, with corresponding death indicator $D_{(1)} = \max\{D_1, D_2\}$. In the illustrative example, these data are 1, 2+, 3, 5, 7+. Calculate the Kaplan-Meier estimate based on this. In the example this gives the survivor function listed in the lower part of Table 14.3. Go through all positive masses on this estimate. In the example, these are 0.2 at 1, 0.27 at 3, 0.27 at 5, and 0.27 for the interval 7+. Suppose at a giving time $t_{(1)}$ there is a contribution $P(t_{(1)})$. This is to be assigned somewhere on the union of the two univariate intervals $(t_{(1)}+, t_{(1)}) \cup (t_{(1)}, t_{(1)}+)$. It will first be split into the three possibilities $t_1 = t_2, t_1 > t_2, t_1 < t_2$, according to the observed frequencies of the data. In the example, at 1, the mass will be assigned to the set $\{t_1 = 1, t_1 < t_2\}$, that is where the single point is. At 3 it goes to the set $\{t_1 = 3, t_1 < t_2\}$, and at 5 to the set $\{t_2 = 5, t_1 > t_2\}$. It will be distributed within the set by the ordinary Kaplan-Meier estimate based on the subset of the data. In the examples, each of these subsets has only a single element, and therefore, the Kaplan-Meier estimate is trivial. For $t_{(1)} = 1$, it places all the mass at 8, leading to a mass of 0.2 at (1,8). For $t_{(1)} = 3$, it places all the mass at 4, leading to a mass of 0.27 at (3,4). For $t_{(1)} = 5$, the Kaplan-Meier estimate places all the mass to the interval (6+,5). One consequence of the interpretation in terms of Figure 5.13 is that the approach works for data on different events.

A simple approach to repair the undefined points is to distribute the mass according to the Kaplan-Meier estimate based on the marginal data, truncated to the set where the mass is supposed to be in. This will be called the marginal filling-in method. This procedure is conservative, that is, it reduces dependence and it turns out that by a refinement of this idea, better performance is obtained (see Section 14.4).

Visser (1996) suggested an approach relevant under order restriction, that is, $T_1 < T_2$. This would for example be the case for recurrent events, or alternatively, for the twin data, one could transform the bivariate time to the time of the first death and the time to the last death within the pair. This approach, illustrated as a multi-state model in Figure 5.14, is perfectly sensible, when the bivariate distribution is symmetric. The example considered in the paper is time to diagnosis of AIDS (T_1) and death (T_2) for children infected. Normally, such data cannot generally satisfy the order restriction, but the data are truncated, so that T_1 is observed, and therefore in the particular data set, the order restriction is fulfilled. The approach requires homogeneous censoring for (T_1, T_2). The data are transformed to $(U_1, U_2) = (T_1, T_2 - T_1)$, which is one-to-one and does not create problems with the censoring under the ordering restriction. When expressed in terms of (T_1, T_2), the approach is identical to the Hanley and Parnes approach. The asymptotic problems with the singly censored observations are elegantly avoided by assuming discrete times, but in practice, the problem is still there.

14.2.2 Heterogeneous censoring

In general bivariate parallel data, we might observe heterogeneous censorings. This means that estimation is much more complicated, depending on the approach. Maximum likelihood estimation is iterative. The methods, which, in fact, are similar to those of univariate interval censoring, can be mathematically translated into linear models for probabilities in a multinomial model. First we have to examine which sets will have positive probability. In the example of Figure 14.2, there will be two sets with positive probability, namely the point of the cross-section of the two single censorings, the point (4,5) and the overlap between the double censoring and one of the single censorings, that is, the univariate interval (6+,5). It turns out that for these data, each of these sets get a mass of 1/2.

14.3   The Dabrowska estimate

An interesting estimate of the bivariate survivor function was suggested by Dabrowska (1988). It was derived by a consideration of bivariate hazard functions. It was found that the function defined in Equation (14.2) is not sufficient to find the survivor function in the bivariate case.

The estimate is as follows. First find the bivariate risk set

$$R(t_1, t_2) = \sum_i 1\{T_{i1} \geq t_1, T_{i2} \geq t_2\}.$$

Then we need the number of bivariate events at each time

$$K_{11}(t_1, t_2) = \sum_i D_{i1} D_{i2} 1\{T_{i1} = t_1, T_{i2} = t_2\}$$

and the number of events for coordinate 1, among those where the second component is alive at time t_2

$$K_{10}(t_1, t_2) = \sum D_{i1} 1\{T_{i1} = t_1, T_{i2} \geq t_2\}$$

and similarly for coordinate 2

$$K_{01}(t_1, t_2) = \sum D_{i2} 1\{T_{i1} \geq t_1, T_{i2} = t_2\}.$$

The quantities are seen relative to the risk set

$$L_{11}(t_1, t_2) = K_{11}(t_1, t_2)/R(t_1, t_2)$$

$$L_{10}(t_1, t_2) = K_{10}(t_1, t_2)/R(t_1, t_2)$$

$$L_{01}(t_1, t_2) = K_{01}(t_1, t_2)/R(t_1, t_2).$$

The marginal survivor functions are found as

$$S_1(t_1) = \prod_{u \leq t_1} \{1 - L_{10}(u, 0)\}$$

$$S_2(t_2) = \prod_{u \leq t_2} \{1 - L_{01}(0, u)\}.$$

These expressions should be interpreted as the usual product integrals, like Equation (2.25). In fact, they are just Kaplan-Meier estimates based on each coordinate separately. At all times without events, the factor is 1 and can be neglected. At times with event, there is a term below 1, which contributes to the estimate. Then the estimate is

$$S(t_1, t_2) = S_1(t_1) S_2(t_2) \prod_{0 \leq u \leq t_1, 0 \leq v \leq t_2} \{1 - H(u, v)\}, \tag{14.5}$$

where H is given by

$$H(t_1, t_2) = \frac{L_{10}(t_1, t_2) L_{01}(t_1, t_2) - L_{11}(t_1, t_2)}{\{1 - L_{10}(t_1, t_2)\}\{1 - L_{01}(t_1, t_2)\}}.$$

It can be seen that Equation (14.5) has a strong interpretation as the product of the marginal survivor functions, modified by the product of H terms, which then describe the dependence.

If we want to assume symmetry, R should be substituted by $R(t_1, t_2) + R(t_2, t_1)$ and similarly K_{11} should be substituted by $K_{11}(t_1, t_2) + K_{11}(t_2, t_1)$. Furthermore, K_{01} should be substituted by $K_{01}(t_1, t_2) + K_{10}(t_2, t_1)$, and $K_{10}(t_1, t_2)$ should be the transpose of the sum.

14.4   The Pruitt estimate

As described above, the non-parametric maximum likelihood approach does not work, because the masses of the single censorings cannot be placed in an appropriate way. Pruitt (1990) suggests a smoothing method, where information is combined over neighborhoods. This is not a truly non-parametric method, as it requires the choice of the bandwidth parameter γ. This parameter will enlarge the set where the estimate is defined, compared to the Hanley and Parnes method.

The approach is based on the observation above that the problem is the singly censored observations. The mass corresponding to these data must be specifically distributed in order for the survivor function to be well defined. The Hanley and Parnes method does not distribute this mass and the Dabrowska method distributes it in a way that fixes the marginal distributions to those obtained by the Kaplan-Meier method. The Pruitt method instead distributes the mass according to a Kaplan-Meier method applied to the observed events in a neighborhood of the observation. The size of the neighborhood is determined by γ. As an example, consider a point censored in the first coordinate (t_1, t_2) with death indicator $(D_1, D_2) = (0, 1)$. This reflects a mass applicable to the set $\{T_1 \geq t_1, T_2 = t_2\}$. The suggested method distributes the mass in this set, according to the Kaplan-Meier estimate applied for the points satisfying $T_1 \geq t_1, t_2 - \gamma \leq T_2 \leq t_2 + \gamma, D_2 = 1$. In the example of Figure 14.1, the only problem is the observation (6+,5). However, whatever value of γ is used, there will be no points satisfying the condition. The requirements for the time values would be satisfied for the point (7+,7+) when $\gamma \geq 2$, but double-censored points and singly censored points in the other direction are ignored. If (7+,7+) was included, the observation (6+,5) would assign its mass to the set (7+,5), just like the Dabrowska method would in this simple case. If there was an extra observation in (8,1), the mass of (6+,5) would be put in (8,5), when $\gamma \geq 4$. In real applications, there will typically be several points satisfying the neighborhood requirement and the mass would be split among the corresponding values of T_1.

Suppose in the example that besides the original points and (8,1), there was an observation (7,1+), singly censored in the other component. If $\gamma =$

Point or set	Hanley and Parnes	Dabrowska
(1,4)	0	−1
(1,5)	0	−1
(1,8)	12	14
(3,4)	16	16
(6+,5)	16	-
(7+,5)	-	16
(7+,7+)	16	16

Table 14.4. Estimates of distributions, for the data of Figure 14.1. Based on Hanley and Parnes method and Dabrowska's method. In multiples of 1/60.

4, this would have its mass evenly distributed between points (7,4) and (7,5), both points being within the neighborhood of (6+,5), suggesting that an event at (7,5) is possible. However, the observation (7,1+) would not influence the spreading of the mass of (6+,5) owing to the restriction of the neighborhood to points with an event in the first coordinate.

In the case of homogeneous censoring, it is possible to evaluate this in a way similar to the Hanley and Parnes procedure, successively distributing the mass along the diagonal and secondly on each ray from the diagonal. In the general case, an EM algorithm is typically used.

A key point is the choice of γ. From a non-parametric estimation point of view, a small value should be used. However, a too small value is not successful in getting points in the neighborhood. As γ increases, more and more points will have non-empty neighborhoods. This increases the set where the survivor function is defined. A large γ will be more efficient, just like any other smoothing method, but at the price of a bias and reduces the non-parametric basis of the approach. In a multivariate survival case, a high degree of smoothing is expected to reduce the dependence.

For asymptotic evaluations to work, γ must go to 0 to avoid bias, but this is also possible. It should just go to 0 so slowly that all neighborhoods will stay non-empty.

14.5 Comparison

Table 14.4 shows the estimated non-zero probabilities under the Hanley and Parnes method and the Dabrowska method for the example of Figure 14.1. They agree for the point (3,4) and the set (7+,7+). The Dabrowska method requires the marginal distributions to fit the Kaplan-Meier estimate based on the marginal data, and therefore it, compared to the Hanley and Parnes estimate, moves mass from (1,4) and (1,5) and gives it to (1,8). As (1,4) and (1,5) have zero mass initially, their mass under the Dabrowska method becomes negative. For the single censoring (6+,5), Hanley and Parnes just gives the mass to this interval, but the Dabrowska method has no mass in the marginal distribution for the interval from 6 to 7 and therefore leads to the same mass's being concentrated on the smaller univariate interval (7+,5). In the table, a hyphen (-) is used to specify that the interval, as such, is not assigned a probability mass. But, we can, as the sets are nested, calculate that Dabrowska's method gives a total mass of 16/60 in the interval (6+,5) and the Hanley and Parnes method has a probability between 0 and 16/60 for the interval (7+,5). The marginal filling-in method applied on the Hanley and Parnes method will also concentrate the mass to the interval (7+,5). As said above, the Pruitt method is unable to distribute the mass of this point because the neighborhood is empty for all values of γ and therefore this method agrees with Hanley and Parnes in this example.

For the heterogeneous censoring example of Figure 14.2, the marginal of the first coordinate gives a mass of 1/2 at 4 and 1/2 to the interval 6+. The marginal of the second coordinate gives a mass of 1 at 5. The only way these relations can be combined is by giving a mass of 1/2 to the point (4,5) and 1/2 to the interval (6+,5). Thus it is exactly the same estimate as derived above by the method of Hanley and Parnes.

The two estimates agree on the diagonal, and this implies that their estimates of the median concordance agree, when the medians are determined by the estimates based on the marginal data. When the Hanley and Parnes method evaluates the median by means of the marginals of the bivariate estimate, there can be discrepancies.

Hanley and Parnes show an example where the observations are known to be ordered so that $T_1 \leq T_2$, but where this ordering is not preserved by the Kaplan-Meier estimate based on the marginal data. We have simplified this example to be the five observations (1,3), (2,4), (3+,3+), (4+,4+) and (5,6). The marginal estimate for the first coordinate puts masses of 0.2 at 1 and 2, and the rest (0.6) at 5. For the second coordinate, the masses are 0.2 at 3 and 0.27 at 4, and 0.53 at 6. This implies that between 4 and 5, the marginal survivor functions have the wrong order. Hanley and Parnes method leads to masses of 0.2 at (1,3) and (2,4) and 0.6 at (5,6), corresponding to the interpretation that the masses of the two double censorings are passed on to (5,6). The marginal estimate corresponding to T_1 agree with the univariate estimate, as it should, as the first coordinate is also the minimum within pairs. The second component disagrees as the marginal of the bivariate estimate corresponds to masses of 0.2 at 3 and 4, and 0.6 at 6. The Dabrowska method gives a mass of 0.2 to (1,3), 0.27 to (2,4), -0.07 to (2,6) and 0.6 to (5,6). All masses satisfy the order requirement, but as some of the masses are negative, the marginal distributions do not preserve the order. Thus, the Hanley and Parnes estimate is superior in this sense. As there are no singly censored pairs, Pruitt's estimate agrees with Hanley and Parnes and the value of γ has no influence.

14.6   Other estimates and extensions

There have been several other estimators suggested. Just a few will be
mentioned and commented upon, but generally the reader is referred to
the original papers for details.

Tsai, Leurgans, and Crowley (1986) presented an estimator based on
a decomposition of the bivariate survivor function. It places mass to the
double events and to the single events with the censoring coming after the
event, and it seems most relevant in the case of homogeneous censoring. It
requires smoothing.

Prentice and Cai (1992) suggested an estimator based on a representation
of the survivor function by a Peano series. This seems to be inspired by
the integrated hazard correlation defined in Section 4.5. It is based on the
covariance between the marginal martingales $N_j(t) - Q_j(t)$ as defined in
Section 2.6.

Lin and Ying (1993) have a simple suggestion for homogeneous censoring.
They suggested

$$\hat{S}(t_1, t_2) = n - 1 \frac{\sum_i 1\{T_{i1} > t_1, T_{i2} > t_2\}}{G(\max\{t_1, t_2\})},$$

where the denominator G is the Kaplan-Meier estimate for the censoring
distribution, that is, with observations $C_i = \max\{T_{i1}, T_{i2}\}$ and indicators
$1 - D_{i1}D_{i2}$. The idea is that the numerator is an estimate for the observed
times, which is then corrected for the influence of censoring by means of
the denominator. Unfortunately, this estimate leads to negative masses.
Furthermore, not all the masses are placed at death times; there can also
be masses, positive as well as negative, at the times of censorings. For the
example of Figure 14.1, the masses are for (1,2) −0.05, for (1,5) −0.125,
for (1,7) −0.375, for (1,8) 0.75, for (2,2) 0.05, for (3,4) 0.25, for (6,5) 0.125
and for (7,7) 0.375. Particularly surprising are the quite large masses at
(1,7) and (7,7), where no events are observed. In this example, the survivor
function is well defined in the whole positive quadrant. More generally, if
the largest time $(\max\{T_{ij}, i = 1, ..., n, j = 1, 2\})$ is a censoring, this will be
the end of the set of definition. Owing to the problems mentioned above,
this estimator is not recommended.

Going from dimension 2 to k implies no further complications from a
theoretical point of view. Equation (14.1) is generalized to a sum of 2^k
terms. Both the Dabrowska estimate and the Hanley and Parnes estimate
are easily generalized. The problem is that we loose the intuition and it
becomes much more difficult to illustrate than a bivariate survivor function. All observations that are not either fully observed or fully censored
will display problems like those of the singly censored observations in the
bivariate case. The idea behind the Pruitt estimate can still be used to
extend the set where the estimate is defined.

Although it is interesting to make this extension, it seems that it is more important to gather experience on the bivariate case, as there are still many aspects that are not clarified.

14.7   Asymptotics

The asymptotic evaluations for the non-parametric case are an order of magnitude more difficult than those of the other approaches treated in this book. Therefore, they are not covered here, but the reader is referred to the papers listed in the bibliography (Section 14.13). However, a few comments will be made. The censoring pattern is important. Generally, independent censoring has been assumed, but it seems that some, but not all, methods can accept process-dependent censoring. An application with process-dependent censoring is presented in Section 14.11.4. With homogeneous censoring, asymptotic evaluations are easier to make and further results can be evaluated.

The estimate by Dabrowska and that of Prentice and Cai have been shown to be asymptotically efficient under independence.

Generally, expressions for the variance are not available. The only variance estimate has been derived for the Hanley and Parnes approach using Greenwoods formula. Otherwise, it has been suggested to use bootstrap methods.

14.8   Graphical illustrations

A non-parametric estimate cannot be interpreted without a way to present it graphically. When we discuss univariate survivor functions, there are just a few ways to illustrate them, giving the survivor function as a function of time. These methods can also be used on the marginal distributions, when we want to illustrate features related to the marginal distribution. This section introduces and discusses various ways to illustrate the bivariate survivor function and features related to the dependence. This turns out to be much more complicated than the univariate case. Unfortunately, there seems to be very little experience on this matter in the statistical literature. Therefore, we briefly present a number of suggestions, and in Section 14.11.1, we apply each method to the twin data set and comment upon the usefulness of each way of presenting the data.

14.8.1   Cuts

The simplest possible way to handle the bivariate time scale is to show $S(t_1, t_2)$ as a function of t_2, for selected values of t_1. It is natural to select 0 as one of the values for t_1 as this gives the marginal distribution for T_2. In this way, we do very little to the original function, but on the other hand, it is also difficult to learn anything from this. Under independence, the curves are proportional, but it is difficult to judge proportionality on a standard illustration. This can be improved by using a log scale for the survivor function, because then independence is transformed into parallellity, but still it may be difficult to judge. This approach is used in Figures 14.6, 14.7 and 14.8.

14.8.2 Conditional on coordinate survival

To make it easier to judge independence, we might modify the cuts by conditioning on $T_1 > t_1$, that is, showing $S(t_1, t_2)/S(t_1, 0)$ as a function of t_2, for selected values of t_1. In this case independence implies that the functions should coincide. It is natural to let 0 be one of the values for t_1, as this gives the marginal survivor curve. The problem with this approach is that typically the functions are close to each other, because we condition with events that are almost the same. The various conditioning events are nested. Therefore, it might make more sense to let the conditioning events be exclusive, see below. This approach is used in Figure 14.9.

14.8.3 Conditional on coordinate interval survival

The suggestion above was basically to compare the survival for persons for which the partner is alive at t_1 to the marginal distribution and when t_1 is small these functions necessarily are close to each other. It might be more sensible to compare those with $T_1 > t_1$ to those with $T_1 \leq t_1$, as these curves will split better. As this requires a figure for each selected value of t_1, we will not do exactly that, but instead group according to the value of T_1. That is, define a set of interval end points $0 = x_0 < x_1 < \dots < x_m = \infty$, and then evaluate the conditional survival of T_2 given the interval containing T_1. The qth curve is then $\{S(x_{q-1}, t_2) - S(x_q, t_2)\}/\{S(x_{q-1}, 0) - S(x_q, 0)\}$, say $H_q(t_2)$, as function of t_2. For the last curve we use that $S(\infty, t_2) = 0$. A practical problem with this approach is how we should select m and x_q. A standard univariate histogram rule of thumb is to choose the number of intervals as $n^{1/2}$. In the bivariate case, this should be modified to $n^{1/4}$, which is typically a small number. The argument of using this number is that it defines a grid, with $n^{1/2}$ cells. In fact, with heavy censoring, it might be sensible to choose an even smaller number. It is not critical that the intervals have the same probability mass, but if there are no natural interval endpoints, we might as well make the intervals have approximately the same probability. This is done by choosing x_q so that $S(x_q, 0) = (m - q)/m$. In practice, we might well prefer a simple value in the neighborhood of this. This approach is used in Figure 14.12.

14.8.4   Three-dimensional plot

As the bivariate survivor function has two arguments, it makes sense to consider a three-dimensional plot. This could be expected to work well, because the function is decreasing in both arguments. The problem with this approach is that we have no experience with judging such functions and it is difficult to read the relevant features in the plot.

14.8.5   Contour curves of the survivor function

For judging such a bivariate function, it is sometimes more convenient to use the contour curves, that is, connect points (t_1, t_2) in the bivariate plane having the same value of $S(t_1, t_2)$. This is very sensitive to the marginal distributions, and for human lifetimes, we see that the contour curves become closer by increasing age. This also implies that it is difficult to evaluate whether the pattern is due to dependence or to marginal distribution. This approach is used in Figure 14.10.

14.8.6   Contour curves after uniform transformation

To modify the previous approach to make it easier to judge dependence, we might transform the marginals to become uniform. In practice, this is done by drawing the contour curves for $S(t_1, t_2)$ as function of $S(t_1, 0)$, say, y_1, and $S(0, t_2)$, say, y_2. Under independence this has a known pattern, as the function equals $y_1 y_2$. This still implies that the curves become closer by increasing age, but this is not as much a problem as we have a fixed standard (independence) to compare with. The independence model is illustrated in Figure 14.4. The value of the median concordance can immediately be read off, as the value at $(1/2, 1/2)$, and then transformed linearly as described in Equation (4.14). This approach is used in Figure 14.11.

14.8.7   Contour curves of the bivariate density

This is the standard way of illustrating a bivariate distribution but seems less sensible for survival distributions. First we do not have an estimate of this function, so some degree of smoothing or grouping is necessary. Secondly, the appearance depends both on the marginal distributions and the dependence, and therefore is a mix of different features.

14.8.8   Bivariate density after uniform transformation

Rather than showing the density function, as in the previous section, it might be easier to understand the results if we show the density when the marginals are transformed to follow the uniform distribution. This is intimately related to the copula approach of Section 13.5. After having

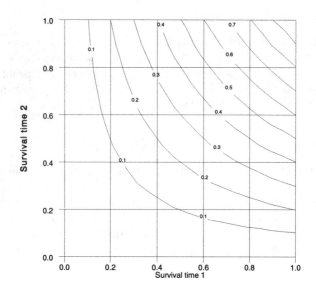

Figure 14.4. Contour curves of the survivor function after uniform transformation. Under independence.

transformed the survivor function, one can either make a splitting into intervals of equal (or approximately equal) length on the probability scale, or smooth the estimate. Only a few intervals are relevant, because otherwise the sampling variation is too high. For standard univariate histograms, there is an old rule of thumb that one can use $n^{1/2}$ intervals. If this rule is applied on the number of bivariate sets, the number of intervals on each axis can be chosen as $n^{1/4}$. Similarly, if smoothing is applied, one should expect to use a rather strong degree of smoothing. This density can then be shown in a three-dimensional plot, or listed in a table (when n is low). This approach is shown in Figure 14.14.

14.8.9 Markov assumption check

All the previous considerations treat the problem as a standard bivariate problem and do not account for the dynamic aspect inherent in survival data. In that frame, we might well ask the question, When one individual has died, is the hazard of death of the other independent of the first time of death? That is, is the dependence time frame short-term or long-term? An alternative formulation of this question is, Is it Markov, when the model is formulated as the multi-state model depicted in Figure 5.12? This will be done in the interval conditioning framework above. Choose an interval endpoint x_q as the time to make the evaluation, say, x_ℓ. Values of 1 and

m are trivial, and should not be chosen. Now evaluate the conditional distribution, for each q, $q \leq \ell$, given $x_{q-1} < T_1 \leq x_q$ and $T_2 > x_\ell$. This is $H_q(t_2)/H_q(x_\ell)$, using the definition of $H_q(t_2)$ in Section 14.8.3. This is only to be considered for $t_2 \geq x_\ell$. Now draw these curves for the relevant values of q as function of t_2. When the Markov assumption is satisfied, these curves should be identical. The whole process might be repeated for other values of ℓ. A low value of ℓ gives only a few curves, with a long definition interval for t_2, but a high value of ℓ gives many curves, but only a short interval to consider them on. The problem with this approach is that it is inefficient. We have to throw information away. It is more efficient to do this directly in a semi-parametric multi-state framework, as exemplified with the twins in Section 6.7.2, but this does require further assumptions, and the aim of this chapter is to avoid making such assumptions. This approach is used in Figure 14.13.

14.9   Quantitative evaluation of dependence

A key problem for the non-parametric estimates is how to extract the interesting information from the large number of survivor function values. The graphical presentations above suffer from fluctuations that might make it difficult to focus on key features. This section considers evaluation by means of a single or a few numerical values. It might seem contradictory to the whole idea, first we derive an estimate based on an extremely large number of points, and then we reduce to a few, but conceptually the same is done in the univariate case where Kaplan-Meier estimates are often reduced to an estimate of the median.

14.9.1   Degree of dependence

For just describing whether there is dependence, the measure best suited for the non-parametric estimate is the median concordance. The dependence measure κ can be found using Equation (4.14). All this requires is interpolation to find the medians of the marginal distributions. An illustration of this approach is in Table 14.9.

Measures like Kendall's τ and Spearman's ρ can, in principle, be evaluated by expressions derived from Equations (4.4) and (4.10), but the problem is that there might be a large mass in some intervals near infinity and a correct way to include these is not available.

14.9.2   Early/late dependence

For more detailed evaluations, we would like to determine whether the dependence is of the early or late type, as introduced in Section 3.2.1.

This can be done by splitting the marginal into fractiles corresponding to third probabilities. That is, find x_{jq}, so that $Pr(T_j < x_{jq}) = q/3$, $j = 1, 2$, $q = 1, 2$. This defines a splitting of the observation space into nine areas, as illustrated in Figure 3.2. Under independence each of these areas has a probability of $1/9$. Under positive dependence, the three diagonal areas have higher probability. Early dependence is obtained when $Pr(T_1 \leq x_{11}, T_2 \leq x_{21}) > Pr(T_1 > x_{12}, T_2 > x_{22})$, and late dependence when $Pr(T_1 \leq x_{11}, T_2 \leq x_{21}) < Pr(T_1 > x_{12}, T_2 > x_{22})$. An illustration of this approach is in Table 14.10.

14.9.3 Short-term dependence

For evaluating whether the dependence is of short-term or long-term time frame, as introduced in Section 3.2.3 and 3.2.4, an even finer resolution is necessary, so that there are 4 intervals instead of 3 as above. Thus define x_{jq}, so that $Pr(T_j \leq x_{jq}) = q/4$, $j = 1, 2$, $q = 1, 2, 3$. This definition may be extended to $q = 0$ or 4, by letting x be 0 and ∞, respectively. That gives 16 probabilities $p_{qm} = Pr(x_{1,q-1} < T_1 \leq x_{1q}, x_{2,m-1} < T_2 \leq x_{2m})$. To evaluate the dependence time frame for individual 2, we should compare the conditional probabilities $r_{qm} = p_{qm} / \sum_{\ell=m}^{4} p_{q\ell}$. This number only makes sense, when individual 1 has died ($q < m$) and is trivially 1 for $m = 4$, so the only ones that can be compared are r_{13} and r_{23}. Short-term dependence is obtained when $r_{13} < r_{23}$, whereas long-term dependence is obtained when $r_{13} \geq r_{23}$. An illustration of this approach is in Table 14.12.

14.10   Model checking

A major purpose of non-parametric methods is to discuss the fit of more specific models. It is, however, less clear how to do this in the bivariate case. Difficulties arise owing to various factors, of which the most important are lack of variance expressions, presence of censoring, and other more technical reasons.

The simplest choice is to pick a single point and compare the specific model with the non-parametric estimate. There are two points that limit the usefulness of this approach. One is that this is very sensitive to the choice of the point. For example, if the point is chosen corresponding to a marginal, say, $(t_1, 0)$, we might observe a perfect agreement if both the specific model and the non-parametric model are identical to the observed marginals. This agreement does not imply that the two estimates agree for other values. The second point is that we do not have an estimate of the variability, making it more difficult to evaluate whether an observed disagreement is important or not.

Another choice is to find the maximum difference between the survivor functions of the two approaches. This, of course, is inspired by the classical Kolmogorov-Smirnoff test for whether an observed distribution agrees with a specific theoretical distribution. Owing to the censoring, the estimate is typically badly determined near ∞, so some modification may be appropriate.

A third choice is some sort of integrated mean square error. This could be weighted in order to concentrate on the survivor function at early times. The main shortcoming is the lack of a variance estimate.

A fourth approach is to take one of the graphical presentations described above and compare it to the similar drawing in the specific model. As a concrete example, Section 14.8.9 describes a graphical way of checking the Markov assumption in a multi-state bivariate model.

Finally, a generalization of the first approach is to evaluate the survivor function at a grid and use this to estimate the probability of a few sets. This approach has been suggested above and used specifically to examine whether the dependence is early or late (Section 14.9.2) or short-term or long-term (Section 14.9.3), but it can equally well be used for examining a specific model. The advantage of this approach is that it brings the probabilities down to a dimension where we can overview the results. In the sections mentioned, the intervals were chosen to have the same marginal probabilities. Whether this should be done for a model checking procedure must be decided according to which assumption is to be checked.

One type of check where this approach is not really useful is for checking the importance of a covariate. We cannot include the covariate in the model, except that we can find an estimate according to the levels of (or a grouping of) the covariate, but comparing just two non-parametric estimates seems to be a difficult task and also unspecific. Instead, it is recommended to include the covariate in one of the models of the previous chapters, like multi-state model, frailty model, or marginal model.

14.11   Applications

14.11.1   Danish twins

The Danish twin data of Section 1.5.1 have been considered using the lifetimes in days. This does, however, demand a large amount of computer memory. Therefore, we also consider the data, grouped both according to years and to months. This means that the events are classified according to the year, respectively, month, they took place. The censorings, however, are changed, because we assume that they survive the whole year, respectively, month, even when they are censored during the period. This is a method that underestimates mortality, and therefore, we should aim at

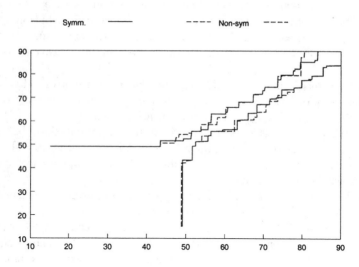

Figure 14.5. Set of definition of the bivariate survivor function, with and without an assumption of symmetry, for Danish twin data, male monozygotic twins. Hanley and Parnes method.

grouping as little as possible. In other words, the monthly-based data are more satisfactory than the yearly data.

A key assumption to discuss is symmetry. As we have no specific knowledge on the numbering of the twins, it makes sense to use the assumption of symmetry. It has several advantages, the most important is that we can discuss twins without needing to introduce a numbering within pairs, and the estimates are invariant to any numbering. Other advantages are that probability masses at each point become smaller, so that the estimate is closer to being continuous. Disadvantages are that it is necessary to keep track of more points as will be illustrated. Furthermore, asymptotic evaluations will be more difficult to perform, and it appears from parametric models (Section 8.11) that asymptotically, there is nothing to gain from the assumption of symmetry.

We will illustrate the methods both with and without an assumption of symmetry. We first consider the male monozygotic twins where there are 1366 pairs, with 1069 deaths happening on 1045 different days. From a bivariate point of view, there are 369 double events and they all happen at different times and 331 univariate intervals, and these are also different. There are 540 months with deaths and 79 years with death, corresponding to deaths in each year category from 15 to 93 years.

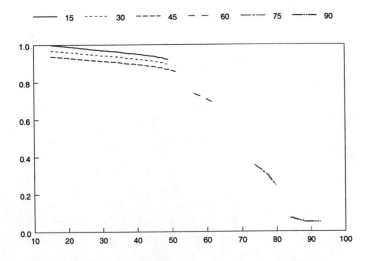

Figure 14.6. Estimate of the bivariate survivor function, with an assumption of symmetry, for Danish twin data, male monozygotic twins, based on grouping into monthly periods. Hanley and Parnes method.

Hanley and Parnes approach

Figure 14.5 shows the set where the estimate can be evaluated, based on monthly data, with and without an assumption of symmetry. The marginal survivor function is well defined up to age 49.1 years where it equals 0.923, under symmetry. Without an assumption of symmetry the first and second marginals are defined up to 48.4 and 49.1 years, respectively where the values are 0.928 and 0.917. Thus the bivariate survivor function is only known in a small set, not even covering the first 10 % of the deaths. It is seen that the assumption of symmetry can both reduce and increase the set, where the function is well defined. With continuous data, the set of definition will be reduced as all observations make to shadows instead of one. On the other hand, ties in the time to the first event may increase the set of definition. Figure 14.6 shows some cuts, the value of the bivariate function $S(t_1, t_2)$ as function of t_2, for selected values of t_1. The values chosen are 15, 30, 45, 60, 75, and 90 years. This is also based on grouping into monthly data. It is clear from this figure that it is a major problem that the estimate is defined on only a small set. One modification to deal with this problem is to group into years instead. This gives, similarly, Figure 14.7. Clearly, the problem is reduced, and the function defined in a larger set, but it is certainly not removed. From these figures, it is very difficult to see whether there is dependence. The fact that the marginals cannot be evaluated se-

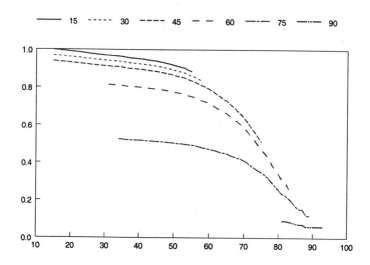

Figure 14.7. Estimate of the bivariate survivor function, with an assumption of symmetry, for Danish twin data, male monozygotic twins, based on grouping into yearly periods. Hanley and Parnes method.

riously limits the usefulness of the approach, because detailed evaluations specifically require an estimate of the marginal survivor functions.

The Dabrowska approach

The similar curves are made for the Dabrowska estimate, assuming symmetry. Figure 14.8 shows the bivariate estimates as cuts, based on daily data. This is automatically defined up to age 93.7 years. The corresponding estimates conditional upon survival to ages 15, 30, 45, 60, 75, and 90 years are shown in Figure 14.9. It is clear already from this figure that the survival function is not always decreasing. This is most marked for the curve among the survivors to age 90 years. The position and size of the masses are first considered. Based on the full data, that is, in days and with and without the assumption of symmetry, Table 14.5 gives a summary on the position of the masses. It is seen here that there is a surprisingly high number of points with negative mass, and that they give an important contribution to the total mass. The assumption of symmetry should stabilize some of these aspects, but comparing the upper and lower part of Table 14.5 rather shows that the assumption leads to be mass being spread at about four times as many points. It seems that generally the total negative masses are reduced, but there are no major changes.

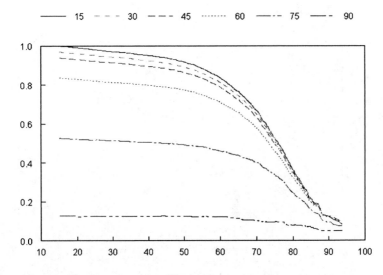

Figure 14.8. Estimate of the bivariate survivor function, with an assumption of symmetry, for Danish twin data, male monozygotic twins, based on daily data. The Dabrowska method.

	No. positive	Pos. mass	No. negative	Neg. mass	Mass at ∞
Males – Non-symmetric					
MZ	51,827	1.343	119,547	−0.453	0.109
DZ	174,919	1.455	401,485	−0.621	0.166
UZ	6,963	1.194	8,177	−0.242	0.048
Females					
MZ	44,424	1.277	80,707	−0.458	0.181
DZ	153,059	1.433	317,784	−0.609	0.176
UZ	10,515	1.329	15,684	−0.382	0.053
Males – Symmetric					
MZ	204,398	1.335	469,287	−0.448	0.114
DZ	681,926	1.521	1,554,770	−0.626	0.105
UZ	27,318	1.233	32,306	−0.262	0.029
Females					
MZ	173,412	1.283	313,012	−0.468	0.184
DZ	594,272	1.433	1,232,076	−0.608	0.174
UZ	41,341	1.333	62,012	−0.387	0.054

Table 14.5. General aspects of position of probability mass for the Dabrowska estimate Danish twin data, with and without an assumption of symmetry.

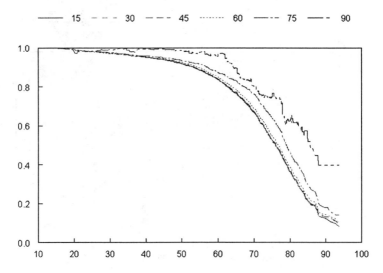

Figure 14.9. Estimate of the conditional survivor function of one twin given survival of the other, with an assumption of symmetry, for Danish twin data, male monozygotic twins, based on daily periods. The Dabrowska method. The curves refer to t_1 being $> 15, > 30, > 45, > 60, > 75$ and > 90 years.

	No. pos.	Pos. mass	No. neg.	Neg. mass	Mass at ∞
Males – Non-symmetric					
MZ	30,570	1.297	65,443	−0.407	0.110
DZ	69,993	1.352	141,779	−0.520	0.168
UZ	6,040	1.184	7,040	−0.232	0.048
Females					
MZ	26,455	1.234	48,495	−0.417	0.183
DZ	65,969	1.343	125,863	−0.521	0.177
UZ	8,862	1.314	12,875	−0.367	0.053
Males – Symmetric					
MZ	73,894	1.256	148,879	−0.370	0.114
DZ	138,268	1.358	259,738	−0.463	0.105
UZ	21,578	1.214	24,958	−0.243	0.029
Females					
MZ	71,722	1.222	133,954	−0.407	0.186
DZ	134,110	1.230	249,630	−0.471	0.176
UZ	29,518	1.305	43,278	−0.359	0.054

Table 14.6. General aspects of position of probability mass for the Dabrowska estimate Danish twin data, grouped into months, with and without an assumption of symmetry.

	Yearly			
Males	No. pos.	Pos. p	No. neg.	Neg. p
MZ	2,129	1.004	2,632	−0.142
DZ	2,350	1.068	2,428	−0.192
UZ	2,319	1.104	1,688	−0.137
Females				
MZ	1,908	0.974	2,768	−0.183
DZ	1,904	1.012	3,212	−0.205
UZ	2,459	1.107	2,130	−0.166

Table 14.7. General aspects of position of probability mass for the Dabrowska estimate Danish twin data, assuming symmetry and grouped into years. p = probability mass.

Table 14.6 gives similar statistics, based on grouping both into months and years. The last column is deleted, as this can easily be calculated as the mass missing after addition of the positive and the negative masses. Comparing months and years in Table 14.7, we see that the monthly data have quite a high number of points with masses. It appears that the problem of negative masses is larger for the daily and monthly data. We cannot see, however, whether the masses are moved a little or are moved far away. If they are moved only a little, we can consider the problem as a local problem. To examine whether this is the case, we take the monthly based estimate and add the masses corresponding to each year. This gives roughly the same results as the estimates based on grouping into years.

Figure 14.10 shows the contour curves found by the Dabrowska approach. Due to the strong dependence on age, it is difficult to judge the degree of dependence.

To avoid the age dependence, Figure 14.11 shows the contour curves after the transformation to uniform marginals. This is now standardized so any deviations from the curves of Figure 14.4 reflect dependence. Clearly, there is dependence. The degree of dependence can be read off at (0.5,0.5) and transformed into the median concordance, as will be done in more detail below. Whether the dependence is most pronounced early or late and whether the dependence is of short-term time frame is not easily seen in this figure.

As an alternative, Figure 14.12 shows the conditional distribution of one lifetime given the lifetime of the other, under an assumption of symmetry. The lifetime that is conditioned on is grouped in six intervals, taken to have approximately 1/6 of the mass. The number 6 was found as the $n^{1/4}$. All evaluations are done on a daily basis. The cutpoints used are 60.3, 70.1, 76.0, 81.0, and 87.5 years. The problem with this approach is that it does not recognize the dynamic aspect of the time, implying that it is not applicable for prediction. If we have to wait for determining one lifetime, the other is probably already observed. This leads to the Markov model

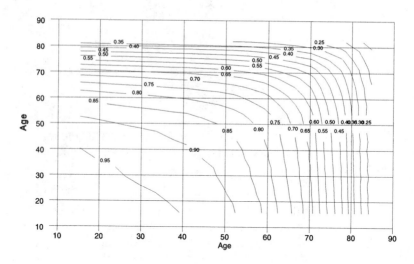

Figure 14.10. Contour curves for the survivor function for Danish twin data, assuming symmetry. The Dabrowska method.

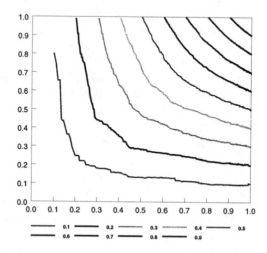

Figure 14.11. Contour curves for the survivor function for Danish twin data, after transformation to uniform marginals, assuming symmetry. The Dabrowska method. Grouped in monthly periods.

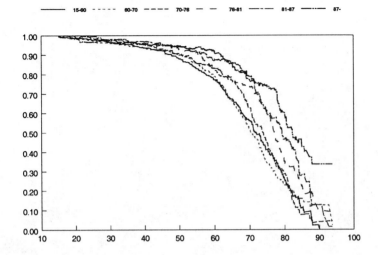

Figure 14.12. Conditional distribution of one lifetime given the other: The conditioned lifetime is grouped in six intervals. Based on data on Danish twins. The Dabrowska method. Interval end points are 60.3, 70.1, 76.0, 81.0, and 87.5 years.

checking (Figure 14.13). The disadvantage of this approach is the great loss of data, most of the probability is excluded from this figure, by the way the data are processed.

For finding the bivariate density after a uniform transformation, the Dabrowska estimate is evaluated for a set of bivariate intervals using a grid, where the marginal probabilities are chosen to about 1/6. It is adjusted for the deviation to 1/6 by dividing with the product of the marginal probabilities. These estimates are then presented in a three-dimensional plots (Figure 14.14). The highest value is 2.22 in the interval near (1,1) suggesting high late dependence.

Pruitt's estimate

This section only considers symmetric models, based on the recorded number of days. Figure 14.15 shows the sets, where the estimate is defined for choices of γ of 1, 3, and 10 years. Even with one-year bandwidth, the set where the estimate is defined is much higher than the Hanley and Parnes method based on data grouped into one-year groups. This is because the Pruitt method uses a neighborhood extending one-year to either side, whereas the grouping method corresponds to asymmetric neighborhoods with a total width of one year. In order to obtain a maximal set of definition a bandwidth of 20 years is needed. This is, of course, because

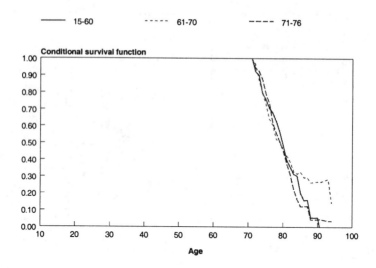

Figure 14.13. Conditional distribution of one lifetime given the other, evaluated at age 76 years. Based on Danish twins data. The Dabrowska method.

there are very few pairs where one twin dies very early (that is, near 15 years of age) and the other dies very old (that is, after 90 years of age). This also implies that if dependence is very high, it can be necessary to choose a rather high bandwidth to obtain a maximal set of definition.

In order to make a figure similar to Figure 14.12, we choose a bandwidth of ten years, as a bandwidth of five years only makes it possible to determine the marginal survivor functions down to 0.20. The conditioning event is split into six intervals, each with an approximate marginal probability of 1/6. In practice this is chosen as the day, where the survivor function crosses multiplies of 1/6. Rounded, the interval endpoints are 60.2, 70.2, 76.1, 81.3, and 87.7 years. The resulting curves are shown in Figure 14.16. The overall conclusion is the same as for Figure 14.12, but with the Pruitt method we obtain monotone survivor functions and therefore they appear much more smooth. Based on this evaluation, the Pruitt method seems preferable.

Figure 14.17 shows the contour curves after the transformation to uniform marginals, similar to Figure 14.11. Overall, the two figures appear much like each other, but the Pruitt method suggests a slightly lower dependence, which might be a consequence of the smoothing performed.

In order to consider whether the estimated dependence becomes smaller by using a larger bandwidth, Table 14.8 shows the age until which the estimated marginal survivor functions are defined, the medians, and the median concordance measure of dependence (κ).

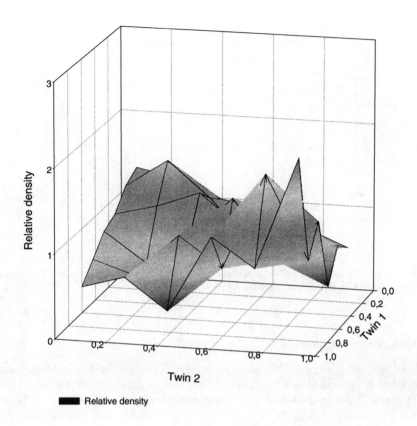

Figure 14.14. Bivariate density after transformation to marginal uniformity. Based on Danish twins data. The Dabrowska method.

γ	Defined until age	Median	κ
1	72.9	> 72.9	-
2	77.8	76.1	0.236
3	85.8	76.1	0.236
5	85.8	76.1	0.236
10	87.7	76.2	0.228
20	89.6	76.4	0.209

Table 14.8. Age until which the marginal survivor function is defined, median and κ for male monozygotic twins, under and assumption of symmetry, based on Pruitt's approach with various bandwidth (γ).

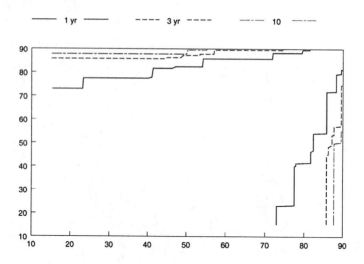

Figure 14.15. Set of definition of the bivariate survivor function, with an assumption of symmetry, for Danish twin data, male monozygotic twins. Pruitt's method using bandwidths of 1, 3, and 10 years.

Quantitative evaluation

The degree of dependence is most easily quantified by the median concordance (see Section 4.4). This is shown in Table 14.9. It appears that grouping into years leads to overestimation of the dependence. Therefore, grouping should be avoided. For monozygotic male twins, there is a surprisingly large difference between the estimates with and without the assumption of symmetry. The medians without the assumption of symmetry are 76.2 and 75.7 years for the two coordinates and 76.0 with the assumption. The Hanley and Parnes approach is not able to evaluate the medians or the median concordance. The Pruitt estimate using the smallest bandwidth to determine the median gives a median of 76.1 years and a median concordance of 0.236. The reason for the difference between this estimate and that of Dabrowska's method (0.261) is not that the two estimates deviate much at the diagonal, but the difference between the two estimates of the median. Even though this difference is only 0.1 year, the survivor function changes markedly along the diagonal.

To evaluate whether the dependence is early or late, we split the distribution into sets with marginal probabilities 1/3. For the monozygotic twins this is illustrated in Table 14.10. Since for the males 1.48 is greater than 1.38, and for the females 1.50 is greater than 1.42, this table suggests that the dependence is late.

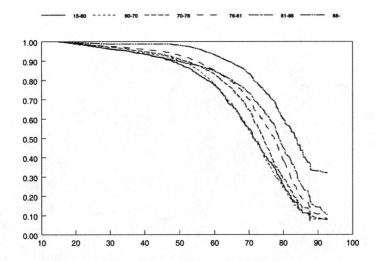

Figure 14.16. Estimate of the conditional survivor function of one twin given survival of the other, with an assumption of symmetry, for Danish twin data, male monozygotic twins. The Pruitt method. The conditioning variable is grouped into 6 groups, t_1 being split according to interval endpoints 60.2, 70.2, 76.1, 81.3, and 87.7 years.

| | Daily | | Monthly | | Yearly | |
	Non-symm.	Symm.	Non-symm.	Symm.	Non-symm.	Symm.
Males						
MZ	0.240	0.261	0.239	0.258	0.259	0.265
DZ	0.090	0.090	0.090	0.087	0.092	0.091
UZ	0.194	0.194	0.210	0.195	0.213	0.207
Females						
MZ	0.143	0.140	0.144	0.144	0.198	0.195
DZ	0.166	0.165	0.167	0.163	0.194	0.191
UZ	0.218	0.232	0.217	0.230	0.225	0.239

Table 14.9. Estimates of median concordance (κ) for the Dabrowska estimate based on Danish twin data, not grouped and grouped into months and years.

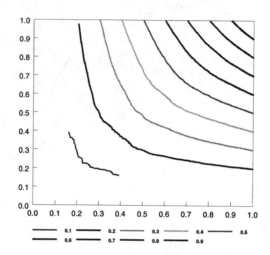

Figure 14.17. Contour curves for the survivor function for Danish twin data, after transformation to uniform marginals, assuming symmetry. The Pruitt method, used with a bandwidth of ten years.

		$(0,x_1)$	(x_1,x_2)	(x_2,∞)
Males	$(0,x_1)$	1.38	0.96	0.66
	(x_1,x_2)	0.96	1.18	0.86
	(x_2,∞)	0.66	0.86	1.48
Females	$(0,x_1)$	1.42	0.85	0.73
	(x_1,x_2)	0.85	1.39	0.76
	(x_2,∞)	0.73	0.76	1.50

Table 14.10. Estimates of probabilities in intervals with marginal probabilities 1/3. Multiplied by 9. Based on the Dabrowska estimate for Danish twin data.

		$(0,x_1)$	(x_1,x_2)	(x_2,∞)
Males	$(0,x_1)$	1.40	0.95	0.67
	(x_1,x_2)	0.95	1.19	0.85
	(x_2,∞)	0.67	0.85	1.48
Females	$(0,x_1)$	1.39	0.86	0.75
	(x_1,x_2)	0.86	1.41	0.73
	(x_2,∞)	0.75	0.73	1.51

Table 14.11. Estimates of probabilities in intervals with marginal probabilities 1/3. Multiplied by 9. Based on the Pruitt estimate for Danish monozygotic twin data and a bandwidth of 3 years.

		$(0,x_1)$	(x_1,x_2)	(x_2,x_3)	(x_3,∞)
Males	$(0,x_1)$	1.39	1.14	0.84	0.63
	(x_1,x_2)	1.14	1.39	0.98	0.50
	(x_2,x_3)	0.84	0.98	1.15	1.04
	(x_3,∞)	0.63	0.50	1.04	1.83
Females	$(0,x_1)$	1.36	1.17	0.79	0.69
	(x_1,x_2)	1.17	0.86	1.25	0.73
	(x_2,x_3)	0.79	1.25	1.41	0.56
	(x_3,∞)	0.69	0.73	0.56	2.02

Table 14.12. Estimates of probabilities in intervals with marginal probabilities 1/4. Multiplied by 16. Based on the Dabrowska estimate for Danish twin data.

A similar table using Pruitt's method is given in Table 14.11. To do this, a bandwidth of three years is used, as the fractiles in the marginal distribution cannot be determined with a bandwidth of two years. The results are similar to those obtained by Dabrowska's method.

To evaluate whether the dependence is short-term or long-term, we split the distribution into sets with marginal probabilities 1/4. For the monozygotic twins this is illustrated in Table 14.12. The conditional probabilities are $r_{13} = 0.57 = 0.84/(0.84 + 0.63)$, $r_{23} = 0.66$ for males and $r_{13} = 0.53$, $r_{23} = 0.63$ for females. In both cases, these values suggest that the dependence is of a short-term time frame. This approach does not allow for evaluation of the uncertainty, so it is not known whether the differences are significant.

14.11.2 Kidney catheter data

The kidney catheter data of Section 1.7.3 have heterogeneous censoring and therefore cannot easily be analyzed by the simple version of the Hanley and Parnes method. Thus, we consider Dabrowska's method. There are 32 events at 29 different times for the first coordinate and 26 events at 23 different times for the second coordinate. This defines a grid of 667 points. From the bivariate point of view, there are 23 double event times and they are all different and 12 singly censored observations and they are all different. The number of points with positive mass is 132. The largest mass is 0.081 and is placed at (185,177), which is a point with a paired event. The number of points with a negative mass is 358. The largest negative mass is -0.028. The total positive mass is 1.191 and the total negative mass is -0.389, and thus the negative mass is substantial. The rest of the mass (0.198) is placed in a neighborhood of ∞. This mass can be placed as univariate intervals or a final bivariate interval. The degree of dependence is evaluated by the median concordance, which corresponds to a value of κ of 0.219, thus suggesting a clear dependence.

14.11.3   Exercise data

The exercise data of Section 1.8.2 is an example that can be used to discuss when not to use the non-parametric methods. First of all, the purpose is to determine the effect of treatment, which shows up as a difference between the coordinates. Without some sort of assumption like proportional hazards or accelerated failure times, it is basically impossible to quantify the treatment effect. Secondly, the dimension of the data is 10 and where it is difficult to illustrate bivariate survival curves, it is intrinsically more difficult in a ten dimensional space. Thirdly, there are just 21 observations in this ten-dimensional space and this is not enough for a non-parametric approach.

14.11.4   Heart transplant data

The data on heart transplants from Stanford of Section 1.9.4 are really longitudinal data on different events. We will try to implement this in a bivariate frame, in order to consider whether this is acceptable. We define T_1 as the time to transplantation and T_2 as the time to death. This means that if a person dies without transplant, we just say that T_1 is undefined (but larger than T_2). One consequence of this is that the marginal distribution of T_1 does not make sense, but the marginal distribution of T_2 does. In the longitudinal frame, we say that dead is an absorbing state, whereas in the bivariate frame, it is process-dependent censoring happening at T_2.

The masses of the Dabrowska estimator are well defined until $t_1 = 309$ days and $t_2 = 1386$ days. In fact, there is a substantial positive mass placed on points $t_1 > t_2$. Summing over t_1 for points $t_1 > t_2$ is fine and reflects the probability of dying at t_2 without having had a transplantation. However, it is not satisfactory that a non-parametric estimate can distribute this mass within such a set specified by a value of t_2. Formulated more generally, it is not acceptable that a non-parametric estimator can supply an estimate in cases, where the actual value is non-identifiable. The conclusion is that the Dabrowska estimator does not work for longitudinal data for different events. Furthermore, it does not accept process-dependent censoring.

The Hanley and Parnes estimate does not give a value for the probability of points with $t_1 > t_2$. Together with the interpretation of the method in terms of Figure 5.13 this implies that the method works for longitudinal data on different events. However, it further cannot estimate the marginal distribution corresponding to the lifetime above $t_2 = 38$ days, which makes it less interesting in practice.

Clearly, these results show that these methods do not automatically handle the fact that when death occurs, the other event (transplantation) makes no sense. For such data, the most sensible approach is the multi-state model, as described in Section 6.7.1.

14.12 Chapter summary

It is beneficial to have a bivariate survival estimate in order to be able to discuss the fit of more specialized models. However, the available suggestions have serious shortcomings. The Hanley and Parnes estimate is a maximum likelihood estimate, but has the problem that it assigns mass to both points and sets, and a consequence of this is that the survivor function is not defined in major parts of the quadrant. This problem can be overcome by Pruitt's method, which, however, includes a choice of bandwidth and a degree of smoothing. The Dabrowska method has the problem that it assigns negative probability masses to some points. As demonstrated in the example, this happens at a very large number of points and the mass is non-ignorable. A further problem that makes us insecure about the approach is that it supplies an estimate for the full bivariate distribution, even when this distribution does not make sense, e.g., for bivariate data for different events with one of the events being death.

The simple version of Hanley and Parnes method requires the censoring to be homogeneous, but allows process-dependent censoring, whereas the Dabrowska method allows general independent censoring. It follows that the Dabrowska method does not work for longitudinal data on different events.

The Dabrowska method gives an estimate of the marginal distribution, which is identical to that determined directly from the marginal data. This is not the case for the Hanley and Parnes method, which instead emphasizes the minimum within pairs. The estimate along the diagonal, that is, $S(t,t)$ equals the Kaplan-Meier estimate based on the data on the first event in each pair. Table 14.13 gives a summary of the properties.

One specific problem is the large number of points to keep track of. It is not recommended to reduce this number by grouping the data, because this can introduce a bias. One should use the best possible resolution and use this for evaluating the probability of the relevant sets.

Property	HP	Dabrowska	Pruitt
Well defined in large set	No	Yes	Yes
Only positive mass	Yes	No	Yes
Choice of bandwidth	No	No	Yes
Marginals = KM	No	Yes	No
Minimum = KM	hom.cens.	hom.cens?	hom.cens.
Explicit	hom.cens.	Yes	hom.cens.
Longitudinal data	Yes	No	Yes

Table 14.13. Properties of non-parametric bivariate estimates. KM=Kaplan-Meier, HP = Hanley and Parnes.

Another problem limiting what we can do with an estimate is the lack of a way to calculate the variability.

Clearly these methods need more consideration and further experience before they can be recommended for routine practical use.

14.13   Bibliographic comments

Many authors, including Hanley and Parnes (1983), Dabrowska (1988), Lin and Ying (1993), Prentice and Cai (1992), Tsai, Leurgans and Crowley (1986), and Visser (1996) have suggested bivariate survival distribution estimates. The method of Pruitt is suggested in a technical report (Pruitt, 1990). The large number of suggestions illustrate that it is a difficult problem and that the final solution may not have been found yet.

A review of the approaches is given by Andersen *et al.* (1993, Chapter 10). A comparison of the approaches by means of simulated data has been done by Pruitt (1993b).

Further asymptotical results for the methods have been found by Dabrowska (1989) and Gill, Laan, and Wellner (1995).

The applications presented here seem to be the first large-scale applications of these procedures.

14.14   Exercises

Exercise 14.1 General concordance

To illustrate the point made in Section 4.4 that concordance should be evaluated at the median, consider the general definition of concordance in Equation (4.12) in a copula model, with $t_{01} = t_{02}$. Evaluate this as a function of t_0 in a shared gamma frailty model. Make the same evaluation in a shared stable frailty model. Make a figure of the functions, choosing the parameters to give $\tau = 0.25$.

Exercise 14.2 Equivariance under increasing transformations

Show that the Dabrowska estimate is equivariant under separate increasing transformations. That is, $Y_{ij} = f_j(T_{ij})$, with f_j an increasing function with $f_j(0) = 0$, as discussed in Table 14.1. Show that the Hanley-Parnes estimate is equivariant, when the functions are independent of j, but not in the general case. Show that Pruitt's approach is not equivariant even in the case of common transformations.

Exercise 14.3 Truncation in Hanley-Parnes approach

Suppose that we have bivariate truncated and censored data. Censoring is assumed homogeneous. Truncation is assumed to happen at a time point v, which is common to the pair members, but may vary between pairs. Describe how the Hanley-Parnes approach can be extended to cover truncation. You may need to assume that the risk set is positive on the diagonal, from time 0 to some time x.

Exercise 14.4 Graphics overview

Which of the figures discussed in Section 14.8 do you find relevant in frailty models and which for multi-state models? Aspects you may consider are the dynamic nature of multi-state models and the reduction of the non-parametric component from two dimensions to one dimension in frailty models (and to two one-dimensional components in the multi-state Markov model).

Exercise 14.5 Flexible piecewise constant hazard model

To avoid some of the problems with the non-parametric approaches, we may consider a flexible parametric model. When the time scales are the same and there is homogeneous censoring, we may consider a piecewise constant hazards model set up in a multi-state structure like that of Figure 5.12. When both individuals are alive, the hazard of death for individual j is $\lambda_j(t)$ for which a standard piecewise formulation is used. When individual 1 has died at time t_1, the hazard of death for individual 2 at time t, ($t > t_1$), is $\mu_2(t, t_1) = \sum_{q,m:q \geq m} \mu_{2qm} 1\{x_{q-1} < t \leq x_q, x_{m-1} < t_1 \leq x_m\}$, with a similar expression for $\mu_1(t, t_2)$. Derive an expression for the survivor function.

Describe precisely the estimated values based on censored bivariate data. What happens if there are no events in a bivariate interval? What is the consequence when a risk set is completely empty? This problem may be handled by using fewer intervals. Do the intervals need to have the same length? Do the intervals for λ and μ need to be the same?

Which problems for the Hanley and Parnes approach and the Dabrowska approach are avoided by this approach? Which problems are introduced?

Exercise 14.6 Bivariate contours

Make figures of the bivariate contours in order to illustrate the point made in Section 14.8.7 and 14.8.8 that dependence in contour curves are best evaluated after transformation to uniformity. Let the marginals be Weibull distributed with parameters $(2.5 \cdot 10^{-11}, 5.28)$ as found in Section 2.2.2 for the Danish population data. Make figures both under independence and for $\tau = 0.25$ for the gamma and stable frailty models. Make similar figures for the Gompertz model with parameters $(8.7 \cdot 10^{-5}, 1.091$ as found in Section 2.2.3 for the same data. Compare to Figures 7.3 and 7.4 for uniform marginals.

Exercise 14.7 Early/late dependence

To obtain a feeling of the degree of dependence one can expect in tables like Table 14.10, calculate the nine probabilities theoretically in a gamma shared frailty model using $\tau = 0.2068$, taken from Table 8.23 on survival of twins. Evaluate also the cross ratio of Equation (7.39). Compare to the non-parametrically estimated values.

Exercise 14.8 Leukemia remission data

Consider the data of Section 1.5.4. Is the censoring homogeneous? Evaluate the Dabrowska, Hanley-Parnes, and Pruitt estimates for these data. What does the hypothesis of no treatment effect say in this frame? Would you recommend this approach for studying the treatment effect?

Exercise 14.9 Stratified estimates

Suppose you have studied the survival experience of a group of monozygotic twins using one of the non-parametric approaches and estimated that κ is 0.25. As a model checking procedure, you consider the two sexes separately and find estimates for κ, which are 0.21 for the males and 0.22 for the females. What is your conclusion based on these calculations and which value of κ would you report as the best description for the dependence in lifetimes of monozygotic twins?

15
Summary

This book has several aims. Of course, on the general level it is to present the multivariate survival data and their analysis. In more detail, it is first to guide the statistician into selecting the most appropriate model for the actual subject matter problem and the actual multivariate survival data set. Second, the aim is to present the available approaches so that they can be used when they are relevant. To judge the relevance, it is important to include a description of the advantages and disadvantages of each single approach. Finally, a more subtle aim is to put all the approaches in a common frame and also describe the similarities between the various data types and approaches.

This chapter first gives a summary of the theory (Section 15.1). As said already in the preface, this book is a toolbox rather than a cookbook. However, Section 15.2 is the closest it comes to being a cookbook. It describes how the analysis of an actual study could run. We list the basic questions needed in order to select the most relevant modeling approach. The applications are summarized in Section 15.3 in order to make the key methodological aspects clear. Finally, Section 15.4 lists some problems that need further work.

15.1   Summary of the theory

Chapters 1 and 3 describe the concepts for multivariate survival data and the probability mechanisms. Such considerations are relevant already before the data are available as they can help in choosing the best design for obtaining data. In the following it is, however, assumed that data are available. Thus the task becomes to consider a specific data set. One should then consider whether the data are parallel (where the number of times is fixed by the subject matter problem) or longitudinal (where the number of times is a consequence of the development of each object under study) (Section 1.4). The data sets are classified into six types (several individuals, similar organs, recurrent events, repeated measurements, different events and competing risks) (Chapter 1, summarized in Table 1.15). In the case of parallel data, it should be considered whether the censoring pattern is homogeneous or not (Section 1.11). Also, it is important to determine whether process-dependent censoring applies. Are there covariates that should be included? What is the purpose of applying the model? Here five different purposes are considered (Section 1.14). The first two consider the effect of covariates, for example, a treatment effect or an effect of some known variable that may influence the risk either directly as a risk factor, or be present for persons with high risk. The reason this is considered as two purposes is that it is important whether this is a common covariate in parallel data (corresponding to constant covariates in longitudinal data) or varying within groups, the so-called matched pairs covariates (Section 1.13). Another possible purpose is to study the dependence present in the data between the components of the multivariate observations. The purpose can also be to evaluate probabilities for some events, even before the study, or conditional on observations for the relevant group or individual. This is called prediction. A final purpose considered is a check of the correctness of the assumptions in a simpler model, that is, model checking.

Then the dependence mechanism should be considered. We have discussed three different types – common events, common risks and event-related dependence (Chapter 3). The relevance of the various dependence mechanisms for the data types was described in Table 3.1. The common risks mechanism corresponds to a random effects model. The event-related mechanism is more of a life history approach. The dependence time frame should also be considered (Section 3.2). Three time frames are treated, instantaneous dependence, leading to several events happening simultaneously; short-term dependence; and long-term dependence. Do we know which type is applicable in the actual case, or do we want to find out?

The various approaches for analyzing multivariate survival data fall into four main categories – multi-state models, frailty models, marginal modeling and non-parametric methods.

The multi-state models (Chapters 5 and 6), are classical models developed for event-related dependence in a longitudinal setting, but owing to their flexibility they are relevant in more general cases as descriptive tools. Traditionally, such models have used a Markov assumption, but they can easily be used more generally. The competing risks model (Chapter 12) is also a multi-state model.

The frailty model and its extensions (Chapters 7–11) are derived as common risks dependence models and thus allow for a random effects interpretation. The first two of these chapters describe the shared frailty model for parallel data, where there are two random effects, a group effect and simple random variation, modeled by the hazard function. This covers first the unspecified frailty, or stratified model (Section 7.1), where there is a parameter for each group. Assuming instead a randomly varying frailty reduces the number of parameters and simplifies the application of asymptotic results, and makes it possible to find the effect of general covariates. The simplest (in some respects) random frailty model is the gamma frailty model (Section 7.3), which can be extended to a general constant shared frailty models (Sections 7.2). In particular, the positive stable model (Section 7.4) offers simple probability results and makes more sense, when covariates are included. Chapter 8 describes how to estimate the parameters of such models, and it also describes asymptotic results. Chapter 9 makes a similar development for recurrent events data. There are many similarities, but also important differences compared to the parallel data. The main differences were described in Table 9.5. Chapter 10 extends the model to more than two random effects. Chapter 11 extends to more complicated dependence structures over time. One line of extension is the independent increments frailty models (Sections 11.1), which lead to instantaneous dependence. Another line is the short-term dependence and approximations to this, described in the rest of the chapter.

Marginal modeling (Chapter 13), is a simple descriptive approach. This is designed for studying the effect of covariates and cannot estimate the dependence. This runs in two versions for parallel data, the coordinate-wise approach and the independence working model. The first makes separate parameter estimates for each coordinate and combines the estimates afterward. The second approach assumes independence for estimation and afterward evaluates an estimate of the variability accounting for the dependence. The approach can gain from a combination with the copula approach (Section 13.6), making it possible to evaluate the dependence. There is a similar approach for recurrent events.

This section gives an outline of how the best model and the best analysis approach are found. The questions to ask before choosing a specific model are listed in Table 15.1, including references to where these questions or answers are discussed.

Finally, the non-parametric approach is a descriptive approach for studying the dependence in the absence of covariates and can be used as a baseline for studying the goodness of fit of specific models (Chapter 14).

The non-parametric approach can only be used for parallel data, whereas the other approaches can be used both for parallel and longitudinal data.

Question	Possible answers	Reference
Type of data	Several individuals	Section 1.5
	Similar organs	Section 1.6
	Recurrent events	Section 1.7
	Repeated measurements	Section 1.8
	Different events	Section 1.9
	Competing risks	Section 1.10
Covariates available	Common	Section 1.13
	Matched pairs	
	General	
	None	
Purpose of study	Common covariate	Section 1.14
	Matched pairs covariate	
	Dependence evaluation	
	Prediction	
	Model checking	
Hazard model	Parametric	Section 2.2
	Non-parametric	Section 2.3
Time scale		Table 1.1
Censoring (parallel data)	Homogeneneous or not	Section 1.11
	Process-dependent	Section 1.11
Truncation	Yes/no	Section 1.12
Dependence mechanism	Common events	Section 3.1.1
	Common risks	Section 3.1.2
	Event-related	Section 3.1.3
Dependence time frame	Instantaneous	Section 3.2.2
	Short-term	Section 3.2.3
	Long-term	Section 3.2.4
	To be determined	

Table 15.1. Questions to consider before choosing a multivariate survival model.

15.2 Course of analysis

The answers to selected questions are used to choose the most relevant approach. The type of data is an extremely important factor and its relation to the four main approaches is described in Table 15.2. This table is partly based on the relevance of the various dependence mechanisms for the six types of data as described in Table 3.1. This is further elaborated on by how the various approaches relate to the probability mechanisms, which are listed in Table 15.3. Owing to some of the detailed questions' being important, the four main approaches are considered as a number of more specific approaches. The relevance of the various approaches for the various purposes is shown in Table 15.4.

Type of data	Multi-state	Frailty	Marginal	Non-parametric
Several individuals	5.3.3	7, 8	13.1, 13.2, 13.6	14
Similar organs	5.3.3	7, 8	13.1, 13.2, 13.6	14
Recurrent events	5.3.1	9	13.4	
Repeated meas.		7, 8	13.1, 13.2, 13.6	
Different events	5.3.2			14.2, 14.4
Competing risks	12			

Table 15.2. Overview of data types and approaches, with references to relevant chapters and sections. Blank means not relevant.

Approach	Common events	Common risks	Event-related
Multi-state	x	(x)	x
Unspecified frailty		x	
Gamma frailty		x	
Shared frailty		x	
Indep. increments frailty	x	x	
General process frailty		x	
Marginal models CW		x	
Marginal models IWM		x	
Non-parametric	x	x	x

Table 15.3. Relevance of the various approaches for the various probability mechanisms. x means relevant; blank, not relevant; (x), that the approach can be relevant for descriptive purposes.

Approach	Common cov.	Matched pairs	Depen-dence	Pre-diction	Model check
Multi-state	x	x	x	x	x
Unspecified frailty		x			x
Gamma frailty			x	x	
Shared frailty	x	x	x	x	
Indep. increm. frailty			x	x	
General process frailty	x	x	x	x	x
Marginal model CW	x				
Marginal model IWM	x	x			
Non-parametric			x	x	x

Table 15.4. Relevance of the various approaches for the various purposes. x means relevant; blank, not relevant.

Approach	Dependence time frame	Complexity
Markov multi-state	Instantaneous or long-term	Low
General multi-state	Any	Low
Unspecified frailty	Long-term	Low
Gamma frailty	Long-term	Medium
Shared frailty	Long-term	Medium
Indep. increments frailty	Instantaneous	Medium
General process frailty	Any	High
Marginal modeling	Not considered	Low
Non-parametric	Any	High

Table 15.5. Dependence time frame for the various approaches and the complexity of the approaches.

The dependence time frame the various approaches assume is shown in Table 15.5. For this evaluation the multi-state models are split into the standard Markov models and the general multi-state models.

A final point to consider is, of course, the complexity of the approach. This subjective evaluation is mainly based on the theoretical background, but also the simplicity of fitting the models, the software available, and also the simplicity of presenting and interpreting the results. Multi-state models, unspecified frailty models, and marginal modeling are of low complexity, whereas the gamma frailty, the shared frailty and the independent increments frailty approaches are of medium complexity; and the general process frailty and completely non-parametric approaches are of high complexity. This is also described in Table 15.5.

For application of the four different main approaches, we can similarly ask relevant questions for each of them. Some are repetitions of the general questions (but with more specific references); others are special to the actual approach.

For the multi-state models, these questions are listed in Table 15.6. First one should consider to which extent one wants to discriminate between the events and the states. Based on this consideration, a state structure can be suggested. Regarding censoring, homogeneous censoring is necessary for a standard application. Process-dependent censoring is generally acceptable. The multi-state approach outperforms the other approaches, when the dependence is of the event-related type, and when the data are for different events. A further advantage is the extreme flexibility of the approach, allowing for very simple models as well as for very detailed semi-parametric models.

For frailty models, the key questions are listed in Table 15.7. The frailty models are particularly sensible, when the purpose is to assess the dependence by means of a random effects interpretation. The choice of frailty distribution, where the book has considered gamma, stable, PVF and log-normal distributions in detail is not listed as a question. Rather this should

Question	Possible answers	Reference
Types of events	Different/Similar	Section 5.3
Types of states		Section 5.3
Type of data	Several individuals	Section 5.3.3
	Similar organs	Section 5.3.3
	Recurrent events	Sections 5.3.1, 5.4.4
	Different events	Section 5.3.2 and others
	Competing risks	Section 5.4.1, Ch. 12
	Complicated	Section 5.3
State structure	Competing risks	Chapter 12
	Alternating states	Section 5.5.6
	Disability model	Section 5.3.2
	Bivariate	Sections 5.3.3, 5.5.3
	Recurrent events	Section 5.4.4
	Other	Section 5.3
Hazard model	Constant	Section 5.5
	Parametric	
	Non-parametric	
Time scale		Example Section 6.7.4
Dependence time frame	Instantaneous	Example Section 5.5.4
	Short-term	Section 5.7
	Markov	Section 5.6
	Long-term (not Markov)	Section 5.7
	To be determined	

Table 15.6. Questions to consider before choosing a multi-state multivariate survival model.

Question	Possible answers	Reference
Type of data	Several individuals	Chapter 7
	Similar organs	Chapter 7
	Recurrent events	Chapter 9
	Repeated measurements	Chapter 7
	Complicated structure	Chapter 10
Covariates available	Yes/no	Section 7.2.7
	Matched pairs	Section 7.1
Purpose of study	Covariate	Section 7.2.7
	Dependence evaluation	Section 7.2.5
	Comparison of dependence	Chapter 10
	Model checking	Chapters 10 and 11
Time of dependence	Early	Section 7.4
	Late	Section 7.3
	To be determined	Sections 7.5 and 7.8
Dependence time frame	Instantaneous	Section 11.1
	Short-term	Chapter 11
	Long-term	Chapter 7
	To be determined	Section 11.3

Table 15.7. Questions to consider before choosing a frailty multivariate survival model.

Question	Possible answers	Reference
Type of data	Parallel data	Section 13.1 and 13.2
	Recurrent events	Section 13.1.1 and 13.4
Censoring	Process-dependent	Section 13.1.3
Covariates	Common	Section 13.1 and 13.2
	Matched pairs	Section 13.2
Dependence model	Frailty	Section 13.6

Table 15.8. Questions to consider before choosing a marginal modeling analysis.

be a consequence of the answers to the other questions, with the gamma model displaying late dependence and the stable model displaying early dependence. For this choice also the covariates are important with only the stable model allowing for proportional hazard functions both in the conditional and the marginal distribution.

For the marginal modeling approach, the key questions are listed in Table 15.8. These approaches are developed to study the effect of covariates. The marginal modeling approach has its main application area for parallel data sets where the dependence is a nuisance and the aim is to consider the effect of covariates. An alternative approach is available for recurrent events. Process-dependent censoring is not acceptable for this approach. The approach can be expanded to model the dependence by the copula-combined approach.

Question	Possible answers	Reference
Purpose	Marginal distribution	Ch. 14 Introduction
	Model checking	Section 14.10
	Dependence assessment	Section 14.9.1
	Early/late dependence	Section 14.9.2
	Dependence time frame	Section 14.9.3
Censoring	Homogeneous	Section 14.1
	Process dependent	Section 14.7
Presentation	Graphics	Section 14.8
	Quantitative	Section 14.9
Coórdinates symmetric	Yes/No	Section 14.11.1

Table 15.9. Questions to consider before choosing a non-parametric approach.

For the non-parametric approach, the key questions are listed in Table 15.9. This approach, which does not allow for covariates, makes most sense, when the aim is to consider the goodness of fit and when more specific models have shown to be misleading.

A somewhat alternative way of summarizing the various approaches is to consider where the main limitations are. Table 15.10 presents some important limitations for each of the four main approaches.

15.3 Summary of the applications

Below some general points on the applicability of the various approaches for the various data sets are described. Only some of the data sets are discussed, as they together illustrate the key features.

15.3.1 Twins

The twin data is a parallel data set for several individuals (Section 1.5.1). Censoring is generally homogeneous and the available covariates, sex, zygosity and the year of birth, are common covariates. In particular, we want to compare the dependence for monozygotic and dizygotic twins. The effects of the sex and year of birth are not interesting in themselves; it is the dependence we want to quantify. If we wanted to study the effects of these covariates, we could as well study singletons. The covariate year of birth is needed to account for the mortality decrease observed over the long calendar time period when studying persons born over a calendar time period of 50 years. The effect of this covariate is a nuisance parameter. The multi-state models are easily applied and give a good fit. The disadvantage of this approach is that the models are purely descriptive, where the frailty models offer an interpretation of the dependence in terms of common unknown risk factors (random effects). The dependence appears to be of a short-term

Approach	Limitation
Multi-state	Homogeneous censoring
	No interpretation in a random effects frame
Frailty	Regression models may have identifiability problems
	Truncation may lead to a non-trivial change
	Complicated dependence structures may be cumbersome
	Short-term dependence complicated
Marginal	Use only for simple parallel data and recurrent events
	Dependence cannot be assessed
	Process-dependent censoring not acceptable
Non-parametric	Estimates have undesired properties
	Cannot account for covariates
	Variance estimate not available
	Difficult to summarize and illustrate the results
	Process-dependent censoring not always acceptable

Table 15.10. Some limitations of the approaches considered.

time frame (although the fit of such models are not significantly better that of the standard models), and thus the standard shared frailty models are not completely satisfactory. General process frailty might make more sense. The completely non-parametric approach is interesting for discussing the fit of the various approaches.

15.3.2   Length of leukemia remission

This is matched pairs drug trial, giving parallel data for several individuals. The patients were matched based on clinical variables and then given either active treatment or placebo. This is described in Section 1.5.4. The aim is to find the effect of the treatment, and the corresponding covariate is of the matched pairs type. The estimated dependence is negative, in conflict with the reasoning behind matching. I believe that, as a more general conclusion, it is rarely advantageous to match persons based on such variables. Even in the most extreme case (monozygotic twins), the dependence in lifetimes is so small that there is no real advantage to making comparisons within pairs. A more useful approach is to record variables known or suspected to influence the time to response, like sex, age, disease severity and center, and include them as covariates in a proportional hazards model. Alternatively, one can stratify according to them. This makes it easier to recruit patients as they are considered individually and we still account for the dependence on these variables.

15.3.3   Exercise data

This is a typical repeated measurements data set, showing parallel data, described in Section 1.8.2. The main interest lies in the effect of the covariates, which are matched pairs covariates. Owing to this, multi-state models are not relevant, and the coordinate-wise marginal modeling approach cannot treat the matched pairs covariates. This data set is easily analyzed by the unspecified frailty model, (the stratified analysis), but some more efficiency can be obtained by a shared frailty model. There is a clear dependence between the repeated occasions. As data cover ten occasions, after four different treatments, it is of interest to examine whether the degree of dependence is the same in all cases (Chapter 10). The models and the analysis thereof is not yet sufficiently well developed to do so in detail, but simple analyses suggests that there is varying dependence between the various responses. Alternatively, the effect of the treatments can be evaluated by the IWM marginal modeling approach.

15.3.4   Kidney catheter infections

This is a longitudinal recurrent events data set, limited to two events per individual. Such a way of reducing the data set is not recommended, as it is impossible to guarantee that it is free of selection effects. The time scale is time since latest insertion, which makes it impossible to use the multi-state models, and the general process frailty. It appears that the purpose is to find the effect of the covariates. The covariates sex and type of disease are common covariates. The covariate age at insertion is not purely common, but differs at most one year between the two spells, and therefore this is in practice a common covariate. It appears that all the dependence is created by the sex, so that when sex is in the model, there is no dependence between the spells. This conclusion, however, was not easy to detect in the proportional hazards frailty model, but emerged by a stratified frailty analysis (Section 8.12.3). Alternatively, the effect of the covariates can be evaluated by the IWM marginal modeling approach.

15.3.5   Epileptic seizures

The epileptic seizure data of Section 1.7.2 is a longitudinal recurrent events data set, where there is a high number of events, but only the number of events in 4 two-week periods are recorded, that is, what we call interval count data. This limits the possible models, but it can be studied by the Poisson overdispersion models of Chapter 9. The purpose is to determine the effect of treatment, accounting for the overdispersion. The simpler evaluations show that there is a clear person variation, but more complex evaluations in Section 11.2.1 show that there further is a random person by time interaction. The treatment effect and its variation can be evaluated in such models.

15.3.6 Amalgam data

This data set, introduced in Section 1.6.2, concerns parallel data for similar organs. However, each dental filling is not made the same time, and the actual time of filling is unknown. This makes it impossible to consider whether there is instantaneous dependence and to evaluate models with short-term dependence. Basically, this limits us to consider constant shared frailty models as described in Section 8.12.4. There are only two covariates available – sex, which is a common covariate, and age, which shows some variation within individuals. Owing to the limited information available, it has been necessary to make the approximation that the age is common for all fillings for a person.

15.3.7 Albuminuria

This data set, described in Section 1.9.1, is a typical life history data set, that is, a longitudinal data set of different events. The only relevant models are the multi-state models. The purpose is to determine the effect of the co-variates known, and to study the progress through the states. Furthermore, it is interesting to discuss whether the time since study start or duration of disease is the most relevant time-scale (Section 6.7.4). Like many other such data, these are really interval censored data and should be analyzed as such. This book does, however, not cover methods for interval censored data. In fact, as the measurements are continuous and the multi-state models can only consider a grouping into a few intervals, normal distribution repeated measurements model might be even more relevant.

15.3.8 Malignant melanoma

This data set described in Section 1.10.2 is a competing risks data set, where we are particularly interested in one cause of death, namely, death of the disease. A number of covariates are available and the purpose is to find out which of these are important for the prognosis. Although it is a multi-state model, which is discussed and treated in Chapter 12, the methods needed are essentially the standard univariate methods of Chapter 2.

15.4 Future development

This book has described many approaches, but there are still many open problems in the understanding and application of these methods. Also, more experience with the methods would be desirable in many cases. This section lists just a few specific problems. For the frailty models, the publicly available software can only handle the shared gamma and lognormal models and cannot evaluate the uncertainty of the dependence. The asymptotic theory is only sparsely developed. More model development and experience is needed for the multivariate frailty models and the short-term frailty models. Also, more generally, it would be desirable with more models showing short-term dependence. Some approaches are suggested in Chapter 11, but they all have some inconveniences that need further study. An accelerated failure-time random effects model would be useful. A model combining genetic theory and survival would be useful. Some problems that such a model could address are additive versus dominant inheritance, competing risks, single loci versus multi-loci dependence, and additive versus multiplicative frailty. Preferably, such a model should be able to handle full pedigree data. For the marginal modeling approach more experience is needed for the combination with the copula approach. For the non-parametric estimates, we need software and more experience with the practical application and presentation of such results.

15.5 Exercises

Exercise 15.1 Heart transplant data

Summarize, in the same way as above, the analyses made for the heart transplant data of Section 1.9.4. Why is a frailty model not applied? Why is a marginal model not applied?

Exercise 15.2 Kidney catheter infections

Why is a multi-state bivariate model not relevant for these data? Would you consider a short-term frailty model?

Exercise 15.3 Tumorigenesis data

Summarize the analyses made for the data of Section 1.5.3. Is there agreement between the results? Did the experiment succeed in reducing the variance by evaluating the effect of the covariate within litters? Why was a multi-state model not applied? Why was a multivariate non-parametric estimate not applied?

Exercise 15.4 Diabetic retinopathy data

Suppose you had the data discussed in Section 1.6.1. What kind of analysis would you apply in order to evaluate the treatment effect?

Exercise 15.5 Recurrent events

Consider the following three types of recurrent events data: fertility data, as described in Section 5.3.1; repeated occurrences of a specified adverse event in a clinical trial; claims to the manufacturer for a given car model during its first years on the market. There are three main approaches to analyzing such data – multi-state models, frailty models, and marginal models. Discuss for each type of data the relevance of each approach. Some aspects, you may consider are to which extent the purpose is to study the mean risk or the differences between objects and whether the dependence is of the event-related or common risks type.

Exercise 15.6 Hypoglycemia study

Suppose you are going to perform a trial of a new treatment of diabetes (versus an existing treatment) with respect to the risk of hypoglycemia. Go through the tables of this chapter and consider the answers to the questions. On the basis of this, choose a design and a way of analyzing the results. Specifically, you should consider the following questions: Would you match patients? Would you use a common observation period? Would you consider all episodes or only the first for each patient?

As background you may use the following information: There is a very large patient variation with respect to hypoglycemic episodes. Run-in and carry-over can last a long time and thus a parallel study is more sensible than a crossover study. Drop-out will happen during a long-lasting trial.

Exercise 15.7 Anesthesia trial

Suppose you are going to design a trial for evaluating the time to unconsciousness for a new drug in two doses, high (H), low (L) versus an existing product in a standard dose (S). This is done in healthy volunteers and in order to have little dropout, it is decided to limit the number of sessions per individual to two. It is known that if unconsciousness occurs, this will usually be within a time period of Δ from the application of the drug. Describe how you would design such a study. All comparisons of H, L and S are judged equally important.

How would you analyze these data? Be precise and consider all questions in the relevant tables of this chapter.

After the analysis, the reviewers come with the following questions: Is the analysis influenced by possible period effects? Would it be more correct to consider the doses relative to body weight? Is an accelerated failure time model more appropriate than a proportional hazards model? Is the dependence in an individual between the two doses of the same drug higher than the dependence between two different drugs? How would you address these questions? As this is considered model checking, you do not need to present results evaluated within a scientifically defendable model.

Appendix A
Mathematical results

The purpose of this appendix is to describe key mathematical and statistical results that are not really survival distributions, but are needed for the study of the properties of frailty models for multivariate survival data. Sections A.3.6 and A.3.7 are less important. They serve the purpose of being alternatives to the main models. The complexity of the expressions in those cases adds perspective to the reason for choosing the simpler models.

A.1 Laplace transforms

The Laplace transform is a function evaluated on the basis of a distribution. The reason this transform is considered here is that it describes exactly the integrals needed for the mixture results of Section 2.2.7 in the univariate case and Chapter 7 in the multivariate case. When the density is $f(y)$, the Laplace transform at s is defined as

$$L(s) = \int \exp(-sy)f(y)dy. \tag{A.1}$$

The integral is over the range of the distribution. An alternative formulation, which does not require the existence of a density is the mean of an exponential function $L(s) = E(\exp(-sY))$, where Y is a random variable from the distribution. In general, there is no guarantee that the integral is finite, except for $s = 0$, where the Laplace transform equals 1. However, in this book, the transform is only evaluated for distributions concentrated on $[0, \infty)$. In this case the integral always exists whenever $s \geq 0$, as all values of the exponential term are bounded above by 1. It may or may not exist for $s < 0$. Also, the function is decreasing. The Laplace transform has many similarities to the characteristic function, but avoids the complex numbers, at the cost of only working for positive random variables, for example, the moments satisfy the relation

$$EY^n = (-1)^n L^{(n)}(0). \tag{A.2}$$

The nth moment exists precisely, when the Laplace transform is n times differentiable in 0. Differentiating the logarithm of the Laplace transform similarly gives the cumulants of the distribution.

Equation (A.2) can be generalized to

$$EY^n \exp(-sY) = (-1)^n L^{(n)}(s). \tag{A.3}$$

The Laplace transform of a sum of independent random variables is easily found, say, $S = Y_1 + \dots + Y_n$. It is

$$L_S(s) = E \exp\{-s(Y_1 + \dots + Y_n)\} = L_1(s) \times \dots \times L_n(s).$$

The Laplace transform can also be defined for a bivariate distribution, say (Y_1, Y_2), as

$$L(s_1, s_2) = E \exp\{-(s_1 Y_1 + s_2 Y_2)\}.$$

A.2   Exponential families

Exponential families are parametric families of distributions, where the observations and the parameters are combined in a particularly simple way. The consequence of this is that very strong results can be derived. For example, all moments exist in the interior of the parameter set, and they can be simply derived from the normalizing constant. Furthermore, simple results are valid regarding existence of the maximum likelihood estimate, which can be found from a set of moment conditions. The reason this family is included here is the close relationship to the Laplace transform. Many common families of distributions are exponential families, like the normal, the binomial, the Poisson, the gamma, the inverse Gaussian, and the negative binomial. Some examples will be considered in Section A.3.

An exponential family is a parametric statistical model, where the density has the form

$$f(y, \theta) = \exp\{(-\theta' t(y)\}g(y)/\varphi(\theta), \tag{A.4}$$

with respect to some measure. Here $t(y)$ is the canonical statistic, which is a, possibly multivariate, function of the observation y, θ is the canonical parameter vector and $\varphi(\cdot)$ is the normalizing constant. The negative sign in the exponential is irrelevant for the definition and can alternatively be put into $t(y)$ or θ. It is included here to make the formula for the Laplace transform simpler. The term $g(y)$ can be left out, in the sense that it can be combined with the measure. We included it here, for two reasons, the measure selected can be a standard measure, Lebesgue measure for continuous data, and counting measure for count data; and secondly, it is intuitively simpler to describe the generation of exponential families (see below). In the case where $t(y) = y$, the family is called a natural exponential family. Also, in cases where $t(y)$ is multivariate, we will say that the family is a natural exponential family in $t(y)$. In particular, when the family is a natural exponential family in $(y, \log y)$, the distribution will have some properties, when used as a frailty distribution. One consequence of the exponential family structure is that the support of the observations is the same for all values of θ. It is assumed that the parameter set is as large as possible, which is obtained by choosing the set

$$\{\theta \mid \int \exp\{-\theta' t(y)\} g(y) dy < \infty\}. \tag{A.5}$$

The normalizing constant $\varphi(\theta)$, considered as a function of the parameter θ is a key function in this theory. In the interior of the parameter set, the function is differentiable and

$$d \log \varphi(\theta)/d\theta_j = -E t_j(Y).$$

On the boundary, the function might not be differentiable and the mean might not exist. Further differentiation of this gives the higher-order cumulants, extending the results for the Laplace transform.

One advantage of the natural exponential families is that the Laplace transform is easily given by means of the normalizing constant. In the simplest case, when $t(y) = y$, the expression is

$$L(s) = \varphi(\theta + s)/\varphi(\theta). \tag{A.6}$$

In the more general case, where $t(y)$ is two-dimensional, $t(y) = (y, t_2(x))$, the expression becomes

$$L(s) = \varphi(\theta_1 + s, \theta_2)/\varphi(\theta_1, \theta_2).$$

Sometimes it will be said that a multi-parameter family is exponential in one parameter. This means that when the other parameters are assumed fixed and known, the family is an exponential family. The advantage of this case is that we can still use some results from the exponential family theory.

Exponential families can be generated when the functions $g(y)$ and $t(y)$ are known, or chosen. This procedure is also denoted exponential tilting. Then the family with the density in Equation (A.4) is obtained by choosing the parameter set given by Equation (A.5). To be specific, we start out by a single distribution for a random variable $Y \geq 0$ with density $g(y)$ and Laplace transform $L(s)$ for $t(y)$. For simplicity, it is assumed that $t(y) = y$. Thus the integral in Equation (A.5) equals $L(\theta)$, implying that an exponential family is defined by

$$f(y, \theta) = \exp\{-\theta' t(y)\} g(y)/L(\theta), \tag{A.7}$$

corresponding to Equation (A.4), with $\varphi(\theta) = L(\theta)$. It follows from the existence of the Laplace function that the largest possible parameter set includes $[0, \infty)$, and that $\varphi(0) = 1$.

A.3   Distribution theory

The aim of this section is to document necessary distribution theory for distributions that are not used as actual survival distributions, but for mixture distributions. This includes gamma, stable, power variance function, and lognormal families. To put these families in perspective, some results for the generalized inverse Gaussian and the non-central gamma distributions are also included.

A.3.1   Gamma distributions

The version of the density that we use is

$$f(y) = \theta^\delta y^{\delta - 1} \exp(-\theta y)/\Gamma(\delta). \tag{A.8}$$

The range of the observations is R_+, and this is also the range for the two parameters (δ, θ). The parameter δ is called the shape parameter. The distribution is denoted gamma(δ, θ). It is an exponential family with canonical statistics Y and $\log Y$. In exponential family layout the density is

$$f(y) = \exp(-\theta y + \delta \log y) \, \{\theta^\delta/\Gamma(\delta)\} \, y^{-1}.$$

If $\delta = 1$, it is an exponential distribution with hazard θ. For $\theta = 1/2$ and $\delta = f/2$, where f is an integer, this is the χ^2-distribution with f degrees of freedom. The relation can be used to evaluate the distribution function in practice, for integer f, as many computer systems have this function. In the general case, the distribution function is given by an incomplete gamma function, see Equation (A.27), as

$$F(y) = 1 - P(\theta y, \delta)/\Gamma(\delta).$$

The distribution of cY for a positive constant c is also a gamma distribution, with δ unchanged, and $\tilde{\theta} = \theta/c$, that is, gamma$(\delta, \theta/c)$. Thus, θ is an inverse scale parameter. If Y_1 and Y_2 are independent, and Y_j follows gamma$(\delta_j, \theta), j = 1, 2$, the distribution of $Y_1 + Y_2$ is gamma$(\delta_1 + \delta_2, \theta)$. A consequence of this result is that the distribution is infinitely divisible. Also the log of a gamma distribution is infinitely divisible; that is, let $W = \log Y$, then the distribution of W is infinitely divisible, but the corresponding distributions are not known. One multiplicative mixture result is that if Y_1, Y_2

are independent, Y_1 has a gamma distribution with parameters $(\tilde{\delta} - \delta, \theta)$, and Y_2 is beta distributed with parameters $(\delta, \tilde{\delta} - \delta)$, then the distribution of $Y_1 Y_2$ is gamma(δ, θ).

The mean is $\mu = \delta/\theta$, and the variance δ/θ^2. Considered as a univariate natural exponential family, i.e., for fixed value of δ, the variance is a quadratic function of the mean, μ^2/δ. Generally, the moments are

$$EY^q = \theta^{-q}\Gamma(\delta + q)/\Gamma(\delta), \tag{A.9}$$

a formula that is valid for all real values of $q > -\delta$. For $q \le -\delta$ this moment is infinite, demonstrating a large tail near 0. Also the mean and variance on the logarithmic scale can be evaluated

$$E \log Y = \psi(\delta) - \log \theta, \ Var(\log Y) = \psi'(\delta), \tag{A.10}$$

where $\psi(x)$ is the digamma function $\Gamma'(x)/\Gamma(x)$. Also mixed moments, including both Y and $\log Y$, can be evaluated in a similar way, for example, $EY^q \log Y = \theta^{-q}\{\Gamma'(\delta + q) - \Gamma(\delta + q) \log \theta\}/\Gamma(\delta)$, still letting $q > -\delta$. The Laplace transform is $L(s) = E \exp(-sY) = \theta^\delta/(\theta + s)^\delta$. The derivatives of this are simply

$$L^{(p)}(s) = (-1)^p \theta^\delta (\theta + s)^{-(\delta+p)}\Gamma(\delta + p)/\Gamma(\delta). \tag{A.11}$$

For evaluating more complicated integrals, one can use the result that for $q > \delta$ and a function $h(y)$, with $E \mid Y^q h(Y) \mid < \infty$, we have

$$E\{Y^q h(Y)\} = \frac{\Gamma(\delta + q)}{\Gamma(\delta)} Eh(\tilde{Y}), \tag{A.12}$$

where $\tilde{Y}$ follows gamma$(\delta + q, \theta)$.

A.3.2 Inverse Gaussian distributions

This is also a distribution on the positive real numbers, and an exponential family with canonical statistics Y and $1/Y$. The traditional parametrization from an exponential family point of view is as

$$f(y) = (2\pi)^{-1/2} y^{-3/2} \psi^{1/2} e^{\sqrt{\phi\psi}} e^{-\phi y/2 - \psi/2y}.$$

Here, however, a different parametrization will be used, to make it fit into the general power variance function family. In this parametrization, the density is

$$f(y) = \delta\pi^{-1/2} \exp(2\delta\theta^{1/2}) y^{-3/2} \exp(-\theta y - \delta^2/y). \tag{A.13}$$

The relation between the parameters are $\phi = 2\theta$ and $\psi = 2\delta^2$. The parameter set is $\delta > 0$, $\theta \ge 0$.

The inverse Gaussian distributions are stopping times in a Brownian motion. Suppose the Brownian motion has drift $\xi \ge 0$ and variance σ^2, the time to reach the value $a > 0$ follows an inverse Gaussian distribution with parameters $\theta = \frac{\xi}{2\sigma^2}$ and $\delta = \frac{a}{\sigma\sqrt{2}}$. If $\xi < 0$, the distribution has a point mass at ∞ and is not in the inverse Gaussian family.

The distribution function is

$$F(y) = \Phi\{(2/t)^{1/2}(-\delta + t\theta^{1/2})\} + e^{4\delta\theta^{1/2}}\Phi\{-(2/t)^{1/2}(\delta + t\theta^{1/2})\}$$

where $\Phi(y)$ is the standard normal distribution function. The distribution of cY, for c a positive constant, is also an inverse Gaussian distribution with parameters $\tilde{\delta} = c^{1/2}\delta$ and $\tilde{\theta} = \theta/c$. Thus the distribution family includes a scale parameter. If Y_1 and Y_2 are independent, and Y_i follows $\text{InvG}(\delta_i, \theta), i = 1, 2$, the distribution of $Y_1 + Y_2$ is $\text{InvG}(\delta_1 + \delta_2, \theta)$. A consequence of this result is that the distribution is infinitely divisible. The distribution of the log of an inverse Gaussian variable is only infinitely divisible if $\theta = 0$.

For $\theta = 0$, it is a positive stable distribution of index $1/2$, and $1/Y$ follows a gamma distribution with parameters $1/2$ and δ^2, and the distribution function reduces to $1 - 2\Phi\{-\delta(2/t)^{1/2}\}$. In this case EY^q exists for $q < 1/2$. For positive θ, all moments, both positive and negative, exist. The cumulants are $\chi_1 = EY = \delta/\theta^{1/2}$, and $\chi_q = \delta(1/2)(3/2)...(q-3/2)/\theta^{q-1/2}$, $q = 2, 3, ...$. Thus the variance is $\sigma^2 = \delta/(2\theta^{3/2})$. Furthermore $E1/Y = (1/2 + \delta\theta^{1/2})/\delta^2$. We can find EY^q for general real q by means of the formulas for the generalized inverse Gaussian distributions, see Section A.3.6. On the log scale, we find the mean

$$E \log Y = \log(\delta\theta^{1/2}) + E_1(2\delta\theta^{1/2})\exp(2\delta\theta^{1/2}), \qquad (A.14)$$

where $E_1(x)$ denotes the exponential integral (see Section A.4.1). The variance of $\log Y$ can be found as the second derivative of a Bessel function, with respect to order

$$Var(\log Y) = h(2\delta\theta^{1/2}), \qquad (A.15)$$

where $h(x) = d^2 \log K_\gamma(x)/d\gamma^2$, evaluated at $\gamma = 1/2$. This can be evaluated by means of Equations (A.30) and (A.31). Also moments of the form $EY^q \log Y$ can be found. Considered as a natural exponential family, i.e. for fixed value of δ, the variance is a cubic function of the mean, $\mu^3/(2\delta^2)$.

A.3.3 Positive stable distributions

A strictly stable distribution is defined by the requirement that the sum of n independent copies of the distribution should have the same distribution as a scale factor times the distribution. Non-strict stable distributions further might need a translation, but we will not consider this possibility here. In mathematical terms, the requirement is that for $Y_1, ...$ i.i.d., there should exist a function $c(n)$ so that

$$c(n)Y_1 =_D Y_1 + ... + Y_n,$$

where $=_D$ denotes has the same distribution as. The function $c(n)$ turns out to have the form $n^{1/\alpha}$, where α is between 0 and 2. This number is called the index of the distribution. For $\alpha = 2$, the normal distribution is obtained. To get a distribution on the positive numbers, it is further necessary to restrict to $\alpha \leq 1$. The distribution has two parameters, α and δ. The Laplace transform is

$$L(s) = \exp(-\delta s^\alpha/\alpha).$$

The derivatives are described under power variance function distributions. The standard case is when $\delta = \alpha$, and will be denoted Posstab(α). Other values correspond to scale transformations of this case. For $\alpha = 1$, the distribution is degenerate at δ, and if $\alpha < 1$, the density is

$$f(y) = -\frac{1}{\pi y} \sum_{k=1}^{\infty} \frac{\Gamma(k\alpha + 1)}{k!} (-y^{-\alpha}\delta/\alpha)^k \sin(\alpha k\pi). \tag{A.16}$$

This expression is a power series in $y^{-\alpha}$, implying that it converges fast for large values of y, and slow for small values of y. For small values of y, it can be approximated by inserting $\theta = 0$ in Equation (A.21).

If Y_1 and Y_2 are independent, following positive stable distributions with the same α and possibly different $\delta_j, j = 1, 2$, the distribution of $Y_1 + Y_2$ is positive stable with the same value of α and $\tilde{\delta} = \delta_1 + \delta_2$. A consequence of this result is that the distribution is infinitely divisible. The distribution of the log of a positive stable variable is also infinitely divisible, but the corresponding distributions are not known.

The distribution of cY, for c a positive constant, is again a positive stable distribution, with the same value of α, and δ exchanged by δc^α. The mean does not exist, for $\alpha < 1$, but the moment EY^q exists for $q < \alpha$, and it equals $(\delta/\alpha)^{q/\alpha}\Gamma(1 - q/\alpha)/\Gamma(1 - q)$. The logarithmic mean equals

$$E \log Y = \alpha^{-1} \log(\delta/\alpha) - (\alpha^{-1} - 1)\psi(1).$$

Furthermore $Var(\log Y) = (\alpha^{-2} - 1)\psi'(1) = (\alpha^{-2} - 1)\pi^2/6$. The qth cumulant $(q > 1)$ of $\log Y$ equals $(-1)^q(\alpha^{-q} - 1)\psi^{(q-1)}(1)$. Also moments of the form $EY^q \log Y$ can be found for real q, $q < \alpha$. For $\delta = \alpha$, the value is

$$EY^q \log Y = \{\psi(1 - q) - \psi(1 - q/\alpha)/\alpha\}\Gamma(1 - q/\alpha)/\Gamma(1 - q).$$

A mixture result that is known is that if Y_1, Y_2 are independent, Y_1 follows Posstab(α), and Y_2 follows Posstab(γ), $i = 1, 2$, the distribution of $Y_1 Y_2^{1/\alpha}$ is Posstab($\alpha\gamma$).

Another mixture result, reported by Williams (1977), is that for $\alpha = 1/n$, n integer, Y has the same distribution as $1/(X_1...X_{n-1})$, where $X_1, ..., X_{n-1}$ are independent gamma variables, where the parameters of X_i are $\delta = i/n$, $\theta = 1$.

A.3.4   Power variance function distributions

This family of distributions is a three-parameter family uniting the above distributions. The distribution is denoted $\text{PVF}(\alpha, \delta, \theta)$. For $\alpha = 0$, the gamma distributions are obtained, with the same parametrization. Some formulas are valid, but many others are different in this case. In any case, the formula for the gamma model is obtained as a limiting case. For $\alpha = 1/2$, the inverse Gaussian distributions are obtained. For $\theta = 0$, the positive stable distributions are obtained. For $\alpha = 1$, a degenerate distribution is obtained, at δ, independently of θ. For $\alpha = -1$, a non-central gamma distribution of shape parameter 0 is obtained. For details on this distribution see Section A.3.7.

The parameter set is $\alpha \leq 1, \delta > 0$, with $\theta \geq 0$ for $\alpha > 0$, and $\theta > 0$ for $\alpha \leq 0$. The distribution is concentrated on the positive numbers for $\alpha \geq 0$, and is positive or zero for $\alpha < 0$. A definition that unites all cases is

$$d \log L(s)/ds = -\delta(\theta + s)^{\alpha-1}.$$

In fact, this definition can be extended to cover $1 < \alpha \leq 2$, but in that case the random variable will be real valued rather than non-negative.

In the case $\alpha > 0$, the distribution can be obtained as the exponential family generated from the positive stable distributions. This means that, as described in Equation (A.7), the density in Equation (A.16) is multiplied by $\exp(-\theta y)$, and renormalized to become a density. That means so that it has integral 1. The factor for the renormalization is derived directly from the Laplace transform. Thus the density is, for $y > 0$

$$f(y) \exp(-\theta y) \exp(\delta\theta^\alpha/\alpha),$$

where $f(y)$ is given by Equation (A.16). In the case $\alpha < 0$, the Γ-term in the density is not necessarily defined, and therefore we can use the alternative expression

$$f(y) = \exp(-\theta y + \delta^\alpha/\alpha)\frac{1}{y}\sum_{k=1}^{\infty}\frac{(-\delta y^{-\alpha}/\alpha)^k}{k!\Gamma(-k\alpha)}.$$

This expression is valid for $y > 0$ and all α-values, except 0 and 1, with the convention that when the Γ-function in the denominator is undefined (which happens when $k\alpha$ is a positive integer), the whole term in the sum is 0. For $\alpha < 0$, there is probability $\exp(\delta\theta^\alpha/\alpha)$ of the random variable being 0. For $\alpha \geq 0$, the distribution is unimodal.

If Y_1 and Y_2 are independent, and Y_i follows $\text{PVF}(\alpha, \delta_i, \theta), i = 1, 2$, the distribution of $Y_1 + Y_2$ is $\text{PVF}(\alpha, \delta_1 + \delta_2, \theta)$. A consequence of this result is that the distribution is infinitely divisible. The distribution of cY_1 is $\text{PVF}(\alpha, \delta_1 c^\alpha, \theta/c)$. Thus the family allows for scale changes, but the change of parameter is not concentrated on a single of the parameters.

When $\theta > 0$, all (positive) moments exist, and the mean is $\mu = \delta\theta^{\alpha-1}$. The variance is $\delta(1-\alpha)\theta^{\alpha-2}$. The qth cumulant $(q > 1)$ is

$$\chi_q = \delta(1-\alpha)(2-\alpha)...(q-1-\alpha)\theta^{\alpha-q}.$$

The moment $E1/Y$ exists generally for $\alpha > 0$, where it is an incomplete gamma function. When $\delta > 1$, the moment can evaluated for $\alpha = 0$, and it never exists for $\alpha < 0$. When $\alpha = 1/n$ for a (positive) integer n, we can further evaluate

$$E(1/Y) = (\delta n)^{-n}\Gamma(n)\sum_{i=0}^{n-1} n^{i+1}\delta^i\theta^{i/n}/\Gamma(i+1).$$

For fixed values of (α, δ), the PVF family is a natural exponential family in θ. Considered as a natural exponential family, the variance is a power function of the mean, $(1-\alpha)\delta^{1/(\alpha-1)}\mu^{1+1/(1-\alpha)}$. For α positive, the power lies between 2 and ∞, and for α negative, the power is between 1 and 2.

For $\alpha < 0$, the distribution is also called compound Poisson, because it can be derived as the sum of a Poisson distributed number of gamma random variables. If N follows a Poisson distribution with mean ρ and $X_1, ...$ are independent identically distributed as gamma(η, ν), then $Y = X_1 + ... + X_N$ (with Y defined as 0, when $N = 0$) follows PVF$(-\eta, \eta\rho\nu^\eta, \nu)$.

The Laplace transform is

$$L(s) = \exp[-\delta\{(\theta+s)^\alpha - \theta^\alpha\}/\alpha]. \tag{A.17}$$

The derivatives are of the form

$$L^{(p)}(s) = (-1)^p L(s)\sum_{j=1}^{p} c_{p,j}(\alpha)\delta^j(\theta+s)^{j\alpha-p}, \tag{A.18}$$

where the coefficients $c_{p,j}(\alpha)$ are polynomials in α, of order $p - j$ given by the recursive formula

$$c_{p,1}(\alpha) = \Gamma(p-\alpha)/\Gamma(1-\alpha), \ c_{p,p} = 1$$

$$c_{p,j}(\alpha) = c_{p-1,j-1}(\alpha) + c_{p-1,j}(\alpha)\{(p-1) - j\alpha\}. \tag{A.19}$$

The first terms are

$$c_{1,1} = 1$$

$$c_{2,1} = 1 - \alpha, \ c_{2,2} = 1$$

$$c_{3,1} = (1-\alpha)(2-\alpha), \ c_{3,2} = 3(1-\alpha), \ c_{3,3} = 1.$$

For some calculations, also the derivatives with respect to α are needed. They similarly satisfy recurrence relations, which are

$$c'_{p,1}(\alpha) = \frac{\Gamma(p-\alpha)}{\Gamma(1-\alpha)}\sum_{j=1}^{p-1}\frac{1}{j-\alpha}, \ c'_{p,p} = 0$$

$$c'_{p,j}(\alpha) = c'_{p-1,j-1}(\alpha) + c'_{p-1,j}(\alpha)\{(p-1) - j\alpha\} - jc_{p-1,j}(\alpha). \quad \text{(A.20)}$$

For α being $1/2$ and -1, the factors can be found explicitly, by means of the formulas

$$c_{p,j}(1/2) = \frac{4^{j-p}(2p-1-j)!}{(p-j)!(p-1)!}$$

and

$$c_{p,j}(-1) = \frac{p!(p-1)!}{(p-j)!j!(j-1)!}.$$

Under the limit $\delta\theta^\alpha \to \infty$, for α fixed, $\alpha < 1$ the distribution is asymptotically normal. A better approximation is the saddle point approximation, which, under the further restriction of $\alpha \neq 0$ is

$$\{2\pi(1-\alpha)\}^{1/2}\delta^{1/\{2(1-\alpha)\}}y^\nu \exp\{-\theta y - \delta^{1/(1-\alpha)}(\alpha^{-1}-1)y^{-\alpha/(1-\alpha)} + \delta\theta^\alpha/\alpha\},$$
$$\text{(A.21)}$$

where $\nu = -(2-\alpha)/\{2(1-\alpha)\}$. This approximation transforms in the same way as the true density under multiplication by c. The approximation is particularly good for y close to 0.

The limit for $\alpha \to -\infty$ is a scaled Poisson. A scaled Poisson is defined as $Y = cQ$, where c is a constant and Q is Poisson, with mean η, say. To obtain convergence under $\alpha \to -\infty$, the mean and variance must converge, in which case,

$$c = \lim \frac{Var(Y)}{EY} = \lim(1-\alpha)/\theta, \eta = \lim \frac{(EY)^2}{Var(Y)} = \lim \delta\theta^\alpha/(1-\alpha).$$

Figure A.1 illustrates the differences between the gamma, the stable and the inverse Gaussian distributions. All the distributions are chosen to have a geometric mean of 1 ($E \log Y = 0$), and a variance of 1 on logarithmic scale, and the figure shows the density of the logarithm of Y. The inverse Gaussian is close to be symmetric, and therefore comparable to the lognormal distributions, whereas the gamma has a large left tail, and the positive stable distribution has an even more important right tail.

A.3.5 Lognormal distributions

A random variable Y is said to be lognormally distributed, when $X = \log Y$ follows a normal distribution. The parameters are the mean (ξ) and the variance σ^2 for X. A number of properties of this family follow directly from well-known properties of the normal distribution. Also, extension to a multivariate distribution is direct. For c a positive constant, the distribution of cY is lognormal with parameters $\xi + \log c$ and σ^2. For c a real constant, the distribution of Y^c is lognormal with parameters $c\xi$ and $c^2\sigma^2$. If Y_1 and Y_2 are independent and lognormally distributed with parameters ξ_1, σ_1^2 and ξ_2, σ_2^2, respectively, Y_1Y_2 is lognormal with parameters $\xi_1 + \xi_2$ and $\sigma_1^2 + \sigma_2^2$. The mean is $EY = \exp(\xi + \sigma^2/2)$. The distribution is infinite divisible.

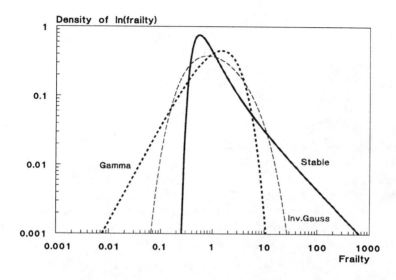

Figure A.1. The density of log Y for gamma, stable and inverse Gaussian distributions with a mean of 0, and variance of 1, measured on the logarithmic scale.

The density is

$$f(y) = \frac{1}{y(2\pi\sigma^2)^{1/2}} \exp[-\{(\log y) - \xi\}^2/(2\sigma^2)]. \qquad (A.22)$$

The distributions make up an exponential family with $\log Y$ and $(\log Y)^2$ as canonical statistics.

The Laplace transform seems difficult to evaluate explicitly. Using classical saddle point techniques, we may approximate the integral $\int \exp(-\kappa(x))dx$ as

$$\kappa''(\tilde{x})^{-1/2} \exp\{-\kappa(\tilde{x})\}, \qquad (A.23)$$

where $\tilde{x}$ is the solution to the equation $\kappa'(x) = 0$. For finding $L(s)$, we set $\kappa(x) = se^x + (x - \xi)^2/(2\sigma^2)$, so that the equation for $\tilde{x}$ is $se^x + (x - \xi)/\sigma^2$ and $\kappa''(x) = se^x + 1/\sigma^2$.

Approximating the derivatives is not more complicated, because the Y^n term in Equation (A.3) just corresponds to a change of the parameter ξ. This is because it is an exponential family with $\log Y$ as canonical statistic. Thus we use $\kappa(x) = se^x + (x - \xi)^2/(2\sigma^2) - nx$, $\kappa'(x) = se^x + (x - \xi)/\sigma^2 - n$ so that $\kappa''(x)$ is unchanged.

For some evaluations, we need the exponential family generated from the lognormal. This will be denoted by LNEF(θ, ξ, σ^2) and is defined by combining Equation (A.7) using $t(y) = y$ with Equation (A.22). From a theoretical point of view, it is not a problem that the normalizing constant $(L(\theta))$ is only given as an integral, but from a practical point of view, it is of course a limitation that we only have an approximation. However, we can still make several observations from the formula. The family is a three-dimensional exponential family with canonical statistics y, $\log y$ and $(\log y)^2$. The distribution of cY is LNEF$(\theta/c, \xi + \log c, \sigma^2)$.

A.3.6 Generalized inverse Gaussian distributions

This distribution is another generalization of the gamma and inverse Gaussian distributions. It does not include the positive stable distributions, except for $\alpha = 1/2$. It can be obtained from the gamma distributions by generating the exponential family with $1/Y$ as canonical statistic. It can be obtained from the inverse Gaussian family by generating the exponential family with $\log Y$ as canonical statistic. It is an exponential family with $Y, 1/Y$ and $\log Y$ as canonical statistics. The density is

$$f(y) = (1/2)(\theta^{1/2}/\delta)^\gamma y^{\gamma-1} \exp(-\theta y - \delta^2/y)/K_\gamma(2\delta\theta^{1/2}) \qquad (A.24)$$

where $K_\gamma(x)$ is the Bessel function described in Section A.4.2. For $\gamma = -1/2$, the inverse Gaussian distributions are obtained, with the same parametrization as used above. For $\delta = 0, \gamma > 0$, the gamma distributions are obtained, but with a different parametrization than used above. We denote the distribution as GIG(γ, δ, θ). The parameter set is, for $\gamma > 0$ that $\delta \geq 0, \theta > 0$, for $\gamma = 0$ $\delta > 0, \theta > 0$ and for $\gamma < 0$ that $\delta > 0, \theta \geq 0$. For $\gamma = 0$, the distribution of $\log Y$ is symmetric.

Moments are easily found, by evaluating the normalizing constant at different values. We find

$$EY^q = (\theta^{1/2}/\delta)^{-q} \frac{K_{\gamma+q}(2\delta\theta^{1/2})}{K_\gamma(2\delta\theta^{1/2})}. \qquad (A.25)$$

If Y is GIG(γ, δ, θ), the distribution of cY is GIG$(\gamma, \delta c^{1/2}, \theta/c)$ and the distribution of $1/Y$ is GIG$(-\gamma, \theta^{1/2}, \delta^2)$.

A.3.7 Non-central gamma distributions

Non-central gamma distributions are directly related to non-central χ^2-distributions. These are obtained as sums of squares of independent normally distributed random variables, with unit variance. If the mean values of the normal variables are all 0, the χ^2-distributions are obtained, but if one or more mean values are different from 0, a non-central distribution is obtained. The standard parametrization of the non-central gamma distribution gives the density

$$e^{-\lambda\theta^\delta}y^\delta e^{-\theta y} \sum_{r=0}^{\infty} \frac{(\lambda\theta)^r y^{r-1}}{r!\Gamma(r+\delta)},$$

where $\lambda \geq 0$ is a non-centrality parameter, δ is the form parameter and θ is the inverse scale parameter in the central case. We will instead use a different parametrization in order to show this as an exponential family. We define $\gamma = \lambda\theta$ and obtain the density

$$e^{-\gamma/\theta}\theta^\delta y^\delta e^{-\theta y} \sum_{r=0}^{\infty} \frac{\gamma^r y^{r-1}}{r!\Gamma(r+\delta)}. \tag{A.26}$$

In this formulation, it is clear that for a fixed value of (γ, δ), it is a natural exponential family with canonical parameter θ. We will denote this distribution as $\mathrm{NCGamma}(\delta, \gamma, \theta)$.

The distribution of cY is $\mathrm{NCGamma}(\delta, \gamma/c, \theta/c)$.

If Y_1 and Y_2 are independent and have parameters $(\delta_1, \gamma_1, \theta)$ and $(\delta_2, \gamma_2, \theta)$, the distribution of $Y_1 + Y_2$ is $\mathrm{NCGamma}(\delta_1 + \delta_2, \gamma_1 + \gamma_2, \theta)$. It follows trivially from this result that the distribution is infinitely divisible.

When the shape parameter converges to 0, the distribution converges to a distribution with a point mass at 0 and a continuous distribution on the positive numbers. Therefore, it is well defined to have a non-central gamma distribution with 0 degrees of freedom.

A.4 Mathematical functions

This section describes the gamma function, the Bessel function, and various related functions needed to do more theoretical evaluations.

A.4.1 The gamma function and related functions

The gamma function is defined as

$$\Gamma(\delta) = \int_0^\infty t^{\delta-1} e^{-t} dt$$

for $\delta > 0$. It satisfies $\Gamma(\delta + 1) = \delta\Gamma(\delta)$.

The incomplete gamma function is the partial integral of the same quantity. Here the version used is the part of the area, from x up to ∞,

$$P(x, \delta) = \int_x^\infty t^{\delta-1} e^{-t} dt. \tag{A.27}$$

This can be evaluated as a power series

$$P(x, \delta) = \Gamma(\delta) - x^\delta \sum_{j=0}^{\infty} \frac{(-x)^j}{(\delta+j)j!}, \tag{A.28}$$

but it converges slowly for high values of δ, and therefore it is an advantage first to apply the partial integration formula

$$P(x, \delta) = (\delta - 1)P(x, \delta - 1) + x^{\delta-1} e^{-x}$$

several times. The power series is best to evaluate for $0 < \delta < 2$. When δ is an integer, it can be described as a finite sum

$$P(x, \delta) = \sum_{j=0}^{\delta-1} x^j \exp(-x)/j!. \tag{A.29}$$

The digamma function is defined as $\psi(x) = \Gamma'(x)/\Gamma(x)$. This is needed for moments on the logarithmic scale because

$$\Gamma'(\delta) = \int_0^\infty (\log t) t^{\delta-1} e^{-t} dt,$$

which is obtained by differentiation under the integral sign.

Other gamma-related functions are

$$J_k(\alpha) = \int_0^\infty e^{-x} (\log x)^k / (1 - \alpha + \alpha x) dx,$$

which we need for $k = 1, 2$, in order to evaluate the Fisher information in Section 8.11.2. No expressions to reduce these are known, and they therefore have to be evaluated by numerical integration.

The exponential integral is the analogue of the incomplete gamma function for $\delta = 0$. We have formulated Equation (A.27) in order to fit the exponential integral

$$E_1(x) = \int_x^\infty t^{-1} e^{-t} dt = \int_1^\infty t^{-1} e^{-xt} dt.$$

This integral is infinite, when $x = 0$ is inserted. It can be evaluated by polynomial approximations (Abramowitz and Stegun, 1965, (5.1.53) and (5.1.56)).

This is generalized to mth order, by

$$E_m(x) = \int_1^\infty t^{-m} e^{-xt} dt.$$

To actually evaluate this function, use first the relation

$$E_{m+1}(x) = \frac{1}{m} \{e^{-x} - x E_m(x)\}.$$

For $0 < m < 1$, $E_m(x)$ is evaluated by the power series Equation (A.28) with $\delta = 1 - m$.

A.4.2   Bessel functions

This function is helpful in order to handle the inverse Gaussian distribution and necessary in order to handle the generalized inverse Gaussian distribution. The general definition of the Bessel function we use is

$$K_\gamma(\omega) = (1/2) \int_0^\infty t^{\gamma-1} \exp\{-\omega(t + 1/t)/2\} dt.$$

In order to calculate it, we use the expression

$$K_\gamma(\omega) = (\pi/2)\{I_{-\gamma}(\omega) - I_\gamma(\omega)\}/\sin(\gamma\pi) \qquad (A.30)$$

for non-integer γ, where

$$I_\gamma(\omega) = (\omega/2)^\gamma \sum_{m=0}^{\infty} \frac{(\omega/2)^{2m}}{m!\Gamma(\gamma + m + 1)}. \qquad (A.31)$$

It does satisfy a recurrence relation

$$K_{\gamma+1}(\omega) = \frac{2\gamma}{\omega} K_\gamma(\omega) + K_{\gamma-1}(\omega),$$

and it is known that $K_{-\gamma}(\omega) = K_\gamma(\omega)$. For the half integer values, there is an explicit expression

$$K_{n+1/2}(\omega) = \{\pi/(2\omega)\}^{1/2} e^{-\omega} \{1 + \sum_{j=1}^{n} \frac{(n+j)!}{(n-j)!j!}(2\omega)^{-j}\} \qquad (A.32)$$

for $n = 0, 1, ...$ For $n = 0$, it reduces to

$$K_{1/2}(\omega) = K_{-1/2}(\omega) = \{\pi/(2\omega)\}^{1/2} e^{-\omega}.$$

A.4.3 Hypergeometric functions

The only hypergeometric function used in the book is the function $_3F_2$, defined as

$$_3F_2(\alpha, \beta, \gamma, \delta, \epsilon, x) = \sum_{m=0}^{\infty} \frac{\Gamma(\alpha + m)\Gamma(\beta + m)\Gamma(\gamma + m)\Gamma(\delta)\Gamma(\epsilon)x^m}{\Gamma(\alpha)\Gamma(\beta)\Gamma(\gamma)\Gamma(\delta + m)\Gamma(\epsilon + m)m!}.$$

$$(A.33)$$

A.5 Bibliography

A classical reference to Laplace transforms and stable distributions is Feller (1971). The PVF model was suggested by Tweedie (1984) and later independently derived by Hougaard (1986a) and Bar-Lev and Enis (1986). The generalized inverse Gaussian distribution is described in detail by Jørgensen (1981). The non-central gamma distribution with zero degrees of freedom was described by Siegel (1979).

Most of the results on mathematical functions are described in Abramowitz and Stegun (1965).

The precision of the Laplace transform approximation to the lognormal distribution was considered by Ducrocq (1996).

Figure A.1 is reproduced from Hougaard (1995), with kind permission from Kluwer Academic Publishers.

A.6   Exercises

Exercise A.1 Variance in an exponential family

Derive explicitly the variance of $t(Y)$ in an exponential family expressed by means of the derivatives of $\log \varphi(\theta)$.

Exercise A.2 MLE in exponential families

Consider a sample $Y_1, ..., Y_n$ of independent observations from a one-parameter natural exponential family. Show that the maximum likelihood equation for θ equals the first moment equation.

Exercise A.3 Information in exponential families

Consider n independent observations from an exponential family given by the density in Equation (A.4). Find the observed information about θ (minus the second derivative of the log likelihood). Show that it is independent of the observations, and thus that calculating the expected information is trivial.

Exercise A.4 Lognormal exponential family

Consider the LNEF family defined in Section A.3.5. Use the fact that cY is in the same family to derive a relation of the normalizing constants. Show how this can be used to derive the Laplace transform of the lognormal distribution based on the Laplace transform for $\xi = 0$.

Exercise A.5 Generalized inverse Gaussian Laplace

Find the Laplace transform of the generalized inverse Gaussian distribution. What is the variance in the distribution?

Exercise A.6 Non-central gamma Laplace

Find the Laplace transform of the non-central gamma distribution by means of Equations (A.6) and (A.26). Check the calculations by inserting $\gamma = 0$ to get the Laplace transform of the gamma distribution, and $\delta = 0$ to get the Laplace transform of the PVF distribution with $\alpha = -1$, but in a a different parametrization. Find the mean and variance using Equation (A.2).

Appendix B
Iterative solutions

Many of the models considered can be fitted by standard software, like SAS or Splus, but there are also a number that cannot. This section describes the standard Newton-Raphson iteration technique and a number of modifications that can be used. The approach is general for solving equations based on differentiable functions, but here the method will be considered in a context of maximizing log likelihood functions. So there is a differentiable log likelihood function given, $\ell(\theta)$, where the argument is vector valued. The dimension of θ is denoted p. The aim is to find θ, so that the value of ℓ is as large as possible. There is an initial value of θ given and this has to be found by other means. At the maximum, the derivatives are 0 and therefore corresponding notation will be introduced. The vector of derivatives is denoted F and the matrix of second derivatives H. This matrix is symmetric. At the maximum, H will be negative definite, that is, all eigenvalues are negative. If there are both positive and negative eigenvalues, the point is not a local maximum, but a saddle point. Most iterative procedures are only known to converge to a stationary point, that is, a point, where F is 0. To make sure that it is a local maximum, one can check that it is a local maximum. This is the case, when all the diagonal elements of H and H^{-1} are negative. If one or more eigenvalues for H are 0, some parameters cannot be identified in this point and the matrix cannot be inverted, as it does not have maximal rank. When the value of θ is not optimal, the matrix H does not need to be negative definite.

B.1   Newton-Raphson iteration

Newton-Raphson iteration is a way of improving an estimate in successive steps. It requires the values of the derivatives and second derivatives, and based on any given θ, it suggests the value

$$\theta - FH^{-1}. \tag{B.1}$$

This updating equation is then applied a number of times, until the successive changes are small. Near the maximum, this procedure is optimal and the error, as measured by F, is squared at each step.

B.2   Extensions and modifications

Often, we want to estimate in a model involving only a subset of the parameters. Then we, of course, only need the derivatives with respect to those parameters. Rather than making a specific program for each set of possible parameters to maximize over, it is easier to calculate all the derivatives and then select the necessary components of F and H. Accordingly, only those components should be updated in Equation (B.1). They can be picked out simply, but sometimes it is convenient to do so by a matrix G, which has p columns and each of the, say q, parameters to maximize over, requires a row with a 1 at the qth place and 0 other places. Then Equation (B.1) is substituted by

$$\theta - G'(GF)(GHG')^{-1}. \tag{B.2}$$

The advantage of this expression is that we keep the same parameter dimension by considering the full parameter.

A further advantage is that it is possible use the approach to introduce restrictions, for example, that two parameters are equal. If, for example, there is a four parameter model, with parameters $\alpha, \beta_1, \beta_2, \gamma$ and the hypothesis of symmetry $\beta_1 = \beta_2$ should be considered and γ is assumed equal to γ_0, the initial estimate should be required to satisfy these relations and then a matrix

$$G = \begin{pmatrix} 1 & 0 & 0 & 0 \\ 0 & 1 & 1 & 0 \end{pmatrix}$$

is used. In this way, γ will never be changed and β_1 and β_2 will stay equal. The reason this works for common β's is that the derivatives calculated by GF and GHG' are exactly the first and second derivatives of the parameters α and β, when we express the original parameter $(\alpha, \beta_1, \beta_2, \gamma)$ as a function $(\alpha, \beta, \beta, \gamma_0)$ of (α, β).

As described above, the procedure does not require the calculation of the log likelihood value, but it is an advantage to do so, to ensure that the likelihood is indeed increasing for each step and monitor the iteration.

Secondly, the value is, in most cases, needed for comparing likelihoods later on. A third advantage is that during program development, one can perform numerical differentiation in order to check that the derivatives are correct.

If the likelihood is decreased or if the suggested change is very large, one can use a smaller step length, that is, multiply the adjustment in Equation (B.1) by a number between 0 and 1. In bad likelihoods, the suggested value can be outside the parameter set, in which case the step length can also be used to preserve the value within the parameter set.

Another way to solve this problem is the Marquardt approach to add some constant to the diagonal of H. In this framework, it should be a negative constant. I find it more convenient to multiply the diagonal by a factor above 1. In matrix language, this means substituting H by $\tilde{H} = H + c \, \text{diag}\{H\}$, where c is a constant and $\text{diag}\{H\}$ is the matrix, which is equal to H on the diagonal and is 0 outside the diagonal. In the univariate case, this corresponds to reducing the step length, but in multivariate parameter problems, this also changes the direction of the parameter modification from the original Newton-Raphson method.

The above modifications are sensible when the diagonal elements of the second derivatives are all negative, because, if c is large enough, $\tilde{H}$ will be negative definite. When the diagonal elements of H are not all negative, we need further methods. Then we have two possibilities, one is to choose a G matrix to select only those coordinates with negative second derivatives. This improves the likelihood and often it moves into a point where the other diagonal elements also become negative. If there still are negative elements, the second possibility, a manual change of the relevant parameters, is needed. In order to examine whether H is negative definite, one might evaluate the eigenvalues, but this might require extra calculations. Therefore, it is suggested to detect this by studying the diagonal elements of H^{-1}. They should also be negative. If they are not, H is not negative definite and a Marquardt approach must be used, with a factor so large that the diagonals of the inverse matrix becomes negative. The method of reducing the step length does not work in this case. Calculating the determinant is not sufficient to check whether the matrix is negative definite, because there could be several eigenvalues of the wrong sign.

Some of these matrices might have a very high dimension and the inversion of a matrix can be time-consuming. The inversion is needed (see Section B.3) in the final step to evaluate the variance of the parameter estimates, by means of $-H^{-1}$, but during the iteration, we can be satisfied with an approximation to the second derivative. The main requirements for the approximation are that it should be simple to evaluate and fast to invert. The suggestion here is to choose a set of mixed derivatives that are approximated by 0. Then the matrix inversion formula becomes

$$\begin{pmatrix} A & B \\ B' & D \end{pmatrix}^{-1} = \begin{pmatrix} A^{-1} + CE^{-1}C' & -CE^{-1} \\ -E^{-1}C' & E^{-1} \end{pmatrix}, \quad (B.3)$$

where $E = D - B'A^{-1}B$, $C = A^{-1}B$, Rao (1972, p. 33). The matrices should be chosen so that A is a diagonal matrix of high dimension, whereas D and thus E have low dimension. Specifically, for the semi-parametric hazard models, the hazard parameters make up the D-matrix and the other parameters make up the A-matrix.

Equation (B.3) can also be used to save memory for large matrices. The second derivatives are symmetric and thus, it is sufficient to evaluate and store the upper triangular part of it. The inverse can be evaluated by recursive application of Equation (B.3), each time letting A be one-dimensional.

B.3   Standard error evaluation

The variance matrix of the parameters is directly found as $-H^{-1}$ in the final iteration in Equation (B.1). For the more general case of Equation (B.2), the variance of the reduced parameter is $-(GHG')^{-1}$, which easily is extended to the variance matrix of the full parameter by $-G'(GHG')^{-1}G$. When G is not of full rank, this matrix will not be of full rank either, but this is not a problem.

When the parameter dimension is large, computer limitations may make it impossible to invert the matrix. The variance matrix for the important parameters may be found by numerical differentiation of a number of profile likelihoods. To be specific, suppose the full parameter θ is split into a one-dimensional parameter θ_1 and the rest, θ_2. From the full likelihood, say, $\ell(\theta_1, \theta_2)$, we find the profile likelihood as $\ell_1(\theta_1) = \sup_{\theta_2} \ell(\theta_1, \theta_2)$. For each θ_1, we find the maximum likelihood estimate of θ_2 as $\hat{\theta}_2(\theta_1)$. The asymptotic variance of $\hat{\theta}_1$ can then be found as $-1/d^2\ell_1(\theta_1)/d\theta_1^2$ evaluated at the estimate $\hat{\theta}_1$. The vector of covariances between θ_1 and θ_2 is found by the formula $d\hat{\theta}_2(\theta_1)/d\theta_1$, also evaluated at the estimate. In practice, this is found by first finding the estimate $(\hat{\theta}_1, \hat{\theta}_2)$ in the full model, with corresponding value of the likelihood of L_0. Then a number, say, ϵ, is added to $\hat{\theta}_1$ and the best fitting value of θ_2, that is, $\hat{\theta}_2(\hat{\theta}_1 + \epsilon)$, say θ_{2+}, is found. The log likelihood value is L_+. Then the variance of $\hat{\theta}_1$ is found as $v_1 = \epsilon^2/\{2(L_0 - L_1)\}$. The covariances are found as $v_{12} = (\theta_{2+} - \hat{\theta}_2)v_1/\epsilon$. It is recommended also to make the evaluations using $\theta_1 - \epsilon$ and take averages of L_+ and L_- for evaluating v_1. The covariance is then found as $v_{12} = (\theta_{2+} - \theta_{2-})v_1/(2\epsilon)$. The advantage of this is that it is less influenced by higher-order terms in the likelihood. This approach gives one row of the variance matrix and can be repeated for all the important parameters in the place of θ_1. Considering all the important parameters, this gives a matrix, V, which is made symmetric by substituting by $(V + V')/2$. This matrix can then be used as a variance matrix evaluated in the usual way.

References

[1] Aalen, O.O. (1978). Nonparametric inference for a family of counting processes. *Ann. Statist.* **6**, 534–545.

[2] Aalen, O.O. (1987). Mixing distributions on a Markov chain. *Scand. J. Statist.* **14**, 281–289.

[3] Aalen, O.O. (1988). Heterogeneity in survival analysis. *Statist. Med.* **7**, 1121–1137.

[4] Aalen, O.O. (1992). Modelling heterogeneity in survival analysis by the compound Poisson distribution. *Ann. Appl. Prob.* **2**, 951–972.

[5] Aalen, O.O. (1994). Effects of frailty in survival analysis. *Statistical Methods in Medical Research*, **3**, 227–243.

[6] Aalen, O.O., Bjertness, E. and Sønju, T. (1995). Analysis of dependent survival data applied to lifetimes of amalgam fillings. *Statist. Med.* **14**, 1819–1829.

[7] Aalen, O.O., Farewell, V.T., de Angelis, D., Day, N.E. and Gill, O.N. (1997). A Markov model for HIV disease progression including the effect of HIV diagnosis and treatment: Application to AIDS prediction in England and Wales. *Statist. Med.*, **16**, 2191–2210.

[8] Aalen, O.O. and Johansen, S. (1978). An empirical transition matrix for non-homogeneous Markov chains based on censored observations. *Scand. J. Statist.* **5**, 141–150.

[9] Abramowitz, M. and Stegun, I.A. (1965). *Handbook of mathematical functions.* Dover Publications, New York.

[10] Allison, P.D. (1995). Survival analysis using SAS System. A practical guide. SAS Institute Inc.

[11] Altman, D.G. and de Stavola, B.L. (1994). Practical problems in fitting a proportional hazards model to data with updated measurements of the covariates. *Statist. Med.* **13**, 301–344.

[12] Andersen, P.K. and Borgan, Ø. (1985). Counting process models for life history data: A review. *Scand. J. Statist.* **12**, 97–158.

[13] Andersen, P.K., Borgan, Ø., Gill, R.D. and Keiding, N. (1993). *Statistical models based on counting processes.* Springer Verlag, New York.

[14] Andersen, P.K. and Green, A. (1985). Evaluation of estimation bias in an illness-death-emigration model. *Scand. J. Statist.* **12**, 63–88.

[15] Andersen, P.K., Klein, J.P., Knudsen, K.M. and Palacios, R.T. (1997). Estimation of variance in Cox's regression model with shared gamma frailties. *Biometrics* **53**, 1475–1484.

[16] Bandeen-Roche, K.J. and Liang, K.-Y. (1996). Modelling failure-time associations in data with multiple levels of clustering. *Biometrika* **83**, 29–39.

[17] Bar-Lev, S.K. and Enis, P. (1986). Reproducibility and natural exponential families with power variance functions. *Ann. Statist.* **14**, 1507–1522.

[18] Bennett, S. (1983). Analysis of survival data by the proportional odds model. *Statist. Med.* **2**, 273–277.

[19] Berg, G.J. van den (1997). Association measures for durations in bivariate hazard rate models. *J. Economet.* **79**, 221–245.

[20] Bichsel, F. (1964). Erfahrungs-Tarifierung in der Motorfahrzeughafpflicht-Versicherung. *Mitteilungen – Vereinigung Schweizerischer Versicherungsmathematiker* **64**, 119–143.

[21] Bjarnason, H. and Hougaard, P. (2000). Fisher information for two gamma frailty bivariate Weibull models. *Lifetime Data Anal.* **6**, 59-71.

[22] Blomqvist, N. (1950). On a measure of dependence between two random variables. *Ann. Math. Statist.* **21**, 593–600.

[23] Borch-Johnsen, K., Andersen, P.K. and Deckert, T. (1985). The effect of proteinuria on relative mortality in Type 1 (insulin-dependent) diabetes mellitus. *Diabetologia* **28**, 590–596.

[24] Brown, W.B., Hollander, M. and Korwar, R.M. (1974). Nonparametric tests of independence for censored data with applications to heart transplant studies. In *Reliability and Biometry: Statistical analysis of lifelength* (eds. F. Proschan and R.G. Serfling), pp. 327–354. SIAM, Philadelphia.

[25] Burridge, J. (1981). Empirical Bayes analysis of survival time data. *J. R. Statist. Soc. B.* **43**, 65–75

[26] Cai, J. (1999). Hypothesis testing of hazard ratio parameters in marginal models for multivariate failure time data. *Lifetime Data Anal.* **5**, 39–53.

[27] Cai, J. and Prentice, R.L. (1995). Estimating equations for hazard ratio parameters based on correlated failure time data. *Biometrika* **82**, 151–164.

[28] Cai, J. and Prentice, R.L. (1997). Regression estimation using multivariate failure time data and a common baseline hazard function. *Lifetime Data Anal.* **3**, 197–213.

[29] Clayton, D.G. (1978). A model for association in bivariate life tables and its application in epidemiological studies of familial tendency in chronic disease incidence. *Biometrika* **65**, 141–151.

[30] Clayton, D.G. and Cuzick, J. (1985). Multivariate generalizations of the proportional hazards model (with discussion). *J. R. Statist. Soc. A* **148**, 82–117.

[31] Clegg, L.X., Cai, J. and Sen, P.K. (1999). A marginal mixed baseline hazards model for multivariate failure time data. *Biometrics* **55**, 805–812.

[32] Cox, D.R. (1972). Regression models and life tables (with discussion). *J. R. Statist. Soc. B* **34**, 187–220.

[33] Cox, D.R. and Oakes, D. (1984). *Analysis of survival data.* Chapman and Hall.

[34] Crowder, M. (1989). A multivariate distribution with Weibull connections. *J. R. Statist. Soc. B* **51**, 93–107.

[35] Crowley, J. and Hu, M. (1977). Covariance analysis of heart transplant survival data. *J. Am. Statist. Assoc.* **72**, 27–35.

[36] Dabrowska, D.M. (1988). Kaplan-Meier estimate on the plane: Weak convergence, LIL and the bootstrap. *J. Mult. Anal.* **29**, 308–325.

[37] Dabrowska, D.M. (1988). Kaplan-Meier estimate on the plane. *Ann. Statist.* **16**, 1475–1489.

[38] Danahy, D.T. *et al.* (1977). Sustained hemodynamic and antianginal effect of high dose oral isosorbide dinitrate. *Circulation* **55**, 381–387.

[39] David, H. and Moeschberger, M.L. (1978). *The theory of competing risks.* Charles Griffin, London.

[40] Drzewiecki, K.T. Ladefoged, C. and Christensen, H.E. (1980). Biopsy and prognosis for cutaneous malignant melanomas in clinical stage 1. *Scand. J. Plast. Reconstr. Surg.* **14**, 229–234.

[41] Ducrocq, V. and Casella, G. (1996). A Bayesian analysis of mixed survival models. *Genet. Sel. Evol.* **28**, 505–529.

[42] Efron, B. (1967). The two sample problem with censored data. In *Proc. 5th Berkeley Symp. Math. Statist. Prob.*, **4**, 831–853. University of California Press, Berkeley.

[43] Efron, B. and Hinkley, D.V. (1978). Assessing the accuracy of the maximum likelihood estimator: Observed versus expected Fisher information. *Biometrika* **65**, 457–487.

[44] Elbers, C. and Ridder, G. (1982). True and spurious duration dependence: the identifiability of the proportional hazard model. *Rev. Econ. Stud.* **XLIX**, 403–409.

[45] Fan, J., Prentice, R.L. and Hsu, L. (2000). A class of weighted dependence measures for bivariate failure time data. *J. R. Statist. Soc. B*, **62**, 181–190.

[46] Fechner, G.T. (1897). *Kollektivmasslehre.* W. Engelmann, Leipzig.

[47] Feller, W. (1971). *An introduction to probability theory and its applications 2, 2nd edition.* John Wiley and Sons, New York.

[48] Fisher, R.A. and Tippett, L.H.C. (1928). Limiting forms of the frequency distribution of the largest or smallest member of a sample. *Proc. Cambridge Phil. Soc.* **24**, 180–190.

[49] Fix, E. and Neyman, J. (1951). A simple stochastic model of recovery, relapse, death and loss of patients. *Hum. Biol.* **28**, 205–241.

[50] Fleming, T.R. (1992). Evaluating therapeutic interventions: some issues and experiences (with discussion). *Statist. Sci.* **7**, 428–456.

[51] Fleming, T.R. and Harrington, D.P. (1991). *Counting processes and survival analysis.* John Wiley and Sons, New York.

[52] Freireich, E.J. *et al.* (1963). The effect of 6-Mercaptopurine on the duration of steroid-induced remissions in acute leukemia: a model for evaluation of other potentially useful therapy. *Blood* **21**, 699–716.

[53] Freund, J.E. (1961). A bivariate extension of the exponential distribution. *J. Am. Statist. Assoc.* **56**, 971–977.

[54] Gail, M.H. (1984). Biased estimates of treatment effect in randomized experiments with nonlinear regressions and omitted covariates. *Biometrika* **71**, 431–444.

[55] Gail, M.H., Santner, T.J. and Brown, C.C. (1980). An analysis of comparative carcinogenesis experiments based on multiple times to tumor. *Biometrics* **36**, 255–266.

[56] Gall, M.-A., Borch-Johnsen, K., Hougaard, P., Nielsen, F.S. and Parving, H.-H. (1995). Albuminuria and poor glycemic control predict mortality in NIDDM. *Diabetes* **44**, 1303–1309.

[57] Gall, M.-A., Hougaard, P., Borch-Johnsen, K. and Parving, H.-H. (1997). Risk factors for development of incipient and overt diabetic nephropathy in patients with non-insulin dependent diabetes mellitus: prospective, observational study. *Br. Med. J.* **314**, 783–788.

[58] Gao, S. and Zhou, X. (1997). An empirical comparison of two semiparametric approaches for the estimation of covariate effects from multivariate failure time data. *Statist. Med.* **16**, 2049–2062.

[59] Genest, C. and MacKay, J. (1986a). Copules Archimediennes et familles de lois bidimensionnelles dont les marges sont donnees. *Can. J. Statist.* **14**, 145–159.

[60] Genest, C. and MacKay, J. (1986b). The Joy of Copulas: Bivariate distributions with uniform marginals. *Am. Statistician* **40**, 280–283.

[61] Genest, C. and Rivest, J.-P. (1993). Statistical inference procedures for bivariate archimedian copulas. *J. Am. Statist. Assoc.* **88**, 1034–1043.

[62] Gill, R., van der Laan, M.J. and Wellner, J.A. (1995). Inefficient estimators of the bivariate survival function for three models. *Ann. Inst. Henri Poincaré* **31**, 545–597.

[63] Glidden, D.V. (1999). Checking the adequacy of the gamma frailty model for multivariate failure times. *Biometrika* **86**, 381–393.

[64] Glidden, D.V. and Self, S.G. (1999). Semiparametric likelihood estimation in the Clayton-Oakes failure time model. *Scand. J. Statist.* **26**, 363–372.

[65] Gompertz, B. (1825). On the nature of the function expressive of the law of human mortality and on a new method to determine the value of the contingencies. *Proc. Trans. Roy. Soc.* 513–585.

[66] Gossiaux, A. and Lemaire, J. (1981). Methodes d'ajustement de distributions de sinistres. *Bull. Assoc. Swiss Actuaries* **81**, 87–95.

[67] Green, A., Borch-Johnsen, Andersen, P.K., Hougaard, P., Keiding, N., Kreiner, S. and Deckert, T. (1985). Relative mortality of type 1 (insulin-dependent) diabetes in Denmark: 1933–1981. *Diabetologia* **28**,339–342.

[68] Green, A. and Hougaard, P. (1984). Epidemiological studies of diabetes mellitus in Denmark: 5. Mortality and causes of death among insulin-treated diabetic patients. *Diabetologia* **26**, 190–194.

[69] Greenwood, M. and Yule, G.U. (1920). An inquiry into the nature of frequency distributions representative of multiple happenings with particular reference to the occurrence of multiple attacks of disease or of repeated accidents. *J. R. Statist. Soc.* **83**, 255–279.

[70] Gumbel, E.J. (1958). Distributions à plusieurs variables dont les marges sont donnees (with remarks by M. Frechet). *C. R. Acad. Sci. Paris* **246**, 2717–2720.

[71] Gumbel, E.J. (1960). Bivariate exponential distributions. *J. Am. Statist. Assoc.* **55**, 698–707.

[72] Guo, G. (1993). Use of sibling data to estimate family mortality effects in Guatemala. *Demography*, **30**, 15–32.

[73] Guo, G. and Rodriguez, G. (1992). Estimating a multivariate proportional hazards model for clustered data using the EM algorithm. With an application to child survival in Guatemala. *J. Am. Statist. Assoc.* **87**, 969–976.

[74] Hanley, J.A. and Parnes, M.N. (1983). Non-parametric estimation of a multivariate distribution in the presence of censoring. *Biometrics* **39**, 129–139.

[75] Hauge, M. (1981). The Danish twin register. In *Prospective Longitudinal Research: An Empirical Basis for the Primary Prevention of Psychosocial Disorders* (eds., S.A. Mednick, A.E. Baert and B.P. Bachmann),Oxford University Press, pp. 217–221.

[76] Hauge, M., Harvald, B., Fischer, M, Gotlieb-Jensen, K., Juel-Nielsen, N., Raebild, I., Shapiro, R. and Videbeck, T. (1968). The Danish twin register. *Acta Geneticae Medicae et Gemellogogiae* **17**, 315–331.

[77] Heckman, J.J. and Honore, B.E. (1989). The identifiability of the competing risks model. *Biometrika* **76**, 325–330.

[78] Hoel, D.G. and Walburg, H.E. (1972). Statistical analysis of survival experiments. *J. Natl. Cancer Inst.* **49**, 361–372.

[79] Hoem, J.M. (1976). The statistical theory of demographic rates. A review of current developments (with discussion), *Scand. J. Statist.* **3**, 169–185.

[80] Hoem, J.M. (1977). A Markov chain model of working life tables. *Scand. Actuarial J.* **1977**, 1–20.

[81] Holgate, P. (1970). The modality of some compound Poisson distributions. *Biometrika* **57**, 666–667.

[82] Holla, M.S. (1966). On a Poisson-inverse Gaussian distribution. *Metrika* **11**, 115–121.

[83] Holt, J.D. and Prentice, R.L. (1974). Survival analysis in twin studies and matched-pair experiments. *Biometrika* **61**, 17–30.

[84] Hougaard, P. (1984). Life table methods for heterogeneous populations: Distributions describing the heterogeneity. *Biometrika* **71**, 75–84.

[85] Hougaard, P. (1986a). Survival models for heterogeneous populations derived from stable distributions. *Biometrika* **73**, 387–396. (Correction **75**, 395.)

[86] Hougaard, P. (1986b). A class of multivariate failure time distributions. *Biometrika* **73**, 671–678. (Correction, **75**, 395.)

[87] Hougaard, P. (1987). Modelling multivariate survival. *Scand. J. Statist.* **14**, 291–304.

[88] Hougaard, P. (1989). Fitting a multivariate failure time distribution. *IEEE Trans. on Reliability* **38**, 444–448.

[89] Hougaard, P. (1991). Modelling heterogeneity in survival data. *J. Appl. Prob.* **28**, 695–701.

[90] Hougaard, P. (1995). Frailty models for survival data. *Lifetime Data Anal.* **1**, 255–273.

[91] Hougaard, P. (1999). Fundamentals of survival data. *Biometrics* **55**, 13–22.

[92] Hougaard, P., Harvald, B. and Holm, N.V. (1992a). Measuring the similarities between the lifetimes of adult Danish twins born between 1881–1930. *J. Am. Statist. Assoc.* **87**, 17–24.

[93] Hougaard, P., Harvald, B. and Holm, N.V. (1992b). Assessment of dependence in the life times of twins. In *Survival Analysis: State of the Art* (eds., J.P. Klein and P.K. Goel), Kluwer Academic Publishers, pp. 77–97.

[94] Hougaard, P., Harvald, B. and Holm, N.V. (1992c). Models for multivariate failure time data, with application to the survival of twins. In *Statistical Modelling* (eds., P.G.M. van der Heijden, W. Jansen, B. Francis and G.U.H. Seeber), Elsevier Science Publishers, New York, pp. 159–173

[95] Hougaard, P., Lee, M.-L.T. and Whitmore, G.A. (1997). Analysis of overdispersed count data by mixtures of Poisson variables and Poisson processes. *Biometrics* **53**, 1225–1238.

[96] Hougaard, P. and Madsen, E.B. (1985). Dynamic evaluation of short-term prognosis after myocardial infarction. *Statist. Med.* **4**, 29–38.

[97] Hougaard, P., Myglegaard, P. and Borch-Johnsen, K. (1994). Heterogeneity models of disease susceptibility, with application to diabetic nephropathy. *Biometrics* **50**, 1178–1188.

[98] Hsu, L. and Prentice, R.L. (1996). On assessing the strength of dependency between failure time variates. *Biometrika* **83**, 491–506.

[99] Huster, W.J. Brookmeyer, R. and Self, S.G. (1989). Modelling paired survival data with covariates. *Biometrics* **45**, 145–156.

[100] Hutchinson, T.P. and Lai, C.D. (1991). *The Engineering Statistician's Guide to Continuous Bivariate Distributions*. Rumsby Scientific Publishing, Adelaide.

[101] Johnson, P. and Hey, G. (1971). A review of the scope for using claims histories of individual policies in risk assessment. *Bulletin Association Royale des Actuaires Belges* **66**, 159–195.

[102] Jørgensen, B. (1981). *Statistical Properties of the Generalized Inverse Gaussian Distribution*. Lecture Notes in Statistics 9. Springer Verlag, Heidelberg.

[103] Kalbfleisch, J.D. (1978). Bayesian analysis of survival distributions. *J. R. Statist. Soc. B* **40**, 214–221.

[104] Kalbfleisch, J.D. and Lawless, J.F. (1985). The analysis of panel data under a Markov assumption. *J. Am. Statist. Assoc.* **80**, 863–871.

[105] Kalbfleisch, J.D. and Prentice, R.L. (1980). *The statistical analysis of failure time data*. John Wiley and Sons, New York.

[106] Kaplan, E.L. and Meier, P. (1958). Non-parametric estimation from incomplete observations. *J. Am. Statist. Assoc.* **53**, 457–481, 562–563.

[107] Kay, R. (1986). A Markov model for analysing cancer markers and disease states in survival studies, *Biometrics* **42**, 855–865,

[108] Keiding, N. and Andersen, P.K. (1989). Nonparametric estimation of transition intensities and transition probabilities: a case study of a two-state Markov process. *Appl. Statist.* **38**, 319–329.

[109] Kendall, M.G. (1938). A new measure of rank correlation. *Biometrika* **30**, 81–93.

[110] Kessing, L.V., Olsen, E.W. and Andersen, P.K. (1999). Recurrence of affective disorders: Analysis with frailty models. *Am. J. Epidemiol.* **149**, 404–411.

[111] Klein, J.P. (1992). Semiparametric estimation of random effects using the Cox model based on the EM algorithm. *Biometrics* **48**, 795–806.

[112] Klein, J.P., Keiding, N. and Copelan, E.A. (1994). Plotting summary predictions in multistate survival models: probabilities of relapse and death in remission for bone marrow transplantation patients. *Statist. Med.* **13**, 2315–2332.

[113] Klein, J.P., Keiding, N. and Kamby, C. (1989). Semiparametric Marshall-Olkin models applied to the occurrence of metastases at multiple sites after breast cancer. *Biometrics* **45**, 1073–1086.

[114] Klein, J.P. and Moeschberger, M. (1997). *Survival Analysis*. Springer Verlag, New York.

[115] Klein, J.P., Moeschberger, M., Li, Y.H. and Wang, S.T. (1992). Estimating random effects in the Framingham heart study. In Survival Analysis: State of the Art (eds., J.P. Klein and P.K. Goel), pp. 99–120. Kluwer Academic Publishers, Dordrecht.

[116] Korsgaard, I.R., Madsen, P. and Jensen, J. (1998). Bayesian inference in the semiparametric log normal frailty model using Gibbs sampling. *Genet. Sel. Evol.* **30**, 241–256.

524   References

[117] Korsgaard, I.R. and Andersen, A.H. (1998). The additive genetic gamma frailty model. *Scand. J. Statist.* **25**, 255-269.

[118] Lawless, J.F. (1987). Negative binomial and mixed Poisson regression. *Can. J. Statist.* **15**, 209-225.

[119] Lawless, J.F. and Nadeau, C. (1995). Some simple robust methods for the analysis of recurrent events. *Technometrics* **37**, 158-168.

[120] Le, C.T. and Lindgren, B.R. (1996). Duration of ventilating tubes: A test for comparing two clustered samples of censored data. *Biometrics* **52**, 328-334.

[121] Lee, E.W., Wei, L.J. and Amato, D.A. (1992). Cox-type regression analysis for large numbers of small groups of correlated failure time observations. In *Survival Analysis: State of the Art* (eds., J.P. Klein and P.K. Goel), Kluwer Academic Publishers, Dordrecht, pp. 237-247.

[122] Lee, L. (1979). Multivariate distributions having Weibull properties. *J. Mult. Anal.* **9**, 267-277.

[123] Lee, M.-L.T. and Whitmore, G.A. (1993). Stochastic processes directed by randomized time. *J. Appl. Prob.* **30**, 302-314.

[124] Liang, K.-Y., Self, S.G., Bandeen-Roche, K.J. and Zeger, S.L. (1995). Some recent developments for regression analysis of multivariate failure time data. *Lifetime Data Anal.* **1**, 403-415.

[125] Liang, K.-Y., Self, S.G. and Chang, Y.-C. (1993). Modelling marginal hazards in multivariate failure time data. *J. R. Statist. Soc. B.* **55**, 441-453.

[126] Lin, D.Y. (1994). Cox regression analysis of multivariate failure time data: The marginal approach. *Statist. Med.* **13**, 2233-2247.

[127] Lin, D.Y. and Wei, L.J. (1989). The robust inference for the Cox proportional hazards model. *J. Am. Statist. Assoc.* **84**, 1074-1078.

[128] Lin, D.Y. and Ying, Z. (1993). A simple nonparametric estimator of the bivariate survival function under univariate censoring. *Biometrika* **80**, 573-581.

[129] Lindeboom, M. and Van Den Berg , G.J. (1994). Heterogeneity in models for bivariate survival: the importance of the mixing distribution. *J. R. Statist. Soc. B.* **56**, 49-60.

[130] Lu, J.-C. and Bhattacharyya, G.K. (1990). Some new constructions of bivariate Weibull models. *Ann. Inst. Statist. Math.* **42**, 543-559.

[131] Madsen, E.B., Hougaard, P. and Gilpin, E. (1983). Dynamic evaluation of prognosis from time-dependent variables in acute myocardial infarction. *Am. J. Cardiol.* **51**, 1579-1583.

[132] Mahe, C. and Chevret, S. (1999). Estimating regression parameters and degree of dependence for multivariate failure time data. *Biometrics* **55**, 1078-1084.

[133] Manatunga, A.K. and Oakes, D. (1996). A measure of association for bivariate frailty distributions. *J. Mult. Anal.* **56**, 60-74.

[134] Manatunga, A.K. and Oakes, D. (1999). Parametric analysis for matched pair survival data. *Lifetime Data Anal.* **5**, 371-387.

[135] Mantel, N., Bohidar, N.R. and Ciminera, J.L. (1977). Mantel-Haenszel analyses of litter-matched time-to-response data, with modifications for recovery of interlitter information. *Cancer Res.* **37**, 3863–3868.

[136] Marshall, A.W. and Olkin, I. (1967). A multivariate exponential distribution. *J. Am. Statist. Assoc.* **62**, 30–44.

[137] Marshall, A.W. and Olkin, I. (1988). Families of multivariate distributions. *J. Am. Statist. Assoc.* **83**, 834–841.

[138] McGilchrist, C.A. (1993). REML estimation for survival models with frailty. *Biometrics* **49**, 221–225.

[139] McGilchrist, C.A. and Aisbett, C.W. (1991). Regression with frailty in survival analysis. *Biometrics* **47**, 461–466.

[140] Moertel, C.G., Fleming, T.R., McDonald, J.S., Haller, D.G., Laurie, J.A., Goodman, P.J., Ungerleider, J.S., Emerson, W.A., Tormey, D.C., Glick, J.H., Veeder, M.H. and Mailliard, J.A. (1990). Levamisole and Fluorouracil for adjuvant therapy of resected colon carcinoma. *N. Engl. J. Med.* **322**, 352–358.

[141] Murphy, S.A. (1994). Consistency in a proportional hazards model incorporating a random effect. *Ann. Statist.* **22**, 712–731.

[142] Murphy, S.A. (1995). Asymptotic theory for the frailty model. *Ann. Statist.* **23**, 182–198.

[143] Müller, H.-G. and Wang, J.-L. (1994). Hazard rate estimation under random censoring with varying kernels and bandwidths. *Biometrics* **50**, 61–76.

[144] Nelson, W. (1982). *Applied Life Data Analysis.* John Wiley and Sons, New York.

[145] Nelson, W. (1995). Confidence limits for recurrence data - Applied to cost or number of product repairs. *Technometrics* **37**, 147–157.

[146] Nielsen, G.G., Gill, R.D., Andersen, P.K. and Sørensen, T.I.A. (1992). A counting process approach to maximum likelihood estimation in frailty models. *Scand. J. Statist.* **19**, 25–43.

[147] Oakes, D. (1982a). A concordance test for independence in the presence of censoring. *Biometrics* **38**, 451–455.

[148] Oakes, D. (1982b). A model for association in bivariate survival data. *J. R. Statist. Soc. B* **44**, 414–422.

[149] Oakes, D. (1989). Bivariate survival models induced by frailties. *J. Am. Statist. Assoc.* **84**, 487–493.

[150] Oakes, D. (1992). Frailty models for multiple event times. In *Survival Analysis: State of the Art* (eds., J.P. Klein and P.K. Goel), Kluwer Academic Publishers, Dordrecht, pp. 371-379.

[151] Oakes, D. (1994). Multivariate survival distributions. *Nonparametric Statistics* **3**, 343–354.

[152] Oakes, D. and Jeong, J.-H. (1998). Frailty models and rank tests. *Lifetime Data Anal.* **4**, 209–228.

[153] Oakes, D. and Manatunga, A.K. (1992). Fisher information for a bivariate extreme value distribution. *Biometrika* **79**, 827–832.

[154] Omar, R.Z., Stallard, N. and Whitehead, J. (1995). A parametric multistate model for the analysis of carcinogenicity experiments *Lifetime Data Anal.* **1**, 327–346.

[155] Ord, J.K. and Whitmore, G.A. (1986). The Poisson-inverse Gaussian distribution as a model for species abundance. *Commun. Statist.-Theor. Meth.* **15**, 853–871.

[156] Paik, M.C., Tsai, W.-Y. and Ottman, R. (1994). Multivariate survival analysis using piecewise gamma frailties. *Biometrics* **50**, 975–988.

[157] Parner, E. (1998). Asymptotic theory for the correlated gamma-frailty model. *Ann. Statist.* **26**, 183–214.

[158] Petersen, J.H. (1998). An additive frailty model for correlated life times. *Biometrics* **54**, 646–661.

[159] Peto, R. (1972). Contribution to Cox, D.R. (1972): Regression models and life tables (with discussion). *J. R. Statist. Soc. B* **34**, 205–207.

[160] Pickles, A. and Crouchley, R. (1994). Generalizations and applications of frailty models for survival and event data. *Statist. Meth. Med. Res.* **3**, 263–278.

[161] Pickles, A., Crouchley, R., Simonoff, E., Eaves, L., Meyer, J., Rutter, M., Hewitt, J. and Silberg, J. (1994). Survival models for development genetic data: Age of onset of puberty and antisocial behaviour in twins. *Genet. Epidemiol.* **11**, 155–70.

[162] Platz, O. (1984). A Markov model for common-cause failures. *Reliab. Eng.* **9**, 25–31.

[163] Prentice, R.L. and Cai, J. (1992). Covariance and survivor function estimation using censored multivariate failure time data. *Biometrika* **79**, 495–512.

[164] Prentice, R.L., Kalbfleisch, J.D., Peterson, A.V., Flournoy, N., Farewell, V.T. and Breslow, N.E. (1978). The analysis of failure times in the presence of competing risks. *Biometrics* **34**, 541–554.

[165] Proschan, F. and Sullo, P. (1974). Estimating the parameters of a bivariate exponential distribution in several sampling situations. In *Reliability and Biometry*. SIAM, Philadelphia, pp. 423–440.

[166] Pruitt, R.C. (1990). Strong consistency of self-consistent estimators: General theory and an application to bivariate survival analysis. Technical report 543, University of Minnesota, School of Statistics.

[167] Pruitt, R.C. (1993a). Identifiability of bivariate survival curves from censored data. *J. Am. Statist. Assoc.* **88**, 573–579.

[168] Pruitt, R.C. (1993b). Small sample comparison of six bivariate survival curve estimators. *J. Statist. Comput. Simul.* **45**, 147–167.

[169] Ramlau-Hansen, H., Jespersen, N.C.B., Andersen, P.K. Borch-Johnsen, K. and Deckert, T. (1987). Life insurance for insulin-dependent diabetics. *Scand. Actuarial J.*, 19–36.

[170] Rao, C.R. (1972). *Linear statistical inference and its applications.* Second Edition. John Wiley and Sons, New York.

[171] Rasmussen, T., Schliemann, T., Sørensen, J.C., Zimmer, J. and West, M.J. (1996). Memory impaired aged rats: No loss of principal hippocampal and subicular neurons. *Neurobiol. Aging* **17**, 143–147.

[172] Ripatti, S. and Palmgren, J. (1999) Estimation of multivariate frailty models using penalized partial likelihood. Research Report Department of Biostatistics, University of Copenhagen.

[173] Royall, R.M. (1986). Model robust confidence intervals using maximum likelihood observations *Int. Statist. Rev.* **54**, 221–226.

[174] Sankaran, M. (1968). Mixtures by the inverse Gaussian distribution. *Sankhya B* **30**, 455–458.

[175] Sargent D.J. (1998). A general framework for random effects survival analysis in the Cox proportional hazards setting. *Biometrics* **54**, 1486–1497.

[176] Sastry, N. (1997). A nested frailty model for survival data, with an application to the study of child survival in northeast Brazil. *J. Am. Statist. Assoc.* **92**, 426–435.

[177] Self, S. (1993). A regression model for counting processes with a time dependent frailty. Manuscript.

[178] Shi, D. (1995). Fisher information for a multivariate extreme value distribution. *Biometrika* **82,** 644–649.

[179] Shih, J.H. (1998). A goodness-of-fit test for association in a bivariate survival model. *Biometrika* **85,** 189–200.

[180] Shih, J.H. and Louis, T.A. (1995a). Assessing gamma frailty models for clustered failure time data. *Lifetime Data Anal.* **1**, 205–220.

[181] Shih, J.H. and Louis, T.A. (1995b). Inferences on the association parameter in copula models for bivariate survival data. *Biometrics* **51**, 1384–1399.

[182] Sichel, H.S. (1971). On a family of discrete distributions particularly suited to represent long-tailed frequency data. In Proceedings of the Third Symposium on Mathematical Statistics, (Ed., N.F. Laubscher), Pretoria, South Africa, 51–97.

[183] Sichel, H.S. (1973). Statistical valuation of diamondiferous deposits. *J. S. African Inst. Mining Metallurgy* **73**, 235–243.

[184] Sichel, H.S. (1974). On a distribution representing sentence-length in written prose. *J. R. Statist. Soc. A* **137**, 25–34.

[185] Sichel, H.S. (1982). Asymptotic efficiencies of three methods of estimation for the inverse Gaussian-Poisson distribution. *Biometrika* **69**, 467–472.

[186] Siegel, A.F. (1979). The noncentral chi-squared distribution with zero degrees of freedom and testing for uniformity. *Biometrika* **66**, 381–386.

[187] Spearman, C. (1904). The proof and measurement of correlation between two things. *Am. J. Psychiatr.* **15**, 72–101.

[188] Spiekerman, C.F. and Lin, D.Y. (1998). Marginal regression models for multivariate failure time data. *J. Am. Statist. Assoc.* **93**, 1164–1175.

[189] Statistical Yearbook of Denmark (1996). Danmarks Statistik.

[190] Sverdrup, E. (1965). Estimates and test procedures in connection with stochastic models for deaths, recoveries and transfers between different states of health. *Skand. Aktuarietidskr.* **48**, 184–211.

[191] Sørensen, T.I.A., Nielsen, G.G., Andersen, P.K. and Teasdale, T.W. (1988). Genetic and environmental influences on premature death in adult adoptees. *N. Engl. J. Med.* **318**, 727–732.

[192] Tawn, J.A. (1988). Bivariate extreme value theory: Models and estimation. *Biometrika* **75**, 397–415.

[193] Thall, P.F. and Vail, S.C. (1990). Some covariance models for longitudinal count data with overdispersion. *Biometrics* **46**, 657–671.

[194] Therneau, T.M. and Hamilton, S.A. (1997). rhDNase as an example of recurrent event analysis. *Statist. Med.* **16**, 2029–2047.

[195] Tsai, W.-Y., Leurgans, S. and Crowley, J. (1986). Nonparametric estimation of a bivariate survival function in the presence of censoring. *Ann. Statist.* **14**, 1351–1365.

[196] Tweedie, M.C.K. (1984). An index which distinguishes between some important exponential families. In: *Statistics: Applications and New Directions.* Proceedings of the Indian Statistical Institute Golden Jubilee International Conference. (eds., J.K. Ghosh and J. Roy), 579–604.

[197] Vaupel, J.W., Manton, K.G. and Stallard, E. (1979). The impact of heterogeneity in individual frailty on the dynamics of mortality. *Demography* **16**, 439–454.

[198] Vaupel, J.W. and Yashin, A.I. (1985). The deviant dynamics of death in heterogeneous populations. In: Sociological Methodology (ed., N.B. Tuma), Jossey-Bass Publishers, San Francisco, pp. 179–211.

[199] Visser, M. (1996). Nonparametric estimation of the bivariate survival function with an application to vertically transmitted AIDS. *Biometrika* **83**, 507–518.

[200] Wassell, J.T. and Moeschberger, M.L. (1993). A bivariate survival model with modified gamma frailty for assessing the impact of interventions. *Statist. Med.* **12**, 241–248.

[201] Wei, L.J., Lin, D.Y. and Weissfeld, L. (1989). Regression analysis of multivariate incomplete failure time data by modeling marginal distributions. *J. Am. Statist. Assoc.* **84**, 1065–1073.

[202] Weibull, W. (1939). A statistical theory of the strength of materials. *Ingeniörsvetenskapsakademiens handlinger* **151**

[203] Weibull, W. (1951). A statistical distribution of wide applicability. *J. Appl. Mech.* **18**, 293–297.

[204] Weier, D.R. and Basu, A.P. (1980). An investigation of Kendall's τ modified for censored data with applications. *J. Statist. Planning Inference* **4**, 381–390.

[205] Whitmore, G.A. and Lee, M.-L.T. (1991). A multivariate survival distribution generated by an inverse Gaussian mixture of exponentials. *Technometrics* **33**, 39–50.

[206] Williams, E.J. (1977). Some representations of stable random variables as products. *Biometrika* **64**, 167–169.

[207] Willmot, G. (1987). The Poisson-Inverse Gaussian distribution as an alternative to the negative binomial. *Scand. Actuarial J.*, 113–127.

[208] Woodbury, M.A. and Manton, K.G. (1977). A random walk model of human mortality and aging. *Theor. Population Biol.* **11**, 37–48.

[209] Xue, X. and Brookmeyer, R. (1996). Bivariate frailty model for the analysis of multivariate survival time. *Lifetime Data Anal.* **2**, 277–289.

[210] Yashin, A.I. and Iachine, I. (1995). How long can humans live? Lower bound for biological limit of human longevity calculated from Danish twin data using correlated frailty model. *Mechanisms of Ageing and Development* **80**, 147–169.

[211] Yashin, A.I., Manton, K.G. and Lowrimore, G.R. (1997). Evaluating partially observed survival histories: Retrospective projection of covariate trajectories. *Appl. Stoch. Models Data Anal.* **13**, 1–13.

[212] Yashin, A.I., Manton, K.G. and Stallard, E. (1986). Dependent competing risks: a stochastic process model. *J. Math. Biol.* **24**, 119–140.

[213] Yashin, A.I., Manton, K.G. and Stallard, E. (1989). The propagation of uncertainty in human mortality processes operating in stochastic environments. *Theor. Population Biology* **35**, 119–141.

[214] Younes, N. and Lachin, J. (1997). Link-based models for survival data with interval and continuous time censoring. *Biometrics* **53**, 1199–1211.

Index